# MENTAL HEALTH NURSING

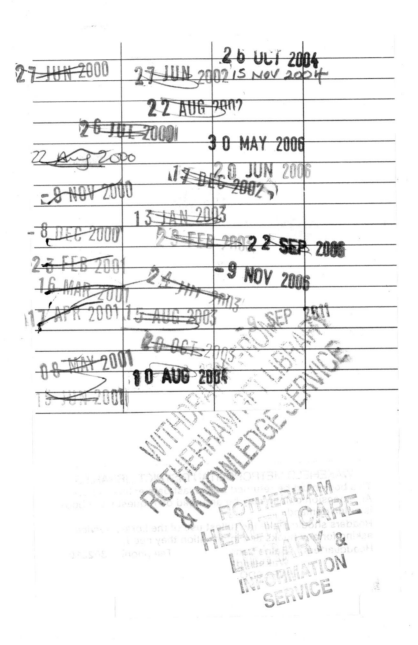

# Mental Health Nursing

## From first principles to professional practice

Edited by

## *Harry Wright*

*Clinical Nurse Specialist in Psychotherapy, The Hazel Clinic, Powys*

and

## *Martin Giddey*

*Senior Lecturer in Social Policy and Course Leader, Postgraduate programme in Mental Health Studies, University of Portsmouth*

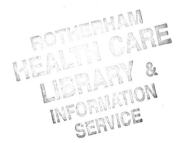
**Stanley Thornes (Publishers) Ltd**

First published by Chapman & Hall in 1993
(ISBN 0-412-41210-1)

Reprinted in 1997 by:
Stanley Thornes (Publishers) Ltd
Ellenborough House
Wellington Street
CHELTENHAM
GL50 1YW
United Kingdom

B-9914

98  99  00  01  /  10  9  8  7  6  5  4  3  2

A catalogue record for this book is available from the British Library

ISBN 0-7487-3282-9

Typeset by Expo Holdings
Printed and bound in Great Britain by Athenæum Press Ltd, Gateshead,
Tyne & Wear

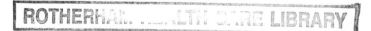

# CONTENTS

# CONTRIBUTORS

PHILIP BARKER
Clinical Nurse Consultant and Honorary
Lecturer at the University of Dundee, Scotland

DAVID CARPENTER
Principal Lecturer, Applied Philosophy and
Medical Law, University of Portsmouth

DAVID B. COOPER
Formerly Senior Nurse Manager, Special
Services, Suffolk

RUTH DAVIES
Senior Tutor responsible for the Therapeutic
Community Course, Institute of Advanced
Nursing Education, The Royal College of
Nursing

GORDON DEAKIN
Senior Education Manager and Nurse
Behaviour Therapist, South West College of
Health Studies, Plymouth

JULIA FABRICIUS
Psycho-analyist in private practice, formerly
Nurse Tutor, Bloomsbury College of Nurse
Education

JEAN FAUGIER
Senior Research Fellow, Department of
Nursing, University of Manchester

MARTIN GIDDEY
Senior Lecturer in Social Policy and Course
Leader, Postgraduate Programme in Mental
Health Studies, University of Portsmouth

CHRISTINE HALEK
Clinical Nurse Specialist in Anorexia
Nervosa, Pathfinder Community and
Specialist Mental Health Service, London

FRANK HARDIMAN
Director of Nursing Developments and
Lecturer, Bethlem Royal and Maudsley
Hospitals School of Nursing, London

SEAMUS KILLEN
Director of Nursing, Mental Health Unit,
Littlemore, Oxford

VIVIEN LINDOW
Mental Health Service Users as Community
Care Providers Project, Social Work
Department, Bristol University

BRENDAN McMAHON
Psychotherapist, Brooklands Community
Mental Health Team, Ilkeston, Derbyshire

RALPH NICHOLS
Doctorial Student,Uniiversity of Portsmouth.

JAMES OSBORN
Clinical Nurse Specialist, Child and Family
Consultation Centre, Mental Health
Foundation for Mid-Staffordshire NHS Trust

MIC RAFFERTY
Programme Manager, Clinical Developments,
Mid and West Wales College of Nursing and
Midwifery, University College of Swansea,
Swansea

GARY ROLFE
Senior Lecturer in Mental Health Nursing,
University of Portsmouth

LINDA ROWDEN
Clinical Nurse Specialist – Psychological
Support 1986–90, Royal Marsden Hospital,
Surrey

JEAN SIMMS
Senior Lecturer in Community Psychiatric
Nursing, University of Portsmouth

HARRY WRIGHT
Clinical Nurse Specialist in Psychotherapy,
The Hazel Centre Powys Health Authority,
Organizer and Tutor: 'A Course in Group and
Family Work'

# PREFACE

The extent and pace of change and development within the mental health services has never been greater than during the last decade. Significantly, these changes and developments have occurred both outside the profession and within. Central government has instigated major changes in health policy, which have had a direct impact on the organization and delivery of nursing care. Professional roles have evolved in ways which have extended and diversified the nature of mental health nursing. Educational developments have emphasized the importance of both theoretical knowledge and clinical competence for qualified practitioners and nurses in training. There is an expectation, from the public at large and from within the profession, that mental health nurses should be skilled and knowledgeable practitioners, who must also be flexible and creative in their work; above all, they must be able to demonstrate – to clients, to employers, and to the general public – that the care they provide is effective.

This new and comprehensive mental health nursing textbook is designed to meet the needs both of qualified practitioners and those following the Project 2000 scheme of nurse training. It is a book for nurses, by nurses. The contributors have been drawn from a wide variety of nursing specialities; each is a specialist in her or his field, whether this is clinical practice, nurse management, teaching, research, or academic enquiry.

The book emphasizes skills, underpinned by a sound knowledge of human psychosocial development, as the basis for effective nursing practice. Thus each section offers theoretical ideas and concepts, together with practical approaches to nursing intervention in a highly integrated way.

The last decade has also been characterized by a radical transition from a service which was once predominantly institutional in nature, to one in which the community is the central location for care and treatment. This text reflects a strong community focus as the starting point for consideration of client need.

Emphasis is placed upon the need for supervision and support for nurse practitioners. This is recognized as having paramount importance by all who have contributed for at least two reasons. Firstly, the nurse is held to be accountable for the work he or she undertakes, and both client and nurse gain from the benefit that skilled supervision of practice affords; unacceptable or unhelpful practices are not allowed to develop, while useful practices are nurtured. Secondly, the work undertaken by mental health nurses can be exceedingly stressful, and it therefore is essential that the nurse has the opportunity to debrief, or to work on client-nurse interactions towards an understanding of the causes of the stress they have induced.

For the first time in a text of this sort, the consumer is given a direct voice. Such is the importance of this perspective that it is given prominence in the opening section of the book. While most of us are already well aware of the greater emphasis given by government to consumer empowerment, this section provides a challenging reminder of the vulnerability of those in distress, and of the risks of abuse and misuse of power by those who society has entrusted with responsibility for their care. It is our intention that the emphasis given to the culture and practice of supervision within mental health nursing should enable nurses to achieve qualities of safe and sensitive practice that will reduce the possibility of such abuse and misuse of power.

The reader will be able to use this text both for rapid reference to specific areas, and to gain an understanding of concepts and therapeutic practices at a deeper level. While a text of this sort will satisfy most of the reader's professional interest in mental health, its coverage is not exhaustive. However, extensive bibliographies and recommendations for further reading provide signposts to the broad literature concerning mental health and nursing.

We would like to end with a quotation from Carl Rogers. It expresses a sentiment which we and the contributors hold as a central and guiding principle to the work of mental health nurses; that, above all, nursing intervention should be characterized by 'an absolute respect for the dignity and integrity of the client'.

# FOREWORD

Mental Health should be everyone's concern. All nursing students will need to be familiar both with the preventative aspects and the treatment issues in this complex and fascinating field. Project 2000 has changed, I suspect forever, the ways in which nurses are taught and, more slowly, the practice of nursing. All of this has implications for student nurses and for qualified nursing practitioners. This book can help both groups.

Various changes in mental health care are immediately obvious. The term 'mental health' has largely replaced 'psychiatry' and this reflects the move towards prevention of mental illness and the promotion of positive health – a move fired in no small measure by mental health nurses. Also, the context of mental health care has changed. In recent years we have seen a shift towards community care. Although the policy of closing down large psychiatric hospitals and of developing care in the community has not always been sensitively handled, the idea of enabling people to remain at home, as far as possible, is here to stay. The emphases on individualized and self care have also developed out of the community focus. These approaches to care are richly represented in this book. Finally, in this short list of changes, Mental Health Nursing, as a distinct branch of nursing has also been changed by Project 2000. In future, all nurses will undergo a period of general training before specializing in mental health care. Again, this book will help in both the common core and in the specialist modules of nursing diploma courses

*Mental Health Nursing* is, by any standard, a huge achievement. It brings together not only up-to-date information about all aspects of the field but it also brings together key writers in the Mental Health arena. For the first time, students, educators, managers and clinicians can find the writings of leaders in the field of Mental Health Nursing, together in the one volume. The result is a vital and challenging text that will be of immense value to a wide range of readers.

Just to turn things on their head for a moment, it is difficult to find anything that has been left out of this book. It covers both societal and psychological aspects of health care, both therapy and nursing skills. It also contains useful and informative examples from practice. These are particularly helpful in illustrating how a particular theoretical construct works in practice. That is vital. For mental health nursing must be a **practical** discipline. There are volumes and volumes written about theories of mental illness and concepts of self, family and society. One of the greatest strengths of this book is that it illustrates how so many of these ideas can be practised by nurses in the mental health field.

From an educational point of view, *Mental Health Nursing* will fill an important gap in any personal or college library. Both lecturers and students will find valuable information on context, dynamics, diagnosis, treatment, self-awareness, interpersonal skills and a wide range of other mental health topics. The editing is such that whilst the experts who have contributed to this book sometimes offer differing points of view – and that is how it should be – the whole book remains easy to read and to refer to. Colleges of Nursing will be quick to adopt this book as required reading and reference in Mental Health branches of Project 2000 courses. But it has applications  far broader than that. *Mental Health Nursing* will also be of immense value to any nurse who has an interest in the psychological and spiritual care of her or his patients. And that should include all nurses.

The editors and the contributors to this book are to be congratulated for having produced a work of this sort. I learned an immense amount from reading it and I know that it will quickly become a standard work in the field of mental health nursing. Read it slowly, refer to it often. There is a huge amount of information contained in these pages. The mental health field is a complicated one and none of the authors glosses over that complexity. Each chapter both stands on its own as valuable guide to the particular topic and also complements its neighbours. Mental health nursing, as a distinct field of nursing, is here to stay and *Mental Health Nursing* contributes enormously to its development.

Philip Burnard,
Director of Postgraduate Nursing Studies,
School of Nursing Studies,
University of Wales College of Medicine, Cardiff, UK.

# PART ONE

# INTRODUCTION

# THE THERAPEUTIC RELATIONSHIP

*Harry Wright*

It is interesting to consider how, when we are together as families, friends, or colleagues, we ordinarily view the difficulties that beset us or those close to us with a sensitive understanding that takes into account our experiences, both past and present. When faced with a client who also is experiencing distress, however, we are tempted to think in terms of 'illness' and 'diagnosis', and the management of the client and his problems. Sometimes this can be appropriate, but it begins to become inappropriate when it serves as a barrier to caring and feeling. Such attitudes can impede the developing relationship between the nurse and those with whom she is working.

When a friend or a loved one is in distress, we offer comfort. We often have an instinctual appreciation of the cause of the upset. We may also have factual knowledge, but sometimes we know something because of how we feel – somehow there has been a communication, often without words, sometimes even without apparent gesture, that tells us how a friend or loved one is feeling; we feel it ourselves.

In the past, mental health nurses were often discouraged by more experienced, qualified nurses from forming what were termed 'personal', 'special', or 'individual' relationships with their clients. We were told we should not become 'too involved' with them. There were many reasons why this advice or instruction was given. Some held the view that any involvement that touched upon the personal feelings of the nurse was bad for

both the client and the nurse, who could no longer be deemed impartial, and consequently could not maintain the detached and objective perspective thought to be necessary to do effective work. Others were concerned for the emotional well-being of the nurse, wishing to discourage an unmanageable quality of distress, which they believed would render the nurse unable to work effectively with the client, or would leave him or her stressed and needful.

Both of these points of view contain elements of the truth: it is possible to become over-involved and to lose a professional perspective; and it is possible for anyone – especially nurses, who have such intense and continuing close relationships with their clients – to become so suffused with their clients' feelings that they may themselves feel overwhelmed.

Today, the nurse is expected to use her own feeling responses in a professional way, in order to gain an understanding of the emotional life of her clients so that she might respond in an appropriate and therapeutic way. This is a hopeful change in perspective, but it brings with it many problems to do with intimacy and trust, which are inherent to the human condition and consequently inevitable, but are not unresolvable.

Our clients are no longer content to be the recipients of helpful, planned interventions – they wish also to be cared for and understood; they do not want just to be able to learn how to manage better – they want to feel better too. This seems entirely predictable and human; is it not what each of us seeks to gain in the personal relationships we form throughout our lives? And yet it is this aspect that has been disregarded for so long by some workers in the mental health field. While it may be important to understand why this should be so, it is more important to discover why the need of care and understanding should be of such a central concern to our clients and to ourselves. If we can resolve these questions, we will have established a sound basis to our nursing practice.

## CENTRAL CONCERNS

At the risk of over-simplifying complex issues, we probably can agree that for most of us our first formative experiences were gained in the arms of the parents or other primary-care givers who held us safely and fed us at the breast or on the bottle. It is this relationship, in its quality, or lack of it, that acts as a template for all our subsequent relationships, throughout the rest of our lives.

If the maternal or other primary relationship was characterized by a continuing, predictable, and caring presence, it is likely we will have grown in trust and developed an ability to maintain equally caring and continuing relationships. Where it was determined by a paucity of care, and an unpredictable and discontinuous presence, then it is likely we will have grown in an atmosphere of uncertainty, doubt, and mistrust, leaving us needful of affection and untrusting of any care we are subsequently offered. Where we have been given the chance to deal with appropriate levels of frustration, disappointment, and anxiety, it is probable we will not become overwhelmed by apparently inexplicable anxieties later in life. If we have been overly protected from experiencing even the slightest worry or discomfiting frustration, or have been left to cope on our own, with inappropriate levels of anxiety, we are more likely to fail to manage frustration, distress, and anxiety as adults.

Over the past decade or so, many models of care have been provided by practitioners and teachers, whose aim it is to enable the nurse to take the whole person into account. We are encouraged to consider the physical, emotional, social, and spiritual well-being of those in our care. Parallels can be drawn here. For example, this is what Winnicott's (1974) model of the good enough mother does moment by moment throughout the formative years of her child's young life. It is not a bad model to hold if we wish to become good enough nurses. Winnicott used the term 'good enough' to acknowledge that we each are human, and consequently prey to human failings. Inevitably, we will not always manage in the best way possible. All we can hope for is to be good enough overall. Of course, with practice, education, and experience we improve, we learn from our own experience, and, sometimes, those of others – we mature, change, and develop throughout the whole of our lives.

This leads to another point that is of central concern to all mental health nurses. Throughout our lives we are offered many chances to re-experience and to rework, under changed circumstances, issues and relationships that remain unresolved from earlier times. That this happens is exciting and hopeful, not least because it gives assurance to those who work with people in distress that the task of helping individuals to change, while difficult, is not impossible to achieve.

How is it that the relationships of infancy and childhood form the foundations upon which all other relationships are built, and yet we also have the chance to rework unsatisfactory experiences in later life? The experience of being human is to be beset by many thoughts, feelings, and impulses that often seem to be opposed. Most of us have had the feeling of being filled with a powerful hatred for someone we know we also love. Such contradictory feelings, this duality, is central to the business of being a person. For most of us, because the foundations upon which we build will be sound enough, we will not be impeded by intrusive or unmanageable levels of uncertainty or a basic mistrust. For a smaller proportion, the foundations will be so shaky that all available time and energy will be spent holding oneself together, so that changes can only be made with the help of committed, experienced others, who are able to understand and withstand high levels of distress and anxiety.

Nursing is not just about techniques, methods, and models: primarily and essentially it is to do with being a person who works with other people at times when they are ill, distressed, or anxious. That is not to say that models and techniques are useless or unimportant; it is simply to recognize that techniques and methodologies are of no value unless they are used appropriately by nurses, who are people first, and technicians or practitioners second.

While this book is full of information on various types of nursing interventions, theoretical models, and therapeutic practices, it is not intended as a recipe book for mental health nursing. While the information is of much potential value to each of us as nurse practitioners, it requires that we are able to bring a human awareness and sensitivity to our work. How, then, do we bring together these three elements of caring – the maternal as a model for good-enough nursing practice; one's humanity; and theoretical or skills-based knowledge – in a way that enhances our work and is helpful to our clients?

## THE CONCEPT OF CONTAINMENT

It is likely that at some point in our nursing careers we will all hear colleagues talking of clients in a disparaging way. All too often, the people with problems we find difficult to understand will be referred to as 'manipulative' or 'attention-seeking'; even senior nurses have been heard to refer to their clients as 'professional patients'. While some people are manipulative or do seek attention, it is hard to believe that anyone would deliberately and consciously make a career out of needing mental health care. What is often neglected is the fact that people become manipulative or attention-seeking because of their need or distress. When nurses use such descriptions they are not so much describing the client as admitting to an inability to understand why they are like this, and disguising their own despairing feelings that they do not know how to help.

People who manipulate may do so because it is hard for them to believe that their needs or wants will willingly be met. The same sort of consideration would apply to people who continuously seek attention. It seems reasonable to assume in a general way that those who so desperately search for acknowledgement are driven by a gnawing doubt that it will be given freely. There is, perhaps, something in their previous experience that leads them to believe that inevitably they will be overlooked. Even when freely given, the recognition they crave so intensely may not seem satisfyingly real, so they doubt it and test it, even to the point of destruction. Such people have to test the recognition to prove it is real, perhaps because they have experienced times when their hopes have been raised, only to be dashed once more. This basic sense of uncertainty and mistrust, despite the goodwill of those who work with them, is what may eventually lead some nurses to use such aggressive and despairing terms as 'manipulator' or 'attention-seeker'.

Often such clients are discharged as being unwilling to accept the help that is offered, or because no effective treatment can be found. There is a current demand that all care should be cost-effective. While this is not a bad thing in itself, it is often interpreted as meaning that treatment should be cheap and brief. In the field of mental health care, cost-effectiveness should be measured over the long term. A period of treatment that lasts for some years of once-weekly or once-fortnightly sessions may prove to be more effective and cheaper overall, especially if we take into account the costs of providing a life-time of short-lived involvements that often offer only limited or superficial change. One consequence is that clients may be readmitted time and again for the same problems.

A good-enough parent helps the child to develop a sense of security, a feeling of basic trust, and an ability to enjoy close relationships through his or her continuing, constant, predictable, and caring presence (Erikson, 1965; Menzies Lyth, 1989a). This takes years to establish. Where there has been some problem, a sense of mistrust will form that will need to be dealt with before it is possible for the individual to begin to be able to believe in himself, and to trust the goodwill of those close to him.

If we examine the personal histories of the clients with whom we work, more often than not we will discover problems to do with early experiences in childhood and infancy, perhaps where there has been a failure in the nurturing relationship; or we will find that the quality of care has been impoverished, or lacking altogether. Such problems cannot be dealt with on a short-term basis, but require the constancy, continuity, and predictability that were missing from the early relationship. We grow through relationships, and we change through their helpful impact; we learn through experience, and our feelings and behaviour are shaped by what we learn.

The parent or other primary care giver 'contains' (Bion, 1970) or 'holds' (Winnicott, 1974) the child by keeping him in her mind and holding him in her arms, through thinking about his needs and striving to understand his experience. She makes sense for him of the many experiences that are new to him, and she withstands his angry, destructive, and frightened feelings.

Similarly, if we are to help our clients, we need to be able to contain them in ways that are similar to a parent holding the child. The nurse may not literally hold her clients in her arms, but she does endeavour to keep them safely in her mind and to think about them, and she strives to understand why they feel and behave as they do. She offers her understanding of what is happening and why in the same ways in which a parent might explain the world to her child. For example, the mother might say to her distressed and angry child, 'Never mind. Did you wake up and I wasn't there, and were you frightened?' The nurse might say to a similarly distressed and angry client, 'You seem angry and hurt. I've noticed you are like this each time I return from a break or holiday. I think you may be angry with me for leaving you.'

Of course, before we can identify this sort of event we have to be involved in an ongoing relationship that allows us the privilege of seeing repeated behaviour. If we are involved in a continuing relationship, whether we spot it or not our clients will invest us with significance and have feelings about us. How are we to cope with the feelings of anger and dislike, jealousy, mistrust, hatred, and affection – all the human feelings our clients have for us and engender in us? The nurse needs containing too.

## HOLDING THE NURSE

Although there has been much valuable work done by many researchers and clinicians (Menzies Lyth, 1989b; Fabricius, 1990; Wright, 1989, 1991) on the need to provide support for nurses working with people in distress, it is still not commonly given. As well, the picture changes from region to region, and even neighbouring localities vary in the provision of support.

If we are to provide the highest standards of care to our clients, we must establish proper and appropriate support systems for nurses at all levels. Regular support and clinical supervision seminars should be provided from the beginning of training and throughout the professional life of each and every nurse. As there is sometimes confusion about differences between support and supervision, and some misunderstanding about what supervision means, it would be helpful to consider these now.

## SUPPORT

The word 'support' tends to be a bit of a catch-all for many kinds of help. Here it is used to describe a quality of awareness and understanding that takes account of the individual experiences of the nurse, and her emotional life as it relates to and is affected by the work she undertakes with those in her care. We know we are touched by the feelings of others – we feel sadness for their hurt, and empathy for their distress. This is an ordinary part of the human condition. Nurses working in the field of mental health come into close and continuous contact every day with those who are experiencing extreme levels of feeling. Consequently, it is necessary to the emotional well-being of the nurse that he or she is given the opportunity to share the feelings with others that such contact engenders.

For example, a colleague, who is an experienced, qualified nurse, spoke of how difficult she sometimes found it to cope with the high levels of anxiety she was left with after her regular contact with a distressed woman client with whom she worked as a community nurse. She found it hard to re-focus her attention at the end of the working day upon her own small child. Her concentration would wander from her daughter, and she would find herself anxiously thinking about her client. The high degree of anxiety her client aroused in her made it difficult for the nurse to give her little girl the quality of attention any child needs. She worried about this too, feeling she was failing both as a mother and as a nurse, believing she should be able to take her client's difficulties in her stride.

The nurse joined a support group of other nurses, which was convened by an appropriately trained and experienced colleague. Over time, this small group of nurses developed sufficient trust in each other to be able to talk openly, if not without some uncertainty, of the problems they found their work caused them. The nurse in question shared her uncertainty with the group, and found others experienced similar distress and feelings of failure. This was a tremendous relief to her and to the others in this support group, each of whom felt they alone could not manage without a struggle. I. D. Yalom (1970), a renowned researcher into groups, calls this phenomenon 'universality', and describes its power to deal with the worry that all feel 'unique in their wretchedness'.

This sort of support, which looks at the experience of the nurse as an individual, is often best provided in small-group situations, as it allows sharing, feedback, and identification (Wright, 1989b), which in turn enable a sense of being safely contained. Such small-group work is of potential value to all mental health nurses, and would be of particular benefit to those still engaged in training, who have yet to discover their individual strengths and weaknesses, skills, and abilities.

## SUPERVISION

This too is a word that is used to mean many different things: some understand it, for example, to refer to the responsibility of the manager to oversee the work undertaken by his or her employees. In this sense it is often given a pejorative connotation whereby the manager 'inspects' or 'judges' the quality of the work of others, criticizes it, and demands improvements.

Here, supervision is used to describe a process of trusting enquiry, which encourages learning to take place and understanding to develop. It can be undertaken in one-to-one situations or in small groups, and can be offered by colleagues who are one's peers, or by a clinician who has training and expertise in supervision. Generally, it is better to arrange for supervision with a colleague who has more experience and who is trained to a higher level than oneself because of the special knowledge that appropriately trained and experienced colleagues can bring. Sometimes this is not possible, and supervision with one's peer-group is then essential.

Supervision differs from support groups in that the aims are different. The support group looks at the feelings aroused in the nurse through her contact with distressed clients, while supervision makes a detailed examination of the work undertaken by the nurse with her client, as the following example shows.

CASE STUDY – A SUPERVISION SEMINAR

A nurse was concerned about the well-being of the six-year-old daughter of one of the families she visited. The mother talked of the night-time terrors that had been happening for the past month or so that awoke the little girl from her sleep, leaving her anxious and drained. Her behaviour at school had deteriorated and she was inattentive, seeming to daydream much of the time. The drawings she made were of frightening monsters that oozed a nasty green slime, and she told her mother and the nurse that she was 'horrible'. The mother and the nurse were at a loss to understand what was happening to the child, who had become withdrawn even at home. The mother could identify nothing that might have affected her daughter in this way.

In the supervision seminar, the nurse was encouraged to ask about the family's past history, subsequently learning that when the little girl was two years old a baby brother of only six months had contracted a virus that had killed him. At the time, the little girl had been extremely jealous of her baby brother, and when he died she had been sent to stay with an aunt for two weeks over the period of the burial. The little girl had not seen her brother before he died, and

did not go to the funeral. The seminar group considered that she may have felt that her jealous wish to be rid of this newly arrived competitor had become fact, and that her angry and jealously destructive feelings had been responsible for his death. The nurse had also noted that the mother was pregnant, and had asked her if she had told her daughter she was expecting another baby. The mother said she had, about four weeks ago. Both the mother and the nurse were stunned by the realization that the announcement coincided with the onset of the little girl's nightmares and withdrawn behaviour.

The seminar encouraged the nurse to talk with the mother about her daughter's anxieties, and to help her to think about how she might help the child to understand that she was not as horrible or as monstrous as she felt. It seems probable that the little girl phantasized that the virus that had caused the baby's death had resulted from the poisonous and destructive feelings that had 'leaked' from her, like the nasty slime that leaked from the monsters she drew.

It took a great deal of courage and skill on the part of the nurse to help the mother to face the feelings that so troubled her little girl; it is not easy for any of us to face feelings of loss, and for a mother, the loss of a child sometimes cannot be borne. Knowing this, the nurse had to first confront the distress caused within herself before she was able to help the mother to face her sorrow, and to understand and ease her little girl's pain and anxiety.

Without the supervision seminar, it is possible that the reasons for the little girl's distress would not have been discovered, and that the nurse would have found it almost impossible to confront the mother. The seminar enabled the nurse to help the mother to understand her child's fears, so she could deal with them through explanation and her continuing love.

## ENDING WITH THE BEGINNING

Throughout this book, the team of contributors describe and elucidate various theories of development, causality, and practice. All have a legitimate place in the broad church of mental health care. Inevitably, the reader will be drawn to a particular way of thinking and working. It would be wrong, however, to suppose that any one perspective is the only truth. Just as it is possible to have several views of the same mountain depending upon where one is standing, one can have several views of people and of their problems and what causes them depending upon a particlar perspective. One might prefer to work, for example, behaviourally, but may feel the interventions will benefit from a psychoanalytic understanding. Another may think analytically, but find that a systems perspective offers a useful was of dealing with the problems that beset some people.

Whichever our predilection, it is important to remember that we are nurses. We have a special role, and we are required to keep in mind the physical, emotional, social, and spiritual well-being of those in or care. We cannot fulfil this responsibility adequately unless we allow ourselves to be reached at an emotional level by our clients. To become good-enough nurses we could do much worse than to model the base of our care upon the good-enough parent. Those with whom we work need the same predictable presence, constancy, and continuity of care that is offered by a parent to her child.

If we are to cope with the stress that the distress of others inevitably causes, then we too need a continuing, constant, and predictable quality of care. While this type of care is recognized by many nurses as being essential, unfortunately it is available to but a few. Such support and supervision should be established as a requirement for all nurses on a regular basis, beginning with training and continuing into and throughout qualified practice. Where it is not provided, then we can form our own groups for peer supervision. If the nurse is safely to contain her clients, she must be safely held herself.

## REFERENCES

Bion, W. R. (1970) *Attention and Interpretation*, Tavistock, London.

Erikson, E. H. (1965) *Childhood and Society*, Penguin, Harmondsworth.

Fabricius, J. (1991) Running on the spot, or can nursing really change?, in *Psychoanalytic Psychotherapy*, 5, 2, Charlesworth & Co. Ltd., Huddersfield.

Menzies Lyth, I. (1989a) Staff support systems: task and anti-task in adolescent institutions, in *Containing Anxiety in Institutions*, Free Association Books, London.

Menzies Lyth, I. (1989b) The development of the self in children in institutions, in *Containing Anxiety in Institutions*, Free Association Books, London.

Winnicott, D. W. (1974) *Playing and Reality*, Penguin, Harmondsworth.

Wright, H. (1989a) *Groupwork: Perspectives and Practice*, Scutari, London.

Wright, H. (1989b) *Groupwork: Perspectives and Practice*, Scutari, London.

Wright, H. (1991) The patient, the nurse, his life and her mother: psychodynamic influences in nurse education and practice, in *Psychoanalytic Psychotherapy*, 5, 2, Charlesworth & Co. Ltd., Huddersfield.

Yalom, I. D. (1970) *The Theory and Practice of Group Psychotherapy*, Basic Books, New York.

# MENTAL HEALTH CARE IN A CHANGING SOCIETY

*Martin Giddey*

In the last decade of the twentieth century, many societies have developed systems of mental health care that provide a range of helping approaches and are available from a number of different sources. Such systems were developed over a long period of time, and have been shaped by a variety of influences, including the ways in which people have understood the nature and causes of mental distress; experience and research related to different forms of care and therapy; and public and professional attitudes to people with mental health problems. The political, economic, and social structures and processes of a society also provide an important context within which such influences make an impact. This context is in itself an important factor in the shaping of the mental health services.

In order to address questions such as 'Why is there currently so much emphasis on community care?', or 'Why do mental health nurses work in a particularly sort of way?', we need not only to examine contemporary influences, but also to turn to history.

## THE EIGHTEENTH CENTURY

At the beginning of the eighteenth century, although the concept of mental illness was unknown, this not uncommon aspect of the human condition – referred to at the time by a variety of terms, including 'madness', 'insanity', and 'lunacy', – obviously existed.

The ways in which mental illness was conceived reflected both the prevailing social ethos, and the limited development of scientific knowledge concerning human physiology and psychology.

Although the statute laws against witchcraft had been repealed by 1736, associations between witchcraft and madness persisted well into the century, and many continued to conceptualize madness in cosmic, mystical, or religious ways. The term 'lunatic', for example, which was in use during this period, implies a disturbance of mind or spirit caused by the influence of the moon. Medical science had little to offer beyond the traditional panaceas of purging and bloodletting. Mental disturbance and moral weakness were often seen as synonymous, and those afflicted were only to be pitied; the insane were at the bottom of a social hierarchy, in a highly stratified society.

While misconceptions and apathy may have characterized general attitudes to mental illness, those affected could nevertheless constitute a public nuisance. And it was only as a result of this that the state engaged with people with mental health problems. If they were also poor, then the Poor Laws were brought to bear; if they wandered from their communities, the vagrancy laws pertained; if their condition lead to criminal behaviour, the criminal law was used.

The state did not address the problem of madness directly, and so people with mental health problems were to be found in prisons, workhouses, and in or near their own homes. Private madhouses were available to only those able to afford the charges. A very few independent institutions for the insane existed, of which the Retreat at York and the Bethlem, formerly known as Bedlam, in London are prominent examples. Almost universally, mentally ill people were confined in conditions of filth, squalour, and cruel restraint.

The Vagrancy Act of 1744 was the first legislation to mention madness. Its provisions directed that lunatics could be apprehended, kept, and maintained, usually in gaol. Growing public concern about cruelty and exploitation in the hitherto unregulated private madhouses lead to the Act for Regulating Private Madhouses, which was passed in 1774. This Act established five important principles in lunacy legislation (Jones, 1972):

1. Licensing by a public authority of private institutions.
2. Notification of the admission of a person alleged to be insane.
3. Visitation by Commissioners, whose method of appointment was prescribed by Parliament.
4. Inspection to ensure humane conditions and the release of those wrongfully detained.
5. Supervision by the medical profession.

## THE NINETEENTH CENTURY

In 1808, the passing of the County Asylums Act, the purpose of which was 'for the better care and maintenance of lunatics, being paupers or criminals in England', created provisions for the building of county asylums. The first of these was completed in Nottingham in 1810, and by the end of the century there were 77 in all, serving almost every district in the country, and housing 74,004 inmates.

Further legislation continued throughout the century. Of particular note is the Lunatics Act (1845), which facilitated the appointment of Lunacy Commissioners. The Commissioners had extensive powers of inspecting, licensing, and reporting on every county asylum and licensed house in the land. The Lunacy Act of 1890 prescribed the precise circumstances in which admissions could be made. It should be emphasized that the County Asylums could only take certified patients.

During the course of the century, a social revolution had taken place. At its beginning, the state hardly engaged directly with mentally ill people at all; by its end, an almost universal system, controlled by a centralized bureaucracy and based entirely on institutional care, had been created. Concurrent with this was at least a partial revolution in approaches to the care of people with mental health problems. Early pioneers in humane treatment had provided evidence that restraint was not only unnecessary, but was usually counter-therapeutic. Social reformers were much influenced by this evidence, ensuring that the physical conditions in which inmates were confined improved progressively, subsequent to the Act of 1845.

## THE TWENTIETH CENTURY

During the first 30 years of the twentieth century two opposing trends were evident. The first was the consolidation of the nineteenth-century system, in which the lunatic asylum was pre-eminent as the state's response to the mentally ill. The size of county asylums grew from an average of 961 beds in 1900 to 1 221 beds in 1930. The second trend was increasing discussion about the need to diversify approaches to care and treatment, and to move away from an exclusively institutional strategy.

In 1915, the Maudsley Hospital was built in South London. The hospital was unique in that it catered only for acute cases of mental illness, had a very large outpatient clinic, and a commitment to teaching and research. All of the patients were voluntary, a fact made possible by the hospital's having no catchment area responsibility.

In 1919 the Ministry of Health was created, but had little responsibility for services for the mentally ill until the Local Government Act (1929) finally abolished the Poor Law Authorities.

In 1918, the annual report of the Board of Control made recommendations suggesting specific measures to avoid closed institutions as the principal resource in the treatment of mental illness. These included:

1. providing short-term inpatient treatment without certification;
2. establishing psychiatric clinics in general hospitals for both outpatients and inpatients;
3. recommending that senior medical staff in asylums should hold the Diploma in Psychological Medicine (DPM);
4. developing outpatient clinics at asylums;
5. providing grants to voluntary societies for the provision of after-care.

The Royal Commission on Lunacy and Mental Disorder of 1924 made a range of recommendations that eventually lead to the Mental Treatment Act of 1930. This Act made provision for treatment on a voluntary basis; further encouraged the development of outpatient clinics; and changed the terminology used to describe mentally ill people, for example, a 'lunatic' was to be known as a 'patient' or a 'person of unsound mind'. The 1930 Act was generally welcomed as enabling patterns of care that were established in the nineteenth century to be brought firmly in line with twentieth-century needs. Further progress and reform were held in abeyance when the outbreak of the Second World War in 1939 required the diversion of resources to the war effort.

The National Health Service (NHS) was established in 1948; the former county asylums were now under the control of the newly created Regional Hospital Boards. Section 28 of the National Health Service Act

empowered local authorities to make provisions for prevention and after-care, but this was permissive rather than mandatory. The split between the provision of specialized mental health care by the health services and after-care by the local authorities was subsequently to cause serious problems with the liaison and co-ordination of services. Mental hospitals were frequently sited outside the catchment areas they served, and, additionally, those catchment areas were not coterminous with local authority boundaries.

Three 'revolutions' in mental health care developed during the 1950s and 1960s (Jones, 1972).

Firstly, the administrative revolution reflected a considerable diversification of provisions. Day-care services, hostels for after-care, and psychiatric units within general hospitals all became commonplace. The regime within district mental hospitals became more open and flexible as a result of open-door policies, shorter admissions, and voluntary treatment. Some innovative centres had begun the process of reform even earlier. Northfield, the first therapeutic community in Britain, had been established during the Second World War, and the Cassell Hospital was re-established on therapeutic community lines in 1948.

Secondly, the legislative revolution began with the report of the Royal Commission on Mental Illness and Mental Deficiency in 1957. The Report's recommendations formed the basis of the Mental Health Act (1959), which repealed all previous legislation in the field of mental health. The Act emphasized the importance of informal voluntary admission, and made provisions for three types of compulsory admission: admission as an emergency, admission for observation, and admission for treatment.

Thirdly, the clinical revolution, also known as 'the pharmacological revolution', was probably one of the most significant developments in the history of mental health care. Phenothiazine drugs, a new form of therapeutic agent, were developed in France in 1952, and by 1954 had become generally available for prescription. The most common of these, chlorpromazine (Largactil), was used extensively in the treatment of schizophrenia. Its therapeutic effect was significantly to reduce or to eradicate the experience of delusions and hallucinations. Such improvements lead both to shorter admissions to hospital, and to the possibility of much more effective rehabilitation programmes. On this basis, in 1961 Enoch Powell, Minister of Health, predicted a 50% reduction in numbers of mental hospital beds within a 15-year period (NAMH, 1961).

In 1959, Dr Russell Barton, a hospital psychiatrist, published a tract in which he argued that many long-term residents of mental hospitals had become doubly handicapped: the primary effects of mental illness were compounded by the secondary effect of loss of individuality, autonomy, and initiative. Such an effect resulted from living in a custodial setting in which the residents have little or no involvement in the determination of their own care and treatment, and few opportunities to accept responsibilities which might prepare them for independent living. Barton's work probably had little impact on admission rates, however, it did prompt a gradual reappraisal, and, subsequently, a slow reform of inpatient regimes.

Social psychology was also an important influence at this time, and contributed further to the development of therapeutic communities, groupwork approaches, and a more sensitive, facilitating role for psychiatric nurses. This influence, combined with social science perspectives of mental hospitals (Goffmann, 1961), also informed radical critiques of institutional care as custodial and repressive. Such critiques were underpinned by the occurrence of a series of scandals concerning the neglect and abuse of patients in mental hospitals and mental handicap hospitals during the 1960s and early 1970s (Martin, 1984).

The 1971 White Paper *Hospital Services for the Mentally Ill* envisaged the decline and eventual closure of mental hospitals within a 15–20-year period. Inpatient services would be transferred to psychiatric units within general hospitals. There was a further commitment to community care, but the report lacked detail as to how such services would be developed.

Further pharmacological progress in the treatment of people suffering from schizophrenia was made during the early 1970s. Phenothiazine drugs were now generally available as 'depot preparations'. Slow-release forms could now be administered by injection, providing a therapeutic effect that could last for up to four weeks. This development substantially mitigated the common problem of lack of reliability in self-administration, and thereby significantly reduced the relapse rate.

Between the turn of the century and the 1970s considerable progress had been made in relation to legislative reform, the efficacy of treatment, and the development of alternatives to institutional care. However, it is notable that inpatient treatment in mental hospitals – an approach largely developed during the middle of the previous century – continued to constitute the principal resource for psychiatric care. It is also notable that policies recommending the diversification of services, made as early as 1918, took almost half a century to develop to a significant extent.

## THE MOVE TOWARDS COMMUNITY CARE

A new impetus in the move towards community care arose from the National Health Services Reorganization Act (1974). The redrawing of health authority boundaries so that they would be coterminous with those of local authorities facilitated collaborative working between authorities. But the Act went further in placing an obligation to undertake collaborative working on health and local authorities. This statutory obliga-tion was further reinforced by Section 22 of the National Health Service Act (1977).

The goals of such collaborative working, insofar as they relate to the field of mental health, were strongly informed by the 1975 White Paper *Better Services for the Mentally Ill*, which emphasized the importance of measures to prevent mental illness; early intervention; support for families; and the provision of appropriate accommodation and social facilities. The White Paper observes that 'the hallmark of a good service is a high degree of local co-ordination'. The approach of local co-ordination was extended to the joint setting of priorities and joint planning by the 1976 consultative document, *Priorities for Health and Personal Social Services* (HMSO, 1976).

Collaborative working would be pursued through the establishment of the Joint Consultative Committees. The DHSS report of 1974 (HRC[74]19) described a general pattern which the Committees were expected to take. Flexible working practices were anti-cipated in relation to local circumstances and changing needs. The limitation of these arrangements was that they made no provi-sion for financial collaboration. Accordingly, the DHSS later published circulars in 1976 and 1977 that made provision for jointly funded, time-limited projects. These projects were administered and planned by Joint-Care Planning Teams, which were comprised of key officers from both health and local authorities.

Concern about the efficiency and effective-ness of joint-funding schemes was reflected in the Comptroller and Auditor General's Report for 1981–2, which questioned whether health authorities in particular were managing joint-finance schemes adequately. This concern was later reiterated by the House of Commons Committee of Public Accounts (1983). A move towards rational planning and administration of jointly financed community care schemes began with

the DHSS *Consultative Document for Moving Resources for Care in England* (HMSO, 1981). The response to the proposals in the document was generally positive.

More detailed and specific arrangements were published in the *Care in the Community Circular* (HMSO, 1983). This made provisions for an initiative which was designed to enable substantial numbers of long-stay hospital patients to be resettled in the community. Most of the patients concerned were from mental illness and mental handicap hospitals. The concept of 'normalization', and the anticipated improvement in quality of life were major rationales upon which the arrangements were predicated. Provisions were made which enabled district health authorities to transfer funds to other agencies in order to support community care pro-grammes and developments. The major recipients were local authority social services departments, but others could include educa-tion authorities, housing associations, and voluntary bodies.

In 1982 the report of the Barclay Committee, which undertook an enquiry into the role and tasks of social workers, sug-gested a form of community care organ-ization based on local 'caring networks'. Relatively small-scale, decentralized services could, it was suggested, be more responsive to local needs. This form of organization was to prove influential in relation to the establishment of locality based mental health centres, and small, geographically based 'patch teams'.

The Mental Health Act (1983) is notable for its almost total failure to acknowledge community care, other than in requiring approved social workers to explore alter-natives to hospitalization.

Most of the official reports mentioned so far had acknowledged, either tacitly or expli-citly, that the concept of community care was valid, desirable, and practicable. Reservations that had been expressed were mostly concerned with the need for greater clarity and more detail in the approaches being used. However, the 1984–5 *Report of the House of Commons Committee on the Social Services* (HMSO, 1985) contrasted sharply with previous complacent views. Section 8 of the Report states, 'The phrase "community care" means little in itself....It has in fact come to have such a general reference as to be virtually meaningless. It has become a slogan with all the weakness that that implies.'

The Report was critical of what it saw as a lack of resources, inadequate organization and planning, and insufficient funding for community care. It expressed concern that the quality of life of those who relied on community care provisions had not improved, and in some cases had deteriorated. It was particularly scathing about the management of needs consequent on the closure of mental hospitals. Section 30 of the Report states:

The pace of removal of hospital facilities for mental illness has far outrun the provision of services in the community to replace them. Putting pressure on authorities to close or run down hospitals without similar incentives or resources to develop alternative services is putting the cart before the horse.

The Report may have had greater impact, since the Social Services Committee had an all-party membership with the greatest number of members drawn from the party in power at the time. Although the Report was unequivocal in the expression of its reservations and criticisms about community care, Jones (1988) has suggested it lacked analytic power, and tended to make general prescriptions rather than identifying precise points for action. Such limitations may have enabled the government in 1985 to publish a response to the Report that basically communicated the message that all was essentially well, and that areas of difficulty were actively being worked with.

The Report of the Audit Commission, *Making a Reality Of Community Care* (HMSO, 1986), was much more precise in its identification of aspects of community care that seemed to be either failing or functioning inadequately. The major aspects were social security policy, organizational confusion, resource allocation, and inadequate staffing. In the summary of the Report, the Commission states:

...joint planning and community care policies are in some disarray. The result is poor value for money. Too many people are cared for in settings costing over £200 per week when they would receive more appropriate care in the community at a total cost to public funds of £100–£130 per week. Conversely, people in the community may not be getting the care they need.

The Report proposed a number of specific measures designed to remove anomalies in funding and organization, and to achieve a more rational apportionment of responsibilities for differing groups of dependent people.

The specificity of the Audit Commission's critique and recommendations made it impossible for the government to accept the Report passively. The National Health Service Management Board was asked by the government to consider the Report. The Board subsequently appointed its Deputy Chairman, Sir Roy Griffiths, to produce a report that would recommend action to be taken in relation to the findings of the Audit Commission.

The Griffiths' Report, *Community Care: Agenda for Action* was presented to the Secretary of State in November 1987. The Report contained four principal recommendations:

1. The appointment of a Minister of State to be responsible for community care.
2. Responsibility for most of the provision, and all the co-ordination of community care for all groups of dependent people to be transferred to local authorities.

3. Increased funding from central government.
4. Powers for local authorities to 'buy in' additional services from both voluntary, private, and other statutory agencies.

Jones (1988) has commented that, 'These basically sensible recommendations ran into a political minefield.' It is notable that the government took four months to publish the Report. It is certain that the government found the Report unpalatable for a number of reasons. Firstly, it reiterated and re-emphasized many of the concerns and criticisms previously published in the 1985 Social Services Committee and the 1986 Audit Commission Reports. Secondly, the proposals would confer a range of additional powers and responsibilities on local authorities at a time when the government had achieved considerable success in attenuating local authority powers. Thirdly, the proposals would require additional spending by both local and central government when the government had already adopted a high-profile policy of minimizing public spending.

There may also have been a subjective element of private disappointment within the government, since Sir Roy's previous report on management within the NHS had been seen as ideologically sound and therefore implemented wholeheartedly.

In January 1989, the government published a White Paper on NHS reform entitled *Working for Patients* (HMSO, 1989). In November of the same year, a second White Paper, *Caring for People* was published (HMSO, 1989). The latter was the government's response to the Griffiths' Report on community care, and it is notable that it had taken nearly two years to produce. The recommendations of both have been combined and encapsulated in the National Health Service and Community Care Act (1990). Many of the provisions of the Act came into effect in April 1991. Broadly, the Act underpins the following principles:

- Health authorities and social services departments will continue to purchase care, but will not always provide it themselves.
- The commercial (for-profit) sector will be encouraged to take a much more prominent role in health and community care.
- The voluntary sector will be expected to play a much greater part, particularly in relation to community care.
- The planning, management, and organization of services will be undertaken more systematically and at a more local level, with the aim of matching needs to resources more effectively.
- Business principles, or 'market forces', will be used wherever possible, with the aim of containing costs and providing better value for money.
- Hospitals or community health departments will be able to apply for 'self-governing trust status', which would provide them with greater autonomy in relation to health authorities.
- The local authority (in effect, social services departments) will be the lead agency in the planning and organization of community care.
- All clients requiring long-term community care will have a specific case manager to assess their needs, and to co-ordinate the services they require.
- Those GP practices which are given control of their own budgets will be able freely to refer clients to whichever agency, service, or personnel will provide the best service.
- No mental hospital or mental handicap hospital will be allowed to close, unless it can be demonstrated that adequate alternative services can be provided locally.

Support for the provisions of the 1990 Act has been far from universal. Various interest groups have expressed reservations about the appropriateness and viability of the new approaches. The National Schizophrenia Fellowship has voiced concern about the extent and pace of the closure of mental hospitals. The MIND organization has expressed concern about the uneven distribution and quality of community resources for people with mental health problems. The Carers National Association is deeply worried about the extent to which informal carers – families, neighbours, and friends – are seen as a central part of the strategy, without being supported by additional resources. Opposition political parties have suggested that the funding of community care initiatives is inadequate, and that some of the reforms, for example the internal market in health care, would be reversed if they were elected to government.

Academic commentators too have offered views that do not wholeheartedly support the new approaches. It has been suggested that inadequate resources have constituted an interim phase in a strategy that seeks to place commercial interests at the centre of community-care provisions (Giddey, 1989). Goodwin (1990) suggest that 'the policy represents a tortuous synthesis of conflicting aims and interests; some that might be supported, and some criticized.' Whatever one's personal views, the NHS Reform and Community Care Act (1990) is a major influence in the developing role of the mental health nurse.

## THE EVOLUTION OF MENTAL HEALTH NURSING

Few of those who cared for the inmates of the Victorian county asylums received any specific or formal training. Their tasks and responsibilities were generally determined by the all-powerful medical superintendents, thus the caring role was much influenced by the medical model. However, the asylum workers, or 'lunatic attendants' as they were then known, not infrequently had other talents which they used to good effect within the institutions, for example, some had agricultural skills, others were craftsmen.

It was not until 1890 that the first formal system of training was instituted by the Medico-Psychological Association (Walk, 1961). When the Nurses Registration Act was passed in 1919, there were provisions for 'nurses trained in the nursing and care of persons suffering from mental diseases' to be included in a supplementary part of the Register. Thus mental health nurses were involved in the system of statutorily controlled professional nursing in Britain from its inception.

Throughout the nineteenth century, and indeed much of the twentieth, the role of the mental health nurse has been centred almost exclusively on the asylum or mental hospital. This has meant that during much of this period the nursing role has been concerned as much with the efficient running of institutions as it has with the provision of appropriate care for clients. Earlier schemes of training had provided a useful knowledge base concerning physical and mental pathology, and many nurses certainly developed excellent observational skills. But the information generated by nursing observations was more likely to be used in arriving at a medical diagnosis or for evaluating psychiatric treatment than in providing a basis for thoughtful, individualized nursing care.

During the middle of this century, various mental health nurses developed an interest in finding a theoretical framework that would help them to make sense of their work with clients. Psychoanalytic principles, particularly those developed by Freud, seemed potentially useful. Adequate training in the use of this model, however, was almost unavailable, and it was in danger of being applied in ways that were crude, simplistic, or inappropriate; the novel *One Flew Over the Cuckoo's Nest* (Kesey, 1962) provides an excellent satire of this.

Nevertheless, these early attempts to find frameworks and concepts that would specifically support nursing in psychiatry can now be seen as formative. Nurses were beginning to find ways of articulating what it was about their role and skills that was discreet from the contribution of other disciplines.

The advent in the 1970s of multidisciplinary team-working provided further opportunities for nurses to convey the value of their work to colleagues from other professions, and to participate in key decision-making processes. This required not only confidence in their own abilities, but the skill to communicate effectively their knowledge, understanding, and professional judgements in the interest of clients.

At Warlingham Park Hospital in 1954 the country's first community psychiatric nursing (CPN) service was established. Initially, the CPNs were largely involved in the follow-up care of clients discharged from hospital, but they also developed programmes of social support in the community. Over the next decade, other areas also developed small-scale CPN services, but, many of the nurses worked in the community on a part-time basis only (Simmons and Brooker, 1986).

The patchy and small-scale provision of CPN services during this period occurred for two reasons. Firstly, psychiatric nursing was still viewed by many as a predominantly or entirely institutional vocation (looking back, this view may seem surprising since general nurses had been deployed in the community as district nurses since the early part of the century); and secondly, other professionals, such as psychiatric social workers (usually employed by hospitals) and mental welfare officers (employed by local authorities), already provided mental health care and support in the community.

The implementation of the Local Authorities Act (1970) lead to the abolition of the role of mental welfare officers, whose responsibilities were assumed by generic social workers, many of whom would have received much less professional training in mental health. Numbers of psychiatric social workers had always been small, and

eventually training in this speciality was discontinued. The demise of these two professional groups created a vacuum in community mental health care, which CPNs were effectively able to fill. The importance of this growing group of specialist mental health nurses was recognized by the authorities responsible for nursing education, and in 1974 the first post-registration training courses in community psychiatric nursing were offered.

The 1970s saw the setting up of well-organized community nursing services in almost all health districts throughout the country. Community psychiatric nurses worked with clients in their own homes and neighbourhoods. At first, CPNs usually accepted referrals only from psychiatrists at the parent hospital, but later they took referrals from a wider variety of sources. Some CPNs undertook specialist post-registration courses, which equipped them with further knowledge, skill, and authority. CPNs were thus often seen as professionals who would take a leading role in recommending or determining the care and treatment clients required.

Today, CPNs work from a wide variety of bases. Some are attached to health centres, GP practices, and child and family guidance clinics. Training courses in community psychiatric nursing are available throughout the UK, and some of these are now linked to academic studies at graduate and postgraduate level.

During the 1980s, the nursing process was introduced, as a framework for the organization and delivery of care, to all nursing specialities, including mental health, in the UK. This enabled mental health nurses to adopt a much more systematic approach to their work; an approach which was also client-centred and holistic. Later, nursing models provided therapeutic philosophies and goals that were specific to nursing, and contributed to the development of a body of nursing knowledge.

## SUMMARY

The 1960s were a period during which mental health nurses struggled to embrace theory and to establish a stronger professional identity. During the 1970s, they played a key part in multidisciplinary working, and extended their role into the community. Throughout the 1980s they organized and evaluated their work in a more systematic way, and many began to acquire additional therapeutic skills. How, then, might we characterize mental health nursing in the 1990s?

This decade has heralded the end of a long era in which institutional care and treatment has been predominant. In addition to working in hospitals, many mental health nurses now work in permanent day-units, travelling day-care services, outpatient clinics, community mental health centres, small locality-based residential homes, and in the homes of clients. As well as being employed by health authorities, they may be employed by social services departments, by voluntary agencies or charitable trusts, and by commercial care organizations. Educational opportunities, whether clinical or academic, continue to expand, and the Project 2000 system of nurse training seeks to prepare nurses for a professional practitioner role.

At a time when traditional structures and patterns of care are being deconstructed, it is essential that nurses are able to speak clearly and cogently about the ways in which quality mental health care can be most effectively organized and delivered. It is also necessary for us to speak with confidence about what nursing has to offer during this period of radical reform. It has never been more important for nurses to advocate with and on behalf of clients, for the health needs of the communities to which we all belong.

It will be some time before the impact upon mental health nursing of the National Health Service and Community Care Act (1990) can be fully assessed. The following questions explore some of the key issues and debates. The questions may provide a basis for personal reflection, for discussion with colleagues, for discussion as an educational activity, or even for a formal debate. You may be able to think of further questions of your own to add to the list. (The abbreviation MHN denotes Mental Health Nurse.)

1. Social services departments are now the leading agency for community care. Does this mean that in future MHNs will only be deployed within acute psychiatric services?
2. The part played in mental health care by informal carers, volunteers, and health care assistants has never been greater. Is this a strategy for deprofessionalizing the service?
3. Under the provisions of the 1990 Act, what skills and knowledge would an MHN require to function effectively as a case manager?
4. Does the concept of an internal market in health undermine the nursing philosophy of an holistic, client-centred approach to care?
5. At a time when the control of budgets and other resources has been given great emphasis, how effectively could you advocate policy changes in the interests of clients?
6. Will management skills eventually be seen as more important for MHNs than clinical nursing skills?
7. How much do you know about the conditions which create mental health, as opposed to those which may create mental distress?
8. Can you justify the title mental health nurse, as opposed to the title/mental illness nurse?
9. Since health and welfare services are subject to considerable political influence, should MHNs become more politically knowledgeable and active?

## REFERENCES

Barton, W. R. (1959) *Institutional Neurosis*, Wright, Bristol.

Giddey, M. N. (1989) Community care and the new right: a social policy analysis: Unpub. postgrad. dissertation, Frewen Library, Portsmouth University.

Goffman, E. (1961) *Asylums: Essays on the Social Situation of Mental Patients and Other Inmates*, Doubleday, New York.

Goodwin, S. (1990) *Community Care and the Future of Mental Health Service Provision*, Avebury, Aldershot.

Jones, K. (1972) *A History of the Mental Health Services*, Routledge, London.

Jones, K. (1988) *Experience in Mental Health: Community Care and Social Policy*, Sage, London.

Kesey, K. (1962) *One Flew Over the Cuckoo's Nest*, Picador, London.

Martin, J. P. (1984) *Hospitals in Trouble*, Basil Blackwell, Oxford.

National Assoc. For Mental Health (1961), annual report.

Simmons, S. and Brooker, C. (1986) *Community Psychiatric Nursing, A Social Perspective*, Heinemann, London.

Walk, A. (1961) The history of mental nursing, *J. Mental Science*, 107, 446.

## POLICY DOCUMENTS

A chronological list (1974–90) of official publications of significance to community care and mental health.

**1974** National Health Service Reorganization Act.
DHSS, Collaboration between health and local authorities: reports of working party: establishment of joint consultative committees, (HRC [74] 19), HMSO.

**1975** White Paper *Better Services for the Mentally Ill*, Cmnd. 6233, HMSO.

**1976** DHSS, *Priorities for Health and Personal Social Services*, HMSO.

**1977** National Health Service Act.
DHSS, *Joint Care Planning: Health and Local Authorities*, (HC [77] 17; LAC [77] 10), HMSO.

**1979** Royal Commission on the National Health Service.

**1981** DHSS, *Care in Action, A Handbook of Policies and Priorities for Health and Personal Social Services in England*, HMSO.

DHSS, *Care in the Community: A Consultative Document for Moving Resources for Care in England*, HMSO.

DHSS, *Report of a Study in Community Care*, HMSO.

**1981–2** Comptroller and auditor general, *Report on Appropriation Accounts*, 1981–2, Vol. 8, HMSO.

**1982** Barclay Committee, *Social Workers: Their Role and Tasks*, Bedford Square Press, London.

**1983** DHSS, *Explanatory Note on Care in the Community*, HMSO.

DHSS, *Care in the Community*, (HC [83] 6; LAC [83] 5), HMSO.

House of Commons Committee of Public Accounts. DHSS, *The Joint Funding of Care by the National Health Service and Local Government*. 8th Report, Session 1982–3, HC160, HMSO.

Mental Health Act.

DHSS, *NHS Management Enquiry* (Griffiths Report), HMSO.

**1985** DHSS, *Progress in Partnership: Report of the Working Group in Joint Planning*, HMSO.

House of Commons Committee on the Social Services, *Community Care: with Special Reference to Mentally Ill and Mentally Handicapped People*. House of Commons Paper 13–1, Session 1984–5, HMSO.

DHSS, *Government Response to the Second Report from the Social Services Committee*, 1984–5 Session, HMSO.

**1986** DHSS, *Collaboration Between the National Health Service, Local Government and Voluntary Organizations: Joint Planning and Collaboration*, draft circular, HMSO.

House of Commons Committee on the Social Services, *Fourth Report: Public Expenditure on the Social Services*, HC387, Session 1985–6. HMSO.

*Government Response to the Fourth Report from the Social Services Committee*, Session 1985–6, Cmnd. 27, HMSO.

Audit Commission, *Making a Reality of Community Care*, HMSO.

**1987** DHSS, *Public Support for Residential Care: Report of a Joint Central and Local Government Working Party*. (Fifth Report), DHSS leaflets.

**1988** Griffiths, R. *Community Care: Agenda for Action, A Report for the Secretary of State for Social Services*, HMSO.

**1989** White Paper *Working for Patients*, Cm 555, HMSO.

White Paper *Caring for People: Community Care in the Next Decade and Beyond*, Cm 849, HMSO.

**1990** National Health Service and Community Care Act.

*Vivien Lindow*

I don't know how it is for other people, but fear lay behind my first visit to a psychiatrist. I was a 19-year-old student.

## CHILDHOOD AND ADOLESCENCE

Growing up. Weeping, fighting my younger sister, who is much better than me, prettier than me. Wetting my knickers through primary school, stealing from the cloakroom, playing on my own. They don't like me. I smell. Mother doesn't like me. I'm sulky.

My parents fight. They hate each other, their hatred is violent. I withdraw into myself. It's my fault. I want to be invisible.

Going to boarding school, getting wobbly breasts and not daring to ask for a bra. Not being given one because my older sister refused to wear one. Eons of embarrassment when I move. Not being given sanitary pads. My period comes. Matron is cross because I have no sanitary pads. I can no more go to a shop and buy them than fly to the moon.

Mother never mentions anything like that. She has her own troubles. She nags me to go for walks. I go for walks. She nags me to go to parties. I go to parties, and hide until it is time to go home. I want to be invisible.

Even as an 18-year-old A-level student in a classroom with girls and a teacher I have known for seven years, in response to a question that I know the answer to I seize up, go red and rigid, and wish the earth would open up and swallow me rather than say the Norman Invasion happened in 1066. I'm afraid to my stomach.

I have a friend, Barbara, and can get on with the others. I am good at exams and get into university. I hope my troubles, including that I don't have a boyfriend and everyone else does, will get solved there.

At university, nothing is solved. I am as unhappy and terrified as ever. More so. Now there are lots of men, men tutors, men students. I want to know how to talk to them, but I can't. Men are angry. Men are violent. Tutorials are the worst hell I've endured so far. I can't speak to these strange men.

I get stuck on page 158 of Warren's *King John*. I sit there staring at it for three days. My psychiatric career is about to begin.

## THE WARD

They send me to the hospital to see a psychiatrist. He is a small man with glasses. He asks me about my periods. Again I wish the earth would open up and swallow me. A strange man. Periods.

He tells me to stay. He says they used to call these places 'asylums'. So I'm a lunatic. Straightjackets.

It's not bad. I ring up Barbara, who has gone to be a medical student in Birmingham, and joke about 'being in the bin'. We arrange to go to Greece by train for a holiday. They let me out. I go to Greece.

## STIGMA

There's more to the stigma attached to being diagnosed and treated as mentally ill than the fact you can never again get a job with an insurance company. It's impossible ever to get a decent job. There are no anti-discrimination laws like there are for criminals after a time. But it's the damage that it does to you inside that's worst.

I certainly felt bad about myself before I went into hospital. I was a miserably frightened young woman who needed some help. But to turn me into a lunatic by putting me into an asylum was ridiculous. It was not the building, which was a single psychiatric ward in Bristol's Royal Infirmary, a general hospital, it was the stigma and the rest of the baggage that our society has attached to seeing a psychiatrist.

The rest of my life has been marked by that. I took on the role of mental patient. I already knew something was wrong with me. Now I knew I was mad. Doctors and nurses were in charge. They would cure me. It was out of my hands.

It is not enough for mental health services to use non-stigmatizing language and attitudes. People arrive for their first appointment with all of society's stereotype of what it means. Ignoring it means that people take it inside themselves. Stigma needs to be addressed directly. If you pretend it's not there, you leave people alone with it.

## ILLNESS AND DIAGNOSIS

One of my worst fears when I became a psychiatric patient was that they would label me 'schizophrenic'. Most people are ordinary citizens when they enter the system, and hold the same prejudices as everyone else.

I never asked my diagnosis, and always talked about depression. I knew, really, because my psychiatrist suggested I should read R. D. Laing's *The Divided Self*, and Laing was a well-known writer about schizophrenia. I also read a textbook by another psychiatrist who treated me, and could tell I fitted into that category.

Suggesting someone is ill is better than suggesting they are bad, as they used to do. However, this is not an illness like measles, a broken leg, or diabetes, and society knows this. Treating emotional distress as an illness has some harmful effects, both physical and psychological, as I found when I received drugs and ECT.

Other harmful psychological effects are a feeling of helplessness, that everyone else is an expert, and that there is something wrong with one's head. Mental health services tend to be very controlling, and one enters a world of secrecy in which one can be compulsorily detained. With these features sapping my confidence and my self-respect, I became less able to live my life, not more.

There is no shred of evidence for the medical view that emotional distress is an illness of the sort we call physical illness. Psychiatrists don't even agree on a definition of, or test for, schizophrenia. They have had enormous resources of time and money to research schizophrenia. The power and money vested in psychiatry and the drug companies makes sure they don't abandon the futile search (Warner, 1985).

Treating distressed people like machines that have gone wrong is degrading and disabling.

## CHRONOLOGY

By the time I was 28 I had been in hospital 10 times. After my first hospital stay things went well for a while, though I remained a very shy person. I never finished my history course. I discovered that alcohol helped me to mix with people. I went to a party, and met the man I was later to marry.

I lived with him. We loved and hated and loved, and we got married. A few weeks after we married Barbara was killed in an accident. That was it. My life fell apart.

If Barbara could die, nothing was safe. She was much better than me. She was a doctor. I should have died. I want to die. Month after month after year of the greatest torture. Life is not worth living. Electric shocks to my head. Several serious attempts to kill myself (what would a cheerful attempt be like?) More hell. Self-hatred.

In and out of hospital. My clothes taken away. Detained under the Mental Health Act, sexually harassed and exploited by staff. Thinner and thinner. Less and less a person.

They kept throwing me out of hospital. A few jobs: Woolworth's assistant, factory hand, invoice clerk. Sometimes a few weeks, sometimes three months. At 28 I was unemployed, unemployable, divorced. The worst hospital and best hospital were yet to come.

## DRUGS

On my first hospital visit they gave me amitriptyline, an antidepressant. I don't know what it did do, but it did nothing at all to help with my fear of other people and my dislike of myself.

The people on the ward helped with that. I got on speaking terms with a young male fellow-patient. The doctors, all men, scared me red. But I remember one nurse. She was kind; she was friendly; she was not afraid of us; she treated us as her equals; she was not mysterious about things.

In the years after Barbara died, I consumed a lot of prescribed drugs. I decided they were making me worse when I was 28. I was taking chlorpromazine, amitriptyline, antihistamine (for its sedative effects), valium and mogadon (both benzodiazepines). Valium came on the market as a new non-addictive wonder drug, as all psychological drugs do. In all the years that I took various antidepressants (it's chance that I finished on the one I started on), no one told me they also contain sedatives. This means I was taking five different sedative drugs every day. In addition, I was taking an amphetamine that my GP thought would help my fatigue.

The drugs used in psychiatry are very strong. Breggin (1983), a psychiatrist, writes:

'The major tranquillizers are highly toxic drugs. They are especially potent neuro-toxins, and frequently produce permanent damage to the brain.'

Warner (1985) gives a good account of the complex matter of major tranquillizers (neuroleptics, anti-psychotic drugs). He suggests there is no case for the routine use of such drugs on everyone who has had a psychotic episode. This is in no way a suggestion that people should be deprived of helpful drugs. Warner also argues that the long-term outcome for those diagnosed as schizophrenic has not improved since the introduction of the anti-psychotic drugs in 1954.

Davis (1991), another psychiatrist, makes it clear in a useful article about psychotropic drugs that since no biological cause of 'mental illnesses' is known, the drugs are not specific cures. He shows that psychiatric drugs in everyday use are introduced without proper trials, are given in far higher than recommended doses, without proper consent, and in mixtures that have never been tested.

Believe the people who take major tranquillizers (neuroleptics, anti-psychotic drugs) when they say that life on them is hell. Sometimes non-compliance to taking drugs is depicted as if it is another irrational symptom of whatever is supposed to be wrong, yet these drugs may damage you forever and are horrible to live with. For example, people can't see straight, feel spontaneously, concentrate, shit regularly, have sex, or sit in the sunshine. They develop tics and all manner of other side-effects. Would you like to live life with a 'chemical personality'? It is only reasonable to want to try life without these drugs.

Some people find a drug that helps them, other people prefer either to do without altogether, or have them in their control to take if needed. The point is, who is in charge? If people want to come off major tranquillizers, support should be available.

I don't know how doctors define the term 'addictive', but I've spent a lot of time in self-help groups with people coming off all types of psychotropic drugs. There is no question that people on anti-depressants become dependent on the sedative content. Talking to people about stopping taking them, it is the first one they crave, not the effect three weeks later. The same with the other drugs, including major and minor tranquillizers.

All these drugs have major effects on the central nervous system. When we stop taking them, it is hellish. The system that has become accustomed to them tries to adjust back. The behaviours that got us defined as 'mentally ill' are a reaction to stress, so our 'symptoms' often come back. Then the doctor says, 'I told you you needed these drugs', and most people get shoved back on them during the withdrawal time. Their system never gets back its level, and the person has no opportunity to learn new ways to cope with stress and fear and guilt, and all the other emotions that the drugs are designed to suppress.

Coming off psychotropic drugs is a different kind of hell, because it is chosen. I don't believe I got over the effects for two years after the last pill, and during that time I needed massive support.

So, what were the effects of drugs in my life? It is impossible to unpick all the strands. No one could go through the torturing experience of deep depression and beyond without trying the anti-depressant drugs. But to keep someone on one after another, mixed up with all sorts of other drugs, is irresponsible. How could I or the doctor judge the effect of any one drug when I was taking all the others?

They had a strong anaesthetic effect on the pain. But as the years went by, I gradually got worse: more anguished, more withdrawn, stranger. Why, then, give more, stronger, drugs? They added to the confusion. When I stopped taking the drugs, at last I discovered that much of the discomfort of my life had actually been caused by them.

They had also masked my dependence on alcohol. With so many drugs, I didn't need much alcohol to achieve my aim, which was to pass out. Occasionally I became worried about the number of prescribed drugs I was on and stopped taking them; my alcohol intake shot up. On state benefits I could not afford this, so I went back on the prescribed drugs.

It was necessary for me to stop all drugs, including alcohol, to find out who was underneath. I found the same shy, frightened woman – considerably damaged by her experiences in the mental health system.

Five years later, it was as though Barbara had died yesterday. I had done no mourning. My grief had been drugged away. Part of the emotional work I had to do to live in the world was that mourning.

## ECT

I do not think the people who had care of me in the mental health system were bad. They were doing their best in an outrageously inappropriate system.

A terrified and benumbed woman went into hospital the second time. I felt a huge guilt that if I hadn't got married Barbara wouldn't have gone on holiday on her own and got killed.

The psychiatrist who was allotted to me was unusual. He was interested in making a relationship with me. He was patient, visited me every day, and started to build up my trust.

This is where I made a major mistake. I trusted him, and for the first time in my life I tried to explain my fears and terrors and feelings to another person. I felt misplaced on the earth, like an alien among human beings.

I have seen my file. He described me as 'pre-psychotic' after the ward round told me that I must have electric shocks to my head.

On paper it was successful. After 'only' three lots of ECT my mood lifted. My memory was a bit odd. If you'd talked to me in the few weeks after having ECT you'd have put me down as a satisfied customer. But all trust in other human beings was gone. All trust in other human beings was gone.

I've written that twice because it was a disastrous thing for me. I started off afraid of other people. A mental health worker said I could trust him. When I told him how I felt he gave me electric shocks to my head.

After that I became silent. I hated myself more, this proved I was guilty. I started trying to kill myself.

The research literature shows that ECT affects the memory, and may well work by brain trauma, making the person forget for a while the reason for their distress: nobody knows how it works (Johnstone, 1989). It certainly has no proven long-term, anti-depressant effects. What is *never* discussed in the literature is the profoundly damaging psychological effects ECT can have.

The first person who was given ECT begged not to be given another shock, and was ignored (Baruch *et al.*, 1978). Since then, countless people have expressed fear and unwillingness to have ECT. But they go on using it. They go on persuading people who don't want it – even people who have had it before, who are making a judgement based on experience.

Please, I beg of you, never try to persuade someone to have electric shocks to their brain if they don't want them. If they are per-suaded to consent, then withdraw their consent, back them up. How can it be ethical to insist that a weeping and unwilling person has electric shocks to their head that have an unknown (to science, not to recipients) effect?

In 50 years, people will look back on this practice as barbaric, as we now look back on bedding down people in straw and attaching them to the wall with fetters. They used to think that was humane treatment too.

## COERCION AND CONSENT

People are unlikely to feel safe in a system where they can be deprived of their freedom. It is not necessary to have been sectioned under the Mental Health Act, as I have, to know about this sanction. People attending any mental health service soon meet people who have been coerced.

If we were treated better and more appropriately, and given choices, we would more often be willing to use the services without legal coercion. In this age of consumerism, it seems strange to apply this term to recipients of services that people can be compelled to use.

Nor are many voluntary patients truly voluntary. Once we know we can be coerced, we often stay to avoid being sectioned. We certainly would not be there if there were a kinder place of refuge, but there are few user-friendly refuges available. In most areas there are no alternatives. Especially if you are poor, and even more so if you are Black (Selig, 1991).

One of the worst aspects of the mental health services is that if a person annoys the staff by not wanting so much medication, or wanting to leave hospital, or by making a complaint about conditions, all other services are withdrawn. This is a not very subtle way of coercing people to do your will, and of punishing them if they do not. People should have the right to opt-out of part of workers' plans without losing all services. This practice is a disgrace; unfortunately, a common disgrace.

## WHAT HELPED?

The beginning of the end of psychiatry for me was a self-help group. I realized that I was getting worse, not better, and that the doctors did not have a cure for what was wrong with me. This was difficult, since they had always treated me as though I was ill. I thought they would make me better, or why did they keep taking me into hospital?

Alcohol plus prescribed drugs rendered me unconscious quickly, which was the only tolerable path. Not that it was really tolerable: I wanted to be dead for five years non-stop, but could not succeed in doing it.

Then I heard of a way out. A friend's boyfriend had joined a self-help network to give up drink and valium. A few months later I hit a further low-spot of despair, and went along to a meeting. I was greeted as an equal. No one prescribed anything, but they said that if I wanted to get off drugs I could come to meetings and find out how they had done it. No one was an expert; they'd all started where I was. Meetings were led in turn, all tasks were subject to election and time-limited, so all members quickly felt owner-ship of the group.

Coming off the drugs was the most difficult thing I have ever done. They had affected my nervous system, and coming off them was as stressful a life event as any other I have experienced. And it went on for so long. I threw up every day – one of the lesser after-effects – for 18 months.

I had to keep away from psychiatry. The workers, trained to make sure that no one expresses any emotion, would not support my effort to live without drugs. My GP wrote prescriptions that I did not take to the chemist: I had to have his sick-notes to get benefits. I could not possibly have worked at this time. Eventually he accepted that I was not taking drugs, and was finding other ways to cope.

Without the drugs I was the person I had been before, plus all the damage of the years on drugs, including the physical adjustment my nervous system had to make to the absence of toxic substances. Plus the psycho-logical damage of being a psychiatric patient; being given electric shocks to my head; being treated as of no account; confined legally and illegally (by having clothes taken away); sexually exploited and harassed by several men who were mental health workers (including a nurse manager, a staff nurse, and the hospital chaplain).

I cannot describe the difference between a self-help group based on mutual respect, and the mental health system where one set of people are the healers and get status and money for it, and another are the 'mentally ill', at the bottom of the hierarchy with less than equal citizenship, stigmatized, no power, barely enough money, seldom respected work, and sometimes no housing.

## LIFE WITHOUT DRUGS

There are times when it is difficult for me to look after myself. At its worst, a few months after I stopped taking the drugs, I couldn't move when I woke up. I would want to turn over and put my radio on, but I couldn't. It might take an hour – which seems like a week when deeply depressed – to move.

Another hour to roll out of bed on to the floor and to put the paraffin heater on. Each action takes a separate, courageous decision. Crawl to the kitchen. Make the decision to fill the kettle; another decision to move to the stove and put it on the gas; and so on.

Usually one wakes in the early hours as it is getting light, after half-an-hour's sleep, having spent the night in indescribable mental anguish, and just falling into a heavy sleep. I have wanted to die many, many times since I gave up psychiatry, but I never wanted to kill myself. Now that I don't allow people to punish me and treat me badly in the name of medicine, the question doesn't arise.

There was in fact some professional help that helped once I had regained charge of my life. I said I would tell you about my worst hospital and my best. The worst was a locked ward of an old 'bin' where there was dried shit on my bedstead, shit in the washbasin. I thought I had gone to bedlam. I was there because after a year of no drugs at all I was in such a deep depression that I couldn't look after myself, and asked again for psychiatric help. I got through this time without taking medication.

I was in the locked ward voluntarily, but even after years of being a psychiatric patient I still had no idea of my right to leave the ward. I was there for assessment to go into an addiction unit run as a therapeutic community. After a few weeks I got this place, and it was the most helpful psychiatric ward I was ever in.

What made it so helpful was the ethos that we were all there to help each other. We had to agree to a written contract before we went in. We could leave at any time. No one took any drugs. The contract said some unusual things, for example 'Free expression of feelings and exchange of views is desired so that we can learn about these reactions between people.' Also, 'The staff do not have all the answers, and they have their problems too. The patient is just as likely as the staff members to find a solution to one of the problems under discussion.'

This last sentence had a galvanizing effect on my evaluation of the contribution I could make. I was in this residential place for over three months, and came home transformed. It was like being brought up again. It was a lesson in love from fellow group and staff members. I carry the things I learned with me still.

Not surprisingly, this regime did not last for long after I left. The NHS is not good at recognizing unconventional effectiveness. This way of working is not popular with doctors, who like to be the experts in charge, and who are threatened when patients become assertive, don't take pills, and look for other solutions. The staff on the unit have the lifelong gratitude of countless people, several of whom I know are still thriving many years later. Now the unit is completely closed.

Since then I have had other help, which has always been democratic in spirit, with me in charge of my part. I have been greatly helped by a transactional analysis group, a gestalt group, and individual counselling. The point is that I have chosen these things, and I use them to enhance my life.

What works for me does not work for everyone. I would like to see genuine choice for all. All the things that helped me can be misused as power-bases for professional people to make service-users conform to their views.

I attend my self-help group twice a week, and I continue to learn in an atmosphere of caring. We are people, and so sometimes argue and hate each other, but what we have in common is far stronger than our divisions. We have no experts; nobody makes a living out of us. We make voluntary (truly) contributions to keep the meetings running, and maintain our independence by not taking money from outside. Most of us get back to work, as I have, which takes care of many aspects of dignity. It works for me.

My GP eventually said that I was the most severely depressed patient he had ever had, and that it was 'a miracle' what had happened. I know many hundreds of people who were, like me, chronic psychiatric patients who have benefited from freedom from mental health services. They tend to try and leave it all behind them; psychiatrists, if they remember us at all, talk about 'spontaneous remission'. This is an insult to the work it takes, another case of professional arrogance.

**REFUGE**

An ideal service for me would be a non-medical place run by people who understand what I'm going through, where I could go for respite when my life is impossible. There would be access to medical and social help as I think appropriate, chosen by me in conjunction with advisers, who would tell me the truth about drug side-effects and other matters. The stereotypes that spring up when we use the word 'asylum' should be remembered when talking about this form of care. In respite care people could be shown they matter by being nurtured.

Mental distress takes many forms, but the person is usually frightened by what is happening, and can be helped by non-frightened people. It is a matter of finding the appropriate level of communication. For example, R. D. Laing writes of how he would read a book or fall asleep to show someone he was not scared of them (Capra, 1988).

You can help by being yourself. That doesn't mean being a super-person, un-scathed by life, not burdened with human troubles some, or most, of the time. It means being an equal person who is there and gives feedback. Honest, non-judgemental feedback, uncontaminated by interpretation, is one of the hardest things to get in this society. The people who showed me this respect, what-ever their training, were the ones who gave me a basis for an independent life.

It is easier to be an expert, to get the comfort and status from that. Nurses who have experience of people in severe emo-tional distress certainly gain an expertise in being there for frightened people. But if you wrap that up in technical mumbo-jumbo, you will create a distance that makes you less helpful. Professional people often have the ability trained out of them just to let people be, just to be there for them and with them.

### COMMUNITY CARE

Some exciting developments in the US and Canada include the user-run places where people can receive support in crisis, as described by Judi Chamberlin (1988), herself a psychiatric survivor.

They closed the mental hospitals earlier than us in the US, and one lesson we should learn from them is that the people with the least need got the most community services. People who decide to be nurses usually want to help people. Perhaps, when you are deciding where to work you would consider targeting your care to those in greatest need, at least for part of your career. Some people experience life-long troubles, and they have traditionally received the worst services.

People who use the services long-term need to be given the power to make choices about the help they get. This may include choosing key workers, therapists, daytime activities, and so on. It seems ridiculous that people are now 'prescribed' sessions of art therapy, when they could use the resources much more cheaply and naturally by going to existing art classes, in groups if they preferred, and retain their dignity in the process.

As well as choice, the attractiveness of services should be considered. If you were feeling you could not continue with life, or were assailed by frightening visions or voices, would you want to use the services currently available?

### WHAT WILL HELP THE MOST?

I wish I could tell you the answer is psycho-therapy for all. I do not believe this. I think there should be many choices, and that each individual will find the thing that helps him or her. Since we are talking about emotional distress and mental anguish, the thing that makes the biggest difference is being treated with care and respect.

Many individuals do have issues they want to explore, either from their past or their present relationships. As long as the power of the therapist is not misused (Masson, 1988), this might be something an individual chooses to do.

It might be much more use to some people to have the salary of one expensive therapist spent on a subsidized lunch club with asso-ciated crèche. If a person cannot afford a varied diet, has little company except small children, or none at all, has no work, a year-in-year-out facility of that sort might be of greater use (Barker *et al.*, 1987; Ramon *et al.*, 1991).

The more that service planning involves service users, the more likely it is that services will be appropriate and effective. This is happening in many places. Beeforth and other service users describe some of the results when this happens. They also give the example of Brighton Users' Charter as a standard for good mental health services. Involving service users in planning and management is one way to prevent the old hierarchies of experts, with the attendant dangers of dependency and social disablement, from moving into the community.

## THE MENTAL HEALTH SYSTEM SURVIVOR MOVEMENT

This movement has gone from strength to strength since the mid 1980s. There are some useful addresses at the end of this chapter. I felt a huge, vast, gigantic outrage at what happened to me in the psychiatric system. It is still happening to many members of my local group, and to other survivors all over the country. Since I have come across this politicized movement (different from the therapeutic self-help movement), I have really learned to speak out. I am interested in doing what I can to improve the mental health system, along with other survivors.

At our first national conference at Edale in 1987, members of Survivors Speak Out agreed a charter of needs and demands:

1. That mental health service providers recognize and use people's first-hand experience of emotional distress for the good of others.
2. Provision of refuge, planned and under the control of survivors of psychiatry.
3. Provision of free counselling for all.
4. Choice of services, including self-help alternatives.
5. A government review of services, with recipients sharing their views.
6. Provision of resources to implement self-advocacy for all users.
7. Adequate funding for non-medical community services, especially crisis intervention.
8. Facility for representation of users and ex-users of services on statutory bodies, including community health councils,

mental health tribunals and the Mental Health Act Commission.
9. Full and free access to all personal medical records.
10. Legal protection and means of redress for all psychiatric patients.
11. Establishment of the democratic right of staff to refuse to administer any treatment, without risk of sanction or prejudice.
12. The phasing out of electroconvulsive therapy and psychosurgery.
13. Independent monitoring of drug use and its consequences.
14. Provision for all patients of full written and verbal information on treatments, including adverse research findings.
15. An end to discrimination against people who receive, or have received, psychiatric services, with particular regard to housing, employment, insurance, etc. (Survivors Speak Out, 1990)

## WHAT NEXT?

Asking a service user to write this chapter is a welcome example of the first demand being met, but it should go further than that. No mental health professional should be trained without people who have used mental health services taking part in the course as trainers. This 'user perspective' should be part of the examined body of learning that all nurses and other workers have to know.

One service-user activity has been organizing conferences. Two such events examined new ways of interpreting, living with and valuing the experience of hearing voices (Romme *et al.*, 1991). Other user-led conferences have looked at major tranquillizers, the experiences of self-injury, and of eating distress. We find that some professionals are keen to learn from us.

Survivor-run advocacy and self-advocacy groups are growing all over the country. These groups allow mental health service users to meet together and speak for themselves, and encourage others to revalue themselves. As part of this movement, I have changed from a nearly mute person to someone who can give talks, has been on national television, argues with psychiatrists (not a rewarding process), and writes what I believe without feeling afraid of being locked up.

It is very exciting. One of the things we are working for is the meaningful involvement of mental health service users in all aspects of managing, running, and monitoring services, as well as taking part in planning. There is a lot going on, and it is wonderful to find mental health workers acting as our allies. We do need help, but the help that has been available so far has often damaged us. We need electric shocks like a hole in the head.

## REFERENCES

Barker, I. and Peck, E. (1987) *Power in Strange Places: User Empowerment in Mental Health Services*, Good Practices in Mental Health, 380–384 Harrow Rd. London W9 2HU.

Baruch, G. and Treacher, A. (1978) *Psychiatry Observed*, Routledge, London.

Beeforth, M., Conlan, E., Field, V. *et al.* (eds) (1990) *Whose Service Is It Anyway? Users' Views on Co-ordinating Community Care*, Research and Development in Psychiatry, 134–138 Borough High Street, London SE1 ILB.

Breggin, P. R. (1983) *Psychiatric Drugs: Hazards to the Brain*, Springer, New York.

Capra, F. (1988) *Uncommon Wisdom*, Harper Collins, London.

Chamberlin, J. (1988) *On Our Own*, MIND.

Johnstone, L. (1989) *Users and Abusers of Psychiatry: A Critical Look at Traditional Psychiatric Practice*, Routledge, London.

Masson, J. (1988) *Against Therapy*, Harper/Collins, London.

Ramon, S. and Giannichedda, M. G. (1991) (2nd edn) *Psychiatry in Transition: The British and Italian Experience*, Pluto Press, London.

Romme, M. and Escher, S. (1991) Heard but not seen, *Openmind*, 49, 16–17.

Russell Davis, D. (1991) The debate on drugs – a personal view, *Openmind*, 49, 10–11.

Selig, N. (1991) Ethnicity and gender as uncomfortable issues, in *Psychiatry in Transition: The British and Italian Experience*, Pluto Press, London. (eds Ramon, S and Giannichedda, M. G.)

Warner, R. (1985) *Recovery from Schizophrenia*, Routledge, London.

## JOURNALS

*Asylum*. A magazine for democratic psychiatry, c/o Prof. F. A. Jenner, 0 Floor, Royal Hallamshire Hospital, Sheffield, S10 2JF.

*Mindwaves*. Journal of Mind's service-user network, see MINDLINK, Useful Addresses.

*Openmind*. MIND's journal. Has user-friendly and user-written articles, from MIND mail-order service below.

## FURTHER READING

*Treated Well? A Code of Practice for Psychiatric Hospitals* (1988), Good Practices for Mental Health and Camden Consortium.

Hutchinson, M., Linton, M. Lucas, J. (1990). *User Involvement Information Pack*, MIND South-east.

*Fit for Consumption? Mental Health Service Users' View of Treatment in Islington (1989)*, Islington Mental Health Forum.

Laing, R. D. (1960) *The Divided Self*, Penguin, Harmondsworth.

Read, S. (1989) *Only For a Fortnight: My Life in a Locked Ward*, Bloomsbury, London.

Sacks, O. (1990) *Awakenings*, Pan, London.

Survivors Speak Out (1990) (2nd edn) *Self-Advocacy Action Pack: Empowering Mental Health Service Users*.

## USEFUL ADDRESSES

Survivors Speak Out.
34 Osnaburgh Street
London NW1 3ND

Mindlink
22 Harley Street
London NW2 2RG
MIND's service-user network.

Astride
Elizabeth Taylor
21 Pasture Close
Wembley, Middlesex
A contact list of mental health service providers who are also survivors, for mutual support.

MIND Mail Order Service
1st Floor, Kemp House
152–160 City Road
London EC1V 2NP
Will send publication list, including videos, how to order *Openmind*, and some of the publications in the references list.

# PART TWO

# UNDERSTANDING PEOPLE – NORMAL HUMAN DEVELOPMENT

# SOCIAL DEVELOPMENT AND SOCIAL GROUP PERSPECTIVES

*Christine Halek*

## SOCIETY: RULES AND NORMS

'Society' is a concept with which we are all familiar but which is extremely difficult to define. Each society is recognized as having a discrete identity, despite being made up of many thousands or millions of individuals, and encompassing a huge number of opinions, attitudes, and behaviours. In order to function, a society has to operate by a series of rules and expectations, many of which are enshrined in, for example, a legal system, or religious or political beliefs. The Ten Commandments are a good example of a set of basic groundrules by which the ancient Jewish people were expected to regulate their attitudes and behaviour.

Of course, the ancient Jewish nation was very small, compared to the huge and complex societies in which we now live. It is not possible to regulate every detail of life in today's society by passing laws or declaring what is acceptable or unacceptable. Thus a large part of our life is governed by a hidden consensus, which leads us to expect certain types of behaviour and consider them normal or acceptable, and to reject others, which are considered deviant or unacceptable (Hilgard, *et al.*, 1979). These 'hidden' norms or rules govern every detail of our lives, from how we greet someone in a social situation, or what we wear on what occasion, to how to judge whether someone is ill or not. They also have a great influence on how we perceive ourselves, especially in relation to

others, and are thus closely bound with our self-esteem.

The norms vary in different social groups, and are not static. For example, it is now considered fairly normal in the UK for people to cohabit if they are not married, although it is still not as acceptable in Britain as in, for example, Sweden. However, it is not simply a case of more people cohabiting that has lead to a change in the norm; there has been a change in attitude towards sexuality and family groupings, and also a change in the behaviour of people within certain social strata. Conflicting norms may coexist within different groups; for example, it may be normal for White British women to leave home in their late teens and early 20s and live independently, whereas those from say, Indian, Italian, or Spanish families would be likely to live at home until marriage.

The norms that exist in society exert a powerful pressure on us. One of the tasks of our families and schoolteachers is to teach us about society's norms and how to conform to them in a way that enables us to be accepted and to function as members of society. Thus we gradually learn about other families and other people, and what sorts of behaviour are acceptable in different situations. We also learn the consequences of not fitting in – sometimes in very rough or cruel ways. For example, being ostracized or bullied by others is a powerful weapon with which to punish those who are unable or unwilling to conform. Another way is to single a person out for his or her differences, and to make fun of or attack them.

Social acceptance thus becomes a very important goal. It is interesting that in adolescence, when the young person is actively resisting the pressure to conform to his family's and society's norms, acceptance by his or her peer group, or a subgroup of it, is of paramount importance. Social acceptance is thought to be a prime motivator in causing people to adapt their behaviour to the norms prevalent in the society or social group they belong or wish to belong to (Argyle, 1982). Those who are unable or unwilling to adapt have a much more difficult time, and may be stigmatized or persecuted for their failure to conform (Goffman, 1963). It may also follow that those who are unable for some reason to conform to society's norms are those most likely to flout them (Bowlby, 1944).

If we look more closely at norms generally, we can see that they are associated with certain spheres of our existence; there are various discrete areas in a person's life, and the norms are different within each area. Intra-psychically, for example, we can theoretically have complete freedom; the main limitation will be what we ourselves consider acceptable to think or feel, which in turn will be limited by the norms of the environment within which we have grown up, – primarily our family and our society. Nevertheless, in our individual sphere we have a freedom to think, for example, that it is acceptable to feel like killing someone, whereas most of us would not carry this feeling over into our social sphere, at least not through our actions. In our families we may be constrained to behave in ways that differ from how we are when with friends, or at work. Family norms can sometimes be freer than social norms, but at other times more restrictive: for example, it may now be socially acceptable for couples to live together openly without being married, yet many people find their families less ready to accept this than today's society.

## ROLES AND STEREOTYPES

The norms we adhere to in society often feel imposed and constraining; they may conflict in many ways with our self-interest and our feelings. Norms may govern the way we dress, speak, and act – particularly in association with our roles. For example, someone in authority will have permission to behave differently from those under his or her authority; men are often expected to behave in different ways from women; older people differently from younger people; one social class differently from another. These roles, which may be allocated to us or chosen by us, can exert a further constraining influence on us, which must be accommodated if we are to adapt successfully to them. However, learning about the norms that are expected of us in different situations can also help us to move freely between roles, perhaps out of a role we do not want or did not choose into a more preferable one (Argyle, 1979), or allowing us to mix with and be accepted by others in a range of different situations.

The pressure to conform is one way in which society ensures its discrete identity and survival. Nevertheless, if we consider the diversity that underlies any society, it seems clear that the 'arrangement' we have for co-existing is subject to many forces that threaten its stability, and that some of the pressure to conform is a reaction to this threat. Such forces are ever-present in the shape of wars, revolutions, abrupt changes of power, and so on. Individual societies manage these forces in different ways, some achieving stability, and others continually subject to fragmentation.

One of the ways we cope with this threat of fragmentation is to divide ourselves into groups. Experiences in large groups show this results partly from a need to belong to a group of like-minded people as protection against the anxiety of being an individual in a huge, undefined mass; and partly as a means for diverse forces to find expression in a controlled way (Kreeger, 1975). Thus people may belong to different groups on the basis of strong belief, – often 'political', to do with allocation of power and position in society – or they may identify with certain groups on the basis of religious affiliation and/or cultural identity, class, education, mutual interest, and so on.

These groups are free to oppose each other or ally themselves with each other, but usually in a ritualized way that does not lead to catastrophe. These destructive forces then become 'institutionalized' as in, for example, the case of political forces in Britain: a public statement by a member of one political party is likely to be countered by someone from another party, or one party usually takes an identifiable stance on any one of a number of issues. Thus, the opposing forces are channelled into safe outlets, which do not threaten the underlying social order.

This sort of ritualized opposition is able to occur because society tends to use stereotypes, which are basically a shorthand way of categorizing someone or something that we all do continuously. Although stereotyping may be useful at times, it also can operate to the disadvantage of individuals and groups, and ultimately to society. An example of this is the apartheid policy in South Africa, by which people are classified by skin colour alone, and power and decision-making has been channelled into the hands of a tiny minority, depriving the country of the use of most of its potential intelligence, creativity, skill, and ability.

Many people are unhappy with this state of affairs, where institutionalized behaviours and attitudes have taken precedence. Challenging social norms, however, is no easy task. Another function of social groupings, then, is to influence society in a way that individuals rarely can. The pressure for change in society is almost always achieved by the banding together of like-minded people to form a group without which the individual's

voice would probably go unheard. Even those individuals who seem to achieve change almost single-handedly can only do so with the approval of many others. Thus we often 'silently' choose people to fulfil certain essential functions in society: to do good, to cause trouble, to make decisions, to cause dissent, and so on. Although many people will be unhappy with the 'choice' of the person to fill such a role, nevertheless, he or she will have been chosen by some sort of majority consensus.

## THE INDIVIDUAL IN SOCIETY

We live virtually our entire lives in social situations. It is almost impossible to think of ourselves without reference to the context in which we live, particularly our relationships with other individuals and groups. Historically, this social context has promoted our survival, and we continue to need to co-operate and coexist in a variety of social groupings and situations.

### EARLY SOCIAL DEVELOPMENT

It is now generally acknowledged that human infants are born with the capacity for socialization (Stern, 1985; Winnicott, 1965). The infant quickly learns to distinguish between his mother or primary carer and other carers, and soon shows a preference for this most important person. He can also make his presence felt from a very early age: when he is able to smile, vocalize, and imitate, he is capable of initiating social interactions of some complexity. Think how difficult it is to resist a baby's or young child's smile: it has a compelling attractiveness, leading most people to respond with a combination of smiling, gazing, and vocalizing, and possibly moving closer to the child. Similarly, a young baby may turn away from his mother, or stop feeding if he wants to end or alter an interaction. The infant is already able to control social interactions, and begins to learn about other people and himself through their responses to him.

The **dyadic**, or two-person, relationship an infant has with his mother or primary carer is likely to form the basis for his future social functioning, particularly as regards intimate relationships and friendships (Bowlby, 1979). The relationship with the mother or carer has at least two important social functions. Firstly, the infant learns that what he communicates to his mother leads to a response from her, which in turn leads him to respond. The infant and the mother will develop their own patterns or rhythms of stimulus and response that will be quite particular to them, and which the infant will carry into all his future relationships (Rayner, 1986). Secondly, the mother's responses give the infant information about himself as well as about her, and from this he will begin to form an impression of what he is like. This process is known as '**mirroring**', and also continues in our relationships with others throughout life (Winnicott, 1967).

This primary relationship is the springboard for many others in life. Most people move on to extend their repertoire of relationships to include father, siblings, peers, people in authority, people needing help, and so on. Some people seek what they missed in the primary relationship; others seek people who can make them feel the same as their primary carer did. Bowlby's work on attachment concluded that children who were securely attached to their mothers were more socially confident and competent than those who were insecure or 'anxiously attached' (Bowlby, 1965). Such social competence, or 'social skills', is essential for successful integration into society in the many different roles which young people and adults are expected to fulfil (Argyle, 1979).

As the child grows up, he is exposed to a variety of different social situations to which he must adapt. There may already be other children in the family, or siblings may soon follow. The child may go to a play-group or nursery school, and from there to more formalized schooling. The role of other children in the socialization process is very important, particularly for dealing with issues of rivalry, competition, sharing, co-operation, and friendship. Playing together, squabbling and fighting are all ways of establishing relationships with a peer group, and of developing a social personality. For instance, some children are leaders and others followers, some are clowns, some are trouble-makers and so on. Such roles can be adopted at an early age. Children who miss out on such experiences for some reason, such as through illness or enforced isolation, are likely to have some difficulty in adolescence or adulthood when it comes to living and working with others (Shaffer, 1982).

In school the child comes face to face with another set of social expectations: imposed discipline and authority. Although these issues will have been met with before, it will usually have been in the context of family and close relationships, whereas the authority of teachers and other adults is more arbitrary and less open to influence. The child has to learn to cope alone, with the possibility of conflict between the family's rules and norms and those of the school environment. He may find this frightening, freeing, difficult, or relatively straightforward, depending on the degree to which he and those around him are able to develop co-operative relationships. He will also learn the consequences of not being able to adapt, whether through punishment, teasing, or bullying. It is often obvious at an early age which children are likely to have problems socializing and forming relationships in later life.

## THE PROCESS OF SOCIALIZATION

The socialization process involves learning how to fit in to social situations while retaining one's own identity. We are all born with innate constitutional factors that help to mould our intellectual development and our personalities, and determine to some extent how we learn. But these can never be separated from the social context within which we develop. The child's capacity for learning is thus governed by his developing intellectual and physical capacities (Piaget, 1955), as well as his environment, the quality of care he receives, and the degree to which he is stimulated to learn – what Winnicott calls 'a **facilitating environment**'.

Within these conditions, the child learns by various methods, such as observation, conditioning (social learning), imitation, and identification. By observing what other people do and the consequences of that, the child learns how to achieve certain things, or perhaps what happens when, for example, you get upset or shout at someone. This is one of the main ways in which children learn about emotional control and expression within the family (Bandura, 1969). Through conditioning, or social learning, the child learns which sorts of behaviour bring rewards or are acceptable (Skinner, 1974). Learning to say 'mama' or 'dada', for example, comes from the child's initial attempts at vocalizing being selectively reinforced or rewarded by his parents. He gradually learns that there are preferred sounds, and that they relate to mother and father. Here, imitation will also have been used to achieve learning. A further example of conditioning might be the use of 'no' to teach the child what is forbidden or dangerous or unacceptable. The things associated with 'no' will be treated differently from other things.

In identification, learning stems from the wish to be like someone, usually, at first, a parent (Skynner *et al.*, 1982). Thus a young child will try to help with the housework, or to play football, or to read books; that is, behave in a way which he associates with the favoured person, as though he can thereby become like him or her. This process of learning by identification is particularly important for the development of gender identity and cultural/racial identity.

## THE CONCEPT OF PSYCHOSOCIAL DEVELOPMENT

The relationship between personality and social functioning has been particularly developed by Erikson (1963, 1980), who believed that the personality develops throughout life through contact with the environment, and that this places certain demands on the person. As we grow and develop, and as society changes, the demands on each person change as well and must be successfully negotiated. Erikson felt that each person has to negotiate a series of stages or 'crises', by which he meant significant turning–points in development, during his or her life. At each of these crises, some challenge has to be faced and overcome if the person is to continue to develop heathily within society, particularly in relationship to other people. Although the stages appear separate and closely related to chronological age and development, in practice they are not exclusive and may have to be negotiated more than once (Clark *et al.*, 1988).

### ADOLESCENCE

Adolescence is an important stage in a person's social development. In many cultures it is celebrated or marked in particular ways, which have a clear social context. In Western societies adolescence has become rather a prolonged affair, brought about by changes in patterns of work practice, education, and the rise of a 'youth culture' (Rutter, 1979). It is still seen, however, as a rite of passage, a stage which the person has to pass through in order to emerge as an adult who can take his or her place in society. In other societies, and in some cultural groups in our own society, what would be adolescence involves an abrupt change of role from child to man or woman, for example, with the consequent assumption of adult responsibilities; biological markers of puberty and sexual development are often used to determine when the child's role changes at this time.

## ADULT SOCIAL FUNCTIONING

The social learning experiences that the child and adolescent undergo determine to a large extent how he or she will function in adult life. By early adulthood we are in a position to interact co-operatively with others in a variety of social roles: some of these will be work or task-oriented, others will be related to our family, and others to close personal relationships. Early experiences may influence our choice of job and our success or failure within it, as well as our choice of partner or friends and hobbies. An only child, for example, who as a child was not particularly outgoing, perhaps finding it difficult to make friends, might choose a job in charge of others, or working in a field where co-operation or teamwork is not particularly important. We might infer that he would find sharing responsibilities difficult. A middle child might be better at negotiating and problem-solving in groups. Of course, things are not so clear-cut, in that a middle child might have been well-integrated or left out, or a person might choose in adult life to tackle areas in which he or she had little chance to succeed when younger. Nevertheless, the person's earlier social learning and functioning will influence his position in adult life (Skynner *et al.*, 1982).

## SOCIAL RELATIONSHIPS

The ability to relate to others in social situations is of great importance for us as individuals, and also for the social groups and societies we belong to. Our social relationships with others revolve around two main areas: work and free time. In many ways these are our links between our individual social development and the society we live in. Those who for some reason do not or cannot participate in the work or the social spheres, may be seriously disadvantaged and marginalized in a distressing way by others. (Goffman, 1963).

## WORK

Work is the means whereby we take an active part in ensuring that society continues to function and to provide us with the things we need. At least that is the idea, although many would say they do not get what they need or want from society. Every job in society fits into an enormously complex organization, which is made up of many interacting systems that shape our society. Thus, our cheques are cleared, our rubbish collected, our food manufactured and supplied, our illnesses diagnosed, and hopefully treated. Our jobs will almost certainly depend on someone else's, and we, in our turn, will be depended upon.

Work is enormously important for our sense of identity (Hunt *et al.*, 1975). When we meet someone new, often one of the first things we find out about them is what their job is. Work gives us a structure and sense of purpose, a clear role and clear responsibilities, as well as money with which to resource the rest of our lives. While not everyone is going to find these things in equal measure in their work, being without work can have serious effects on a person's mood and self-esteem. It can also affect his or her opportunity for social contact and necessary stimulation. The lack of money and security that often goes with being unemployed makes such things even more problematic, and causes increased worry and stress. Maintaining good physical and mental health in these circumstances is often very difficult.

Work is usually the arena within which we develop our public selves, where we continue to learn about dealing with authority, leadership, assuming roles – all the things we began to learn early in life (Argyle, 1979). The person who is not able to work – maybe because they did not learn enough about these things when young – is not able to continue to develop in this way, and becomes less likely to find work and opportunities to develop. The person finds him or herself in a vicious circle, which can be very difficult to get out of.

Most jobs form part of what are called social systems, that is, the job exists regardless of the individual characteristics of the person employed to do it (Argyle, 1979). This means it is always necessary to adjust the fit of a person to a job. Because the job is usually less flexible than the person, the person may have to compromise certain aspects of his or her personality or behaviour to fit in. Personality also accounts for the type of work we choose: for example, nurses prefer to work with people. Some prefer to work in isolation, and others as part of a team (Peek *et al.*, 1975).

PLAY

Play, or leisure, is the time outside our work which is ours to do with as we wish. For many people such time may seem to be taken up with family or other responsibilities, but when we talk about leisure in a social context, we are thinking about how people function in relatively unstructured situations, where their roles and responsibilities are less clear. The lack of structure can cause particular problems for those people who do not have a clear sense of their own identity or social roles. Particularly important aspects of leisure time are making friends and belonging to groups.

Friendship combines durability and intimacy, and is one of the most important of our social relationships (Argyle, 1982). It is normal to have friends who play different roles in our lives and with whom we share differing degrees of intimacy. Some people make long-lasting friendships, others less so. Some people have great difficulty making friends.

In order to make friends, we first have to come into contact with people. We then find ourselves attracted to certain people, and if we like them, we continue to interact with them. In this way we set up an attachment in which increased interaction leads to greater liking. Friends are usually people with whom we have some similarities, such as common interests or a shared background.

As the greatest part of initial attraction is non-verbal, and non-verbal behaviour is different in different social groups, we are usually attracted to people of our own cultural background or social class, although this is by no means inevitable (Schaffer, 1982). We also seek a certain level of self-disclosure with others with which we feel comfortable. Like our early relationships in our family, these relationships operate by a complex and sensitive set of feedback cues by which we regulate our interactions (Bowlby, 1979). These make up what we usually call social skills (Argyle, 1979). People who have poor social skills have difficulty making friends, and as with the unemployed, miss the opportunity to further develop the necessary skills needed to make and maintain friendships. Friendships that go wrong can be affected by a person's earlier experiences of relationships, particularly of intimacy.

The other main area of social functioning is belonging to certain groups that have an essentially social function, rather than being task-orientated, like work. Thus, even though they may involve a task, the groups are basically organized to promote social relationships, enjoyment, relaxation, or as a vehicle for sharing a common interest or set of values. Some people feel much more comfortable with group activities than others; some may find themselves in an organizing or leadership role, others in a more passive role; some may tend to avoid group activities. These roles may coincide with those adopted in our work lives, or may be quite different (Goffman, 1963).

PRIVATE AND PUBLIC SELVES

The interface between our private and our public selves is managed by a sophisticated system of self–management, which, if we are fortunate, we acquire as we grow and develop in childhood and adolescence (Goffman, 1963). Our social functioning is all the time based on our private selves, which in turn receives feedback from our social selves. Most of us are aware of a discrepancy between the self we present to others and that which we present to close friends and partners. Sometimes the interface breaks down or cannot be adequately managed.

Just as norms govern the functioning of society as a whole, they also dictate the extent to which we can show our private selves to others. This is particularly true at work or in relation to authority. For a lot of people in Britain, these norms affect emotional expression, especially in relation to gender and position. If you are in a position of authority you are constrained, especially as regards the expression of things like vulnerability and anxiety. The position is more difficult if you are a man. Desiring power and being ambitious, however, may present problems for women. This has far more to do with society's norms and expectations than with individuals' own wants or abilities. An awareness of these norms and expectations, and the degree to which they constrain or enable us in our various roles in life is essential if we are to find our place in society (Hunt *et al.*, 1975).

## SOCIAL FUNCTIONING AND MENTAL HEALTH

Appropriate social functioning and integration are seen as markers of good mental health; the main way a person is recognized as being mentally ill is when his behaviour becomes abnormal or socially unacceptable. Equally, re-integration, or acceptance back into society, depends largely on being able to function within the norms expected by society. Thus, a person does not have to be well, but he has to behave as though he were well. If he can achieve this, people will assume he is well. This emphasis on 'visible' health can be problematic for people with psychological problems, as well as for those who are physically disabled or different in some way, that is their non-conformity is evident (Goffman, 1963).

## CONCLUSION

In looking at the whole area of mental health it is crucially important for us as nurses to understand the social context in which the person has developed and to which he will probably need to return. Indeed, many would say that social functioning is the yardstick by which mental health is to be 'measured'.

## REFERENCES

Argyle, M. (1979) *The Psychology of Interpersonal Behaviour*, Penguin, Harmondsworth.

Argyle, M. (1982) Social behaviour, in *Psychology and People*, (eds A. J. Chapman and A. Gale), Macmillan, London.

Bandura, A. (1969) *Principles of Behaviour Modification*, Holt, Reinhart & Winston, London.

Bowlby, J. (1944) Forty-four juvenile thieves: their characters and home life, *International J. Pyschoanalysis* 25; 19–52.

Bowlby, J. (1965) *Childcare and the Growth of Love*, Penguin, Harmondsworth.

Bowlby, J. (1979) *The Making and Breaking of Affectional Bonds*, Tavistock, London.

Clark, E. and Keeble, S. (1988–9) *The Developing Person*, South Bank Polytech. Distance Learning Centre, London.

Erikson, E. H. (1963) *Childhood and Society*, WW Norton & Co, New York.

Erikson, E. H. (1980) *Identity and the Life Cycle*, WW Norton & Co., New York.

Goffman, E. (1963) *The Presentation of Self in Everyday Life*, Penguin, Harmondsworth.

Goffman, E. (1963) *Stigma*, Penguin, Harmondsworth.

Hilgard, E. R.; Atkinson, R. L. and Atkinson, R. C. (1979) *Introduction to Psychology*, Harcourt, Brace Jovanovich, Inc., New York.

Hunt, S. and Hilton, J. (1975 ) *Individual Development and Social Experience*, George Allen & Unwin, London.

Kreeger, (1975) *The Large Group, Dynamics of Therapy*, Maresfield Reprints, London.

Peek, D. and Whitlow, D. (1975) *Approaches to Personality Theory*, Methuen, London.

Piaget, J. (1955) *The Child's Construction of Reality*, Routledge & Kegan Paul, London.

Rutter, M. (1979) *Changing Youth in a Changing Society*, Nuffield Provincial Hospitals Trust.

Schaffer, H. R. (1982) Social development in early childhood, in *Psychology and People*, (eds A. J. Chapman and A. Gale) Macmillan, London.

Skinner, B. F. (1974) *About Behaviourism*, Jonathan Cape, London.

Skynner, R. and Cleese, J. (1982) *Families and How to Survive Them*, Methuen, London.

Stern, D. N. (1985) *The Inter-Personal World of the Infant*, Basic Books, New York.

Winnicott, D. W. (1965) *The Maturational Processes and the Facilitating Environment*, Hogarth Press, London.

Winnicott, D. W. (1967) Mirror-role of mother and family in child development, in *Playing and Reality* (1980) Penguin, Harmondsworth.

Winnicott, D. W. (1973) *The Child, the Family and the Outside World*, Penguin, Harmondsworth.

*Julia Fabricius*

The term 'psychodynamic' implies that psychic, or mental, processes are dynamic as opposed to static: they involve movement and force. A psychodynamic interpretation always contains the idea that an individual's behaviour and subjective experience are the outcome of a conflict, usually largely unconscious, between opposing forces in the mind.

Psychodynamic psychology is essentially an intraperson, or, more specifically, an intrapsychic, psychology. This is in contrast to, for example, behavioural psychology, in which behaviour is regarded as the outcome of forces in the environment acting on the individual; or social psychology, in which behaviour is explained by reference to interpersonal or intergroup processes. The discipline within which psychodynamic psychology has been set out is psychoanalysis.

## THE DEVELOPMENTAL POINT OF VIEW

Psychodynamic psychology is *par excellence* a developmental psychology. In any individual, the mental conflicts and the method of dealing with them are considered to have a history that goes back to birth. The final balance of forces in the mind at any point in the life of an individual will be the result of both constitutional and experiential factors. Either of these can change at any stage of life, but the crucial period in which a person's usual or habitual state of equilibrium is set is from birth to five years.

Psychodynamically speaking, how the mental conflicts in these early years are resolved remains an integral part of the structure of the adult mind. The proverb 'the child is father to the man' is highly applicable; or, as it has been put by two British psychoanalysts, contained in every adult mind there is 'the child within' (Sandler and Sandler, 1987).

Sigmund Freud (1856–1939) was the first to describe the mental life of adults in terms of psychodynamics and in terms of its childhood origins. Interestingly, it was from examining mental processes in adults that Freud first formed his hypotheses about childhood development. Freud described only one child case, Little Hans, in which he did not treat Hans directly but advised the boy's father (Freud, 1925). Later, psychoanalysts working directly with children, for example Freud's daughter Anna, confirmed many of his findings and added to them. Just as Freud made inferences about childhood from working with adults, some psychoanalysts working with children, notably Melanie Klein (1882–1960) and her followers, have put forward new hypotheses about mental processes in early infancy.

## THE NATURE OF THE MIND

Before developmental processes can be described in detail, we need to understand what it is that develops.

From a psychodynamic perspective, the individual's mind consists of two main components: the sensual, sexual, and aggressive drives; and the part through which these drives operate – or which denies them operation – and which relates to the world.

Freud described the mind thus in his well-known **structural model** (1923), in which he called the first component the **id**, and the second the **ego**. It is important to emphasize that this is only a model – a way of describing something that is abstract in concrete terms in order to make it easier to think about. It does not mean the mind literally consists of entities called the id and the ego.

THE ID AND THE EGO

The id is the part of our mind where the drives are represented. These drives are intimately connected with the physical body and its functions. In the mind, these physical drives are represented as wishes and impulses. If left to its own devices, the id would operate entirely on what Freud called **the pleasure principle** by which wishes would be instantly gratified; if this could not be done by realistic means, it would be done by hallucinatory or delusional ones. There is no such thing as delay, logic, or rational thought.

The ego, by contrast, operates to a much greater extent by what Freud called **the reality principle**. The ego is the part of our mind that considers the consequences of our actions – for example, that an action motivated by the id might lead to the loss of love or disapproval, or physical danger. The ego, as the 'executive' part of the mind, has different courses of action open to it: it may carry out the wishes of the id immediately; or it may instigate a delay, a total ban, or some sort of compromise by which the wishes are only partly gratified, in the interests of reality. However, the ego is always the servant of the id, as well as of reality. Freud used the metaphor of a horse and rider: the id, as the horse, is a powerful animal; the rider, ego, may only have a semblance of control by partly going where the horse wants.

Within the ego there is a substructure called the **super-ego.** This is a part of the ego, which is formed by identification with our parents and their authority. It is the part of the mind that judges our thoughts and actions, which can make us feel either approved of and loved, or disapproved of and punished. Often it is the super-ego which will not allow the ego to carry out the wishes of the id (page 97).

An important element in this theory of the mind is that much mental functioning takes place unconsciously. The wishes of the id, and the approval or disapproval of the super-ego are only experienced consciously in so far as they are mediated through the ego. This means they may only be known to us consciously in a form that is altered from the original. Even much of the activity of the ego takes place unconsciously.

Freud's structural model was created to aid thought about something (the mind) that cannot be seen. Remembering this can help to make the model less difficult to understand, and less dry than it otherwise might be.

Another aspect that can help the newcomer get to grips with Freud's theory is the English translation of German terms. Freud's English translator used Latin terms – 'id' and 'ego' – for the German *Das Es* and *Das Ich*, meaning, in English, 'the it' and 'the I'. The English translation in fact gives a much better sense of the meaning: the 'it', or id, contains the irrational; and the 'I', or ego, mediates between the id and the world outside. In common English usage one might say, for example, 'I don't know why *I* did that, *it* just came over me.'

THE STRUCTURAL MODEL AND DEVELOPMENT

Although Freud's book *The Ego and The Id* was not published until 1923, many of his ideas about development were published much earlier. One of the main sources is *The Three Essays on the Theory of Sexuality* 1905, in which he was concerned solely with the development of drives, or instinct. At that stage, although Freud had described reactions against drive expression, and spelled out the operation of the pleasure and reality principles, he had not formulated his ideas about the ego, and so could not describe its development. To some extent, the task was left to his successors, some of whom gave greater emphasis to the id development, and some to the ego. But as the preceding section has made clear, the two go hand in hand: each has its own developmental pathway, but neither is independent of the other.

In health, and with what the psychoanalyst Donald Winnicott called a 'good-enough environment' (1960), there will be progression in the development of both structures. If things go wrong, there can be a **fixation** at particular points, or a **regression** to earlier stages that had previously been surmounted. When things go well, development involves a progressive recognition of reality, and an increasing ability to 'own' all of one's personality.

## FREUD'S VIEW OF DEVELOPMENT

Freud's theory of development grew over nearly 40 years, and changed considerably in his life time. In such a brief summary as this, inevitably some of his ideas will be telescoped together, and explained only briefly.

Freud believed that young children are essentially sensual beings. The body and the feelings created by its functioning are a source of pleasure. When a wish arises to repeat a pleasurable sensation, independently of the bodily function that introduced it, it produces a drive.

Freud's early theory is one of **libido** development. He saw libido – Latin for wish or desire – as a non-specific sensual drive for bodily gratification, which at different stages of development becomes centred on particular bodily zones, and which is the forerunner of adult sexuality. Preoccupation with the more infantile zones never disappears completely – it may persist in normal adult sexuality, as in using the mouth for kissing, in perverse sexuality, and in other ways.

## THE ORAL STAGE AND THE BEGINNINGS OF THE REALITY PRINCIPLE

For Freud, the newborn infant is a bundle of drives and needs ruled entirely by the pleasure principle. He thought the infant is essentially autoerotic, that is, directed to gratify needs in himself without any desire for, or awareness of, other people. The fact that another person is essential for the infant's survival is at first of no relevance to him, since he does not yet operate by the reality principle.

The infant is biologically programmed to suck in order to live. Freud thought this leads to the mouth becoming the principle libidinal zone in early infancy; sucking and mouthing become aims in themselves, independent of the infant's need for nutrition. This can be seen clearly in babies, and also in many adults where eating, drinking, or smoking is done other than for reasons of hunger or thirst.

Hunger is intolerable for the infant. Because he lives by the pleasure principle, he must try to satisfy his drives immediately. In normal circumstances, his screaming and writhing will result in him being given a feed; if he has to wait, he may suck his finger or the corner of a blanket, and thus be temporarily quieted. Freud believed the infant was able to fantasize that the finger or blanket was the nipple or bottle teat. Again, the vestiges of such a mechanism can be seen in many normal adults, who in times of deprivation may fantasize that they have what they want.

Even for the infant, however, such a manner of satisfying needs will not work indefinitely, and even the most attentive mother will not at all times be able to satisfy her baby quickly enough. In this way the infant becomes aware of reality, or as Freud (1911) put it:

It was only the non-occurrence of the expected satisfaction, the disappointment experienced, that led to the abandonment of this attempt at satisfaction by means of hallucination. Instead of it, the psychical apparatus had to decide to form a conception of the real circumstances in the external world and to endeavour to make an alteration in them. A new principle of mental functioning was thus introduced; what was presented in the mind was no longer what was agreeable but what was real, even if it happened to be disagreeable.

This is the beginning of mental functioning, in which there can be the toleration of delay in impulse satisfaction, reality testing, and, above all, rational thought. It is learned only gradually throughout childhood; even in adults pleasure-principle functioning persists to some extent, if only in dreams and fantasies.

## THE ANAL STAGE

The anal zone becomes the focus of sensual pleasure at the time in which the child is learning bowel control. The passage of faeces can cause pleasurable sensations in the anal mucous membrane. The issue of potty-training can also become a battleground between child and caretaker, with children refusing to empty their bowels when and where the adult wants. The toddler's battle for autonomy is carried out in other areas of life as well.

For the young child, the faeces are part of his own body, and can represent his first gift to the adult. Adults seem to recognize this too, in their frequent expressions of, for example, 'Do a nice poo for mummy!' As Freud said, 'By producing them [faeces] he can express his active compliance with the environment, and, by withholding them, his disobedience.' (Freud 1905). In adults, traces of such issues can be seen in such character traits as meanness and stubbornness. Freud

also postulated that from being a gift, faeces can come to mean 'baby'; young children often develop sexual theories in which babies are conceived by eating, and are born through the bowels.

## THE PHALLIC STAGE

Although very young infants can be observed to touch their genitals, given the opportunity the genitals do not become a main source of sensual pleasure until a child is about three years. At around this time it is common for children of both sexes to become aware of genital sensation during urination, bathing, or through accidental contact, and for them to deliberately reproduce this sensation by masturbation. In addition, many children of this age of both sexes take pleasure in exhibiting themselves – being naked, running and jumping, showing off – all activities that have a phallic origin.

## THE OEDIPUS COMPLEX

This is a centrepiece of psychoanalytic theory. Freud first wrote about the Oedipus Complex in 1900, and adhered to his ideas about it throughout his life. All subsequent psychoanalysts, although they might disagree about the timing or the exact nature of the Oedipus Complex, have thought that it is of fundamental importance in development.

Freud named the Oedipus Complex after the hero of the Greek myth. The Delphic oracle had predicted that Oedipus would kill his father and marry his mother, and due to an unfortunate set of circumstances this prediction came true (Graves, 1955). Freud found that all of the adults he worked with showed evidence of a more or less deeply buried attachment to the parent of the opposite sex, and hostility towards the parent of the same sex. He thought this originated from sometime between the third and fifth years, and speculated that the theme had become embedded in Greek myth and also in other literature, for example, in Shakespeare's *Hamlet*, because it struck a universal chord for humanity.

In ideal circumstances, the Oedipus Complex is eventually given up, but as with other developmental stages, traces of it nearly always remain, although usually largely unconsciously. In the boy, hostility and aggressive wishes directed towards the father are overcome both by fear of the father, who is bigger and stronger, and by the child's love for him. In particular, the boy fears his father might punish him by castration, a belief that may be stimulated by the discovery that a girl does not have a penis. This sounds a very primitive idea, but the mind of the child is in fact at a primitive stage of development in which a talion morality of 'an eye for an eye' is held. In a normal family, for the child who also loves his father greatly, such thoughts are troubling, puzzling, and thus usually unconscious or only partly conscious.

Because of this conflict in feelings, the little boy gives up his ambition to take his father's place with his mother, and in so doing internalizes his father; he accepts his father as both an internal and external authority, and thus the super-ego is formed. Thereafter, incestuous desires are forbidden from the child's mind, and the whole affair is lost from conscious memory. It is important to emphasize that the super-ego represents the loving, supporting aspects of the parents as well as their more severe aspects. Some of the child's own aggression may be attributed to this internal figure, and indeed people with particularly severe super-egos often have not had severe parents in reality.

In the girl, Freud believed the situation to be more complicated. For her, the discovery of the male's penis can lead to envy and a feeling of inferiority, leading to hostility towards the mother for not giving her the wished-for penis, and a turning towards the father. For many girls, Freud thought the wish for a penis of her own gives way to the wish for a man's penis and the wish for a baby, but in some the original **penis envy** may, more or less unconsciously, persist: 'Whereas in boys the Oedipus Complex is destroyed by the castration complex, in girls it is made possible and led up to by the castration complex.' (Freud 1925).

Many psychoanalysts have since questioned and revised Freud's ideas about girls. Most now think the little girl is not just a 'failed boy', but has an early and innate sense of femininity. Nevertheless, in the unconscious mind, different truths can coexist. It is certainly true that in some girls and women envy of men and a masculine form of striving is an issue.

## LATENCY AND PUBERTY

At the age of five or six, the repudiation of the Oedipus Complex and the wishes associated with it brings about a period of **latency** in drive development – a pause in the evolution of sexuality. There is a desexualization of the child's interests and relationships, the emergence of such feelings as shame and disgust, and a growth of **sublimations**, in which sexual energy is diverted towards intellectual development.

At puberty, the sexual drives reawaken. The adolescent's task is to loosen his bonds with his family, and to achieve a non-incestuous genital aim. This period of development may often entail a degree of reworking of earlier conflicts, particularly the Oedipal.

## ANNA FREUD'S VIEW OF DEVELOPMENT

Freud, a Viennese Jew, came to London with his family in 1938, dying a year later. His daughter Anna (1895–1980), originally a teacher, had trained as a psychoanalyst in Vienna, and had started to work with children. In London during the war she set up the Hampstead War Nurseries, which later became the Hampstead Clinic, and after her death in 1984, the Anna Freud Centre.

Freud's early theory had been mainly about the development of drives, or id development. Anna Freud was particularly interested in ego development, and in the relationship between id and ego development.

## THE CONCEPT OF DEVELOPMENTAL LINES

From her work with both normal and disturbed children, Anna Freud mapped out a number of lines of development, each line describing a continuum from a state of dependent, irrational, drive-determined being, to one of increasing self-mastery. To quote Anna Freud (1966):

> Such lines – always contributed to form the side of both id and ego development – lead, for example, from the infant's suckling and weaning experiences to the adult's rational rather than emotional attitude to food intake; from cleanliness training enforced on the child by environmental pressure to the adult's more or less ingrained and unshakable bladder and bowel control; from the child's sharing possession of his body with his mother to the adolescent's claim for independence and self-determination in body management;

On the developmental line 'from sucking to rational eating', for example, Anna Freud describes the following stages:

1. Being nursed at the breast or bottle; interference with need satisfaction caused by, e.g., hunger periods or forced feeding, set up the first, and often lasting, disturbances in the positive relationship to food.
2. Weaning, initiated either by infant or by mother. If by the latter, and especially if carried out abruptly, the infant's protests may have an adverse effect on the normal pleasure in food.
3. The transition from being fed to self-feeding, with or without implements;

'food' and 'mother' still being identified with each other.
4. Self-feeding; disagreements with mother about what and how much will be eaten, table manners, etc.; craving for sweets as a substitute for oral suckling pleasures; food fads and disgust as a result of newly acquired reactions against anal interests.
5. Gradual fading out of the equation food= mother in the Oedipal period; irrational attitudes towards eating now determined by infantile sexual theories, e.g., fantasies of impregnation through the mouth.
6. Gradual fading out of the sexualization of eating and increase in the rational attitude to food; earlier experiences being decisive in shaping the individual's tastes, habits, preferences, aversions and addictions in later life.

A child's progress through the stages of a developmental line is easily affected by illness or other upset. A sick or distressed child may often lose his previously secure bladder control, for example, or revert to babyish eating. This is described as **regression**. Regression to a more immature way of functioning can often be seen in adults when they are ill or troubled in some way, and it is a common way of temporarily coping with difficulties. It is often to some extent enforced on sick people in hospital, by, for example, putting them to bed, feeding them, and making decisions for them, and nurses should be careful not to do this more than is necessary or appropriate.

## OBJECT RELATIONS AND THE INTERNAL WORLD

With the increasing interest in the ego and its development, many psychoanalysts became interested in the way the world – and particularly the people in it – is represented in the mind. This representation can be described as the internal world, which exists in the mind of a person and may or may not bear much resemblance to the real external world.

Some terminology is needed here. In psychoanalytic literature, people are often referred to as **objects**, and thus relationships with people as **object relations**. The reason for this is not because people are considered to be inanimate, but to distinguish the object from the subject. A person also has a relationship with, and a mental representation of, himself, which is extremely important. Such phrases as 'the external world', 'the internal world', or 'the object world' in psychoanalytic writing all refer to a world of people – inanimate objects having minimal relevance in psychoanalytic discussion.

It was pointed out earlier that Freud thought the newborn infant related only to himself and had no awareness of external objects. Of course there are people in the infant's external world – his parents and others – but in his subjective, internal world, Freud thought there were not. Many psychoanalysts today do not agree with this.

Joseph Sandler, a British psychoanalyst who for a long time was a leading member of staff at the Hampstead Clinic, has written extensively about the development of the internal representation of self and objects. He described the representational world thus (1962):

> The representational world might be compared to a stage set within a theatre. The characters on the stage represent the child's various objects, as well as the child himself. Needless to say, the child is usually the hero of the piece.

This state of affairs, Sandler says, comes about only gradually. At first, the child's representational world contains only crude images of pleasures and unpleasures, and it is only slowly that he learns to distinguish self from not-self, and to establish a representation of his boundaries.

Later, there may be different self-representations, such as 'self-as-I-would-like-to-be', or 'ideal self'. If the ideal self representation is very different from that of the actual self, a person may become depressed. Similarly, a representation of actual self that is identical to, and merges with, that of ideal self, might lead to self-satisfied, uninsightful, manic behaviour (Joffe *et al.* 1965).

Once clear boundaries are established between self and object representations, either may be altered on the basis of the other. The self-representation may be made a bit like that of the object by a mechanism called **identification**, or some aspect that in reality belongs to the self may be included in the object representation, which is called **projection** (page 81). During early development and beyond, there is a tendency to identify with loved and admired aspects of objects, and to project disliked aspects of oneself on to objects. By such means, the internal, subjective world can come to have a rather different form from the external world. Never the less, the internal world is still subjectively real to the person who experiences it, even though the internal and external reality may differ.

Representations are also formed of relationships between self and object, for example, 'mother being loving to me', or 'father being severe to me', so that feelings become represented as states that occur in relation to people, and in particular contexts (page 97).

## MELANIE KLEIN'S VIEW OF DEVELOPMENT

Melanie Klein (1882–1960) was born in Vienna, and studied psychoanalysis in Budapest and Berlin. From 1926 she lived and worked in London. Many of Klein's views differed considerably from those of Anna Freud, and indeed there was, and to some extent remains, quite a lot of disagreement between their followers. However, many psychoanalysts of all persuasions believe that Melanie Klein made a most important contribution to the theory of development, even if they do not agree with some aspects of what she said.

Klein's particular interest was in very early psychic development – the first six months of life. Some agree with much of what Klein said but disagree that it occurs so early. Klein differed from both Sigmund and Anna Freud in that she believed that from birth the infant has the beginnings of an ego, and that he also has an awareness of objects, albeit a primitive one. Another characteristic of Klein's work is that she put particular emphasis on hate and aggression. Following Freud's later theory, she believed this was innate, present from birth, and that it could be directed towards either the self or objects.

Klein described two major phases of early development, which she called the **paranoid-schizoid position** (1946) and the **depressive position** (1940). She used the word 'position' rather than phase or stage to indicate that these are mental states that to some extent persist throughout life, and can be moved in and out of according to circumstance and state of health; they are not stages that are achieved once and for all. As with many psychoanalytic terms, it helps if one tries not to be dismayed by the jargon, but to understand the underlying ideas.

## THE PARANOID-SCHIZOID POSITION

The term 'schizoid' means split. Klein used it because she believed that immense anxiety arises in the weak ego of the newborn baby, due to the opposition of the two main instinctual drives, love and hate. The innate hate experienced is too much for the child's fragile ego to tolerate at first, and so it splits into a part that loves and a part that hates. Because the object cannot be both loved and hated, in the mind it is divided into two objects – one loved and one hated. This is known as **splitting**. The infant's hate is projected on to the hated object, so the experience is one of a hateful object, rather than of a hated one. Because of this projected hate, the object becomes feared as a persecutor, and hence the term 'paranoid'.

What this means is that when the baby has good, comforting experiences – for example a good feed – he feels the object is entirely and ideally good. When he is hungry or in pain, however, his experience is not of a lack of something good, but of being attacked by something or someone bad. Klein described this in terms of the child experiencing a 'bad breast' that attacks him, and a 'good breast' that feeds and comforts him – rather than one mother, who cannot always fulfil his needs instantly.

## THE DEPRESSIVE POSITION

If conditions are favourable over the first three to six months of life and the child receives loving care, the ego gradually becomes stronger and the child is more able to tolerate its aggressive impulses without splitting into good and bad objects. The infant increasingly feels his good impulses and objects are stronger than the bad, which allows his projection to lessen. His paranoid fear decreases, and both ego and object gradually become more integrated.

Klein defined the depressive position as the phase of development when the infant recognizes a whole object – a mother who is both loved and hated. This leads to mourning for the lost ideal object, and a feeling of guilt for the infant's own aggression, which he feels has destroyed it; hence the term **depressive**. It is thus the stage at which concern can be felt for someone else. That the child may also experience weaning – a real loss – at around this time, may play a part in the development of these feelings.

Klein thought that this state in infancy is a precursor to all future states of mourning and depression. It can lead to a desire to make amends by reparation; or, alternatively, to defensive movement back into the paranoid-schizoid position; or to the **manic denial** that there has even been a loss, or that it matters. These fluctuations occur in everyone to some extent throughout life.

The paranoid-schizoid position is a psychotic one in that reality is not acknowledged, but it is not uncommon to meet people who, while not psychotic, split their world into all good and all bad. In reality, most situations and relationships have both good and bad aspects, and we have mixed feelings as well. The ability to acknowledge this and to live with it is an achievement of the depressive position.

The following vignettes may help to illustrate these ideas.

> John, a first-year student nurse, on several occasions became angry in classes where the tutor tried to pick up students comments about how difficult and upsetting work on the wards could sometimes be. He would furiously accuse the tutor of being negative and of making the students depressed. The work, he said, was never depressing.

This could be understood as John using the mechanisms of splitting, **idealization**, and denial, which are characteristic of the paranoid-schizoid position. The wards and the patients were idealized, with a complete denial that there was ever anything upsetting about the work. The tutor, on the other hand, became the all-bad persecutor. John was unable to maintain his precarious state of mental equilibrium by this means: at the end of his first year he made a suicide attempt, and left nursing shortly afterwards.

> Sally, another first-year student, was able to talk with guilt and great distress about an old woman she was nursing. The patient was confused and incontinent, and constantly demanded attention. Sally spoke of how awful she felt because at times she hated the patient for being as she was. Such feelings caused conflict and guilt in Sally because she cared about the woman and wanted to give her the best care.

Sally was experiencing the mixed feelings and guilt characteristic of the depressive position. With the help of the tutor and the class, she was able to understand that having feelings is not the same as acting on them, and was able to become more accepting of her feelings.

## PHANTASY AND INTERNAL OBJECT RELATIONS

Melanie Klein and her followers saw the internal world as more than a representational one. They believe that the infant constructed an inner world in, what feels to him to be, a very active and almost concrete way by using **phantasy** (which has, as will be seen, a different meaning from 'fantasy').

Phantasies are closely associated with instinctual drives and bodily processes, but their creation is a function of the ego. For example, an infant sucking at the breast might phantasize that he is actually incorporating the breast, so that he then feels he has a good object inside himself. Similarly, a hungry, raging baby might feel his screams and hunger pain are actually the bad breast attacking him, and that he has a bad, attacking object inside him. Klein believed that in this way an individual constructs an internal world of objects which, although largely unconscious, feels very concrete and real.

## THE CONTRIBUTION OF DONALD WINNICOTT

Donald Winnicott (1897–1971) was both a paediatrician and a psychoanalyst, and used his vast experience of mothers and babies to deepen and develop his psychoanalytic ideas. Winnicott placed particular emphasis on the function of maternal care in infancy, a function which he described under the general terms of **holding**. By holding, Winnicott meant not only the physical holding that the mother or mothering person gives to the baby, but also a mental function whereby the mother acts as a container and executor for the baby's peremptory and unorganized drives and needs. Winnicott (1960) says of holding that it:

> Protects from physiological insult. Takes account of the infant's skin sensitivity – touch, temperature, auditory sensitivity, visual sensitivity, sensitivity to falling and of the infant's lack of knowledge of anything other than the self. It includes the whole routine of care throughout the day and night, and it is not the same with any two infants because it is part of the infant and no two infants are alike. Also it follows the minute day-to-day changes belonging to the infant's growth and development, both physical and psychological.

The mother's holding allows the infant's experience to become gradually more integrated, and in time he develops some self-holding, self-regulating function, or ego function of his own.

For a time the maternal holding gives the baby an experience of omnipotence – a sense that he really does function by the pleasure principle, that he only has to have a wish in order for it to be met. Of course, for the child's own executive function to develop, a gradual disillusionment from this belief is necessary.

A mother who can provide this holding must be, in Winnicott's phrase, **good enough**. A 'too good' mother, who continues to meet every need of the child almost before it is felt does not allow the child to learn to interact with reality. Of course, it is not possible to be that good, but some mothers have difficulty allowing a developing child to take on increased autonomy.

However, a not good enough mother and lack of holding can lead to an experience of terrible anxiety, which Winnicott termed 'nameless dread', and a lack of integration. Winnicott thought that such experiences could lead to psychosis; and physical death if bad enough, or, alternatively, to the development of what he called a **false self**. This is a part of the self which acts as a caretaker, beneath which the **true self** with its possibilities for spontaneity is deeply buried. Adults who have developed a false self may be dimly aware of living behind a shell, of not being real, of futility, and of a lack of spontaneity.

Winnicott thought the ability to give good enough mothering requires a special state in the mother which he called **primary maternal preoccupation**. This develops during pregnancy, and lasts for several weeks after the birth of the child. In this state of intense involvement with the baby, unborn and then born, the mother is able to identify with the baby to such a degree that she can understand his needs and provide the right thing at the right moment. Winnicott suggests that this state is almost an illness, but one which is necessary for the baby. The mother is withdrawn from many of her other concerns because of it, and to do this she needs someone else, usually the baby's father, to manage some of those for her.

Winnicott frequently described the care of mentally sick people as similar to the maternal holding of very young infants. It is certainly often part of the function of the nurse, when someone has physical and mental needs which for the time being they cannot meet themselves.

## CONCLUSION

It will have become apparent that the psychodynamic perspective on development is not a unified one. There are, of course, many other psychoanalytic writers than those presented here, who may add to what has been said, but complicate it further.

How should the reader deal with such a complexity of ideas? He or she should approach the subject eclectically and with an open mind, using different ideas where and when they seem applicable or helpful in the understanding of people and their problems. It is sometimes possible to see that different theories are describing similar phenomena by means of different models or metaphors. For example, Figure 1.1 shows a diagrammatic representation of one way in which different theories can be integrated (Wright, 1989).

In summary, two principles can be emphasized. Firstly, what is being considered when talking about the psychodynamic perspective on development is the development of the mind – an entirely subjective and abstract phenomenon. The mind can never be seen – only the effects of its functioning are available for study. Thus to discuss it involves hypothesis and inference. That much mental functioning takes place unconsciously adds to this difficulty greatly. The second principle is that although mental development is under the right circumstances steadily progressive, there

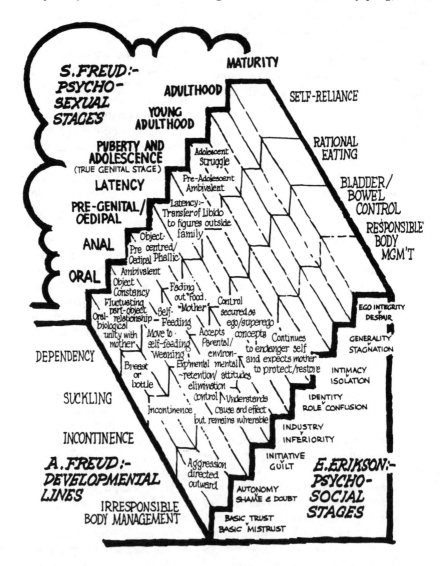

**Fig. 1.1** An interrelating view of developmental theories

is what Sandler and Joffe have called 'a tendency to persistence in psychological function and development'. This means that earlier modes of function are seldom deleted from the record. They may be well buried beneath later and more mature modes, but they are still there, and under circumstances of stress or illness the individual may regress to using them.

## REFERENCES

Freud, A. (1966) *Normality and Pathology in Childhood*, Hogarth, London.

Freud, S. (1905) *Three Essays on the Theory of Sexuality*, SE VII, Hogarth, London, and Vol. 7, Penguin, Harmondsworth.

Freud, S. (1911) Formulations on the two principles of mental functioning, SE XII, Hogarth, London.

Freud, S. (1923) *The Ego and the Id*, SE XII, Hogarth, London, and Vol. II Penguin, Harmondsworth.

Freud, S. (1925) The dissolution of the Oedipus Complex, SE XIV, Hogarth London .

Freud, S. (1925) Analysis of a phobia in a five-year-old boy SE X Hogarth, London, and Vol. 8, Penguin, Harmondsworth.

Graves, R. (1955) *The Greek Myths 2*, Penguin, Harmondsworth.

Joffe, W. and Sandler, J. (1965) Pain, depression and individuation, in *From Safety to Super Ego* (J. Sandler, 1987), Karnac, London.

Klein, M. (1940) Mourning and its relation to manic-depressive states, in *Love, Guilt and Reparation*, Hogarth, London, and Virago, London.

Klein, M. (1946) Notes on some schizoid mechanisms, in *Envy and Gratitude*, Hogarth, London, and Virago, London.

Sandler, J. (1962) The representational world, in *From Safety to Super Ego*, Karnac, London.

Sandler, J. and Joffe, W. (1967) The tendency to persistence in psychological function and development, in *From Safety to Super Ego* (J. Sandler, 1987), Karnac, London.

Sandler, A. M. and Sandler, J. The past unconscious, the present unconscious and the vicissitudes of guilt, *Intl. J. Psycho-Anal.*, 68, 331–41.

Winnicott, D. (1960) Primary maternal preoccupation, in *Through Paediatrics to Psycho-Analysis*, (D. Winnicott, 1975) Hogarth, London.

Winnicott, D. (1960) Ego distortion in terms of true and false self, in *The Maturational Process and the Facilitating Environment* (D. Winnicott, 1965), Hogarth, London, and Karnac, London.

Winnicott, D. (1960) The theory of the parent-infant relationship, in *The Maturational Process and the Facilitating Environment* (D. Winnicott, 1965) Hogarth, London, and Karnac, London.

Wright, H. (1989) *Group Work – Preparation and Practice*, Scutari, London.

## FURTHER READING

Freud, S. (1916–17) *Introductory Lectures on Psycho-Analysis* SE XV and XVI, Hogarth, London, and Vol. 1, Penguin, Harmondsworth.

Segal, H. (1973) *Introduction to the Work of Melanie Klein*, Hogarth, London, and Karnac, London.

Wollheim, R. (1971) *Freud*, Harper Collins, London.

# COGNITIVE ASPECTS 6

*Philip Barker*

Freudian theory represented a major landmark in modern psychology, and bridged the gulf between early twentieth-century science and more traditional views of the human psyche. Psychoanalytic thought sought to explain the intrapsychic workings of the mind by reference to unconscious processes, which were assumed to be the primary determinants of human behaviour.

Although cognitive developmental theory is a more recent school of thought, it is linked to psychological theorists who were contemporaries of Freud. Its roots probably lie with William James, the American psychologist, who was much influenced by Darwin. James believed that mental processes evolved like other physical processes. His work emphasized the role played by consciousness in human adaption to the environment. This later became known as **functionalism** (Evans, 1981). A less direct influence came from Gestalt psychology, which proposed that the whole is greater than the sum of its parts (Kohler, 1930). The Gestalt school, which was prominent in pre-war Germany, was disrupted by the rise of Nazism. It had, however, already made a significant contribution to studies of perception and learning, both of which were to figure strongly in later cognitive models of human development.

## COGNITIVE PROCESSES

The term 'cognition' is often assumed to refer only to thinking. In fact, it refers to the process by which we handle knowledge, and to the faculty of knowing (Watson, 1976). But it may also be understood through the metaphor of 'gnomon' – the pin of a sundial which 'measures the heavens from shadows' (Gregory, 1987). This is an apposite metaphor for cognition, which translates all human experiences into a 'shadow' that is cast in the human memory.

Cognition therefore entails attending, perceiving, thinking, and remembering. The adult is the person he is because of his genetic inheritance; his environmental experiences; his personal needs and motivations; and the way in which he contrues the world about him. It has been suggested that at least five types of cognitive processes exist (Guilford, 1959):

1. Recognition of, or sensitivity to, the environment.
2. Retention or collection of information.
3. Divergent thinking, or the ability to conjure up hypotheses or courses of action as part of problem-solving.
4. Convergent thinking, or integrating divergent ideas into a unified plan.
5. Decision-making, or making firm decisions for action on the basis of convergent ideas.

People who experience difficulties in any one of these areas may be described as having a cognitive impairment. It is clear that people do not all interpret their worlds in the same way at all times; for example, the difficulty adults and children experience in understanding each other's view of the world is essentially a cognitive problem. Similarly, much of the 'incomprehensibility' of mental illness (*sic*) is related to the specific cognitive processes involved in the construction of different disorders.

SPEAKING YOUR MIND

Voltaire is reputed to have written that 'thought depends absolutely on the stomach, but in spite of that, those who have the best stomachs are not the best thinkers'. In the 200 years since Voltaire, progress on the psychological understanding of cognition has been slow; thinking is often referred to as the 'mysterious concept which everyone understands but no one can explain' (Bourne *et al.*, 1971). With the decline of behaviourism – which rejected the study of thought because of its 'mentalistic' associations – and the emergence of the computer and artificial intelligence, the objective study of mental processes has re-emerged as a vital force in psychology.

The study of cognition is tied inextricably to language development, an area beyond the scope of this chapter. Suffice it to say that how humans form mental images and concepts is central to any theory of language acquisition. Cognitive development addresses the process by which humans use language to problem-solve and think creatively. Human beings can only speak of knowing who they are because of the richness of their language.

## THE FUNCTIONAL CENTRE OF THE PERSON

The cognitive developmental model is arguably the linchpin of all the developmental theories. Psychodynamic, family, and social models all describe potential influences upon the development of the person, which can only be realized through cognition. When major problems in the area of cognitive functioning are experienced, as in profound intellectual impairment, or after major neurological trauma, some would argue that such

individuals are 'people' but not 'persons', emphasizing the relative nature of the concept of autonomy (Benson, 1983).

A significant degree of cognitive capacity appears to be necessary to make sense of the world outside, as well as of the self within. All newborn babies are human beings by virtue of a discrete biological classification; they are people, not animals. It could be argued that a certain kind of development is necessary to translate the human baby into a person. Children who have suffered profound neurological impairment might, for example, be viewed as non-persons by virtue of their difficulty to respond cognitively to their environment. Similarly, people who are beginning to lose their grasp of where, and perhaps who, they are – as in some forms of brain damage or dementia – may also be losing their personhood. Descartes's famous dictum, 'I think, therefore I am', might have a negative corollary: without cognition, the person does not exist. This does not mean, however, the individual is any less human; the definition of humanity involves a different set of criteria.

This description of cognitive development overlaps significantly with psychodynamic explanations (Chapter 5) in terms of the construction of the self, and with social and group perspectives (Chapter 4) in terms of information-processing and social learning. Cognitive developmental theory also is influenced by evolutionary theories. Humans appear to differ from their closest animal relations in terms of the richness of their cognitive processes. People use their memory to recall and to reconstruct past experiences; to generalize from those past experiences by imagining ('what might have happened if...'); and can construct fantastic events in their minds – situations which have never happened, which might be possible, or may be wholly impossible. People also use their cognitive processes to filter, manipulate, or otherwise sort, massive amounts of information coming from the environment. By sorting, the brain identifies pieces of information that will or will not be attended to. Many animals, such as dogs and cats, as well as primates, appear to 'think' in the sense that they behave in ways that suggest the outcome of problem-solving. Some primates even appear to possess a sense of 'self'. Humans, however, appear to be the only animals who enjoy the richness of cognition described above. The variety and intensity of these cognitive experiences have helped us to split the atom and land on the moon; they also have helped to devastate our own lives and speed the destruction of our own planet. Cognition, therefore, can be used as an adaptive force; this was the original area that interested William James. (The negative use of cognition, which can be either intentional or unconscious is described in Chapters 11 and 13.)

## INVENTING AND EXPLAINING

This section deals with aspects of normal human development; this chapter discusses some aspects of the role of cognition in the development of the person. Given cognition controls everything the person experiences, our discussion can only be superficial. It should not be forgotten, either, that cognitive science also is developing. Increasingly, it is recognized that no single model can unravel the mysterious workings of the mind. The complexities of personhood, and the riddle of how we can be all we can be, should not be underestimated.

The French philosopher Jean-Paul Sartre observed that people make themselves up as they speak. Similarly, people use their cognitive processes to make sense of their world, defining it and themselves in their own unique terms. Although the concept of cognitive processes is well accepted, a range of different theoretical models have been developed to explain the development of the person. Here, two major theories, which emphasize development in children and adolescents, will be discussed as preparation

for what can go wrong in human development (Part Three).

## PIAGET: A STRUCTURE MODEL

The development of the person is a life-long process. The earliest indications that cognitive development is taking place occurs soon after birth; at around three months, primitive reflexes begin to disappear as the infant develops greater voluntary control of vision, muscular co-ordination, and memory. The infant gradually develops a relationship with the world by acquiring visually directed reaching and the ability to orient, at the same time he uses other senses to explore the world. Language, which is closely related to cognitive development, plays an increasingly important role in the direction of the child's behaviour, and by the end of the first year, the child will begin to make meaningful sounds.

This development process, which continues throughout childhood, can end for some people at an appropriate cut-off point, when, for example, boys become men, fulfilling the requirements of their cultural stereotype. Others may continue to grow and develop, experiencing major shifts in attitude, acquiring new skills, searching the heights of their capabilities, for the rest of their lives. Abraham Maslow described this form of continuous development as 'self-actualization', whereby people become all they possibly can be; a process which, naturally, is a life-long venture.

If development ends at the point of death, where does it begin? The beginnings of the person lie in childhood. The development of the child is a socialization process (Chapter 4). As children grow to become adult members of their society, they are required to go through a process of change. The child develops specific characteristics by using discrete psychological mechanisms to bring about the changes required. These characteristics become part of the child's developing cognitive structure, as he interacts developmentally with the world.

The child is not *tabula rasa*. The world does not simply act upon the child. Rather, from his earliest days the child interacts with the world. Even very young infants can distinguish complex patterns from simpler forms, and the crawling infant has already mastered his perception of depth and height. As the child develops he appears to proceed through discrete stages, reaching different levels of functioning at which different types of interaction with his world are possible.

The most famous description of these developmental stages was provided by Jean Piaget, the Swiss developmental psychologist, who, from the early 1920s until his death in 1980, explored the role of cognition in the child's developing interaction with his world. Piaget's theory aimed to explain the changes in thinking style that occurs along the developmental path from birth to adulthood. His theory was influenced strongly by existing biological models, which saw human development as a process of adaption. Piaget's developmental model was presented in four overlapping phases that emphasized the active nature of the child's relationship with his environment. Within this relationship the child used his natural, innate cognitive powers to adapt himself to his environment.

Piaget assumed that these cognitive processes existed within an innate structure, which allowed the child to organize the information he collected about his world in order to make sense of it. The development of the child's ability to organize such information, and the behaviour which was produced, reflected his intelligence. 'Intelligence' was a term for the internal organization of information related to adaption. In Piaget's view, this did not develop at random. Instead, every act of cognition was related organizationally to all other acts of cognition. Development involved an interactive, integrated, and coherent pattern. In this sense, Piaget was an early example of a systems theorist (page 72).

## THE DEVELOPMENTAL STAGES

The four stages of development are commonly equated with chronological age (Table 6.1). However, Piaget acknowledged that these developmental milestones could vary from person to person, and even from culture to culture. Although development is continuous, each of Piaget's stages involve quite distinct and different schemes of thinking. The distinguishing feature of the cognitive model of development, expressed mainly through Piaget's research, is the emphasis upon the child's understanding of the world, rather than his emotional reaction to it.

### Stage 1

In Stage 1, the infant develops basic reflex movements into action sequences, at the same time increasing his understanding (cognition) of the effect of his behaviour on his environment. The young infant uses reflexes, such as sucking, to collect information about his world. Such actions are not deliberate attempts at understanding, but are automatic reflex actions. Gradually, children begin to explore their world non-reflexively, often engaging in stereotyped, repetitive movements, which can give rise to longstanding habits, such as holding the nose while sucking the thumb (Piaget, 1952). Piaget called such exploration 'circular reactions'.

This sensori-motor stage commonly runs from birth to around 18 months, during which time the child develops concepts without the use of thought as adults know it. The child

**Table 6.1** Piaget's developmental model

| | |
|---|---|
| **Stage 1** | Sensori-motor period (birth–18 months) |
| **Stage 2** | Pre-operational thinking (18 months–6 years) |
| **Stage 3** | Concrete-operational thinking (7–12 years) |
| **Stage 4** | Formal-operational thinking (adolescence–adulthood) |

uses his available cognitive structures, or mental powers, to collect information about his world, a process Piaget called 'assimilation'. The more information the child collects, the more complex become his cognitive structures. This modification of the child's earlier cognitive structure Piaget termed 'accommodation', indicating the manner in which the child's thinking adapts to meet the demands of his environment.

Towards the end of his first year, the child begins to develop an understanding of the world outside of himself. For example, the young infant will not look for a toy that has been covered up, which to him 'disappears', while he watches. A few months later, however, he will begin searching for the hidden toy, having acquired the internal organization necessary to develop the concept of object permanence, or that things continue to exist even when he cannot sense them. The development of object permanence, and concurrently of language, frees the child from the exclusive here-and-now existence of early infancy, where the child only knows what is immediately experienced, and where he is wrapped up in a limited experience of himself.

## Stage 2

Once the child begins to consolidate his language, he is able to represent internally the world that exists independent of him externally. Once he possesses language, though not necessarily speech, the child can learn through instruction and interaction, instead of simply through sensori-motor learning. In Stage 2, the child begins to develop thinking structures without being aware that he is actually doing so. This pre-operational phase, which usually begins around 18 months, involves the evolution of representative or symbolic thinking, which is essentially intuitive.

The development of symbolic function occurs mainly in play, where it is integrated with the acquisition of language. The child begins to use symbols to represent objects or actions, for example, he may use a stone to represent a sweet (object); or will put a doll to bed (action), representing sleep. In neither case does the child confuse the symbol with reality.

Three other characteristics – **egocentrism**, **animism**, and **artificialism** – are also central to this phase of development.

Very young children, for example, around three-years old, find it difficult to understand situations they have not yet experienced directly. Some psychologists have argued that the children in Piaget's studies found certain problems difficult because they did not make much sense of them. In Piaget's view, such children attached highly private meanings to public meanings, unaware that others did not necessarily share their interpretation. As the child gained more social experience he would come to realize this, and would modify his so-called 'egocentricity'.

At this stage, the child also shows a tendency to attribute life to inanimate objects. This use of animistic thought is focused upon objects that are considered important by adults, such as cars. As he develops, the child comes to acknowledge that only specific elements, such as the wind, possess a life of their own. Similarly, the child assumes that all of creation is a result of human endeavour, since this is all that he knows. The sun is lit by a match, or dogs are made by people to watch over the house. The idea that anything might not be artificially created is inconceivable.

At this stage, the child's thinking is dominated by his immediate perception of events. If water in a glass is poured into a taller container, the child will assert there is more water. Similarly, if one of two equal balls of modelling clay is re-modelled into a sausage shape, the ball is now larger than the other. When the water and clay are returned to their original containers or shapes, to the child they become the same again. Because the child does not yet possess adult problem-solving capacities, he uses **syncretic reasoning**, trying to reconcile conflicting beliefs. The child's ability to make such an analysis of external events, albeit incorrectly, demonstrates the existence of mental processes. He remains dominated, however, by the external fact that, for example, one glass is taller than another, rather than by a conceptual understanding that amounts of water remain the same.

## Stage 3

In Stage 3, logical methods develop: the child begins to figure out the meaning of events, using informational observations and mental representation. This is the **concrete-operational phase** of childhood, extending usually from seven to twelve years. When faced with apparent contradictions between what he sees (perceptual) and what he thinks should be the case (logical), the child draws upon his internal logical structures to resolve the difference. The child who has reached Stage 3 has developed the concept of conservation; he appreciates that although things appear to change, they remain the same; this child knows that the amount of water in the tall and in the squat glass is the same.

In this phase the child also acquires the class-inclusion concept. For example, if a number of wooden beads are shown, most of which are brown and a few white, the child can recognize both that the beads are wooden, and that there are more brown than white ones. If he is asked if there are more brown than wooden ones, a younger child will reply 'yes', the reason being that there are only a few white ones. He will repeat this answer, even when reminded that all the beads are wooden. Young children, and even adults, may be confused by the way the question is asked. If emphasis is given to the word 'wooden', this may draw attention to the distinguishing characteristic.

## Stage 4

In Stage 4, the child proceeds to more advanced, adult thought. Until now, the child has relied on his relationship with reality. In the final stage of development, as the child passes into adolescence, he begins to think abstractly and hypothetically. Now he can symbolize information, form hypotheses ('if this…then that'), and use concepts without necessarily having had direct experience of them. If told that 'John is shorter than Phil; John is taller than Bob; who is the tallest of the three?', the child who can reason abstractly will determine that Phil is the tallest without seeing or even imagining them. This stage marks a divorce in the child's thinking from concrete reality, and is called the **formal-operational phase**. It is characteristic of adolescence and beyond, and sees the full balance of cognition established. No further need for structural changes in the person's thinking style is necessary.

It is worth noting that Piaget's investigation of this developmental phase focused upon the adolescent's use of logic applied to physical scientific experiments. Other researchers have shown that the ability to solve such scientific problems is not common to all adolescents, or even to all adults, however, they may be able to use the same logical, hypothetical, and abstract forms of reasoning when applied to other problems.

## PIAGET RECONSIDERED

Piaget's theory assumes that the development of human thinking progresses through stages that involve qualitatively different thinking styles. Children do not simply learn more and more facts as they grow up – there are changes in the way they think.

Two important disputes surround Piaget's theory. First, the idea of discrete stages suggests that development is not continuous. Piaget acknowledged that the borderlines between one stage and another could be blurred, however, he paid less attention to the fact that some children might display attainment of a particular stage in one aspect of his thinking, but not in another. Also, under certain conditions older children may show a regression in their thinking style. An alternative view is that the stages of cognitive development exist as dominant tendencies, rather than as absolute milestones.

A second criticism relates to the age-old nature-versus-nurture debate. Piaget has been criticized for paying too little attention to the influence of teaching and training on intellectual development. This does not mean he believed that maturation, or development without specific practice experience, alone could explain cognitive development. Indeed, Piaget argued that most of the child's cognitive structures were constructed by the child; only assimilation and accommodation were present at birth. His critics argue that this underplays the importance of innate characteristics. An alternative view is that all normal children only develop along the same course if inherited structures guide their cognitive functioning (Gelman *et al.*, 1983). It may be that Piaget offered a valuable description of cognitive development, but revealed little of the factors that cause such development (Wright *et al.*, 1972).

## KOHLBERG: SEXUAL IDENTITY AND MORAL DEVELOPMENT

Piaget also developed a theory of moral development that was similar to Freud's notion of the introjection of parental and societal rules and standards (Chapter 8). Whereas Freud assumed that the super-ego was acquired from others, Piaget claimed that the child's autonomous morality came from his spontaneous efforts to organize his own moral code. The American psychologist Lawrence Kohlberg, who was working during the mid-1960s and the late 1970s, extended Piaget's theory to cover the development of sexual identity, and some aspects of personality such as morality, both emphasizing cognitive factors.

## GENDER DEVELOPMENT

Kohlberg recognized that children were not only learning about the physical world as they developed, but also were acquiring concepts about their own bodies and other people. As children learn that objects have permanence, they also discover that people continue to exist even when they have disappeared from sight. Four-year-old children might believe that a live cat wearing a dog mask has become a dog, or that if the whiskers are removed from a picture of a cat it becomes a dog, but by seven years the same children know that once a cat, always a cat. At this age, children also learn about gender constancy, or, once a boy, always a boy.

It does not appear that this learning process, through which children discover what can change and what is immutable, can be speeded up. Exposing children to, for example, information about sex differences does not help them to tell the difference between boys and girls; cognition must develop sufficiently to allow the child to see those anatomical differences as unchanging characteristics, which are used to group people into the classes of men and women.

Once children discover their identity, they begin to want to do things that are consistent with that gender. Kohlberg believed that the identification of what were considered 'male things' rather than 'female things', was determined by sexual stereotypes. Within a traditional family Kohlberg believed a boy will model himself upon his father. He will not learn or even want to become masculine because his father, who he might love or hate, is masculine. He will imitate his father, or other adult males, because they are males. It is important to note that Kohlberg did not believe that a previous emotional relationship, or indeed any reward or sexual drive, was necessary for this imitation to take place. Although Kohlberg's theory carried a male bias, as did all psychological models up to the 1960s and early 1970s, he acknowledged that the same principle applied to girls. Once a girl has acquired gender constancy, she will begin to imitate her mother, or other adult female figures.

MORAL DEVELOPMENT

Kohlberg also examined the development of moral reasoning, which be classified in six stages across three levels (Table 6.2) (Kohlberg, 1976).

## Level 1 – preconventional

At this level, the child can distinguish between right and wrong and good and bad, but does not interpret them in terms of social standards of conduct. The two stages at this level involve obedience to a superior power or prestige accompanied by a fear of punishment, and a naively egoistic orientation according to which a right action involves satisfying one's selfish needs and occasionally the needs of others, Stage 2 involves an instrumental relativism, since rules are followed only when they are in the child's immediate interest.

## Level 2 – conventional

At this level, the person's moral judgements are influenced by expectations: what he thinks his family, social group, or society at large, expect him to do. At Stage 3 the good boy/girl view of the world is paramount – there is a strong need for approval, to please others, and to conform to stereotyped values. At this stage the mutuality of relationships is emphasized: the development of trust, loyalty, respect, and gratitude. At Stage 4, this is replaced by a felt need to do one's duty, show respect for authority, and support the social order. Here, the child begins to recognize the need to contribute to his social group, to institutions (like the school), and to wider society.

## Level 3 – post-conventional

Moral judgements at this level transcend individual authority or conformity to group pressures. The person acknowledges social rules and conventions, but gives emphasis to the underlying values or guiding principles. Kohlberg acknowledged that many people do not reach this level of development. At Stage 5 the person defines duty in terms of contracts, and the need to avoid violating the will or rights of others. The person is aware that most values and rules are relative – part of the social contract to membership of a particular social group. Non-relative values, like life and liberty, are recognized as universal.

At Stage 6, moral behaviour is rationalized in terms of principles of choice, involving the need to be logical and consistent. Concepts such as justice, human rights or the dignity of the individual can be defined as part of a social contract, for example by a repressive totalitarian regime. The person who has reached Stage 6 will challenge such 'laws' on the rational grounds that they violate fundamental, logical principles: the universal ethic.

Kohlberg's developmental theories overlap with the social developmental model. Whereas Piaget emphasized the child's cognitive

**Table 6.2** Stages of moral development

| Level 1 | **Preconventional** | |
|---|---|---|
| | Stage 1 | Punishment and obedience orientation |
| | Stage 2 | Instrumental relativism |
| **Level 2** | **Conventional** | |
| | Stage 3 | Good girl/boy orientation |
| | Stage 4 | Law and order orientation |
| **Level 3** | **Post-conventional or principled** | |
| | Stage 5 | Social contract orientation |
| | Stage 6 | Universal ethical principles |

construction of his relationship to the physical world, Kohlberg's focus on sexuality and morality extended this to aspects of the social environment. Although controversy exists as to whether or not Kohlberg's stages are as fixed as he suggests, some evidence supports the view that moral judgements do develop across stages and across different cultures (Snarey, 1985).

Kohlberg's developmental theories were biased towards studies of males, who formed the basis of his model; females were interviewed only later, once the model was established. In terms of gender development, males and female were distinguished largely by power; he saw power and aggression as intrinsic to the gender models for males, nurturance and dependence, for females. Kohlberg did add, however, that all children would imitate people who were powerful and prestigious.

The ramifications of the gender model are complex, and are complicated further by the important psychological critique stemming from the Women's Movement (Rohrbaugh, 1981). A similar problem existed in Kohlberg's elaboration of the moral development theory: the model was built to around the responses of adolescent males: when females were interviewed later they appeared to function at a lower stage of moral development. One of Kohlberg's female colleagues challenged this finding, arguing that all developmental theories – from Freud through Erikson and Piaget to Kohlberg – had persistently misrepresented women (Gilligan, 1982). She argued that development theories had over-emphasized the acquisition of 'rule-governed' behaviour. The outstanding characteristics of women, such as showing care for and sensitivity towards the needs of others, would mark them as deficient in terms of moral development.

Similarly, the strong Peace and Green Movements of the post-1960s have been characterized by concerns which might appear more driven by law and order, community support, etc. (the conventional level) rather than necessarily self-chosen (Stage 6) ethical principles. The 1980s also witnessed the emergence of new female models who appear to have broken the mould of traditional models of female development. Such changes, which derive from wider societal shifts, have enormous implications for absolute developmental theories such as Kohlberg's.

## COGNITIVE DECLINE IN ADULTHOOD

Although Piaget did not study cognitive changes in adulthood, other researchers have shown that, for example, cognitive functioning may regress with advanced age (Papalia *et al.*, 1973). The significance of these findings is unclear. To some extent, poorer performance on Piagetian-type tasks may involve a loss of attention, a feeling that such tests are undignified or silly, or simply a lack of practice in completing schoolroom-type problem-solving. In general, however, with age there often comes a decline in some cognitive functions, especially memory. Some older people, however, continue to perform well on cognitive tests despite a decline in sensory capability and reaction time.

## OVERVIEW

'Cognition' is an umbrella term under which function a number of mental processes – among them perceiving, recognizing, conceiving, judging, and reasoning. The cognitive developmental model is concerned with the way humans develop the means by which they structure their experiences, make sense of them, and transform environmental stimuli into useable forms of human information. The complexity of such processes should not be under-estimated. This chapter deals only with some aspects of cognitive development. The complete story, including the acquisition of language and the neurological structure of mental life, is a vast canvas beyond the scope of this introduction.

This chapter has described how as children grow they develop concepts which help distinguish between themselves and other elements within their natural and social environments. They also develop ways of explaining, to themselves and others, their relationship to the environment: constructing rules which guide their behaviour, both as children and later as adults.

The development of the organizational structure, or network, which builds upon already accumulated information, is sometimes called a 'schema' (Neisser, 1976). Such schemata are the mental models which we use to map, or give shape to, the world which lies beyond our selves. As the person develops new information, or experiences are encountered which do not fit the existing schema, the child must either reject the information as wrong or irrelevant, or else must reorganize the schema to accommodate the new material. The process by which children revise their schema, in the light of new information, provides the cognitive link with adulthood, where the person may continue to revise indefinitely these mental maps.

Some humanistic therapies have popularized ideas, such as finding oneself. This, and the related therapeutic practice, is far removed from the scientific territory of cognitive theory. Finding oneself does, however, suggest that the person is lost, and that some form of mental map will be necessary for the therapeutic process to be successful. Cognitive theorists would argue that all change in adulthood, like the developmental changes of childhood and adolescence, are fundamentally cognitive: as people change they revise their mental models of themselves and the world.

Strong links exist between cognitive developmental theory and some of the mental health problems discussed in later chapters. Some mental disorders appear to involve faulty information processing: information which comes from the environment (input) is processed through various stages (storage), resulting in specific patterns of behaviour (output). If some fault occurs at any of these three stages (input/storage/output), the person will experience a functional (i.e., behavioural or emotional) problem. Other problems appear to involve faulty schemata, especially where specific belief systems cannot accommodate information that challenges the basic schema. As a result, the person may develop a thinking style that is not adaptive, and which fails to help them to function effectively within his or her natural environment.

Any attempt to explain what it means to be human requires a number of separate levels of explanation. In this chapter we have dealt with only some aspects of one level: how the person computes the information that comes from the natural and social environment. The effect of the family and other social experiences represent other levels, as indeed do the genetic and biological underpinnings of the human experience. As we discover more about the complexity of the human brain, we move closer to the final irony: that our hearts may, after all, lie in our heads.

## REFERENCES

Benson, J. (1983) Who is the autonomous man? *Philosophy* 58, 223, 17.

Bourne, L. E., Ekstrand, B. R., and Dominowski R. L. (1971) *The Psychology of Thinking*, Prentice-Hall, New Jersey.

Evans, R. B. (1981) Introduction: the historical context, in *William James' Principles of Psychology*, Harvard Univ. Press, Cambridge, Mass.

Gelman, R. and Baillargeon, R. (1983) A review of some Piagetian concepts, in *Mussen's Handbook of Child Psychology, Vol. 3 Cognitive Development* (4th edn) (eds H. J. Flavell and E. M. Markman), Wiley, Chichester.

Gilligan, C. (1982) *In a Different Voice: Psychological Theory and Women's Development*, Harvard Univ. Press, Cambridge, Mass.

Gregory, R. L (ed.) (1987) *The Oxford Companion to the Mind*, Oxford Univ. Press, Oxford.

Guilford, J. P. (1959) The structure of intellect, *Psychological Bulletin*, 53, 267–93.

Kohlberg, L. (1976) Moral stages and moralization: the cognitive-developmental approach, *Moral*

*Development and Behaviour; Theory, Research and Social Issues* (ed. T. Lickona), in Holt, Rinehart & Winston, New York.

Kohler, W. (1930) *Gestalt Psychology*, Bell, London.

Neisser, V. (1976) *Cognition and Reality*, Freeman, San Francisco.

Papalia, D. E., Salverson, S. M., and True, M. (1973) An evaluation of quantity conservation performance during old age *International Journal of Aging and Human Development*, 4, 103–9.

Piaget, J. (1952) *The Origins of Intelligence in Children*, International Univ. Press, New York.

Snarey, J. R. (1985) Cross-cultural universality of social-moral development; critical review of Kohlbergian research, *Psychological Bulletin*, 97, 202–32.

Watson, O. (1976) *Longman Modern English Dictionary*, Longman, London.

Wright, D. S., Taylor, A., Davies, D.R. *et al.* (1972) *Introducing Psychology; An Experimental Approach*, Penguin, Harmondsworth.

## FURTHER READING

Flavell, J. H. (1963) *The Development Psychology of Jean Piaget*, Van Nostrand, New York.

Ginsburg, H. and Opper, S. (1969) *Piaget's Theory of Intellectual Development: An Introduction*, Prentice-Hall, New Jersey.

Johnson-Laird, P. N. (1988) *The Computer and the Mind: An Introduction to Cognitive Science*, Harper Collins, London.

Kohlberg, L. (1969) Stage and sequence: the cognitive-developmental approach to socialisation, in D. A. Goslin *Handbook of Socialization Theory and Research*, Rand McNally, Chicago.

Maslow, A. (1962) *Towards a Psychology of Being*, Van Nostrand, Princeton.

Piaget, J. (1967) *Six Psychological Studies*, Vintage Books, New York.

Rohrbaugh, J. B. (1981) *Women: Psychology's Puzzle*, Abacus Edition, Sphere, London.

# FAMILY ASPECTS

## 7

*James Osborn*

Despite all experiments, human society has never found a better way to raise its young then within the family. (B. Bettelheim, 1987)

Yet when we are considering society from any other view than the economic, we can all see well enough that of all its institutions, the family is after all the institution that matters the most. It is at once indispensable as a means to all the rest and in a sense an end in itself...the strongest emotions, the most enduring motives, the most universally accessible sources of happiness are concerned with this business of the family. (E. F. Rathbone, 1924)

Far from being the basis of the good society, the family with all its narrow privacy and tawdry secrets is the source of discontent. (E. R. Leach, 1968)

As can be seen from the above quotes, there are strongly contrasting opinions about the value of family life. What the quotes all share, however, is the appreciation of the importance of the family, not only from the wider societal perspective, but also from that of the individual.

The understanding of a person cannot be complete without an understanding of their context. In the large Victorian psychiatric institutions, the patients – as they were then called – were removed from their context, treated, and then either rehabilitated or institutionalized. One of the benefits of the current community-orientated mental health service is that it provides a greater opportunity for nurses to understand clients within their current context: the ability of a chameleon to change its colouring is perplexing without the capacity to see the background that necessitates this change.

While an appreciation and understanding of context and client is important, more important still is an awareness of the interactive process by which each is influenced by the other. A person is responsible in part for creating their context, and their context is responsible for creating the person. As the anthropologist Gregory Bateson (1972) said, 'No man is "resourceful" or "dependent" or "fatalistic" in a vacuum. His character, whatever it be, is not his but is rather a characteristic of what goes on between him and something or somebody else.'

Bateson develops this idea further in his attempt to develop a definition of mind. He considered that a total concept of mind for an individual needed to be extra-cerebral:

Consider a man felling a tree with an axe. Each stroke of the axe is modified or corrected according to the cut face of the tree left by the previous stroke. This self-corrective process is brought about by a total system tree-eyes-brain-muscles-axe-stroke-tree, and it is the total system that has the characteristic of mind.

In our Western European culture, health problems are still largely defined on an individual basis. High-technology medicine and nursing practices have led to the development of technical interventions aimed at the individual. In considering the promotion of health, and in particular mental health, it makes sense to widen our horizons and include the family as a vital part of the process of understanding a person and their extra-cerebral mind. This is of even greater importance when the culture of an individual and their family differs from that of the nurse and the organization providing the health care.

## IS THERE SUCH A THING AS A 'NORMAL' FAMILY?

There is much talk about the appropriateness of certain types of families. Changes during the last century in family configuration have placed emphasis on the structure and composition of families: single-parent, re-constituted, nuclear, extended, foster and adoptive all define types of family structure. This rich variety of structures, which has developed from the more traditional extended and nuclear families, has lead to concerns being expressed about the strength of the modern family, as well as suggestions that certain types of family are 'normal', and others are not.

Alteration in types of family structure can be understood as the family or individual attempting to adapt to particular influences. The wide variety of family structures, like genetic mutations, are the foundations for the possibility of successful adaptations to changing circumstances. In a rapidly changing world, a structure that appears ideal at a particular time may not necessarily be appropriate in the future. The rise of the nuclear family in Western cultures has been very much a twentieth-century phenomenon, and, as we reach the end of the century, it is apparent that this structure itself is undergoing adaptation. A recent study of family types in the UK illustrates this clearly (OPCS, 1989):

- Couples with children – 50%
- Couples without children – 11%
- Single parents – 14%
- One person living alone – 15%
- Two or more families sharing accommodation – 5%
- Others – 5%

If one considers that the family provides genetic material, early nurturing, development through childhood and adolescence, experience of intimate relationships, inter-generational relationships, and support and stability, it becomes possible to consider such multiple processes as being the essence of family life. A new definition of the family, therefore, could be the organization of people who provide and receive these essential developmental experiences.

In a rapidly changing industrialized society such as ours it is not surprising that continuity in membership and structure has lessened, and a wide variety of configurations of people are attempting to provide the essential processes that we call family life. Changes occur in what families are expected to provide, for example, many functions of the family with regard to education have been supplanted by the state (Halsey, 1986). When considering normality it may thus be more useful to examine the quality of experiences considered appropriate to healthy development, rather than the composition of the family that is providing these experiences.

## THE STRUCTURE OF THE FAMILY

A useful way to gain an understanding of an individual's family is to construct a **geneo-gram,** or family tree. Murray Bowen, one of the pioneering family therapists, was influential in introducing this concept into clinical contexts. Relationship patterns are represented diagrammatically, and a map is compiled that includes the names and ages of all family members over at least three generations (Figures 7.1 and 7.2).

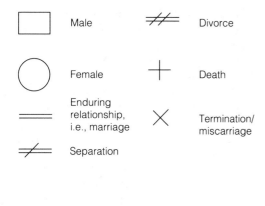

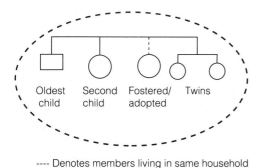

---- Denotes members living in same household

**Figure 7.1** Geneogram symbols

If the subject of the geneogram has children, then at least one generation either side of the subject is included. Dates of significant events such as births, deaths, marriages, divorces, separations, and adoption are noted, as well as any other events which have a significant impact on family development.

The compilation of a geneogram can often be an efficient method of gathering a great deal of information in a short period of time, as the experience of creating a geneogram will indicate (page 76).

Virginia Satir, one of the early family therapists, likens the family to a mobile. If you touch a mobile, you can observe the sequence of movements that occur. Parts of the mobile are affected differently depending on how they are connected to each other. Similarly, the 'connections' between family members result in 'movement' in an individual, producing 'movement' throughout the family. While a family does not have strings or wire, the connections are formed by the nature of the relationships between the members. These relationships are not fixed, and can alter in intensity.

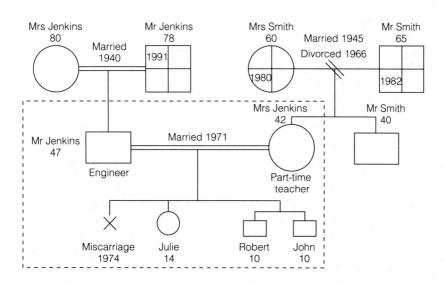

**Figure 7.2** Family tree example

Sit back and think for a moment: if you were to create a mobile that represented your family at this stage in its development, how would it look? What sort of movement would it be making? What form would the connections between the members take?

## THE LIFE-CYCLE OF THE FAMILY

The family life-cycle is a way of conceptualizing the different stages in the development of a family. The nature of the connections between the development of individuals illustrates this. For example, when the youngest child leaves home, the parent(s) are no longer involved in child-rearing on a daily basis. For a couple, this means a change in their relationship as they have more time to spend together. A similar process occurs when a partner retires from full-time work. As change occurs in one aspect of family life, it results in a change in other areas also. Each family's development is of course unique, and, as we have already discussed, not necessarily continuous; however, there are events in family life that are common to many families. A stereotypical family life-cycle is shown in Table 7.1 (Carter *et al.*, 1980).

As well as the common life events there are other circumstances, such as divorce, illness, unemployment, and remarriage, which can occur in families and will alter the direction of life-cycle development of a particular family. Rappaport (1969) describes the nature of all these stages as 'critical transition points in the normal expectable development of the family life-cycle'; and Solomon (1973) found that psychiatric and medical symptoms tend to become more apparent at transitional stages of life-cycle development.

Often transition points are marked by developmental events that involve the loss or acquisition of a family member. However, developmental changes also can produce the loss of a particular type of relationship, and the acquisition of a new form of that relationship. When the last child leaves the parental home, for example, aspects of the parent-child relationship will change; a change will also occur in the marital relationship, as the couple can find themselves living alone for the first time in 20 years. There follow a few vignettes that illustrate issues of family life-cycle development.

Carol is a single parent who lives with her two sons aged nine and five. She separated from their father when pregnant with the youngest, following regular episodes of physical violence by him. Carol has become isolated from adult contact as most of her energy and income goes on caring for the children and running the house. She has a good relationship with her children, and has enjoyed the experience of motherhood despite the lack of support. Her youngest son has just started school, and she is now in a position where it is financially worthwhile to consider returning to part-time employment. At present Carol finds the time during the day passes slowly, but feels apprehensive about returning to work.

Mr and Mrs Williams have been married 25 years. Their eldest daughter has left home, and her first baby is due shortly. Their son is 17 and has just started work. They have both enjoyed the experience of being parents, and were closely involved in their children's development. Mr Williams and his son shared common interests, as did Mrs Williams and her daughter. Both parents miss the relationships they have enjoyed with their children, and experience the house as being much quieter. The opportunity to spend more time in each other's company has been a challenge they have not yet successfully overcome. Differences between them, which went largely unnoticed or unresolved due to the demands of parenting, are now becoming more apparent. This tends to

**Table 7.1** Typical family life-cycle

| Family Life-Cycle Stage | Emotional Process of Transition: Key Principles | Second-Order Changes in Family Status Required to Proceed Developmentally |
| --- | --- | --- |
| Between families; the unattached young adult. | Accepting parent-offspring separation. | Differentiation of self in relation to family of origin. Development of intimate peer relationships. Establishment of self in work. |
| The joining of families through marriage. The newly married couple. | Commitment to new system. | Formation of marital system. Re-alignment of relationships with extended families and friends to include spouse. |
| The family with young children. | Accepting new members into the system. | Adjusting marital system to make space for children. Taking on parenting roles. Re-alignment of relationships with extended family to include parenting and grandparenting roles. |
| The family with adolescents. | Increasing flexibility of family boundaries. | Shifting of parent and child relationships to permit adolescent to move in and out of the system. Refocus on midlife marital and career issues. Beginning shift toward concern for older generation. |
| Launching children and moving on. | Accepting a multitude of exits from and entries into the family system. | Renegotiation of marital system as a dyad. Development of adult relationships between grown children and their parents. Realignment of relationships to include in-laws and grandchildren. Dealing with disabilities and death of parents. |
| The family in later life. | Accepting the shifting of generational roles. | Maintaining own and or couple functioning and interests in face of physiological decline. Exploration of new familial and social-role options. Support for a more central role for middle generation. Making room for the wisdom and experience of the elderly. Supporting the older generation without over-functioning for them. Dealing with the loss of spouse, siblings and other peers, and preparation for own death. Life review and integration. |

result in them attempting to re-involve their children in their lives. As Mr Williams becomes more involved, with his son, his wife becomes more involved with her daughters. The encouragement of dependence and discouragement of independence begins to cause conflict between the son and his parents, as he feels his individual needs are being subjugated.

Mrs Jenkins is 80 years old. Her husband died 18 months ago. She has one son and three grandchildren. She enjoyed a satisfying relationship with her husband, and they shared many interests together. Since his death she has spent more time with her son and his family, who visit frequently. During her husband's illness Mrs Jenkins lost contact with several of her friends. Although her physical health is good, she is reluctant to develop new social initiatives as this seems unfamiliar her. Her oldest grand-daughter has recently been struggling with adolescent issues, and will usually call on Mrs Jenkins for support and a shoulder to lean on when she is having difficulties with her own parents. This usually results in Mrs Jenkin's son visiting as a consequence. He resents the way his mother sticks up for his daughter, and occasionally accuses her of undermining his authority. He has been offered a pro-motion at work, which would require a geographical move that would cause con-siderable disruption to the family.

### ASSESSING LIFE-CYCLE ISSUES

Any individual will be influenced by his or her stage of family life-cycle development. How can this be assessed? The geneogram (page 76) is a good starting place as it pro-vides a current map of family relationships.

Once the geneogram has been drawn, con-sideration of the life-cycle changes that have recently taken or are about to take place for particular family members becomes possible. How have these events produced changes for other family members? What are the emo-tional processes involved? Other devel-opmental events, such as a new career, retirement, leaving home, and what aspects of the relationships are altered by such events can all be considered, as well as geographical moves, illness, divorce, or marital conflict.

It can be useful when a linking statement about the experience of one family member and its effect on another can be made, for example, 'The divorce of my parents has brought me closer to my mother, but has created a greater distance between me and my father.'; or, 'Since my younger brother has left home, I visit my mother more regularly.'

Closeness and distance may be useful criteria to assist in identifying life-cycle stages. Which relationships are getting closer and which more distant? What relationships or forms of relationship are being lost or gained? How does the level of dependence and independence change between family members? What development processes are bringing this about?

The family life-cycle is a way of charting and describing the transitional points in family development. The challenge to the family is to find an adaptation that promotes the healthy development of individual mem-bers, while preserving cohesion and stability.

### CHANGE AND STABILITY

Bateson was one of the first people to use the models of **systems theory** and **cybernetics** as a method of gaining greater understanding about family functioning. From these theories comes the notion that living systems such as the family have two essential and apparently contradictory functions: one is to provide the stability and security essential for devel-opment; the other is to adapt and change in order to facilitate development.

Maruyama (1968) defines two types of change. **Deviation-amplifying processes** are those processes by which change results in other changes, which in turn amplify the original area of change. In systems theory jargon this process is also known as **morphogenesis.** If we go back to the vignette of Mrs Jenkins we can see how this process operates. The more conflict that occurs between Mr Jenkin's son and his daughter, the more frequently she visits her grandmother. The result is an increase in the conflict between father and daughter, which in turn encourages Mrs Jenkins to support her granddaughter. This results in further conflict between Mr Jenkins and his daughter, who in turn spends more time with her grandmother. The changes are amplified as the sequence progresses, and, if they were to continue, it could end up with the daughter moving in with her grandmother.

The concept of the vicious circle is another example of this process. The process itself, however, should not be seen as either negative or positive, as its consequences depend upon the particular circumstances prevailing and the belief system of the observer. Falling in love is a more pleasant example of this process.

The other type of change process identified by Maruyama is **deviation counteracting.** Here, a change occurs that results in further change, which results in the original change being counteracted with a return to the original state. Changes that are perceived as a threat to stability will result in the activation of processes that act to return the system to a stable state. This is also known as **morphostasis,** or **homeostasis.** For example, the effect of the daughter spending increasing time with her grandmother could also have a stabilizing effect. If seen from the perspective of Mrs Jenkins, it would provide her with an opportunity to feel needed and fulfilled at a time of great personal loss, and would reduce the effect of the grief she feels for her husband's death.

The complexity of interactional sequences in families is such that it challenges our conventional cause-effect thinking. It is useful to think in terms of constant processes that have circularity as a feature, and have no beginning or end except for the observer who dares to make an arbitrary definition.

Transitions in life-cycle development result in a change in a previous pattern of behaviour that may have appeared stable. The pressure for change and development in a family will occur both from within, in terms of the individual's developmental needs, and also from without, in terms of the pressures from society to conform to expected norms of behaviour. This pressure for change can produce the experience of instability before the transformation to the next stage of life-cycle development takes place, where a new balance is achieved around relationships that have adapted.

## MINUCHIN'S STRUCTURAL PERSPECTIVE

Salvador Minuchin (1974), a pioneering family therapist, says that family structure is 'The invisible set of functional demands that organizes the way in which family members interact.' The family structure needs to be able to adapt as development occurs in the family life-cycle, responding to internal and external pressures for change, and adapting to meet new circumstances, while continuing to provide continuity for its members.

Minuchin was influential in the development of structural family therapy, which defines some of the important aspects and processes occurring in families. The family is seen as comprising of different parts or **subsystems,** each of which can be formed by generation, sex, interest, or function. Each person belongs to a number of different subsystems in which they learn different skills. For example, it is possible simultaneously to be a grandmother, wife, mother, daughter, older sister, younger sister, aunt, and daughter-in-law. Readers could usefully reflect upon the different subsystems to which they currently belong; consider also the different interactions, skills, and experiences that are occurring within these subsystems.

## BOUNDARIES

Experience in some subsystems may be important in preparation for membership to future systems. Each subsystem is contained by a theoretical boundary, which defines who shall be in the subsystem and how members should behave, both within the subsystem and in their relationships to other sub-systems: an older child who begins to tell her sister what to do may be reminded either by her sister or parent that her role is that of sister, not parent. In another family, a rule may be established that in the absence of a parent the older child assumes some parental authority over younger children. In this case the child joins the parental subsystem on a part-time basis.

In order for the particular interpersonal skills and relationships required in each subsystem to be developed, it is necessary for there to be freedom from interference from other subsystems. For example, if a parent intervenes every time siblings are in conflict, they may be slow to develop the negotiating skills that will be useful to them in their peer-group relationships in other settings.

Similarly, if children intrude into aspects of their parents' marital relationship, this can restrict its development. Minuchin believes that the clarity of boundaries is a useful parameter for the evaluation of family functioning, requiring that the rules that govern the behaviour of members of subsystems are explicit and well-defined. The issue of who does what, and the membership of and structure of the subsystems is less important than the consistent agreement about the performance of these roles. It is possible, for example, for a parental subsystem to include a child, providing responsibility and authority are well defined. However, if one parent objects to this and the child only joins in that parent's absence, then the boundary is less well defined.

Minuchin sees the two types of family boundary that exist at extreme ends of a continuum ranging from 'rigid' to 'enmeshed'. Rigid boundaries result in little exchange of information between subsystems as a result of rules about communication. Consequently, each subsystem has difficulty responding to the needs of members of other systems. The old saying, 'Children should be seen and not heard' is an example of a rigid boundary between intergenerational subsystems. Unfortunately, such rigidity means that a child experiencing difficulty would need to exhibit considerable levels of distress before the parent would become sufficiently aware to respond. When we describe a relationship as being distant, this often refers to the less permeable nature of a rigid boundary.

At the other end of the scale is the enmeshed, or diffuse, type of boundary. This occurs where there is a poor or ineffectual boundary between subsystems. Consequently, the rules for membership and function of the subsystem are not well defined. High levels of involvement occur between the subsystems, and difficulty in one subsystem, i.e., in the parental relationship, immediately activates the concern of the whole family. This can result in everybody being preoccupied with other people's business, leading to interference in subsystem development. The individual's sense of self is reduced, and the perceived differences between one family member and another are slight. Often children intrude into marital subsystems, and families of origin may also become drawn in.

Another consequence of an enmeshed subsystem is that it removes or flattens the hierarchical power differential that exists between parent and child subsystems. Issues of who is in charge become confused, and members may become involved in performing roles that are inappropriate to their level of individual development.

Between these two extremes is the middle range, where there are tendencies towards either enmeshed or rigid boundaries, but not to an excessive degree. This allows the protective functions of a family to be activated, as well as enabling the subsystems the degree of privacy and self-containment they require; thus the roles and functions unique to that subsystem are able to develop.

## THE FAMILY AND MODELLING PROCESSES

In comparing a new born baby with a young adult, it may seem miraculous how in just 20 years an individual grows not only in the physical sense, but also in terms of their repertoire of behaviours, skills, and experiences. How do we learn all these skills, abilities, and qualities? Can you remember how and when you were taught to show affection to people? How did you learn the rules that govern the different intimacies that are appropriate to different relationships? Unlike academic learning, most of this learning to live in the world is acquired unconsciously through a process known as **modelling**.

We all have within us an internal model or map of the world that guides us in the enormously complex and often unconscious processes we engage in constantly. This model is constructed by the process of modelling. The model is created through experiences, often repeated over time, which give us a way of making sense of the world and our relationship to it.

The family is influential in terms of the modelling process and in providing the models upon which we draw. For example, take a simple behaviour such as giving someone a cuddle. How did we learn to do this? If we were cuddled as babies and young children, then we have experience of receiving cuddles. It is likely we were encouraged to give as well as to receive cuddles, and how we do this today will reflect our own experience of being cuddled. We will also have learned the rules about cuddling, and the conditions in which it is deemed appropriate behaviour. There will be a belief held at a family and individual level about cuddling, for example,

cuddling is a good thing to do. This will influence identity formation: 'I'm a cuddly person'; 'Ours is a cuddly family'. There may also be myths created about aspects of cuddling, for example, if you cuddle boys too much they become 'sissies'. There may also be family traditions about cuddling: 'We only cuddle at Christmas and birthdays.' Cuddling is a small piece of behaviour, but as can be seen, enormously complex as well.

When you consider all the other understandings we have developed in our model of the world, it becomes apparent there is need of a method of prioritizing, sorting, and categorizing these into a workable structure that can act as a guide to our conscious and unconscious behaviour, and as a way of understanding and interpreting our experiences in the world. Each individual's development is enormously sophisticated, and almost a unique culture in itself; the family is the major agent in the transmission of such a culture, and each family's culture is also unique.

While the modelling process is continual, the individual's early experiences influence the direction the process takes in the future: a building is started by the laying of a foundation, which determines the size, shape, and direction of its future in terms of height and structural variation.

## A PERSONAL EXPERIENCE OF MODELLING

In order to understand the effect of modelling on family development in a more personal sense, it is useful to consider our own experiences in family life. Below are some suggestions to help you in this process. If you have not constructed your own geneogram yet, you will find it helpful to do so now (page 69).

1. Pick ten adjectives you consider best describe yourself, for example, caring, affectionate, jealous. It is possible to have attributes that seem to conflict, as there may be different contexts in which the qualities show themselves.

2. Now identify the members of your family who you think were most influential in your developing these qualities.
Remember to use 'family' in the widest sense of the word.

- How was each quality demonstrated to you as you were growing up?
- Did you experience them in different ways during different stages of your life?
- How did you experience them when you were 5, 10, 15, 20 – up to your current age?
- How do you think these attributes will be demonstrated in the future by yourself and the members of your family?
- Can you give some examples with regard to each attribute and each current family member?

There is considerable pleasure to be gained from the transmission of positive experiences to our children that remind us of pleasant memories from our own childhood. However, the strong influence of modelling is most apparent when we find ourselves continuing to act in ways that remind us of characteristics of our family, even when we consciously wish to do things differently.

## COMPILING A GENEOGRAM

Start with a large piece of paper (flip-chart paper is ideal). Use 'family' in the widest sense of the word. Refer to page 69 for an explanation of the symbols to be used, an example of a family tree. You can also practise taking another person's geneogram by doing this exercise with a colleague. Always respect people's privacy when compiling a geneogram, and allow them to decide how much information they wish to reveal.

## REFERENCES

Bateson, G. (1972) *Steps to an Ecology of Mind*, Ballantine, New York.

Bateson, G. (1979) *Mind and Nature*, Harper Collins, London.

Bettelheim, B. (1987) *A Good Enough Parent*, Pan, London.

Bowen, M. (1978) *Family Theory in Clinical Practice*, Jason Aronson, New York.

Carter and McGoldrick (1980) *The Changing Family Life Cycle*, Gardner Press, New York.

Halsey, M. (1986) *Change in Society*, Oxford Univ. Press, Oxford.

Leach, E.R. (1968) *A Runaway Word*, BBC Publications, London.

Maruyama, (1968) The second cybernetics: deviation amplifying mutual causal processes, in *Modern Systems Research for the Behavioural Scientist* (ed. W.Buckley), Aldine, Chicago.

Minuchin (1974) *Families and Family Therapy*, Tavistock, London.

OPCS (1989) Labour Force Surveys (1987), Series LFS No. 7, HMSO, London.

Rappaport, R. (1969) The state of crisis: some theoretical considerations, in *Crisis Intervention: Selected Readings* (Parad and Caplan), Family Service Assoc. of America, New York.

Rathbone E.F. (1924) *The Disinherited Family*, Hodders, London.

Satir V. (1988) *The New Peoplemaking*, Science and Behaviour Books, California.

Solomon, M. (1973) Developmental premise for family therapy, *Family Process*, 12, 179–88.

## FURTHER READING

Bateson, G. (1972) *Steps to an Ecology of Mind*, Ballantine, New York.

Bateson, G. (1979) *Mind and Nature*, Harper Collins, London.

Bettelheim, B. (1987) *A Good Enough Parent*, Pan, London.

Dell (1985) Understanding Bateson and Maruyama: toward a biological foundation for the social sciences, *J. Marital and Family Therapy*, 11, 1–20.

Hoffman (1981) *Foundations of Family Therapy*, Basic Books, New York.

Minuchin (1974) *Families and Family Therapy*, Tavistock, London.

Satir, V. (1988) *The New Peoplemaking*, Science and Behaviour Books, California.

# PART THREE

# UNDERSTANDING PEOPLE – PROBLEMS OF DEVELOPMENT AND HEALTH

# DEVELOPMENTAL STAGES AND PRESENTING PROBLEMS

## 8

*Julia Fabricius*

In Chapter 5 a resume was given of the psychodynamic perspective on development. A general picture of the mind as consisting of two parts was described: a representation of the sexual and aggressive needs and drives; and an executive element – the part of the mind through which the needs and drives operate, or which denies them operation, and which relates to the world.

Earlier modes of functioning and states of mind are seldom 'deleted from the record', but tend to persist, even if well buried beneath later and more mature modes. One of the manifestations of things going wrong may be evidence of a fixation at, or regression to, a developmental conflict from an earlier stage of life (page 46 ).

## UNCONSCIOUS PSYCHIC CONFLICT

To try to make the idea of unconscious conflict clearer, two examples from Chapter 5 will be looked at in more detail.

The Oedipus Complex (page 47), involves a conflict between, on the one hand, the boy's love for his mother and wish to have her to himself by getting rid of his father; and, on the other hand, both his love for his father and his fear that his father might retaliate for desiring his mother. In normal circumstances the fear – particularly the boy's castration anxiety – together with his love causes the boy to give up his incestuous desires, and he loses all conscious memory of them.

Unconsciously, however, such desires may persist. Many sexual/sensual and aggressive wishes from early childhood may suffer the same fate: the part of the mind called the ego, sometimes at the behest of the super-ego, finds them unacceptable and incompatible with life in the real world, and they are removed from consciousness, by a mechanism Freud called **repression**.

When a conflict exists between the child's love and hate for the same person, it may be resolved in a rather different way. Melanie Klein believed that the ego uses a splitting mechanism, together with projection of the child's hate. In the child's mind there seems to be two separate people: a perfect, idealized one, and a bad, persecuting one.

Repression, splitting, and projection are examples of different types of **defence mechanism**. With repression, a more mature type of defence mechanism, what is repressed remains in the mind, albeit unconsciously. With splitting and projection, the ego aims to get rid of the aggression both from the subject and from the idealized object by attributing it to a split-off, bad object. These are much more primitive defence mechanisms. In time, most people develop a stronger ego, which can tolerate the co-existence of love and hate for the same object.

## THE UNCONSCIOUS, REPRESSION, AND DEFENCE MECHANISMS

Freud's structural model of the mind (1923) superseded, but never completely replaced, an earlier, topographical, model (1900) in which he described the mind in terms of three systems, as shown in a simplified form in Figure 8.1.

A model is a way of describing something abstract in concrete terms in order to make it easier to think about. Thus, there is no reason why one should not make use of each of Freud's models, together with any others that seem helpful, as and when appropriate.

In Freud's topographical model of 1900, he regarded the **system unconscious** as existing deep within the mind, and the **system conscious** at the surface. Mental content can pass from one system to another, but a censor in the system preconscious does not allow certain sexual and aggressive thoughts to leave the system unconscious. The forbidden thoughts are kept in the unconscious by the force of repression. Sometimes the forbidden thoughts find a way through to consciousness, but only if the censor has managed to disguise them well enough for them to be

unrecognizable. This it does by the use of defence mechanisms.

Freud's topographical model illustrates the dynamic nature of the mind more clearly than his structural model. The thoughts and wishes of the system unconscious are constantly pushing upwards towards consciousness and action; the force of repression is constantly pushing them down, and trying to ensure that they remain unconscious.

## THE NATURE OF THE UNCONSCIOUS

How can the nature of the system unconscious, or the unconscious, be known? By definition, what is unconscious cannot be known directly. However, inferences can be made by observing manifestations of the unconscious in everyday life – dreams, speech, actions, symptoms – in which derivatives of the unconscious have, as it were, slipped past the censor. Using the psychoanalytic technique, in which the subject reports all thoughts, feelings, fantasies, and dreams as they come to mind, without conscious censorship (known as **free association**) the censored material can to some extent be deciphered, and a great deal can be inferred about the unconscious.

While the content of unconscious thoughts will be specific to an individual according to his personal history, some general statements can be made about its nature (Freud, 1900, 1915).

Freud called rational thought secondary process; secondary, because it only develops after pleasure-principle functioning starts to be given up. Because unconscious thoughts do not come into direct contact with consciousness and the external world, they are not subject to the rules of reality and rationality, and are formed under the quite different, illogical rules of what Freud called the **primary process**. These are briefly as follows:

1. Thoughts in the unconscious are all wishes or wishful impulses forbidden to consciousness.

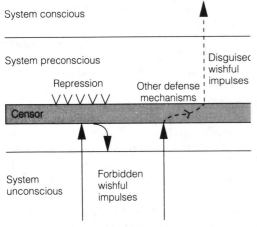

Figure 8.1 Freud's Topographical Model (slightly modified)

2. Childhood wishes especially become fixated in the unconscious.
3. In the unconscious, a wish and its gratification are the same thing, so, for example, guilt can be felt for a wish as if it had been gratified. This can be seen clearly in children, who tend to feel their wishes are omnipotent.
4. One thing can be represented by another, and will be considered to be the equivalent. This can occur through symbolization or when the two are associated in some way that may be extremely illogical.
5. A thought and its opposite can be considered to be the same.
6. Time does not exist.

These characteristics of the unconscious not only enable ideas to proliferate in the dark of the system unconscious, but are sometimes used by the censor in the interest of disguise. For example, an image in a dream may stand for something different than what is outwardly apparent. In jokes and puns the meaning can be seen more easily because the conscious mind can excuse the forbidden thought as 'only a joke'.

## DEFENCE MECHANISMS

The dynamic nature of the mind means that unconscious thoughts are ever forcing upwards, and require a counterforce to keep them down. This counterforce is **repression**. In Freud's earlier writing, the term 'repression' and 'defence' tended to be used synonymously. Later, particularly when there came to be greater interest in ego functioning, defence mechanisms other than repression were described. These ideas were particularly developed by Anna Freud (1936). It is important to emphasize that the defence mechanisms occur unconsciously – the person does not use them in a conscious or deliberate way.

Repression is an all-or-nothing defence mechanism. When it fails, it leads to what Freud called 'the return of the repressed'. Some of the other defence mechanisms make a more economic use of force by allowing the repressed to return in a way that is acceptable to consciousness. Below is a resume of some of these defence mechanisms:

**Reaction formation** Assuming a conscious attitude that is in diametrical opposition to the unconscious wish, for example, being very mild instead of very aggressive.

**Displacement** Attaching the wishful impulse to a different object, for example, wishing to kill the boss instead of one's father, or kicking the cat instead of the real object of one's fury.

**Projection** Attributing one's unacceptable impulses to another, e.g., 'He hates me' instead of 'I hate him'. This mechanism is used in paranoia.

**Identification** Assuming an attribute of another person. To a large extent, it is by this means that the personality is built, but identification can be used as a defence. For example, a bereaved person sometimes identifies with an aspect of the person who was lost. Anna Freud also described a mechanism she called 'identification with the aggressor', which can be seen, for example, in a child smacking his teddy after he has been smacked himself; more sinisterly, it has been described in concentration camp prisoners treating other prisoners in a cruel way.

**Undoing** Attempting to dismiss the existence of past actions and thoughts, usually in a magical way. This mechanism is found in obsessive/compulsive behaviour, where the person feels compelled to think a thought or carry out some action, such as handwashing, in order to undo a forbidden thought.

**Isolation** Isolating certain thoughts or behaviour so their link with the rest of the person's mental life is broken. This mechanism is also characteristic of obsessional behaviour.

**Rationalization** Giving an explanation for an action or thought that appears reasonable, but is not the true unconscious motive.

**Sublimation** Using unconscious drives towards the achievement of creative and socially acceptable aims. This is the basis of all truly creative (free and not bound by rigid defences) achievement.

## WHAT GOES WRONG?

Unconscious wishes, defence mechanisms, and psychic conflict are ubiquitous; human nature and human development being as they are, such phenomena are inevitable, normal, and often a result of healthy development. What, then, is their connection with ill health?

An important principle in the psycho-dynamic understanding of ill health is that there is no abrupt cut-off point between normality and illness. However, there are various ways in which the manifestation of unconscious conflict can cause difficulty and distress, and this can occur for a variety of reasons.

Firstly, the unconscious impulse may be particularly strong due to either innate or developmental factors, and overcome the defences. This might just lead to behaviour that is considered antisocial but does not bother the subject, but often the desires and impulses – whether acted on or not – cause considerable distress and confusion to the subject.

Secondly, the defences may be particularly weak, due to constitutional or developmental factors. Sometimes they may be weakened temporarily by illness or life circumstances.

Thirdly, the defences in general, or a particular defence, may be too strong and rigid, leading to a general inhibition of spontaneity and inner freedom, or to a particular difficulty if a particular defence mechanism is involved. Obsessional diffi-culties, in which the defence mechanisms of undoing and isolation, together with reaction-formation, are used to excess have already been mentioned. Another example given was projection, which, if used excessively, can lead to paranoia.

## NEUROSIS AND SYMPTOM FORMATION

Unless repression is absolute and complete – or totally lacking, an unusual state of affairs likely to lead to psychosis – the result of the conflict between the unconscious, wishful impulse and the defensive counterforce is what Freud called a **compromise formation**, whereby the impulse and the defence are satisfied by the same outcome. A compromise formation may be manifested by a dream, fantasy, artistic creation, accident, lapse of memory, slip of the tongue, or a joke (Freud 1900, 1901, 1905).

An example of a compromise formation would be a person in psychotherapy who is unaware of her unconscious aggressive impulses towards the therapist. The client speaks extremely quietly, such that the therapist has a difficult and uncomfortable time trying to hear, and continues to do this even though the problem has been pointed out several times. What is occurring is the simultaneous operation of reaction formation against the aggressive impulse – speaking quietly instead of shouting – and expression of the aggressive impulse – the therapist is treated to a difficult and uncomfortable time.

Sometimes the compromise formation may be expressed through the development of symptoms and of **neurosis**, which has been defined as: 'A psychogenic affection in which the symptoms are the symbolic expression of a psychical conflict whose origins lie in the subject's childhood history; these symptoms constitute compromises between wish and defence.' (Laplanche and Pontclis, 1973).

Symptoms may become manifest in a wide variety of ways, for example in bodily feelings and complaints, mood changes, fears of a general or specific nature, or compulsive or distressing thoughts. The symptom is only a manifestation of the underlying problem; removing the symptom by such means as reassurance or by hypnosis or a behavioural programme will not remove the underlying cause. This can only be done by the subject becoming conscious of and understanding the true meaning of the symptom.

**Anxiety**, both conscious and unconscious, is a common feature of neurosis. Freud's ideas about the nature of neurotic anxiety changed considerably, but by late in his life he had come to see it as a signal, a state created in the ego by the threatened return of the repressed, and indicating that defensive efforts must be increased if the ego is not to be overpowered by the wishes of the id (Freud, 1926). Below is a clinical example of a neurosis.

## CASE STUDY – JANE

The parents of Jane, aged four and one-half, asked for psychotherapeutic help for their daughter. Jane, an only child, was having difficulty separating from her parents. She was reluctant to leave her mother to attend half days at school, and often did not want to go to parties or play with other children. She also suffered from night fears, possibly bad dreams, although she was not very specific about this, which on most nights caused her to go to her parent's bed and spend the rest of the night with them.

Jane was a bright little girl who was quickly able to convey to her therapist through both play and talking the nature of her concerns and preoccupations. One of these was with marriage and babies: she played many games in which she got married, pregnant (a doll pushed up the front of her dress), and gave birth. After a few weeks, Jane spontaneously told her therapist that she intended to marry her daddy. When asked what would happen

to mummy, she said, 'Well, I'll marry mummy then.' This led to the therapist being able to discuss with Jane how difficult she found it to be in a family of three, and to feel left out of her parents' special relationship.

Another of Jane's preoccupations was with fierce animals. She played many games in which, for example, lions roared and ate up people and other animals. Sometimes crocodiles were in the sea surrounding child and therapist, who had to keep their feet up on the boat in order to be safe. Babies and baby animals had particularly to be protected from these attackers. Over time, Jane's therapist was able to talk to her about the 'roaring-lion part of Jane'. This gradually enabled Jane to dare to be the one manipulating the lion, and even for the lion to eat up the therapist in a very satisfactory way, starting at the feet and working up, until she was entirely eaten. Previously Jane had always instructed the therapist to 'make the lions roar', playing no active part in the game herself. The change showed that she had become able to own her aggressive feelings, and even to risk showing them, albeit in play, towards a person who was important to her.

It gradually became clear that Jane unconsciously feared that the reason her parents had not had more babies was because her own voraciousness and aggression had used up all the resources and destroyed the potential for more children. This became abundantly clear in a game in which she gave birth to a baby – the doll – which then was suddenly and alarmingly turned into a lion and thrown into the rubbish bin. Jane then instructed the therapist to lift her up so she could sit on a high shelf where she would be safely out of the way while the therapist made the lion/baby roar and eat the therapist up.

The lion/baby had a number of different meanings, which over time child and therapist were able to understand together. It represented Jane herself as the voracious aggressive child she unconsciously felt she was, with the eaten-up therapist representing the mother. It also stood for Jane's potential rivals thrown in the rubbish bin. Finally, it was clearly a retaliatory figure, which Jane feared might either dump her in the bin or attack her. As she became more aware of these previously unconscious feelings, Jane was able to leave her mother and enjoy school. She no longer feared either for her mother's safety from her own aggressive wishes, or that she would be abandoned in retaliation.

The source of Jane's aggression was not only to do with potential future babies as rivals. It also concerned Jane's envy of her mother's grown-up sexual body, her ownership of father, and her ability to produce babies. This painful feeling would become apparent when, for example, Jane would first admire pictures in a book of *The Little Mermaid*, who in fact had rather an adult-looking body, and then say she hated the mermaid and wanted to scribble aggressively over the pictures. Similarly, Jane would briefly admire a dress worn by the therapist and then either want to scribble on it, or say she wanted it. She sometimes turned the therapist's skirt back to reveal her petticoat, and then said that she wanted that as well. This wish for the therapist's underclothes was understood as a wish for her body, and when the therapist spoke about this, Jane became more open about wanting to have 'titties' and the ability to make babies, and about her envy of both her therapist and her mother.

Jane expressed great curiosity about whether the therapist had a husband, offering the opinion that if she did he probably looked like a frog. If things should be so unfair that the therapist had a husband and Jane did not, then Jane was certainly not going to let this husband look like a handsome prince. Jane also expressed quite openly a wish to have her father's 'willy', saying on more than one occasion that when he died she was going to cut if off and have it herself.

All the above issues came together after about three months, when Jane told her therapist a frightening dream of two crocodiles and a witch. Together they understood the two crocodiles to represent the crocodile parts of Jane, who wants her mother's two breasts, both in voracious greed and in order to have a grown-up body herself; and the witch, who rides a broomstick, as the witch part of Jane, who wants her father's penis, taking it from both him and her mother. At the same time, the crocodiles and witch were frightening manifestations which Jane felt would bite her back for having such awful thoughts. They could be understood as the beginning of a super-ego.

It is important to emphasize that Jane's disturbing thoughts and wishes were unconscious. Jane was an ordinary little girl and was deeply attached to both her parents; all young children have these sorts of thoughts. The trouble for Jane came when she repressed the thoughts, and the repressing force was not strong enough. The threatened return of the repressed caused her great anxiety and symptom formation. Her symptoms, of bad dreams and going into her parents bed, were a compromise formations. Her fear of crocodiles and witches was due to an externalization of her own aggressive wishes on to the crocodiles and witch, and she also displaced her fear of retaliation from her parents on to those creatures. At the same time, her symptoms served her wishes: to separate her parents; to replace one or other, especially her mother; to be close to their sexual bodies; and to prevent any more babies. As Jane's communications became understood, first by her therapist and then by herself, her night fears lessened and she became able to regularly sleep the whole night in her own bed.

The example given has been of a neurosis in childhood. An important point is that childhood conflicts, if undetected, remain in the unconscious, and evidence of them may appear much later in life. One might hypothesize that Jane might have developed problems as an adult to do with envy and rivalry with other women. Whatever the manifestations of the adult difficulty, the ultimate underlying conflict is always a childhood one.

## DISTURBANCE IN EARLY DEVELOPMENT

Jane's disturbance, although having roots in several periods of development, mainly originated in the **Oedipal period**. Some disturbances are known to originate much earlier.

In 1917, Freud focused his attention on two conditions that he called mourning and melancholia. He noticed that mourning following loss was in many ways similar to melancholia, which today is called depression, despite the fact that there had often been no apparent loss in melancholia. Freud also noted the frequent occurrence of self-reproach, self-blame, and guilt in melancholic people, and how they often seemed to gain satisfaction from these feelings.

These observations led Freud to the idea that there had indeed been a loss for the melancholic, but one of which he/she was unaware. The loss might have been in the form of a rejection rather than a death. The melancholic deals with this loss by identifying with the lost object; there is in fact some satisfaction in the self-hatred, in that it represents a hatred of the lost other.

This way of identifying with an object, rather than relating to it, is an early mechanism, perhaps related to a phantasy of orally taking the object inside oneself. Certainly in some depressed people a history of early deprivation and loss is found. Bowlby (1969, 1973) wrote extensively about the effects of early maternal deprivation on later patterns of attachment and reaction to loss. Robertson (1958) described the devastating effects on young children in hospital if they are separated from familiar care-givers for more than a short time. It was this that played a major part in changing the previous practice of restricting visiting in children's wards to the present-day one of encouraging a child's family to spend as much time as possible with him in hospital. Ideas about mourning and depression around the time of weaning were also developed by Melanie Klein (Chapter 5).

Psychodynamic theories of development have also been used in the understanding of **psychosis** and of psychotic aspects of the personality. Manifestations of psychosis include loss of reality sense, lack of insight, and such phenomena as delusions and hallucinations (page 130).

Freud was aware that psychotic manifestations are sometimes the result of very early developmental failure. It fell to later psychoanalysts to achieve clearer understanding about the primitive mechanisms involved (Bion, 1967; Rosenfeld, 1965). The American psycho-analyst. Otto Kernberg (1967) has given a systematic description of the symptomatic and developmental features of the so-called **borderline personality** disorders – disturbances of early development that include psychotic features but are not florid psychoses. They include the following:

1. Evidence of poor ego development, shown by such features as poorly developed reality testing, poor impulse control, and a paucity of sublimations.
2. Possibility some signs of manifest primary process thinking.

3. Excessive use of primitive defence mechanisms such as splitting and projection.
4. At times, poor differentiation of the mental representations of self and object.

Nurses often come into contact with people with borderline personality disorders. Often they are people who appear outwardly normal but have rather disturbed, 'difficult' behaviour, and there is a tendency for nurses and other staff not to like or to understand them. They are indeed difficult to understand, but it is important to remember that beneath the apparently normal surface the person may be struggling with a primitive and undeveloped level of mental functioning.

## TREATMENT

The method of treatment of psychodynamic disturbance is the same as the method of investigation. Neurosis is the result of the persistence of childhood conflicts, which exert an effect but are not known because they are unconscious. The key to their undoing is for them to become at least partly conscious. The sufferer can then gradually see that the impulse that he unconsciously fears is the re-working of a past wish, and that the defences he is using against it are outmoded and unnecessary. To gain such insight is a difficult task: all the forces that originally set up the defences are used in a vigorous resistance to the process of understanding. However, within the psychoanalytic setting, such understanding can often gradually be gained.

The tendency humans have to repeat and to constantly re-work new editions of old unconscious conflicts is on the side of psychoanalytic treatment. It means that the analyst or therapist and the treatment situation will also be used in this way. Thus the sufferer and the analyst will in time have before them a new version of the neurosis, which they can then study and come to understand together. This is known as the **transference** (Chapter 20).

## REFERENCES

Bion, W. R. (1967) *Second Thoughts*, Heinemann, London.

Bowlby, J. (1969) *Attachment and Loss* (Vol. 1), Hogarth, London, and Penguin, Harmondsworth.

Bowlby, J. (1973) *Attachment and Loss* (Vol. 2), Hogarth, London, and Penguin, Harmondsworth.

Freud, A. (1936) *The Ego and the Mechanisms of Defence*, Hogarth, London.

Freud, S. (1900) *The Interpretation of Dreams*, SE IV, V, Hogarth, London, and Vol. 4, Penguin, Harmondsworth.

Freud, S. (1901) *The Psychopathology of Everyday Life*, SE VI, Hogarth, London, and Vol. 5, Penguin, Harmondsworth.

Freud, S. (1905) *Jokes and their Relation to the Unconscious*, SE VIII, Hogarth, London, and Vol. 6, Penguin

Freud, S. (1915) The unconscious, in SE XIV, Hogarth, London, and Vol. II, Penguin

Freud, S. (1917) Mourning and melancholia, in SE XIV, Hogarth, London, and Vol. 11, Penguin.

Freud, S. (1926) Inhibitions, symptoms and anxiety, in SE XX, Hogarth, London, and Vol. 10, Penguin.

Kernberg, O. (1967) Borderline personality organization, *J. Amer. Psycho-Anal. Assoc.*, 15, 641 – 85.

Laplanche, J. and Pontalis, J. B. (1973) *The Language of Psycho-Analysis*, Hogarth, London, and Karnac, London.

Robertson, J. (1958) *Young Children in Hospital*, Tavistock Publications, London.

Rosenfeld, H. (1965) *Psychotic States*, Karnac, London.

## FURTHER READING

Freud, S. (1909) Analysis of a phobia in a five-year-old-boy, in SE XX, Hogarth, London, and Vol. 8, Penguin, Harmondsworth.

Malan, D.H. (1979) *Individual Psychotherapy and the Science of Psychodynamics*, Butterworth, London.

Rycroft, C. (1972) *A Critical Dictionary of Psycho-Analysis*, Penguin, Harmondsworth.

*As Chapter 7 – 'Family Aspects' – will be referred to in this chapter, it would be helpful to the reader to read that chapter first.*

## James Osborn

You are sitting down for an exam. You turn over the paper to discover that some of the questions are on subjects you have never heard of. What do you do? You decide to leave them for now, and search for a question you think you know about. As you begin to answer it, however, you become aware that the knowledge you have is faulty: it is not sufficient to answer the question, and some of your inaccuracies further complicate your attempt to understand what is going on.

Time is ticking away. At last you see a question you can answer. You are still struggling; it is important to do well. Giving up crosses your mind, but this seems an extreme option. Staring blankly at the page distracts you briefly, but your attention is then drawn back to the text. Possible options pass through your mind.

Suddenly you realize what is needed. You decide to discover what the gaps in your knowledge are, and begin to identify what you need to learn in order to achieve success. You stop the clock, and slip from the room to begin the remainder of your journey towards greater understanding.

Coping with family life is in some ways similar to the difficulties in coping with the examination just described. Knowing what to do usually depends upon having previously gained useful experience and information. When this is absent, incomplete, or distorted,

'finding the right answers' to family needs and problems can seem a daunting task.

### THE WIDER CONTEXT

Families need certain circumstances to function well, including the socio-economic context in which they exist. Erica de'Ath (1988), a family therapist, challenges professionals working with families to consider the importance of these external factors: 'To what extent should the provision of material needs and concern with housing, education, or social policy be considered therapeutic?'.

The level of support and encouragement, and the facilitation of appropriate conditions for successful family life to flourish, will be determined by the values of society – vital factors in determining the health of family members.

The family provides us with the learning and socialization vital to our successful development. Some parts of our model of the world that are derived from our family may be unpleasant or unhelpful; we will also have differing degrees of awareness about this. In a study of middle-class children, the social psychologists Bandura and Walters (1959) found that children imitated the anti-social behaviour shown by their parents. It was also found that marital discord and spouse abuse provided a model for children's behaviour (Gelles, 1980).

When we are aware of and accept responsibility for our model being insufficient, we usually state our desire to change in the negative, for example, 'I wish I didn't lose my temper so much.' It is harder to state this in the positive, and to see, hear, and feel ourselves performing the desired behaviour at some time in the future. Often in families the message received is not the one that was intended; many of us have had those sorts of misunderstandings. As Bandura *et al.* (1959) say, 'Effective learning requires adequate generalizations and sharp distinctions'.

Sometimes the way we are taught something conflicts with the object of the lesson. For example, a parent who physically punishes a child for aggressive behaviour does not provide an alternative model, and confirms the child's model of aggression. 'Do as I say, not as I do' is an ineffective method of communicating an idea.

Bateson *et al.* (1972) offer an extreme example of the confusion and craziness that incongruent messages can create. In the following, R. D. Laing (1965), who pioneered work in Britain on the family dimensions of mental health problems, illustrates this in a family interchange:

**Mother**: 'I don't blame you for talking that way. I know you don't really mean it.'
**Daughter**: 'But I do mean it.'
**Mother**: 'Now, dear. I know you can't help yourself.'
**Daughter**: 'I can help myself.'
**Mother**: 'Now, dear. I know you can't because you're ill. If I thought for a moment you weren't ill, I would be furious with you.'

Johnson *et al.* (1956) noted similar patterns in the communications of families where a member was diagnosed as having schizophrenia:

When these children perceived the anger and hostility of a parent as they did on many occasions, immediately the parent would deny that he was angry and would insist the child deny it too, so that the child was faced with the dilemma of whether to believe the parent or his own senses. If he believed his senses he maintained a firm grasp of reality; if he believed the parent he maintained the needed relationship but distorted his perception of reality.

Often parents, with the best of intentions, seek to avoid repeating their childhood experiences with their own children. Sometimes an over-compensation occurs, as when parents who had an excessively strict upbringing act in an extremely indulgent way towards their children. Lacking an appropriate model for limit-setting, rather than be punitive they seek to avoid any possibility of this occurring. At other times to their surprise and horror, parents find themselves repeating unhelpful patterns of behaviour because they have no alternative models to draw on. The difficulty parents have in distinguishing between their own needs and those of their children is much greater when the needs of both are of a similar quality, as the following shows:

A father who had been physically abused by his foster father found that whenever his son threw a temper tantrum, he would give in to him. He assumed his son was experiencing a similar degree of distress as he had experienced in his own childhood. This was also a protective response, as it meant the father was unlikely to risk an argument, which could result in his becoming over-punitive. His irritation at his lack of control and at his son's power led him to resent his son, and he began to avoid him when he could. In turn, his son increased his demanding behaviour, possibly as a way of trying to re-engage his father. When the conflict between the two escalated, his wife would intervene and calm the situation down, this led to marital conflict, as each was critical of the other's way of handling their son. The conflict between the parents created anxieties for the child, who began to think he was to blame for his parents' arguments, and his temper-tantrums consequently would increase.

Cyclical patterns of interaction such as this are examples of the **deviation-amplifying** and **counteracting loops** described in Chapter 7.

## MODELLING AND CHILD ABUSE

It is apparent that experiences such as abuse, neglect, and deprivation frequently result in people developing mental health problems, not only in terms of the immediate effect, but also in the way in which the experience influences a person's model of the world and their future behaviour. Many people who have experienced abuse have significant emotional adjustment problems as adults. This is due to a combination of factors, such as experiencing developmentally inappropriate and traumatic experiences; the loss of security and trust; and the powerlessness, which can create feelings of anxiety, fear, and helplessness.

## FAMILY LIFE-CYCLE PROBLEMS

### INAPPROPRIATE BEHAVIOUR AND INTERACTIONS

The continuation of behaviour and interactions that were appropriate to an earlier stage of the cycle but are no longer required will occur when one, or possibly more, members of the family fail to acknowledge that life-cycle development has occurred or should occur: 'Symptons emerge when the family structure or adherence to past structure lags behind the developmental needs of members.' (Terkelsen, 1980).

In the example presented in Chapter 7, Carol, a single parent, is faced with the task of sending her youngest son, Tony, to school. She has developed a close and extremely protective relationship with him, and is reluctant to let him out of her sight; she worries that harm may come to him, or that he may not be able to cope without her. Her anxieties are so great that she has difficulty preparing him in a positive way for school, and when her son reacts with anxiety, she responds by protecting him and keeping him at home.

Thus the pattern of dependent child and protective mother – which was an entirely appropriate form of relationship at one stage – becomes counterproductive now that a new level of independence is expected of the boy. He senses her anxiety, and responds by being anxious also. This behavior is then reinforced by the mother, who protects her son from the focus of the anxiety, the school.

It is possible that in some circumstances this type of problem can be resolved by a simple matter of education, in terms of what forms development needs to take. In other situations, it will also be necessary for the family to develop new ways of interacting that are appropriate to that stage. In the case of Carol, it is unlikely that ignorance of developmental stages is a factor, as she has already successfully enabled her older son to attend school without any problems. In order to deal with the problem, she would need to find new ways of helping her son to deal with his anxieties, and also to resolve her own concerns about letting him go to school. It may be that beliefs are relevant in this situation; for example, if Carol believes that because of Tony's early separation from his father, she has to be extra protective towards him, this will influence her behaviour. She may need to allow herself to give up some of the unhelpful guilt she experiences in relation to past events. Another way of considering Carol's dilemma is that she is experiencing a loss in the previous pattern of relationship with her son, while, possibly due to benefit regulations and lack of employment or leisure opportunities, she is unable to make any meaningful new experiences. Thus the process of change becomes more difficult for her.

Single parents do face particular challenges. In research on single-parent families experiencing problems, it was found that isolation from family support was disastrous, and that 'Symptomatic single-parent families are those cut off from their kinship networks by migration and urbanization.' (Morawetz *et al.*, 1982).

## DIFFICULTIES INHERENT TO A PARTICULAR STAGE

There are particular challenges that occur at certain stages of the family life-cycle, for example, the negotiation of increasing independence and responsibility between parents and adolescent children; or the adjustment a couple makes to the arrival of their first child.

In the example of Mrs Jenkins in Chapter 7, she is faced with the challenge of adjusting to the loss of her husband and rebuilding her life. Although the death of her husband was an expected event, Mrs Jenkins nevertheless devoted much of her time and energy to caring for him. The change in her lifestyle will be considerable, in an emotional as well as a practical sense.

Other families may find themselves in situations such as serious illness, divorce, disclosure of incest, unemployment, unplanned pregnancy, or reception of a family member into local authority care. Such events will not have been prepared for, and the family may not have previous experience of dealing with such situations successfully. These unexpected changes test the flexibility of a family's response to change much more than the expected stages; 'an unexpected transition is also triggered when there is a surprise variation in the way that an expected event occurs, such as when an adolescent declares himself gay...' (Burnham, 1986).

Migration is a major life-cycle event. In particular, problems can occur as a result of 'significant stresses arising out of a family's historical experiences of discontinuities in environment of origin as well as in adaptation to Britain.' (Lau, 1986) The experiences of many of the Vietnamese families who came to Britain is a good example of this. When the links with the extended family are weakened,

and a family is isolated from its ethnic community, it may be more susceptible to life-cycle stresses than other families.

It is important to understand the different ways in which families address life-cycle issues, as Lau (1986) states:

> In traditional hierarchical families the separation issues are handled completely differently from those in Western European nuclear-type families. Individuation and personal autonomy are seen as less important than preserving harmonious family relationships. With all families it is important to understand the meaning and function of disturbing symptoms to the family, its cultural group and wider social network.

## PROBLEMS OCCURRING AT THE POINT OF TRANSITION

In Chapter 7, the balance between change and stability as a dilemma for families was discussed. In the example of the Williams family, the gradual moving of the last child away from home produced a crisis in that the difficulties in the marital relationship became more apparent when the demands of parenting decreased. Mr and Mrs Williams became concerned that their relationship could deteriorate to the point of separation. This led them to actively seek to reinvolve themselves with their children, so that a previous degree of stability could be maintained.

This solution will probably have limited effectiveness because it interferes with the developmental needs of the children to individuate and separate from their parents. In fact, it produces conflict between the younger son and the father, which tends to unite the parents in the struggle with their son. The parent-child conflict may also be easier to manage as it is intergenerational rather than marital, and poses less of a threat to the cohesion of the family.

An American study (Hines, 1989) of poor Black families showed that their life-cycles were compressed into a short time-span, which allowed them less time to complete the particular developmental tasks of each stage. Such families also experience more unpredictable life-cycle events, such as unemployment, illness, and death, which require further adaptation. Experiences such as these make it harder for families to consolidate their growth, and developmental tasks that are left incomplete can create difficulties in the future. An example of this is when a young person is unable to achieve a sufficient degree of separation from his or her family of origin. While this may not create problems at the time, eventually it may in future interfere with the successful development of an intimate relationship.

## NURSING INTERVENTIONS AND FAMILY RESPONSES

Nurses need to remember that any intervention that is designed to benefit an individual will also have repercussions for the family. What will the nursing intervention be designed to achieve? It could enable the family system to achieve a form of stability; or it could assist in enabling a transformation.

> Mr and Mrs Williams both begin to drink alcohol more heavily in an attempt to drown their sorrows. Mrs Williams begins to experience feelings of depression and agoraphobia, as Mr Williams becomes angry and aggressive towards her. Mrs Williams takes an overdose of paracetamol, and is treated at the accident and emergency department. She is then admitted to a psychiatric inpatient unit. Mr Williams feels guilty and shocked by his wife's behaviour. The children rally round and endeavour to support their mother. After a few days, Mrs Williams is discharged home, and referred to the community psychiatric nurse.

Here, the marital conflict has been reduced and the family reports no particular problems. The CPN continues to visit the family – but what direction should her work take?

The emergence of behaviour that is defined as psychiatric symptoms can be seen as the members of a family system demonstrating their difficulty in making a life-cycle transition. If the symptoms alone are treated, without reference to the family aspects of the problem, this probably will provide a degree of stability whenever the family system reaches a point that threatens change of some form, a pattern that could continue indefinitely.

An attempt to understand the significance of symptoms in terms of their effects upon family relationships would assist in a more complete understanding of the challenge the family faces. The likelihood of offering a more appropriate solution that assists the family to achieve change, and brings a new form of stability, is thereby increased. However, if nursing interventions concentrate on the difficult marital relationship, this may appear threatening to the family, who may be cautious about such an approach.

The task for the nurse is to intervene in a way that assists the system in achieving a degree of stability, and then to assist the family in working towards the changes they wish to make. This may involve enabling them to discover the interactional nature of some of their difficulties, and agreeing on the changes they need to make.

If the nurse uses a model of therapy that does not include the family dimensions of a problem, she will probably consider solutions the family would not desire. For example, if Mrs Williams were to be seen for individual psychotherapy, or was offered assertiveness training to assist her in expressing her dissatisfaction, this could result in an increase in conflict, which may be perceived as threatening: 'Administering continuous therapeutic inputs to one family member who is experiencing relationship difficulties, frequently serves to disrupt the relationship system in unpredictable and often destructive ways.' (Gurmann *et al.*, 1978).

## CHOOSING THE MOST ECOLOGICAL FORM OF INTERVENTION

An important starting point is to assess the relevance of life-cycle issues to the presenting symptoms.

First, identify which of the three types of life-cycle difficulty referred to earlier appears most appropriate to the problem presented. Consider the interactional aspects of the presenting problem. The symptoms of an individual do not occur in isolation, and are better understood as part of a complex form of communication. The work of Boscolo and Cecchin – co-developers of the Milan School of Family Therapy – in hypothesis development and the understanding of circularity is an excellent example of this approach (Boscolo *et al.*, 1987).

The following questions need to be addressed:

1. How will the nursing interventions affect family relationships?
2. What will be the consequences for the client in following a particular form of treatment?
3. If the family is not directly involved in the treatment process, how will other family members react to it?
4. In what way are the family participating in the treatment process?
5. Are there resources they have that can be utilized?

Unless these questions are successfully addressed by the nurse, it is likely that treatment will be less successful as the family may prefer to pursue their own favoured solutions, or may actively seek to undermine the proposed work. Even if these problems are overcome, the client's relationship with his or her family will be altered in a way that could be detrimental to the client in the long run: 'Change extracts a price and raises the question as to what the repercussions will be for the rest of the system. To ignore these repercussions is to act out of ecological ignorance.' (Papp, 1983).

## MARITAL CONFLICT

When a couple enters into a partnership, each partner brings with them their experiences from their family of origin, and together they form a new family. Each partner will retain a loyalty to their family of origin, who may or may not support the relationship. A new relationship is in a sense the merging of two family styles and the support of the families of origin will be helpful. One advantage of arranged marriages is that they presuppose support for the relationship from the families of origin.

In situations where there are children from previous relationships, the task becomes more complex, as the children may also wish to maintain loyalty to the previous family, and may see the arrival of a step-parent as a potential threat. It is reasonable to expect that conflict will occur in a marital relationship due to the nature of the complex tasks involved in its maintenance. In some families it is resolved successfully, in others it is not.

Anthropologist and psychologist Gregory Bateson (1958) presented a model for understanding such conflict in his work on **schismogenesis**, which he defined as 'a process of differentiation in the norms of individual behaviour resulting from cumulative interaction between individuals'. He observed that there are complementary exchanges of behaviour that reinforce each other, for example, when one partner's dominant behaviour results in the other's submissive response, resulting in further dominant behaviour, and so on. The other type of exchange, which he called 'symmetrical', is when the behaviour exchanged is of the same type: if one partner is critical, this produces a critical response, which leads both to be more critical, and so on. The escalation can develop over time, and eventually results in a change in the nature of a relationship as the differences are amplified.

In certain circumstances, there are checks in the escalation of schismogenic processes, which Bateson termed **restraints**. In a marital relationship, the need for mutual dependence may act as a restraint on differentiation that threatens the relationship. In some marital relationships there is a continually acting restraint that checks these processes of differentiation. In situations where this restraint is lost – as in the case where a child leaves home, or a partner retires, or an elderly relative dies – the marital relationship can be thrown into crisis. This may lead either to the development of a new form of constraint, or the transformation of the relationship into a new form, which could involve the couple staying together, or separating.

It is worthwhile considering the ways in which mental health problems may become a restraint on differentiation in a relationship. **Triangulation** is the term used to describe the process whereby a third person becomes involved in the detouring of conflict between two others. Minuchin *et al.* (1978), in his work with families with an anorexic member, has noticed similar patterns occurring where the symptomatic behaviour of one family member reduces conflict between two others. Hoffman (1981) describes the triangular relationships that occur in families that produce severe psychiatric disorders:

> These triangles obliterate generational lines, confuse appropriate boundaries between family sub-groups, and subvert the family hierarchy as prescribed by a given culture. At the same time, they are associated with families so rigidly organized as to make any changes in organization problematic, especially changes associated with the growing up of the children.

Haley (1980) provides an excellent example of therapeutic work with the families of young people diagnosed as experiencing psychotic illness. He understood the bizarre and irrational behaviour of the young person to be their response to a developmental dilemma in that they had difficulty in successfully individuating from the family, as, should they achieve this, the parental relationship would undergo a crisis. They become involved in a complex sequence of behavioural interactions that restore a stability of sorts to the family system.

When considering marriage and mental health problems, it is worth noting that marriage produces higher levels of mental health for men, but an increase in mental health problems for women (Gore *et al.*, 1978). Skinner (1987) suggests that the power imbalance between men and women is largely responsible for this: '... there is an essential imbalance in the power position of men and women, and their relationships with each other will always be affected by that fact.' It is important for nurses to remember this in their therapeutic relationships. Nurses need to be aware of the way that gender issues affect their practice. Feminists express concern at the fact that many therapeutic relationships consist of male therapist and female client.

## INTRAFAMILIAL ABUSE

Family perspectives on intrafamilial sexual abuse have emphasized mother-daughter role-reversal, and the breaking of the generational boundary between the abuser – commonly father or stepfather – and victim – commonly daughter. There also is an increased risk of child sexual abuse occurring in a family that is isolated from the environment and avoids the differentiation of roles between its members; enmeshed family relationships are often a feature of families where child sexual abuse is committed (Alexander, 1982).

The incestuous relationship has been described as serving a conflict-avoiding or regulating function with regard to the parental relationship (Furniss, 1984). The emphasis in such families on morphostasis at the expense of morphogenesis means that intervention has to be at the level of changing the family structure in order to prevent the reoccurance of abuse, and to assist the victim in their recovery.

A report by the CIBA Foundation (1984) described intrafamilial sexual abuse as a 'manifestation of family pathology'. Feminist critics (Driver, 1989) point out that many mothers are unaware of ongoing sexual abuse. Uncles, grandfathers, and brothers abuse, and many men who sexually abuse children within their own family also abuse children to whom they are not related. Driver also argues that child sexual abuse is an integral part of patriarchal family life, where men – as heads of households with unquestioned rights of access to other family members – produce a situation where sexual abuse can continue to occur. Other writers comment on 'the dominance maintained by men's organization of and control over the structural systems that constitute the society we live in. For example, health, legal, welfare... and familial systems.' (Waldby *et al.*, 1989).

Waldby *et al.* also describe the family dynamics of incest as the playing out of a power relationship, and look at the connections between this and the broader operation of patriarchy. The issue of maternal collusion – either conscious or unconscious – with child sexual abuse is seen as dysfunctional, in the sense of the lack of personal power due to some women's dependence on men for their survival: 'The family is dysfunctional in that the power distribution is so unequal that one person persecutes, one is victimized and a third remains a helpless bystander.' (Waldby *et al.*, 1989); or, as Incest Survivors (1981) put it, 'Incest is the sexual abuse of power.'

Family perspectives on child sexual abuse are important in its prevention and treatment, but it is important that the responsibility for the abuse remains with the abuser, and that the rights and needs of the survivor are given priority. One of the difficulties in our current thinking about sexual abuse is due to the distinction created between perpetrator and victim. It may be preferable to think in terms of the abused as a victim, but allow the perpetrator to be a victim/perpetrator. This could lead to more constructive responses to the problem, which should include the provision of appropriate treatment for sexual offenders as well as for their victims.

There is broad agreement on the psychological effects of sexual abuse (Driver, 1989):

> Sexual abuse causes children moral confusion and leads them to confuse their needs with the desires of the abuser and deprives them of the safety in which to explore their own identity so they can develop as a balanced integrated whole.

In cases of physical abuse, it is more common that families have rigid generational boundaries. Thus factors such as the lack of awareness of developmental stages of children, poor models of parenting, and marital conflict will be relevant. There is often a difficulty in establishing a close relationship with a child, which results in a parent becoming excessively punitive and not responding to the child's distress. Often the child's behaviour will be defined as naughty or deviant, and thus punishment appears an appropriate solution. A more complex understanding of a child's behaviour is often required, which suggests alternative solutions likely to promote a healthy resolution to the problems that occur between children and their parents. Interactional models of understanding behaviour are more appropriate than defining the problem as belonging to the individual child. This enables parents who abuse to consider their part in the process, and to take greater responsibility for change. Symmetrical and complementary behavioural exchanges can be clearly observed in the escalation of behaviour, leading to serious abuse. While considering abuse, it is also important to acknowledge the extent of spouse abuse, partner abuse, and abuse of the elderly – the latter usually occurring at the hands of their carers.

## MAKING THE DIFFERENCE

Watzlawick (1990) states that:

> Well-functioning systems distinguish themselves by greater flexibility and a greater repertoire of rules [while] sick or conflict-ridden systems have few and rigid rules. Pathological systems do not have adequate meta-rules, i.e., rules for changing rules. This implies that such a system will be unable to cope with a situation for which its rules (its behavioural repertoire) are inadequate, while at the same time it is incapable either of generating new rules or changing the existing rules in such a way that the problem can be solved.

Satir (1988) found that no matter what the presenting problem was there were certain characteristics of families experiencing difficulties: 'Self-worth was low. Communication was indirect, vague and not really honest. Rules were rigid, inhuman, non-negotiable and everlasting. The family's link to society was fearful, placating and blaming.' In her work with families she aimed to help them to change these four key factors. When families were 'vital and nurturing' she found that 'self-worth is high. Communication is direct, clear, specific and honest. Rules are flexible, human, appropriate and subject to change. The link to society is open and hopeful and based on choice.'

Finally, as Satir has also stated, 'The changes all rest on new learnings, new awareness and a new consciousness. Everyone can achieve this.'

## REFERENCES

Alexander, P. (1982) A system theory conceptualization of incest, *Family Process*, 24, 79–88.

Bandura, S. L. and Walters, P. D. (1959) *Adolescent Aggression*, Ronald, New York.

Bateson, G. (1958) *Naven*, Stanford Univ. Press, California.

Bateson, G. *et al.* (1972) Toward a theory of schizophrenia in *Steps to an Ecology of Mind*, Ballantine, New York.

Boscolo *et al.* (1987) *Milan Systemic Family Therapy: Conversations on Theory and Practice*, Basic Books, New York.

Burnham, J (1986) *Family Therapy: First Steps to a Systemic Approach*, Tavistock Publications, London.

CIBA Foundation (1984) *Child Sexual Abuse Within the Family*, independent report.

De'Ath, E. (1988) Families and their differing needs, in *Family Therapy in Great Britain* (eds E. Street and W. Dryden), Open Univ. Press, Milton Keynes.

Driver, E (1989) Introduction, in *Child Sexual Abuse, Feminist Perspectives* (eds E. Driver and A. Droisen), Macmillan, London.

Furniss, T. (1984) Conflict avoiding and conflict regulating patterns in incest and child sexual abuse, *Acta Paedo-Psychiatra*, (Vol. 50), *European J. Child and Adolescent Psychiatry*.

Gelles, R. J. (1980) A profile of violence towards children in the US, in *Child Abuse: An Agenda for Action*, (eds Gerbner *et al.*) Oxford Univ. Press, Oxford.

Gore and Tudor, (1978) Adult sex roles and mental illness, *American J. Sociology*

Gurmann and Kniskern (1978) Deterioration in marital and family therapy, *Family Process*, 17.

Haley, J. (1980) *Leaving Home*, McGraw Hill, New York.

Hoffman, L. (1981) *Foundations of Family Therapy*, Basic Books, New York.

Incest Survivors Campaign (1981) Breaking the silence, in *Women Against Violence Against Women*, (eds Rhodes and McNeill), Onlywomens Press, London.

Johnson *et al.* (1956) Studies in schizophrenia at the Mayo Clinic; Observations on ego functions in schizophrenia, *Psychiatry*, 19.

Laing, R. D. (1965) Mystification, confusions and conflict, in *Intensive Family Therapy* (eds Boszormenyi-Nagy and Framo), Harper Row, New York.

Lau, A. (1986) Family therapy across cultures, in *Transcultural Psychiatry*, (ed. J. L. Cox) Croom Helm, London.

Minuchin, *et al.* (1978) *Psychosomatic Families: Anorexia Nervosa in Context*, Harvard Univ. Press, Cambridge.

Moore Hines, P. (1989) Family life-cycle of poor Black families, in *The Changing Family Life Cycle*, (eds Carter and McGoldrick), Gardner Press, New York.

Morawetz and Walker, (1982) *Brief Therapy with Single Parent Families*, Brunner Mazel, New York.

Papp, P. (1983) *The Process of Change*, Guildford Press, New York.

Satir, V. (1988) *The New Peoplemaking*, Science and Behaviour Books, California.

Terkelsen, K. (1980) Towards a theory of the family life cycle, in *The Family Life Cycle: a Framework for Family Therapy* (eds Carter, McGoldrick) Gardner Press, New York.

Waldby *et al.* (1989) Theoretical perspectives on father-daughter incest, in *Child Sexual Abuse, Feminist Perspective*, (eds E. Driver and A. Droisen), Macmillan, London.

Walrond-Skinner (1987) Feminist therapy and family therapy, in *Ethical Issues in Family Therapy* (eds Walrond-Skinner and Watson), Routledge, London.

Watzlawick (1990) *Munchausen's Pigtail or Psychotherapy and Reality*, Norton, New York.

## FURTHER READING

Axline, V. (1964) *Dibs, in Search of Self*, Pelican, Harmondsworth.

Boscolo *et al.* (1987) *Milan Systemic Family Therapy, Conversations on Theory and Practice*, Basic Books, New York.

Burnham, J. (1986) *Family Therapy: First Steps to a Systemic Approach*, Tavistock Publication, London.

De Shazer, (1991) *Putting Difference to Work*, Norton, New York.

Haley, J. (1976) *Problem-Solving Therapy*, Harper and Row, New York.

Haley, J. (1980) *Leaving Home*, McGraw-Hill, New York.

Hoffman, L. (1981) *Foundations of Family Therapy*, Basic Books, New York.

Hudson O' Hanlon and Wiener-Davis (1989) *In Search of Solutions*, Norton, New York.

Satir, V. (1988) *The New Peoplemaking*, Science and Behavior Books, California.

Watzlawick, (1990) *Munchausen's Pigtail or Psychotherapy and Reality*, Norton, New York.

*Christine Halek*

We have looked at ways in which the family situation, particularly as regards issues arising out of transitional points in the family life-cycle, may impede the healthy development and psychological functioning of the individual. So far, we have focused on the immediate family situation – a cross-sectional view, as it were. There is, however, another way of looking at the individual in the family, and that is in terms of the history of the family, and the influences of previous generations on the person's present situation.

## THE PROCESS OF INTERNALIZATION

The concept that a person's influence is not restricted to the span of his lifetime or to the extent of his physical presence is not particularly notable: it is built in to the structure of many societies and religions, as well as into our own psychological functioning. Just because someone dies or goes away does not mean they cease to be a part of our internal world (Skynner *et al.* 1983).

The process of **internalization**, whereby we take in and carry with us significant people in our minds and memories, is recognized as playing a vital role in our ability to survive separation and loss (Bowlby, 1979). For example, if as a baby my mother supported me in my attempts to explore the world, by giving me freedom and comforting me when things did not work out, as an adult I will be able to take on new challenges and survive disappointments in the same way as my mother helped me to, only now I do not need

her to be there because I have internalized those supportive aspects of her.

Unfortunately, it is not only the positive aspects of people that are internalized. For example, if my mother disapproved of or was anxious about my taking on new challenges, such internalized attitudes may lead to my punishing myself for taking risks, or being too afraid to do so. These internalized beliefs and attitudes are felt to be mine, and relate to a time when I needed my mother's help or approval to do things. If they remain unconscious, and I am not aware of them coming from my mother, I will not be able to discover whether as an adult I am really like her, or whether I have a different capacity to take on challenges. The process of discovering how such internalized beliefs and attitudes impair healthy development and functioning is one of the main tasks of the dynamic psychotherapies and psychoanalysis.

### THE SUPER-EGO

This process of taking in, or **introjecting**, and internalizing aspects of another person's beliefs and attitudes towards oneself is one of the main ways in which our parents' influence remains with us even after they have died. Freud (1923) thought the process of internalizing aspects of our parents led to the development of a conscience and to moral concepts of good and bad, or, to use his terms, to the development of a **super-ego**. The super-ego puts limits on the self (ego), making judgements on our thoughts, feelings, and behaviour, and helping to control primitive impulses from the **id**. For example, we are all familiar with the feelings behind the thought, 'I could have killed him', and we often entertain quite wild or violent thoughts towards others. However, we do not act on them because we know it would be inappropriate or morally wrong, or likely to lead to punishment. It is the super-ego that helps us to remain in control of our feelings in a useful way. At other times, however, the wrong things are labelled as being bad, and we are prevented from wanting things like love and attention, or sex – not because anyone is now telling us they are bad, but because we have internalized, and are telling ourselves, that they are bad. If the ego cannot sort out the conflicts between the id and superego, mental ill health may result (Chapters 5 and 8).

## THE INFLUENCE OF GENERATIONS

Internalization is one way in which we are influenced by earlier generations, particularly by our parents. When we are considering the handing down of beliefs and attitudes from one generation to another, it becomes clear that our parents' beliefs and attitudes are also shaped by what they have internalized from their own parents, who also have their own families of origin, and so on. This transmission of beliefs and attitudes down the generations can exert a powerful influence on an individual; it is one of the main ways whereby a family maintains a discrete identity across several generations, despite losing members and adding new ones (Liebermann, 1979).

### MYTHS AND LEGENDS

The ways in which these extended transgenerational influences are transmitted are several. One way is via family myths and legends, which subtly convey the rules of the family to successive generations, and can be equally subtly altered to fit the current family

situation. In fact, it is likely that each person will maintain a slightly different version of the same story, which will reveal how he sees himself within the family and how important it is to him (Byng-Hall, 1979).

Pincus *et al.* (1978) define family myths as secrets or unconscious beliefs and attitudes, which, in being accepted by successive generations of the family, can determine responses and behaviour in certain situations. They see legends as those stories which convey to each generation the rules and obligations of life. Although they are indirect statements of the rules, legends are conscious and the family is aware of their existence. Myths, on the other hand, are secret and hidden, and yet may shape the actions and beliefs of individuals profoundly.

Byng-Hall (1987) gives an interesting account of one of his own family legends and its relevance for him. He is a descendant of a notable sea-faring family, with at least one famous admiral among its ranks. The legend he presents, over 200 years old, concerns a less illustrious forebear who, when faced with overwhelming odds in a sea battle, withdrew without fighting, was branded a coward, and shot. From this legend, Byng-Hall learnt that catastrophe was inevitable when faced with such odds: either way you died; he also learnt that cowardice was the worst sin. By finding out more about the history which gave rise to the legend, he discovered that in fact the whole operation had been bungled by those in command, and that his ancestor, far from being a coward, had shown enormous courage, and had been made the scapegoat for the failure of the operation. This new information meant that cowardice was no longer an issue, and that catastrophe was not necessarily the only outcome of such a situation. Unravelling the legend not only gave Byng-Hall a chance to put the record straight, but also helped him to understand how some of his own beliefs and attitudes had been shaped by the story – or that the way the legend had evolved was a reflection of his family's beliefs and attitudes handed on to him.

The way in which such beliefs and attitudes affect each individual begins in the mother-infant relationship, by the infant building up a picture of himself from the way he and his mother interact. Through this process, called **mirroring**, the infant receives a 'reflection' of himself from his mother's responses to him (Miller, 1983). For example, if the infant is angry at being kept waiting when hungry, and shows this by refusing to feed initially, his mother may either be patient and understand that he is angry; she may panic and think she has done something wrong; or she may be angry with him. From her response the infant in turn may judge his anger to be acceptable, or frightening, or deserving of punishment.

The process of internalization leads the infant to take in his mother's responses to him and make them his own, so that the infant will, for example, avoid being angry with his mother because it seems to upset her and is damaging to their relationship, which in turn upsets him. In this way he comes to see his anger and that of others as dangerous, hurtful, and to be avoided – rather than as a healthy response to some hurt or deprivation.

Unconscious processes such as these are the basis of individual and family mythology, and are carried through into adult life. While legends are fairly accessible, myths may be more difficult to get at. Like legends, they are self-perpetuating, as in this example, largely through the unconscious choice of partners who have a similar mythology to our own (Skynner *et al.*, 1983). This in fact strengthens the power of the myth in the family.

Sarah is a woman who is easily hurt, and because of this is particularly afraid of her own power to hurt. She perceives John, her husband, as unable to tolerate hurt, but capable of hurting her. He is in fact a reflection of herself; each has chosen a partner who mirrors a part of their internal world. They are both very sensitive, and suffer at each other's hands because it is impossible to live closely with another person without hurting them, albeit unintentionally. Each mis-understanding may be experienced as a deliberate hurt. Each becomes more hurt by the other and, because they are sensitive, they become increasingly fearful of their capacity to hurt each other. They tend to avoid emotional closeness to minimize the risk of getting hurt.

With this couple, the myth may be that neither John nor Sarah could openly tolerate being hurt by each other, or that they have already hurt each other so badly they could never recover if this became known in a conscious way. They may also end up believing themselves to be more and more potentially damaging to the other. Whatever the reasoning, the myth of hurt and hurting is never tested out in reality, and so it remains a very powerful force in the relationship, and may be passed on to the children, who may, for example, learn that they must never do anything to hurt their parents because it would be catastrophic; or they may feel themselves to be potentially destructive or damaging, as their parents do. Unless the myth is challenged, it will be transmitted down the generations, and continue to affect family members' responses to each other and to outsiders. It is when such family mytho-logy becomes intolerable or too restrictive for a family member and needs to be changed that mental health problems may result.

FAMILY PATTERNS

Another way in which transgenerational influences can be seen in families is in repeated patterns of behaviour, which become typical or the norm of the family (Dare, 1979). These patterns may be easily seen to an outsider, but less obvious to the family members concerned. They can take many forms, and can affect either all members of the family, or only those in certain positions in the family, or in certain relationships to others.

In the family of the late President Kennedy, there are a large number of tragic events or early deaths. On closer scrutiny, these have affected particularly the eldest sons in the family. One suggestion is that there may be particularly high expectations and stresses on the eldest sons, which cause them to expose themselves to high levels of risk. Among the younger generations of eldest sons there are signs that these strains are beginning to tell, and several of them have had drug problems or serious illness. The patterns of stress could be seen as coming from the expectations and experiences handed down in the family through the generations (McGoldrick *et al.*, 1985).

A well-known phenomenon is when an unpleasant or traumatic experience in childhood is repeated with one's own children, despite it being something which one would wish to avoid repeating (Rutter *et al.* 1976). The following example illustrates this.

Jenny is a young woman who had been given up by her mother for adoption as a young child. The adoption was not successful, and when she was a teenager Jenny traced her mother and attempted to live with her for a time. Her mother, however, who had a partner who was not Jenny's father, was not interested in her, and the relationship soon broke down. Jenny eventually married a man who was jealous and possessive. After the birth of their daughter, Jenny became very depressed and had to be admitted to hospital. She was given the option of bringing her daughter with her, but decided to leave her with her husband, who took the child to his own parents. After she left hospital, Jenny's husband

refused to allow her access to their daughter, saying she was unfit to care for her. Jenny left her husband for another man, and became pregnant again. Her daughter was put on a care order, and was housed with foster parents.

We can see how Jenny unwittingly repeated with her daughter the experience she herself had undergone, and which had been very traumatic for her. Although we can assume there were complex reasons for her depression and admission to hospital, the similarities are striking.

Another way in which patterns in families are repeated is by the forging of a bond between two individuals. Quite often this is done by naming; for example, when a child is named after a favoured aunt or a brother. In some families there is a long tradition of names handed down from one generation to another. Thus a particular figure who was important to the family or to an individual is 'reincarnated' in another (Liebermann, 1979). Along with the name, however, may come a host of roles, characteristics, and attitudes that may be hard to live up to, as the following illustrates.

Roger's sister Sally died from leukaemia when she was six and he was nine, leaving him an only child. Later, when Roger married and had a daughter, she was named Sally. Roger was always very anxious about her, and idolized and indulged her. When she was 16, Sally developed mild anorexia nervosa. Roger was terribly worried, and took her to many doctors, convinced that she was in danger of dying. In family therapy the link between Sally and his sister was made. Sally was able to express her fear of leaving her father as she felt he could not cope without her. Roger was able to recognize that his feelings about Sally growing up and leaving home were not the same as those he had experienced when his sister died. Through therapy, Sally was given permission not to be like Roger's sister, and when she left home to go to university, she began to use her second name, Annette, as her forename.

Sometimes this bond or identification of one individual with another becomes a more direct replacement. Deaths in families are often quickly followed by births (Pincus *et al.*, 1979). In many cases this can be constructive, and help the family to accommodate the death more easily; at other times, the child can be expected to fill the gap left by the dead person, so the family does not have to experience the loss of certain qualities or attitudes seen to reside in the dead person. For example, a child born to a woman whose mother has recently died may unconsciously be expected to provide the mother with love and a sense of specialness she can no longer get from her own mother, particularly at a time when she might most need that. The child will have to adapt quickly to the mother's needs, rather than having its own needs met (Miller, 1983).

Such a child might be seen to have the makings of a good nurse because of an ability to put himself second; however, he will have no chance to learn about himself, his needs and how to deal with them, or to be loved for himself. He may grow up to have difficulties in managing his feelings and making relationships, and may adapt a role whereby other people's well-being seems to depend on him, and his own well-being on his ability to make things go well for others. The stresses of such a role, and of managing the conflicts between his own needs and those of others, can manifest themselves in a variety of mental health problems.

Transgenerational influences do not always originate within the family; there are always powerful social and cultural influences brought to bear on an individual's development. As a vehicle for passing on these influences down the generations, however, the family is probably unrivalled (Elliot, 1986). Each of us assimilates these diverse influences in our own generation and hands them down to the next. This sense of tradition and history is one of the ways by which we feel we belong, and from which we develop a sense of our own identity, thus many people are fascinated by the study of their own families, and pursue this through genealogy. However, at times our identity can feel swamped or threatened by such transgenerational beliefs and attitudes, and the ensuing conflict can be difficult to manage.

While we are all subjected to these demands more or less subtly, it is particularly evident in the children of immigrant families, who may have to juggle two completely different sets of hopes, beliefs, attitudes, and expectations, deriving from the family's loss of their history, and the hope invested in their new home and in the future. The children may have to function in two or more completely different social roles, with different expectations, rules, languages, dress, foods, and so on. The resultant intergenerational conflict can have serious consequences for mental health (El-Islam *et al.*, 1986).

Less obvious conflicts and pressures transmitted down the generations can have equally serious ramifications, depending on the individual's ability to tolerate and resolve conflict – which he or she also will have learnt from his family of origin, in combination with his basic personality makeup. This explains why children subjected to similar pressures respond in very different ways: one may identify with his family's way of functioning, while another may reject it completely. Often these phenomena can skip a generation, with grandparent's attitudes, beliefs and difficulties being especially important. It seems possible that unresolved conflicts with their own parents are handed on by adults to their own children to be sorted out, or not, in the next generation. For example, it is not uncommon to find mental health problems developing at the time of the death of a grandparent. Often the importance of such transgenerational transmission is lost when problems develop and an individual comes for help – another reason for involving families in the assessment and treatment of mental health problems.

## REFERENCES

Bowlby, J. (1979) *The Making and Breaking of Affectional Bonds*, Tavistock, London.

Byng-Hall, J. (1979) Re-editing family mythology during family therapy, *J. Family Therapy*, 1, 103–116.

Byng-Hall, J. (1987) Family legends: their significance for the family therapist, in *Family Therapy* (eds A. Bentorim *et al.*) Academic Press, London.

Dare, C. (1979) Psychoanalysis and systems in family therapy, *J. Family Therapy* 1, 137–51.

Elliot, F. R. (1986) *The Family: Change or Continuity?* Macmillan, London.

El-Islam, M. F.; Abu-Dagga, S. I.; Malasi, T. H. *et al.* (1986) Intergenerational conflict and psychiatric symptoms, *British J. Psychiatry*, 149, 300–6.

Freud, S. (1923) The ego and the superego, SE XIX, and Vol. ll Penguin, Harmondsworth. Hogarth Press, London.

Liebermann, S. (1979) *Transgenerational Family Therapy*, Croom Helm, London.

McGoldrick, M. and Gerson, R. (1985) *Geneograms in Family Assessment*, W. W. Norton & Co.

Miller, A. (1983) *The Drama of the Gifted Child*, Faber, London.

Pincus, L. and Dare, C. (1978) *Secrets in the Family*, Faber, London.

Rutter J. and Madge, N. (1976) *Cycles of Disadvantage*, Heinemann, London.

Skynner, R. and Cleese, J. (1983) *Families and How to Survive Them*, Methuen, London.

Williams, P. (1989) *Family Problems*, Oxford Univ. Press, Oxford.

# STRESS AND DISTRESS

## 11

*Philip Barker*

It is often assumed that stress is a twentieth-century problem. It is more accurate to say that its description and definition is relatively recent. Modern people try to escape the hustle and bustle of their urban lifestyles in much the same way as their ancestors tried to escape extinction by wild animals, starvation, or extremes of temperature: our lives today are no more stressful than those of our prehistoric ancestors. Paradoxically, although modern life is by and large easier than that of any previous generation, if a modern stress problem exists, it is a function of the artifical world we have created to make our lives easier. Modern woman and man have hardly changed at all in their reactions to stress, be it animal, environmental, or high-tech. However, the responses to environmental threat that were at one time useful for our ancestors are often inappropriate for us; our natural bodily defences may be our undoing.

## THE DIMENSIONS OF STRESS

Stress is commonly assumed to be an emotional reaction. More correctly, stress is a specific kind of biological reaction, which can be expressed emotionally. Most emotional expressions, whether pleasant or unpleasant, are short-lived experiences. When emotional arousal is present for a prolonged period, or when it reaches a very high level, this reaction is described as **stress**. Although hard to imagine, some researchers would argue that an excess of either pleasant or unpleasant events can be stressful. Here, stress will be viewed from this objective position: how prolonged or high levels of emotional reaction – pleasant or unpleasant – can have a damaging effect.

Stress is always present in some form: it is necessary for survival. If people are not sufficiently aroused to the dangers of driving, crossing the road, lighting a fire, and so on, injury or death might result. Stress *per se* is not therefore something to be avoided. Selye (1976) emphasized the need to distinguish between positive, or 'eustress' (derived from the Greek, *eu* meaning 'good'); and negative, or 'distress' (from the Latin *dis* meaning 'bad'). This chapter deals almost exclusively with the concept of distress. For simplicity's sake, the term 'stress' will be used throughout, since it has become commonplace to use it when distress is concerned.

## THE CAUSE CONTINUUM

What causes distress? The simplest explanation involves the ideas of overload and underload. If a person is stimulated beyond the level at which (s)he is able to respond, the person will become distressed. Alternatively, if the person is inadequately stimulated, this also will produce distress. For example, workers faced with multiple tasks and insufficient time in which to complete them become excited at first; gradually experience difficulties in thinking straight; lose their sense of judgement; and finally their initiative wanes. They become distressed as a result of stimulation overload. Alternatively, prisoners placed in solitary confinement easily become distracted; find it difficult to keep their mind on any one thing; become bored; and finally also lose their initiative. These people are distressed by stimulation underload. Similarly, some people appear to possess a small appetite for enjoyment, and may become tired and ready for bed when others are ready to celebrate until the early hours of the morning.

STRESSORS

It has become commonplace to assume that different types of stress exist, for example, emotional stress, flying stress, sleep-deprivation stress, and so on. Stress can originate from a wide range of sources. Selye (1976) identified 21 possible classes of 'stressor or conditioning agent', each class containing numerous factors. Included were the effects of trauma, drugs, hormones, diet, physical agents, athletics, climate, occupation, and physiological states. The body's reaction to any or all of the factors can either be positive or negative. Our interest here is with negative reactions: what can go wrong in the body's reaction to the outside world – reactions that can have a major bearing on health.

**Major stressors: the big bang**

A number of researchers have developed life-events scales that attempt to measure the stress effects of different events on the individual (Holmes *et al.*, 1967; Sarason *et al.*, 1979). Most important studies of life-change events have involved large samples of the general population, rating the perceived severity of different events, for example, on a scale of 0–100. From such studies, general principles have emerged regarding the relative severity of different life-change events, such as the death of a spouse, pregnancy, sexual difficulties, or changing to a new school or neighbourhood.

It is unsurprising that people generally perceived the death of a spouse and divorce as the most stressful life-change events. It is

**Table 11.1** Stress value of life events

| | |
|---|---|
| Death of spouse | 100 |
| Divorce | 73 |
| Marital separation | 65 |
| Death of close family member | 63 |
| Detention in jail | 63 |
| Major personal injury/illness | 53 |
| Marriage | 50 |
| Fired from work | 47 |
| Retirement | 45 |
| Pregnancy | 40 |
| Sexual difficulties | 39 |
| Major change in financial state | 38 |
| Death of close friend | 37 |
| Change to different line of work | 36 |
| Mortgage foreclosure | 30 |
| Son/daughter leaving home | 29 |
| Outstanding personal achievement | 28 |
| Start/end of formal schooling | 26 |
| Trouble with boss | 23 |
| Change to new school | 20 |
| Change residence | 20 |
| Major change in eating habits | 15 |
| Holiday | 13 |

worth noting that tables of life-change events, such as the popular Holmes and Rahe (1976)(Table 11.1), include both negative and positive events. Holidays, successes at work, sports, or school, financial windfalls, even pregnancy, can all be stressful. Some events, such as moving to a new neighbourhood, might include both positive events – better facilities, enhanced status – and negative – disorientation, loss of existing friends and neighbours. The type of life-change events covered by the traditional life-events schedules, popular among life assurance companies for obvious reasons, are examples of major stressors.

**Minor stressors: the dripping tap**

Some forms of stress are more insidious. A dripping tap or a trickle from a stream leaves its mark over time: each drip, although individually insignificant, wears down the surface upon which it lands. A Chinese sage observed that although a single grain of corn made no sound, a bushel made an enormous crash. This is an appropriate metaphor for insidious stress. Where disorders cannot be explained by single traumatic events, the explanation may lie in the ceaseless repetition of 'insignificant' events. Selye (1956) observed that even 'trying to remember too many things is one of the major sources of psychological stress' (the reader may well appreciate this particular form of the 'dripping tap').

In this way, everyday events can top-up a person's stress level until they feel over-stressed. Failure to respond to the alarm in the morning may begin the stressful day. When the shower runs either too hot or too cold, stress points begin to accumulate. Your partner has finished the last of the shampoo and you have an important interview ahead; rushing through breakfast, you gulp coffee and cram some toast into your mouth; you forgot to iron a fresh shirt/blouse last night and waste several minutes searching for a clean one; the iron, when found, has a loose connection; you leave home, but driving off you notice you are low on petrol; queuing at the garage, drumming your fingers, you watch the minutes tick by, feeling your adrenalin surging.

People often claim it was just one of the days, or that they got out of bed on the wrong side. The reality often is that people create stress potential by failing to anticipate problems or by failing to plan ahead. Such everyday stressors can be described as minor, but may accumulate, assuming mountainous proportions. The individual's ability to cope with, or, more importantly, the attitude expressed towards, the stress event is of paramount importance. Failure to deal effectively with minor stressors may represent a major stressor itself.

### Special events

In addition to everyday events, stress also comes in the form of special events – usually extreme physical or psychological demands. Exposure to such events may be brief or prolonged: fire, rape, or a road accident may all be brief in duration; combat, occupation during wartime, the consequences of natural or unnatural disasters, or kidnap and hostage situations may all be of longer duration. The psychological consequences of such events have recently been classified as **post-traumatic stress disorder**; an acknowledgement of the severe, traumatizing nature of such events.

## THE MANIFESTATION OF STRESS

### THE AUTONOMIC NERVOUS SYSTEM

Stress can be measured by monitoring the reactions of the body, in particular the function of the autonomic nervous system. While the central nervous system (CNS) controls our reactions to our environment – driving off when the traffic light turns green; applauding at the end of a play – the autonomic nervous system (ANS) produces more automatic responses to environmental events – increasing our heart rate when faced by an assailant, or dilating the pupils to allow more acute vision when searching for an escape route.

Figure 11.1 illustrates the sympathetic and parasympathetic divisions of the ANS. The sympathetic division emanates from the middle of the spinal cord, and helps the body respond actively to threat; the parasympathetic group, emanating from the top and bottom of the cord, slow down the body to allow energy rebuilding and repair work to take place.

Both divisions operate constantly, and both are involved in reacting to stress. When a person becomes anxious, for example, the sympathetic division may produce some of the traditional signs or emotional arousal, such as increased heart rate and elevated blood pressure, dilated pupils, hyperventilation, dryness in the mouth. At the

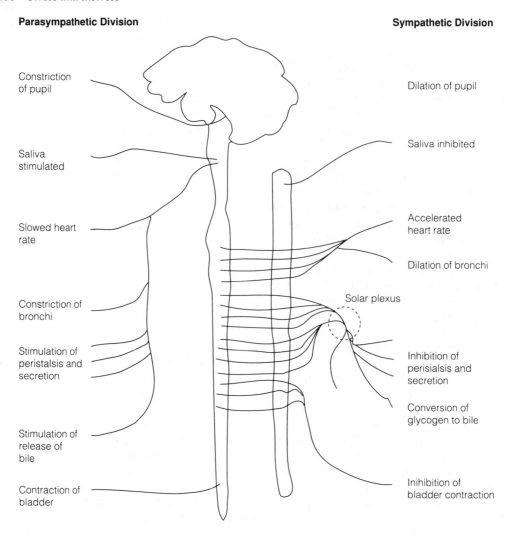

**Parasympathetic Division**

Constriction of pupil

Saliva stimulated

Slowed heart rate

Constriction of bronchi

Stimulation of peristalsis and secretion

Stimulation of release of bile

Contraction of bladder

**Sympathetic Division**

Dilation of pupil

Saliva inhibited

Accelerated heart rate

Dilation of bronchi

Solar plexus

Inhibition of perisialsis and secretion

Conversion of glycogen to bile

Inihibition of bladder contraction

**Figure 11.1** The autonomic nervous system

same time, the parasympathetic division may stimulate increased peristalsis, shown by an upset stomach or diarrohea. In high stress situations, especially when the person is in danger, the sympathetic division dominates. In low-stress situations, such as rest or relaxation, the parasympathetic division is dominant. For most of our waking day we occupy a middle ground between high and low stress, where the sympathetic and parasympathetic divisions are more balanced.

GENERAL ADAPTION SYNDROME

Stress can create or contribute to a number of mental health problems, as well as some overt physical disorders. The body reacts to stress in much the same way as it responds to more basic forms of threat: by the activation of the primitive defence mechanisms of the ANS. Reactions to stress differ little from the primitive fight-or-flight mechanisms. Selye (1974) described the three-stage process – or the 'general adaption syndrome' – involved in the stress reaction.

At the first level, the body responds in a very general way to the stressor through the activation of the sympathetic division of the ANS. All of the body's defences are brought into play, in a stage called 'alarm and mobilization'.

At the second level, if the stress continues the body tries to adapt to the stressor, focusing its resources to deal with the source of the stress. This optimal biological adaption phase is called 'resistance'.

The third stage is the natural outcome of prolonged stress. Here, the body loses its ability to cope, and the result may be complete breakdown or even death. This final stage, called 'exhaustion and disintegration', is the result of the body having expended much of its resources on dealing with a specific stressor in stage two, at the same time leaving itself weak and almost defenceless to deal with other, more minor stressors that might appear.

SPECIFIC STRESS REACTIONS

Specific kinds of stress appear to produce specific kinds of physiological reaction. Stimuli that cause anxiety or provoke anger increase gastric activity, heart rate, blood pressure, muscle tension, and respiration (Schwartz, 1977). However, the possible changes in heart rate, for instance, can vary depending upon whether or not the stressor requires the individual to ignore or attend to environmental stimuli. Doing mental arithmetic (ignoring), and studying an action-replay (attending) produce different heart-rate changes. This reaction has been described as **stimulus specificity**: different stimuli produce different ANS reactions.

The kind of stress reaction depends not only on the nature of the stressor, but also on the characteristics of the individual. Genetic factors and learning make significant contributions to the kinds of stress reactions, which tend to be generalized from one situation to another. Some people tend to show one kind of physiological reaction, others favouring a different class. This explains why some people always show increased heart rate and other cardiovascular changes under stress conditions, while others exhibit tension and other muscular reactions. These reactions have been described as **individual response specificity.**

There is an apparent contradiction between stimulus and individual response specificities: if one kind of stressor produces a specific response, how can individuals vary in their response? The answer lies in the parallel action of the sympathetic and parasympathetic divisions. In stimulus specificity, gastric activity tends to increase in response to anger, and decrease with anxiety. However, some people may show only a small increase in gastric activity, while showing greater changes in heart rate. People we might label 'cardiac reactors' are demonstrating the influence of individual response specificity over stimulus specificity.

THE ROLE OF FEEDBACK

The concept of **feedback** is central to an understanding of how the body reacts to stress. When we are subjected to stress, the CNS recognizes this and, for example, raises the blood pressure or increases the heart rate. This turning on of a specific response, or peripheral organ, is similar to a thermostat turning a heater when the temperature in a room falls below a certain level. This is called feedback. When the blood pressure or heart rate, for example, reaches a certain level, the organ sends back a return message – or **negative feedback** to the CNS, – which produces the turn-off or lowering of the blood pressure/heart rate. When you sit down to eat, your nervous system turns on your gastric juices to assist the eating process. When you have eaten enough, your stomach feeds back to the CNS, turning off the gastric secretions (Figure 11.2).

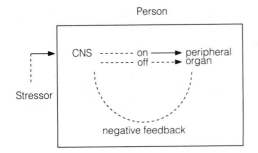

**Figure 11.2** The function of the negative feedback loop

Schwartz (1977) suggested that when this kind of regulation fails (**disregulation**), diseases can develop, as in hypertension or ulcer. Disregulation can occur at one of four stages:

1.  When the person is placed under such high degrees of environmental demand that the internal negative feedback must be ignored, which can result in an overworking of some part of the system. For example, in combat, or during a prolonged crisis.
2.  When the person is 'programmed', either genetically or through learning, to ignore the negative feedback. This faulty CNS information processing appears to be the case with people who, for example, drive themselves towards heart attacks, or eat themselves towards obesity.
3.  When the specific organ is unable to respond to the instructions of the CNS. Such malfunctioning can occur either through genetic inheritance or disease.
4.  The internal negative feedback loop fails to make the 'return call' to the CNS. Some people may be born with, or may develop, defective structures within specific organs, resulting in impaired negative feedback.

**A MODEL OF STRESS**

Having discussed briefly what kind of events might present as stressors, and how the body responds to stress, we shall now consider some views on why people respond to stress in the way they do.

PHYSIOLOGICAL THEORIES

Various theories have been presented to explain vulnerability to stress. Among them, the **somatic-weakness theory** relates specific psychophysiological disorders to a weakness in a particular organ. Asthma might be related, therefore, to a defective respiratory system, this weakness being the result of genetic structure, earlier illness, or dietary habits. The **specific-reaction theory** suggests that people respond differently to stress due to genetic programming. This would explain why some people tend to respond to similar stressors by an overactivity of gastric secretions, leading to ulcer, whereas others increase their blood pressure, resulting in hypertension.

To keep the body in a healthy state, the sympathetic and parasympathetic divisions of the ANS need to be balanced. Although the sympathetic division can overact in order to deal with threat, usually this is short-lived: the parasympathetic division eventually re-stores the balance once the threat has passed. In terms of natural evolution, the body was designed to overact and relax/repair in short bursts, threats from the natural environment being transitory in nature. The evolutionary theory proposes that the evolution of the brain has resulted in our ability to perceive danger and threat, often for extended periods of time, where none exists. Anger, regret, and worry all stimulate the sympathetic division, and the resultant arousal can last for long periods. Evolutionary theorists argue that the body simply cannot cope with the physiological storms created by the highly evolved nervous system, some people developing physical or mental stress-related disorders as a consequence.

Although the explanation of stress-related disorders is as yet in its early stages, much evidence exists to link genetic structures to the onset of specific disorders. It is well known that certain stress-related physical disorders, such as ulcers, run in families, and that mental disorders, such as schizophrenia and manic-depressive disorder, have important genetic links. Such arguments are, however, as yet tentative. What is clear is that stress is a necessary trigger in the causation of stress-related disorders, and it may well interact with an individual who is genetically predisposed to develop one form of stress-related disorder or another.

## PERSONALITY TYPES

An association between specific personality traits and negative reactions to stress has long been recognized. The **Type A/B theory** (Friedman *et al.*, 1974) is the most important explanation.

Personality Type A is described as the person who does most things quickly – eating, walking, talking, and often completing other people's sentences. This personality also is very competitive, works long hours, on a range of tasks at once, finds it difficult to relax and do nothing, and reports a general dissatisfaction with life.

By contrast, personality Type B takes life and work at a more leisurely pace, is more concerned to work *with* people, reports a high degree of life-satisfaction, and tends to concentrate on one thing at a time. Type A personalities are recognized as being coronary-prone individuals: several studies have shown them to be more than twice as likely to experience coronary problems, compared with Type B personalities (Cooper *et al.*, 1981). However, only around 14% of Type A individuals will actually suffer heart attacks.

There is some evidence that competitiveness may be the most significant factor. Type A individuals appear to over-react to competition stress, showing increases in blood pressure, adrenaline secretion, and heart rate – even when competing in computer ping-pong or mental arithmetic (Glass *et al.*, 1980; Williams *et al.*, 1982).

## PSYCHODYNAMIC THEORIES

Psychodynamic theory has long viewed physical disorders, such as gastric ulcer, cancer, hypertension, and so on, as a function of psychological dysfunction. Such disorders are caused by the same mechanical faults that produce anxiety, depression, and other mental disorders (Chapter 8).

Psychodynamic theorists argue that stress-related disorders (organ neuroses) stem from early psychosexual developmental disturbance. Physical symptoms function as **defence mechanisms**, warding off anxiety by keeping the underlying conflict from consciousness.

As to why people 'choose' one form of stress-related symptom, such as hypertension, rather than another, such as gastric ulcer, it is suggested that the symptom reflects **regression**. Disorders involving the gastrointestinal tract, such as obesity, ulcers, or anorexia, might involve the oral stage of development; colitis, the **anal stage**. In the oral stage the infant derives maximum pleasure from sucking and feeding; in the anal stage, the experience of pleasure shifts to elimination. Alexander (1950) argued that, for example, people with gastric ulcers were exhibiting a repressed longing for parental love in childhood, the individual relating, symbolically, the continual readiness of the stomach to receive food to parental love, causing the overactivity of the ANS and the stomach.

Unexpressed hostility was the basis for Alexander's 'anger-in' theory, which he also used to account for hypertension. Although some research shows that hypertension patients score highly on measures of anger or hostility, such data were collected after the onset of the disease, and cannot therefore be used to support the view that anger caused the disorder. Other theorists have emphasized the role of family interaction in stress-related disorders. Such a view may, however, only illustrate the fact that certain disorders tend to run in families, arising perhaps from some genetic base.

Although much contemporary research supports the view that physical, stress-related disorders involve psychological processes, some psychodynamic theories tend to over-interpret the evidence.

## BEHAVIOURAL THEORIES

Until fairly recently, it was assumed that the responses of the ANS were wholly involuntary: they could not be controlled in any way by the person. As a result, behavioural theorists tried initially to explain **disregulation** by using Pavlov's classical conditioning paradigm. If the natural autonomic response, for example, of sneezing through the inhalation of dust were paired repeatedly with some neutral stimulus, such as a school-bag, then the school-bag might become the precipitant of sneezing attacks (Bandura, 1969). Other theorists suggested people could 'use' their symptoms as a way of avoiding unpleasant situations, such as going to work or school.

Dworkin *et al.* (1979) proposed that because aggression was stimulated in some people who belonged to cultures that discouraged overt displays of aggressive behaviour, anger could be inhibited through hypertension. Specific disorders like high blood pressure might become reinforcing as a means of avoiding the expression of inappropriate behaviour, like anger and aggression.

All of these theories assume that a predisposition already exists to one form of physiological disorder or another, reflecting the **diathesis-stress paradigm**. This model states that specific genes or gene combinations lead to a predisposition, or diathesis, towards a disorder. If this predisposition combines with certain kinds of environmental stress, the abnormal behaviour, associated with the disorder, will result.

In the late 1960s, experimental studies with laboratory animals began to show that heart rate and blood pressure could be controlled by the animal (Frazier, 1966; Miller, 1969). Rats even showed an ability to dilate and constrict the blood vessels in different ears at the same time (DiCara *et al.*, 1968). The development of biofeedback training fitted neatly into the feedback theory of disregulation: if people had lost their natural capacity to regulate the ANS, through learning they could be retrained with biofeedback.

More recent **cognitive-behavioural theories** – involving an interaction between information processing and related actions – suggest that the stress-response is more complex. People who are able to predict stress events cope better than those who are put under stress without warning. In the Second World War, Londoners living through the Blitz experienced high levels of anxiety, but fewer stress reactions than people living in rural areas who were bombed unexpectedly. Memory and expectation appear to play an important role in the stress response. Bandura (1977) has shown that people's expectations, based on how they coped in the past, are important in determining how they will cope in response to future stress events. Many stage performers, such as actors, musicians, ballet dancers, consistently experience high levels of anxiety, or stage fright, before a performance, which does not detract from their performance.

When people are subjected to prolonged stress, as in combat, or following disasters, they are unable to escape from the high levels of anxiety experienced in the way that actors can by performing well. Prisoners-of-war and hostages may have to face daily the prospect of dying, or receiving some other form of punishment. Their inability to take constructive action to deal with this special form of stress has been described as **learned helplessness.**

Seligman (1974) first showed that animals subjected to inescapable electric shocks soon stopped exhibiting distressed reactions and began to accept the shocks passively. Many simply lay down in corners, exhibiting what Seligman saw as a 'sense of helplessness'. Under such continual high-stress conditions, the animals became anorexic, or vomited their food, lost weight, and showed marked changes to their skin and hair condition. Post-mortems showed changes in the brain which were thought to be the result of the high-stress conditions. People subjected to similar conditions involving inescapable noise or insoluble problems show similar helpless reactions.

A major revision of Seligman's initial theory is considered central to the explanation of disorders such as major depression, where the same helplessness in the face of adverse circumstances may be present (Abramson, *et al.*, 1978). Feminist writers also have supported the theory of learned helplessness as a way of accounting for the pathological anxiety, social coping problems, and high levels of depression found in women (Chesler, 1972).

The psychic numbing often shown by prisoners-of-war or disaster victims – a metaphorical retreat or withdrawal from the stressful environment – may represent the only form of escape open to people in such circumstances. The emotional blunting shown by people in high-stress conditions may also be related to the virtual extinction of all pre-existing reinforcement: floods, famine, fire, etc. wipe out many, if not all, the things which were important for the person. It is unsurprising that people in such circumstances should become withdrawn or depressed.

## THE SOCIOCULTURAL MODEL

A more recent and provocative set of theories has emerged from sociologists, who argue that many physical and mental diseases/disorders result from the pressures of industrialization and culture. Simeons (1961) suggested that the natural autonomic reaction to perceived threat (the fight-or-flight response) was discouraged by the process of cultural evolution. Instead, people have increasingly been encouraged to reason with their enemies; to resist passively; to 'keep their cool'. In animal experiments, Weiss (1976) showed that rats that were given electric shocks to their tails would instinctively fight with each other. Rats that were shocked in groups and subsequently attacked one another developed less gastric problems than rats that were shocked alone with no one to attack. Weiss suggested that the freedom to make aggressive responses might prevent stress-related illness.

The increase in divorce rates, one-parent families, and general poverty are other factors that have been used to explain stress-related disorders. Much evidence exists to suggest that social support is a significant buffer against stress-related illness, and is an important element in recovery (Silver *et al.*, 1980; Sklar *et al.*, 1981). It is also important to note that the prevalence of stress-related disorders once was much greater in men than in women; this ratio is steadily decreasing, perhaps because women now are exposed to much the same kinds of stress as men.

## THE DIATHESIS-STRESS PARADIGM

Many of the mental health problems referred to in other chapters cannot be explained simply in terms of the effects of factors inside or outside the person. A more likely explanation is that some interaction has taken place between a predisposition towards certain diseases or disorders – or **diathesis** – and environmental events, or stress.

Diathesis is most commonly assumed to refer to some constitutional predisposition, perhaps of a biological or biochemical nature. It can also mean any tendency which a person might have to behave in specific ways as a reaction to stress: the specific ways in which an individual might interpret stress events, as in learned helplessness. Similar cognitive styles may form part of the diathesis-stress paradigm in, for example, depression, schizophrenia, and obsessive-compulsive disorders.

The diathesis-stress paradigm may explain why some people who are exposed repeatedly to extreme traumas recover from their ordeals apparently unscathed. People who develop serious mental disorders like schizophrenia have inherited a physiological predisposition which places them at a disadvantage. It seems apparent, however, that some form of extreme or prolonged stress is necessary to interact with that predisposition, subsequently producing the symptoms of the disorder.

THE BIO-PSYCHOSOCIAL MODEL

Stress can be best defined as the physiological and psychological responses to excessive stimulation. Most often, but not always, this is of an unpleasant nature. Increasingly, it is recognized that many problems of health can best be explained by reference to the interaction of biological, psychological, and social processes (Figure 11.3). Stress originates in the environment, taking the form of a stress-event (stressor). The stress-reaction occurs finally in the sympathetic division of the ANS. The stress process, however, is mediated through psychological and social processes, which represent the person's world.

Some psychological processes, such as beliefs, attitudes, thinking style, and so on,

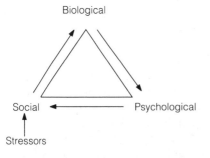

Biological

Social

Psychological

Stressors

**Figure 11.3** The bio-psychosocial model.

increase the perceived threat of a stressful situation. The effect of genetic programming might produce specific kinds of neurological organization that might increase the likelihood of dysfunctional beliefs, thinking styles and so on, which might be the case, for example, in schizophrenia. The same is true of certain social processes. The organization of some families, cultures, occupational settings, etc. may increase the effect of naturally occurring stressors, or produce specific stress-events of their own. The stresses stemming from deadlines, performance-related pay, examinations, and general success or failure are social processes of key importance.

No one part of the bio-psychosocial triangle can explain the occurrence of stress-related disorders. The genetic and biological influences that predispose the person to certain physiological responses are unlikely to be the sole cause. Similarly, the myriad psychological processes occurring before, during, and after a stress event do not adequately explain the resulting stress reaction. And the social context, important though it may be as an example of the stress-environment, does not account for the resultant stress. The interaction between all three seems to be the most reasonable way of explaining how stress reactions develop, although in different individuals the effect of one part of the triangle may be more important than in others. If one imagined looking at this triangle from the other side, one would find the same three processes involved in the treatment of the disorder: manipulation of the biology of the person through drugs, diet, and so on; the psychological state through one psychotherapy or another; and the social context through social support, and other forms of social engineering.

**STRESS-RELATED DISORDERS**

Most examples of the stress-related disorders noted so far involve physical diseases: asthma, coronary heart disease, gastrointestinal disorders, and so on. These were described by Selye (1976) as 'diseases of adaption'. Although the exact nature of the relationship of stress events to all such physical disorders remains unclear, it can be safely assumed that such disorders are influenced significantly by stress. The specific effect of stress events upon the immune system is an exciting departure in stress research, much of it focused upon the development of different forms of cancer. The psycho physiological origins of more and more physical disorders are being uncovered, as stress research becomes more sophisticated.

It is more difficult to be precise about the role of stress in mental disorders. Selye (1976) suggested this was the result of the overlapping nature of psychiatric diagnosis: it is often difficult to distinguish clearly one diagnosis from another. Despite this, it is clear that stress plays a part in the creation of a number of mental disorders, although this varies greatly from one condition to another.

Although many psychoneurotic disorders are assumed to be stress-related, unequivocal objective evidence – in the form of actual physiological disturbance, such as raised ACTH or cortisol secretion – is often hard to pinpoint. Among the disorders commonly believed to be stress-related are: anxiety states, autism, war neuroses, post-traumatic stress syndrome, stuttering, some motor disturbances, headache and backache, and anorexia and bulimia. Selye argued that due to the difficulty in classifying such disorders accurately through bio-physiological tests, almost any psychosomatic derangement could be classified as psychoneurotic, or vice-versa.

Schizophrenia and manic-depressive psychosis are widely accepted as disorders with a strong genetic basis. However, they cannot be entirely controlled by genes or they would show identical rates in identical-twin studies, which has not been shown to be the case. Schizophrenia occurs in identical twins in as few as 40% of cases. Increasingly, it is accepted that environmental stress pre-cipitates the first psychotic episode, and plays a significant part in subsequent relapses. The studies of expressed emotion (EE) in schizophrenia, and of life events in mania are important landmarks in the search to identify the specific factors that might precipitate psychotic breakdown.

Finally, a range of other neuropsychiatric or psychosomatic disorders appear to implicate stress. Parkinson's disease can be aggravated by psychogenic stress; epileptic attacks are more likely if the person suffers from sleep deprivation, emotional arousal, or intellectual over-exertion. And, although as yet unclear, stress appears to play some part in retrograde amnesia, insomnia, multiple sclerosis, and Huntington's chorea.

## SUMMARY

Stress can be described as an imbalance within the psychophysiological system of the person, which occurs as a complex response to environmental events. Short-lived stressful experiences are part of everyday life for all people. When stress reactions become more prolonged, however, a chronic stress state develops, which can play a major role in the development of both physical and mental health problems.

The physiological reactions shown by people in response to stress are identical to those shown by animals placed under threat, either in their natural habitat or under experimental conditions. These reactions involve the ANS, which is responsible for taking care of the body, both in terms of defending it against environmental threat and assisting the restoration of balance, repair, and recovery. Human responses to modern stress events have not changed from the days of fight-or-flight to avoid extinction in prehistoric time. The major change is that humans are now able to create new forms of stress by use of the highly evolved CNS, which can also see threat even when none exists.

Although the basic fight-or-flight mechanism was appropriate for our prehistoric ancestors, it is largely inappropriate in the modern world. When under stress at work, for example, it is neither appropriate to run away or to hit back at the boss. People placed in high-stress situations need to develop new mechanisms for coping with such events.

The past decade has seen a significant recognition of the importance of various self-management approaches, which involve, among other elements: the development of self-relaxation, planned exercise routines, balanced diets, time-management, and social-support networks. People who experience high stress levels need to balance their biological state through diet, exercise, relaxation, and so on; their psychological state through the acquisition of more adaptive attitudes, thinking styles, and other forms of psychological self-regulation; and their social state through the maintenance or development of support networks, the use of disclosure or confidantes at times of high stress, and the rational balance of work and leisure time.

The failure to develop such coping mechanisms can result in a stress-related disorder. Although the nature of the link between stress and illness is still unclear, it is accepted that prolonged stress suppresses the body's immune system. When this natural defence collapses, no resistance to infection is possible, and the regulatory function of many other body systems is impaired.

Stress events come from every corner of our everyday lives: from the most minor interpersonal hassle to the organized chaos of urban life. It should not be forgotten, however, that stress events can be both positive and negative; too much success, excitement, and happiness can be as disabling as many distressing experiences. It is probably the case that in a world dominated by the change ethic we have paid too little attention to helping people to cope with change. Progress may only be a good thing when you are ready for it.

Stress provides two valuable illustrations of what can go wrong with health. Ever since Descartes it has been assumed that the mental and physical worlds of the person – the mind/body split – are separate. Stress-related disorders are prime examples of the interaction between mind – in the form of the CNS and ANS and body – in the form of the viscera and their supportive physiological systems. Mind and body interact constantly to produce the person: one without the other is not a credible idea.

The treatment of stress-related disorders has also illustrated the need for a broader systems approach. Any effective treatment needs to address not only the effect of stress but the stress events at source. The benzodiazepine revolution of the 1960s is one example of merely treating the effect, of tranquillizing people who are unable to cope with the pressures of contemporary society. Valium – affectionately, or ironically, known as 'mother's little helper' – failed to help people attain the necessary balance in their lives; offering a drug-dependency problem for many who failed to develop alternative stress-coping responses. Curing the disorder by, for example, tranquillization, will not necessarily make the person healthy. Indeed, illness in any form may serve an important adaptive function by informing the person that something is wrong in their lives; something needs to be changed. If that something is not attended to, stress may reappear in some other form, affecting a different mental or physical process.

## REFERENCES

Abramson, L. Y.; Seligman, M. E. P.; and Teasdale, J. D. (1978) Learned helplessness in humans, Critique and reformulation. *J. Abnormal Psychology*, 87, 49–74.

Alexander, F. (1950) *Psychosomatic Medicine*, Norton, New York.

Bandura, A. (1969) *Principles of Behaviour Modification*, Holt, Rinehart and Winston, New York.

Bandura, A. (1977) Self-efficacy: toward a unifying theory of behavioural change. *Psychological Review*, 84, 191–215.

Chesler, P. (1972) *Women and Madness*, Doubleday, New York.

Cooper, T., Detre, T., and Weiss, S. M. (1981) Coronary-prone behaviour and coronary heart disease: a critical review. *Circulation*, 63, 1199–1215.

DiCara, L. V. and Miller, N. E. (1968) Instrumental learning of vasomotor responses by rats: learning to respond identically in two ears. *Science* 159, 1485–6.

Dworkin, B. R., Filewich R. J., Miller N. E. *et al.* (1979) Baroreceptor activation reduces reactivity to noxious stimulation: implications for hypertension. *Science* 205, 1299–1301.

Frazier, T. W. (1966) Avoidance conditioning of heart rate in humans. *Psychophysiology*, 3, 188–202.

Friedman, M. and Rosenman, R. H. (1974) *Type A Behaviour and Your Heart*, Alfred Knopf, New York.

Glass, D. C. *et al.* (1980) Effect of harassment and competition upon cardiovascular and plasma catecholamine responses in Type A and Type B individuals. *Psychophysiology*, 17, 453–63.

Holmes, T. S. and Rahe, R. H. (1967) The social readjustment rating scale. *J. Psychosomatic Research*, 11, 213–8.

Miller, N. E. (1969) Learning of visceral and glandular responses. *Science*, 163, 434–45.

Sarason, I. G. and Speilberger, C. D. (eds) (1979) *Stress and Anxiety* (Vol. 6), Hemisphere, Washington, D.C.

Schwartz, G. E. (1977) Psychosomatic disorders and biofeedback; a psychobiological model of disregulation, in (eds J. D. Maser and M.E.P. Seligman), *Psychopathology: Experimental Models*, Freeman, San Francisco.

Seligman, M. E. P. (1974) *Helplessness: On Depression, Development and Death*, Freeman, San Francisco.

Selye, H. (1956) *The Stress of Life*, McGraw-Hill, New York.

Selye, H. (1974) *Stress Without Distress*, Lippincott, Philadelphia.

Selye, H. (1976) *Stress in Health and Disease* Butterworths, London.

Silver, R. L. and Wortman, C. B.(1980) Coping with undesirable life events, in (eds. J. Garber and M. E. P. Seligman) *Human Helplessness: Theory and Applications*, Academic Press, New York.

Simeons, A. T. W. (1961) *Man's Presumptuous Brain: An Evolutionary Interpretation of Psychosomatic Disease*, Dutton, New York.

Sklar, L. S. and Anisman, H. (1981) Stress and cancer. *Psychological Bulletin*, 89, 369–406.

Weiss, J. M. (1976) Somatic effects of predictable and unpredictable shock. *Psychosomatic Medicine* 32, 397–408.

## FURTHER READING

Barker, P. J. (1990) Professional stress, in *Developing Your Career in Nursing*, (ed. D. F. S. Cormack) Chapman & Hall, London.

Langer, T. S. and Michael, S. T. (1963) *Life Stress and Mental Health*, Macmillan, London.

Lazarus, R. and Folkman, S. (1984) *Stress, Appraisal and Coping*, Springer, New York.

# EATING AND APPETITE

## 12

*Christine Halek*

Disturbances of eating, appetite, and weight are not uncommon when people have mental health problems. Some people may believe their food has been poisoned; some may be too overactive to eat adequately; some may be too miserable to eat. We can easily recognize that such disturbances are symptoms of more fundamental problems. There are some disturbances of eating and appetite however, where the food–related problems seem to be primary and not related to some other disorder. These disturbances are usually called the eating disorders, and are grouped together with psychosomatic disorders because both the mind and the body are involved in the picture presented by the sufferer.

The most common disorders nurses come across are anorexia nervosa, bulimia nervosa and obesity. In each of these, weight, weight perception, eating, and appetite are disturbed in different ways, but they all have in common the fact that food and/or weight become central in a person's life, and can occupy all or nearly all his or her thoughts. The problem can also be held to be responsible for the individual's difficulties and failures in life generally.

A good deal of research has been done to establish whether there is a physical basis for such disorders. While it is clear there are genetic and familial factors that are important, and given that disturbed behaviour is accompanied by biochemical changes, it seems these disorders are indeed similar to the eating problems described above in that they are symptoms or manifestations of underlying difficulties.

Such difficulties are often hidden even to the sufferer, and become masked by the disorder, which acts as a decoy. By the time a person comes for help, their problem is clearly related to food, weight, and eating, and it is difficult to track down the underlying problems. Usually it is only by resolving the eating disorder that such problems can be experienced again. However, as the problems are usually perceived as more difficult for the sufferer to cope with than the eating problem, this can lead to relapse or resistance to treatment. The decoy effect can make treatment very difficult, as getting better is likely to mean feeling worse, as far as the sufferer is concerned.

In order to understand why people develop eating disorders, and what the underlying problems might be, we need firstly to consider the developmental and socio-cultural aspects of eating and weight, together with biological and physiological perspectives on hunger and appetite, and the role of the body in relationships.

## FEEDING AND EATING IN DEVELOPMENT AND SOCIALIZATION

The role of food in individual and social development is central: it is essential for growth and life, and being fed is for most of us one of our earliest and most intimate experiences. The cry of a hungry baby is impossible to ignore, and the sight of malnourished children can provoke guilt and pain. Initially, a baby is absolutely dependent on those who feed him, both physically and emotionally. The interaction between the mother or carer and the suckling child is the child's first relationship with another person. A great deal depends on this. Children with feeding problems can have a difficult start in life, and lose out on the pleasurable and comforting associations many of us have with food, as well as the satisfactions to be had from good relationships (Bowlby, 1965; Winnicott, 1973).

The importance of eating is mirrored in society. Different cultures and peoples are associated with certain types of food, and often these foods persist in a community even when it has been assimilated into another. Feasting traditionally marks many social transactions, such as births, weddings, funerals, and visits, and is one of the main ways in which families and friends come together. Food can be used as a gift, or as a way of placating enemies. It can signify wealth or power – business lunches contain many of these elements. Food is used sym-bolically in other ways too, as in wedding ceremonies, where a couple may feed each other, or in religious rites. Attitudes to food, eating, and fasting vary with religious beliefs and customs. Food may be good, bad, pure or impure. Some societies may have abundant food; others may be deprived. All of these aspects of food and eating can play a part in the individual's relationship to food (Gilbert, 1986; Garrow, 1988)

The way an individual's relationship to food develops is thus partly determined by his own biological and psychological develop-ment, and partly by his development in his family and the society or religious group to which he belongs. As a child grows up, eating changes from being bound in a two-person relationship, towards a larger, family arena – and from there to peer-groups and a wider society.

Children soon learn that food is one of the main things over which they have any choice or control, and refusing food can be a

powerful thing to do in one's family. Food fads and dislikes are common in young children and are usually soon overcome, although for some they persist. Similarly, some children are poor eaters and others have hearty appetites. The family dining table can become the setting within which family rules and patterns are laid down. The period during which a Western child is taught table manners can be frustrating and unenjoyable for all concerned. Many children may be rewarded or punished by being giving sweets or being refused them. Food can become the vehicle for powerful transactions that stand for or mirror relationships, whether those that exist, or those that are missing (Buckroyd, 1989).

Preferences for certain foods and eating patterns are often culturally specific. Things we might find unpalatable may be considered delicacies in other cultures. In Western society it is normal to eat several times a day, usually at fixed times, and to eat fairly regular amounts. Such patterns vary from country to country, and are partly a function of abundant food supply – we know there will be enough food whenever we want it. In other societies, where food is scarce or has to be found, gorging is normal when food is abundant, as is restriction when there is a shortage. In societies, such feasts are characterized by eating enormous amounts of food (by our standards) in contrast to a normally monotonous and sparse diet (De Garine, 1972). Eating patterns that are unusual for us can become features of what we call eating disorders.

## BIOLOGICAL AND PSYCHOLOGICAL ASPECTS OF HUNGER

The amount a person eats at a given time is a result of several conflicting factors, among which we may identify at least three: hunger, appetite, and restraint. Hunger is a drive to eat, which can be reliably caused in any normal animal or human subject by an energy deficit... Appetite is a drive to eat food which is palatable in that particular situation... Finally, a person who experiences hunger or appetite for a food may not eat it as a result of restraint, arising from a belief that for some reason (such as politeness, or the need to avoid obesity) it would be wrong to eat that food (Garrow, 1988).

Hunger is largely biologically determined, and is the result of physiological changes in the body that signal the need for more food. If our eating and body weight were governed by hunger alone, it is likely we would maintain a fairly constant weight without ever being over or underweight. If we look at animals in the wild we can see this is so, unless there is a drought or other food shortage.

Being hungry is for most of us an unpleasant experience; babies seem to find it agonizing. For those of us who live in affluent societies, hunger is usually accompanied by the expectation that it will be satisfied. When we are hungry, certain things seem to happen: firstly, we become more aroused and alert, as though on the lookout for food; secondly, we think about food more, and often we may fantasize about what we are going to eat, which may sometimes help us to put up with our hunger for a while. (Segal, 1973).

Hunger also has psychological dimensions and correlates. Hunger, satiety, desire, and fulfilment go together. For humans, as we have said, human contact and eating are bound together, such that they can be easily confused. Some mothers will feed their babies whenever they appear to be in need or distressed, and it seems likely that it is the combination of food and contact that soothes the baby; baby monkeys, deprived of comforting contact, will not feed, even if they are hungry (Harlow, 1958).

In adulthood, this link between eating and human contact persists, for example, many adults eat when they are lonely and deprived of contact. On the other hand, refusing food, even when hungry, can be used as a way of asserting oneself, and can give a sense of power and control, something dieters may be able to identify with. Refusing food may also paradoxically reduce loneliness, which is symbolized by need or hunger. In the same vein, giving into hunger can bring relief, but also feelings of self-indulgence, desire, and lack of control, particularly if other concerns, such as social or moral pressures, are brought to bear on the way we eat.

Remaining in a state of hunger will bring about physical and psychological changes. If a person does not eat in response to feelings of hunger, the body will draw on its energy stores to keep functioning, causing the person to lose weight. In some cases, this becomes extreme and leads to starvation. As the biological aspects of hunger continue to operate, no matter how thin the person, he or she will remain in a state of arousal, and will search for food. If food does become available, it will be eaten slowly and made to last as long as possible.

In a state of hunger, the body tries to economize on energy use by shutting down as far as possible, and for quite some time normal biological functioning may be largely unaffected. Psychologically, the person will be increasingly preoccupied by food, even dreaming about it, to the exclusion of everything else, and thinking becomes increasingly simplified and concrete (Keys, *et al.* 1950). It is important to remember that many of these behaviours, which are associated with anorexia nervosa, are a direct result of starvation, rather than being particular to the disorder.

## APPETITE

Appetite is a more complex concept than hunger, and difficult to define. Appetite causes us to choose certain foods in preference to others, but it is not the same as liking or disliking certain foods; it is more a question of 'what you fancy'. It follows that appetite is unlikely to feature where there is rarely any choice of food, or where hunger overrides it. However, appetite can override hunger too, and partly explains why many of us continue to eat when we know we are full or no longer hungry. We just cannot resist another slice.

Appetite is partly based on habit and past experiences with food. It is also influenced by emotions and needs, which are only loosely connected with nutritional needs. We can observe how a person's appetite changes when they are depressed or angry or anxious. In Christian societies, appetite has also been endowed with moral significance, asceticism being a virtue, and greed a sin. Other so-called appetites, such as lust, ambition, or the desire for revenge, are similarly coloured. Certain foods have been endowed with 'sinful' qualities. 'Good' foods are those that keep you slim and healthy; 'bad' foods are those that every dieter desires but knows they should not have, or which are said to lead to disease or even death. Such attitudes are culturally determined, and relatively transient in society.

## WEIGHT AND SHAPE

Biologically, weight is directly related to what we eat versus our energy needs: anyone who under or over eats is betrayed by their body. Whereas in many societies being overweight is seen as a symbol of wealth and security, in Western society today it is undesirable to be overweight, especially for women. This seems to be related to increasing affluence, not only in society as a whole, but within societies. In the US and the UK, obesity is significantly more common among working-class populations, especially in women, and the pressure to be slim increases for women in higher social classes, whereas for men it is somewhat more acceptable to display one's prosperity through one's body (Stunkard, 1986).

The other important role of weight is related to growth. Puberty is weight-related, and triggered when a certain weight is reached in relation to height. For girls, this is usually 40–45kg (88–99lb) (Crisp, 1980). At this point, growth in height stops. For both sexes, puberty means a change in shape, but for girls it is probably more noticeable and carries different consequences than for boys. Boys' bodies become larger and stronger; girls' become curvier and fatter, women having a higher proportion of body fat than men. Girls start their periods; boys have nocturnal emissions. Both become more sexually attractive and mature, girls lacking the physical strength and power of the boys.

The basic body shape you end up with is not under your control. If you mature later, you are likely to be taller, but that is all. Nevertheless, societies develop their own concepts of what constitutes an ideal physique, and in Western society many people, especially adolescents and young adults, spend many years trying to mould their bodies to fit this ideal, or feeling dreadful because they do not match up to it. The reasons behind this are very complex, but may include: a fear of being unacceptable as one is; a need to display control over one's body, and hence over oneself in general; a desire to control sexual attractiveness; a need to be perfect; and difficulty in coming to terms with one's adult self and one's identity. Such attitudes have now become the norm, such that up to 70% of young girls diet to lose weight (Balding, 1988).

Adolescence is a period when one's relationship to one's body is particularly difficult. Suddenly the young person becomes very conscious of his or her body, its functioning, its shortcomings, and its attractiveness. Cognitive development also takes off and becomes more abstract, so that one becomes more aware of an emotional and spiritual part of oneself that is not bodily, but which seems to exist within the body and which has to be communicated by means of the body. One's body is definitely oneself; other aspects may be less easy to define.

For some people, the process of learning who they are in relation to others and how to deal with life becomes very entangled in their bodily existence, and problems that are not essentially physical can nevertheless only be communicated in a physical way. Eating disorders would seem to be one attempt to solve such dilemmas. These problems become more acute in adolescence, because this is the time when one moves towards independent living. Eating and weight disorders are more likely to arise during adolescence and young adulthood, but this does not mean that young children and older people do not have such problems.

We can now consider the signs and symptoms of the eating disorders with a deeper understanding of surrounding issues, which may be quite complicated. Eating disorders usually develop or become problematic in adolescence and young adulthood, for reasons we have touched on, although taking a careful history may reveal difficulties in childhood and infancy. Anorexia nervosa and bulimia nervosa particularly affect women and are rare in men, and more women seek help for obesity, although it is a common disorder in men too.

## ANOREXIA NERVOSA

Anorexia nervosa means a loss of appetite for psychological reasons. It is a very inaccurate name, as sufferers do not lose their appetite, and strictly speaking have a weight disorder. The anorexia nervosa sufferer strives to be an abnormally low weight because of a fear of normal weight, known as a weight phobia or a fear of fatness. This fear is accompanied by a variety of behaviours and eating patterns that lead the sufferer to be abnormally thin – below 85% of expected weight for age and height – although she may claim she is grossly overweight.

The change in body weight is accompanied by endocrine changes, which show themselves in amenorrhoea (loss of menstrual periods) in females, and loss of libido and sexual functioning. The weight loss may be achieved by reduced calorie intake (abstinence and/or vomiting); dehydration (vomiting, laxative/diuretic abuse, fluid restriction); or extensive exercising. Usually a combination of these are used. The sufferer may be ravenously hungry and does not lose her appetite, but she will resist her body's demands for food.

The effects of being in this state of starvation may be among others, over-activity, poor sleep, a obsessive preoccupation with food, a flattening of emotions, and changes in thinking and personality. If she is unable to resist her hunger, the sufferer may give in to episodes of bingeing, followed by vomiting to avoid absorbing calories, which only increases hunger. This dietary chaos can cause physical complications, especially in conjunction with dehydration, such as serious electrolyte imbalance, oedema, and damage to the gastrointestinal tract. The majority of complications will remit if the sufferer is able to gain weight again in a controlled way and eat normally.

---

ANOREXIA NERVOSA

Loss of weight or failure to gain weight leading to a weight less than 85% of that expected for age and height.

Endocrine disturbances, particularly loss of menstrual periods (amenorrhoea) in females.

Characteristic fear of normal weight and shape which persists even when the sufferer is very emaciated.

---

Anorexia nervosa is a powerful disorder, and causes great distress to sufferer's families. It is often seen as a way for the sufferer to communicate powerful feelings of anger and hopelessness to the family, who may have been unable to help their child to grow through adolescence to adulthood in a satisfactory way. The disorder prevents sufferers from fully engaging in life and taking on the demands and responsibilities of adulthood; instead they regress biologically and emotionally, remaining at home and needing to be 'fed', while refusing to 'feed'. It is often difficult to engage the sufferer in treatment, and she may maintain there is nothing wrong.

## BULIMIA NERVOSA

Bulimia means 'ox-hunger', and refers to the binge-eating episodes characteristic of this disorder. In bulimia nervosa, normal hunger and appetite regulation is overridden, which in almost every case is achieved initially by over-restraint in the form of dieting, particularly by carbohydrate restriction.

This deregulation soon spills over into periods of out-of-control eating, which become regular and frequent. During these binges, the sufferer consumes a large number of calories, usually in the form of carbohydrate-rich foods. After bingeing, she will attempt to avoid gaining weight as a result of eating so much, usually by vomiting, but sometimes by periods of fasting and/or exercise, or by dehydrating herself with laxatives or diuretics. During the binge, the sufferer feels out of control, and afterwards feels extremely distressed and ashamed by her behaviour. She will also express a fear of becoming fat, and disgust or extreme dislike for her body. The bulimia nervosa sufferer is usually an average weight for her age and height, although she may see herself as being much fatter. She may experience physical complications similar to those for anorexia nervosa, including amenorrhoea.

---

BULIMIA NERVOSA

Regular and frequent periods of uncontrolled eating during which a large number of calories is consumed, usually in the form of carbohydrate-rich food (bingeing).

The periods of bingeing are interspersed by attempts to mitigate the fattening effects of the ingested food, usually by vomiting, but also by fasting, laxative abuse, exercise, etc.

The sufferer experiences marked guilt and shame after a binge.

The sufferer is very dissatisfied with her body weight and shape.

---

Many sufferers of bulimia nervosa have a previous history of anorexia nervosa (the reverse is uncommon), and there are obvious similarities between the disorders. However, sufferers of bulimia nervosa are more likely to ask for help themselves, and they are thus easier to relate to, although they are likely to form intense, demanding, and muddled relationships. In anorexia nervosa, sufferers try to escape their needs and their inability to cope with life by appearing to get rid of them altogether; in bulimia nervosa, the needs and engagement with life are there, but cause a chaotic reaction expressed through disturbed eating patterns. The deregulated eating seems to mirror deregulated emotions and impulses. If the eating can be controlled, there is a real or imagined risk that the chaos will come out in other ways, such as cutting, suicidal behaviour, drinking binges, drug use, promiscuity, or shoplifting. Something has gone wrong with the sufferer's ability to interpret and manage her own needs and feelings, and it is this she needs help with.

## OBESITY

Obesity is the most common of all the eating disorders and is the result of a higher calorie intake than is required by an individual to meet his energy requirement. Although it is usually seen as a medical or dietetic problem, it is generally accepted that there are cognitive and emotional factors that lead a person to overeat and become obese and/or fail to lose weight despite an expressed wish to do so. There is a growing interest in obesity as a mental health issue requiring a psychological approach to treatment (Orbach, 1978; Gilbert, 1989).

Obesity that can have consequences for health and well-being is usually defined as being above 130% of the expected weight for height. This weight will result usually from periodic bingeing or sustained overeating for a period of time, without any compensating behaviour which would prevent weight gain. Unfortunately, research suggests that a period of dieting may be necessary to reduce weight, and simply reverting to a normal diet may be insufficient (Garrow, 1988). Complications of obesity can include cardiac and circulatory problems, gastrointestinal problems, mobility, and respiratory problems.

Although obesity is not regularly treated by mental health professionals, and differs from anorexia nervosa and bulimia nervosa in that it is more common and more evenly distributed between the sexes, there are similarities. Eating and weight can become similarly dominant in the sufferer's life, along with a preoccupation with food. Obesity is not considered desirable in our society, and relationships with others thus may be altered. There is, for instance, the common misperception that fat people are more likely to be jolly. Self-esteem and sexual attractiveness may be adversely affected, and a sufferer's lifestyle can become quite limited, depending on the degree of obesity. It is likely that many obese people could benefit in these areas from psychological approaches to their problems. Furthermore, increased appetite and consequent weight gain are fairly common side-effects of many psychotropic drugs, and therefore many of the people we care for as nurses may need help to avoid or to deal with obesity resulting from their treatment (iatrogenic obesity).

## OTHER DISTURBANCES OF EATING AND APPETITE

Preferences for unusual combination of foods or for eating certain foods at times when they are not usually eaten are common in pregnancy. It is not clear why this happens, but it is usually a temporary phenomenon. It is also something that children and adolescents try out for fun or for effect. Potentially more serious is pica, which is an appetite for things not normally considered edible, such as paper and paint. In the 1950s and 1960s this was regarded as serious because of the high lead content of paint, and some children suffered irreversible brain damage as a result of chewing lead-based paints. It is usually regarded as a behavioural problem, and although it can be serious and sometimes accompanies mental handicap, it can also be a transitory phenomenon.

Another problem which is not uncommon is psychogenic vomiting. This occurs when a person vomits for no apparent physical reason, nor for any reason to do directly with avoiding weight gain or food ingestion. It can occur in children, perhaps in the context of school refusal or difficulties at school, and also in association with mental disturbance or disability. As an isolated symptom in adults it is usually indicative of stress or some other underlying problem.

It is worth remembering that many people may suffer from eating and weight problems which may not reach pathological proportions, but which may still cause concern to them. It is likely that the reasons for such problems are not dissimilar, albeit less disturbing, than those one would expect with a serious eating disorder, and counselling or other psychological or behavioural management may still be appropriate for those with such problems.

## REFERENCES

Balding, J. (ed.) (1988) *Young People in 1987*, Health Education Authority, Exeter.

Bowlby, J. (1965) *Child Care and the Growth of Love*, Pelican, Harmondsworth.

Buckroyd, J. (1989) *Eating Your Heart Out*, Optima, London.

Crisp, A. H. (1980) *Anorexia Nervosa: Let Me Be*, Academic Press, London.

De Garine, I. (1972) The socio-cultural aspects of nutrition. *Ecology, Food and Nutrition*, 1, 143–63.

Garrow, J. S. (1988) *Obesity and Related Diseases*, Churchill Livingstone, Edinburgh.

Gilbert, S. (1986) *Pathology of Eating: Psychology and Treatment*, Routledge, London.

Gilbert, S. (1989) *Tomorrow I'll Be Slim*, Routledge, London.

Harlow, H. F. (1958) The nature of love. *J. American Psychology* 12, 673–85.

Keys, A., Brozek, J., Ebert, M. H. *et al.* (1950) *The Biology of Human Starvation* (2 vols), Univ. of Minnesota Press, Minneapolis

Orbach, S. (1978) *Fat is a Feminist Issue*, Paddington Press, London.

Segal, H. (1973) *Introduction to the Work of Melanie Klein*, Hogarth Press, London, and Karnac, London.

Stunkard, A. J. (1986) The control of obesity: social and community perspectives, in *Handbook of Eating Disorders* (eds K. D. Brownell and J. P. Foreyt) Basic Books, New York.

Winnicott, D. W. (1973) Close up of mother feeding baby, in *The Child, The Family and the Outside World*, Pelican, Harmondsworth.

## FURTHER READING

Brownell, K. D. and Foreyt, J. P. (eds) (1986) *Handbook of Eating Disorders*, Basic Books, New York.

Bruch, H. (1974) *Eating disorders: obesity, anorexia nervosa and the person within*. Basic Books, New York.

Crisp, A. H., Jonghin, N., Halek, C. *et al.*, (1989) *Anorexia nervosa and the wish to change*, St. George's Hospital Medical School, London.

Dally, P. and Gomez, J. (1980) *Obesity and Anorexia Nervosa: a Question of Shape*, Faber, London.

Duker, M., Slade, R. (1988) *Anorexia nervosa and bulimia: how to help*, Open University Press, Milton Keynes.

Garner, D. M. and Garfinkel, P. E. (eds), (1985) *Handbook of Psychotherapy for Anorexia Nervosa and Bulimia*, Guildford Press, New York.

Lawrence, M. (1983) *The Anorexic Experience*, Women's Press, London.

Palmer, R. (1980) *Anorexia nervosa*, Penguin, Harmondsworth.

Russel, G. F. M. (1970) Anorexia nervosa: its identity as an illness and its treatment, in *Modern Trends in Psychological Medicine*, (ed. J. Price) Butterworth & Co., London.

Selvini-Palazolli, M. (1974) *Self-starvation*, Chaucer, London.

*Philip Barker*

This chapter deals with major mental health problems. The assumption will be made that such problems are synonymous with forms of mental disorder. This comparison is important: although the definition of what exactly constitutes major forms of mental disorder is unclear, the notion of major mental health problems is even less clear. In general, however, the reader can assume that major equates with severe: this includes people suffering from some forms of psychotic or personality disorder; the latter group might also include other forms of extreme behaviour, such as aggression and anti-social action. People affected by other mental health problems would also be included in this group: in particular, severe forms of depression that are non-psychotic. To give the reader an opportunity to share the perspective of medical diagnosis that is commonly accepted, the descriptive terms used by psychiatrists will be used.

Psychoses and personality disorders are commonly accepted as examples of major mental disorder. The weakness of this concept is that it suggests that all other forms of mental disorder are minor. The terms 'psychotic' or 'personality disorder' are umbrella, catch-all titles that simplify complex states in an attempt to make them more understandable. As we shall see, a range of different psychoses and personality disorders can be described. It is important also to acknowledge that such terms reflect our professional view of a person's behaviour and experience. Although we talk about people suffering from this or that disorder, this only means we have classified their experience, or our experience of them, in a particular way.

The classifications used in this chapter derive in part from the International Classification of Diseases (ICD 9), which is used in the UK, and the Diagnostic and Statistical Manual (DSM 3), which is used in the US. These two systems offer definitions, for example, of what is – or is not – a psychosis. It should be borne in mind that these manuals offer no assistance in clarifying the experience of the person with the disorder. They are useful, therefore, for helping us to find out in what way one person appears to resemble another; it is nursings task to discover in what way people differ from one another.

## MAJOR MENTAL DISORDER

What constitutes a major form of mental disorder? The traditional approach has focused attention on diagnosis. Most psychiatric texts suggest, for example, that psychoses are the most severe of all forms of psychological disorder. In one sense this is correct: a psychosis can involve the severest disruption of normal psychological processes. This does not mean, however, that all people so disrupted are necessarily disturbed by their experience. At the same time, some people with so-called minor disorders, such as anxiety or depression, may be sufficiently disturbed to attempt suicide. Such people may also make greater demands on mental health services. So how should major, or severe, mental health problems be classified?

An attempt was made recently in the US to clarify what is meant by 'severe and persistent mental illness' (Schinnar *et al.* 1990). It was assumed for many years that the most severe examples of mental illness were to be found in hospitals. As the emphasis on care shifted to the community, the definition of severity became broader; people with severe and persistent disabilities resulting mainly from mental illness became the seriously mentally ill. Schinnar and his colleagues studied 17 such definitions. Each classified severity in different ways. As a result, different estimates of the size and nature of the problem were revealed. Difficulty continues to exist in the US, as in this country, in gaining agreement as to how exactly serious/severe/major mental disorder should be defined.

It seems clear that major mental disorders are those that have a disabling effect upon the person over a long period. A suggested definition is that a major mental health problem is present when:

- the person's ability to pursue work or career opportunities or domestic life is partially or completely impaired;
- the person's ability to function socially is impaired;
- the symptoms of the disorder continue to distress or handicap the person;
- the person has a continuing need for support or treatment.

In general, such a disabling state is likely to be caused by the kind of conditions discussed in this chapter. The reader should be aware, however, that some people with so-called minor disorders also will meet the criteria above. There is a danger of dismissing some people as the 'worried well' for the simple reason they are not suffering from a psychosis (Clare, 1991). The effect of a disorder upon the person may be more important than the name of the disorder itself.

## THE BIO-PSYCHOSOCIAL MODEL

In considering the presentation of the major mental disorders from a bio-psychosocial perspective, the reader might ask what might be happening internally within the person in terms of biological and psychological events, as well as externally in the form of various social, interpersonal processes.

The bio-psychosocial (Figure 13.1) represents a broad, open-ended view of mental disorder. The model is a triangle. Each point represents possible influences on the person, and each interacts with influences, or is influenced by, the other points of the triangle.

The model acknowledges that many, if not most, disorders are influenced by certain biological process. All people are to some extent a function of their genetic programme: hair colour and intellectual faculties are two examples of personal characteristics derived from the genetic programme. The person is therefore born to be a certain kind of person. These biological processes do not, however, explain how the infant becomes a person, or indeed what kind of person the adult will become. Such biological processes interact with specific, wide-ranging, social processes, represented by the person's family in particular, and all other social, interpersonal contacts, in general. These social factors play a major role in providing a context within which the biological self learns to become a certain kind of person. It would be argued, for example, that although a child might be born with strength, agility, or natural speed, she or he needs a specific kind of social environment in order to turn these natural

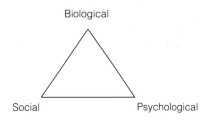

**Figure 13.1** The bio-psychosocial model

assets into those of an athlete. We shall assume that people are neither born nor made into different manifestations of mental disorder; rather, that the interaction of certain innate structures with other environmental processes lead to the possibilities of a disorder.

Why say 'lead' and not 'cause'? The answer is a complex one. It appears that the person plays some part in influencing both the social environment and the basic characteristics of his or her constitution. The psychological processes, which are the third part of our triangle, can play a vital part in determining the outcome of both biology and environment. The biological processes provide a base for the development of certain forms of psychological functioning: how we think, our belief systems, and how we act upon these. Thinking style, attitudes, and values are, however, influenced greatly by our social environment. It is clear, however, that once people have acquired certain values, thinking styles, and so on, these can be used to influence the social and biological environment of the person. Exactly how this happens is not clear. If we did not accept that this happens, however, we would be assuming that people were the mechanical outcome of the interaction of nature and nurture, and that the person had no effect on the conduct of his or her life. This is inappropriate for describing severe forms of mental disorder, which should be viewed merely as different forms of human 'being'.

The major mental health problems are not a true group; perhaps the only feature they have in common is the concept of severity. For this reason each class of disorder will be discussed in general, identifying the key features. Then the presentation typical of that group will be discussed, summarizing the relevant theoretical explanations. To simplify the discussion, these major problems will be classified in terms of affect (mood), cognition (thinking style and content) and behaviour. Although most major mental disorders involve a complex of affective, cognitive, and behavioural disturbance, one of these headings gives the various disorders their characteristic features.

## THE MAJOR DISORDERS OF AFFECT

The term **affective disorder** is used universally to classify mental health problems where a disturbance of mood is the main feature. Where mood is flattened, the disturbance is called depression; where it is elevated, the condition is described as mania. Affective disorders are best understood as a continuum of severity, ranging from the mildest forms of everyday unhappiness (dysphoria) at one extreme, to severe forms of depressive psychosis at the other. Included along this continuum are depressions associated with the life-cycle, such as post-natal depression and depression in older people, as well as manic-depressive psychosis, where the two extremes of emotion alternate.

The prominent feature of any affective disorder is a change in vitality. The depressed person experiences a slowing of the thinking processes, accompanied by emotional changes, sadness and feelings of emptiness predominating. At the same time, changes occur in the loss of natural drives for eating (anorexia) and sexual activity (libido). Where the person is manic, these features are reversed: both thinking and motor behaviour speeds up. The manic person's mood is predominantly excited, elevated, or fanciful. In some cases mania occurs as a specific affective disorder. Most commonly it alternates with depression, as in manic depressive psychosis.

## DEPRESSION

Unhappiness is an ordinary human experience, especially when associated with some form of unpleasant life event. The melancholy associated with such events passes with time. In some cases the person is left with a legacy of understanding, or psychological growth. In this sense, some forms of unhappiness can offer positive contributions to human development. Pathological depression involves similar feelings, which may appear to others to be an exaggerated response to ordinary life events. These feelings disrupt the person's life, and may pass, only to recur fitfully. In some cases the affective disturbance re-creates the pain of the initial disturbance with every recurrence. The singular pain of depression is its outstanding characteristic.

Depression can occur either alone or as an alternative to mania. The experience of depression is identical in both cases. The person's mood can range from mild sadness to profound melancholy. Mild to severe anxiety or apprehension can also be present. Loss of appetite, often with a lack of taste for food, leads to weight loss. In a small number of cases the person may go on eating binges. The person may be indifferent to usual interests, and may be acutely aware of feelings of inertia, lack of motivation, and physical tiredness. In severe examples the person may experience a slowing of speech, thought, and actual movement. In other cases the person may experience also feelings of anxiety, restlessness, and agitation. In either case, the person may find it difficult to concentrate: even simple tasks requiring decision-making and planning may prove too difficult, due to the disruption of normal cognitive processes. Some people also report emotional numbness and are unable, much to their distress, to feel for others.

Variation in mood is the predominant feature. This is often reflected by a disturbance of natural rhythm, especially in the early stages of the disorder: the person feels worst on awakening, gradually improving during the day. Sleep is disrupted, but this may be partly due to dietary changes that arise from appetite loss. Although the depth and onset of sleep may be affected, early morning wakening is the most prominent feature.

Psychological features also vary in severity. Exaggerated feelings of worthlessness, guilt, and hopelessness can extend to delusions of guilt, poverty, punishment, catastrophe, and nihilism. Paranoid ideas and ideas of reference may also be present. Suicide, which is associated strongly with severe depression, stems from feelings of hopelessness. Suicidal action is most common on entry to, or exit from, a deep depressive phase. When the person is severely depressed, suicide is unlikely, largely because it requires so much effort, both of thought and action.

## MANIA

The main characteristic of mania is an experience of euphoria. The person feels a sense of heightened energy, well-being, and enthusiasm. Speech is rapid and discursive, the person often fleeting from one subject to another, often in an amusing fashion. The person's thinking may be easily distracted: when coupled with exaggerated activity, this results in failure to complete tasks. In hypomania the person may tax friends and colleagues greatly by forceful organization of the environment. As mania heightens, grandiose schemes may be undertaken, incurring financial embarrassment or disruption of the person's affairs, or those of the family. Need for sleep appears to decline, as more time is devoted to planning and executing increasingly grandiose schemes. At this level sexual disinhibition may be evident. Exhaustion can result from overactivity, and diminishing self-care can, on rare occasions, be fatal.

In some cases the mania alternates with depression, in a so-called mixed affective state. Although the person appears excited and over enthusiastic, questioning easily reveals an underlying depressed mood, which gives a nightmarish quality to the person's life.

### Classification of the depressions

A wide range of diagnostic systems are used to define affective disorder. Where depression is profound and related to no obvious life events, it may be described as endogenous: it is assumed that the depression arises from within. Other forms of depression which appear to be related to specific life events (such as unemployment, bereavement, relationship difficulties) may be described as exogenous or reactive, stemming from outwith the person.

This way of dividing depression into two classes is called a **binary classification**. Similar classifications exist in the distinction between primary and secondary, and psychotic and neurotic depression. These diagnoses, which allocate affective disorders to one of two classes, stem from Kraepelin's original view that there were only two forms of depression: psychogenic, or reactive, depression, and manic depressive insanity (sic). The distinction between psychotic and neurotic types of depression developed in the US (Levitt *et al.* 1983), whereas in the UK, a different view was held. Lewis (1934) argued that depression was one illness, ranging in severity from minor forms apparently related to life events at one end, to the severest form of manic depressive disorder at the other.

A diagnostic approach has developed in recent years that distinguishes between people who experience only depression (**unipolar** or **major depression**), and those who experience both depression and mania (**bipolar disorder**). However, people who suffer only from recurrent bouts of mania are also diagnosed as bipolar. Research suggests that these are two distinct forms of affective disorder.

Major depression is one of the commonest forms of mental disorder; it affects 8–11% of men, and 18–23% of women (Weissman *et al.*, 1978). It is also more evident in the lower socio-economic groups (Hirschfield *et al.* 1982). Bipolar disorder occurs equally in men and women in around one percent of the population.

Differences also exist in the symptoms of depression in these two groups. When de-

pressed, the bipolar group person is likely to sleep more and to feel lethargic. Unipolar depression is characterized by insomnia and agitation. The first episode of bipolar depression is likely when the person is younger (on average around 28). Unipolar depression begins later (around the mid-30s). Two further distinctions are evident: bipolar disorder tends to run more in families than major depression; lithium carbonate, which is effective in the treatment of depression in bipolar disorder, is not in major depression. These differences support the view that unipolar and bipolar disorders are quite distinct forms of affective disorder (Depue *et al.*, 1978)

The major problem of the unipolar/bipolar distinction is that it does not allow for the great variety of affective disturbance evident in people with depression. Some people with bipolar disorder only show mania; others alternate rapidly from mania to depression, or may experience both at the same time in a mixed affective state. Major depression embraces a wide range of affective disturbance, including people who are depressed by specific life events; those where age appears significant, such as depression in middle-age, or old age; those where hallucinations and delusions accompany the depressed mood; those who improve when their life improves; and those who remain depressed – melancholic – even when something good happens. This dual classification also fails to distinguish between people who have a short-lived but severe affective disorder, and those who experience a long-lasting affective disturbance.

EXPLANATIONS OF AFFECTIVE DISORDER

**Genetics**

Genetic studies show that where bipolar disorder occurs in an identical twin, the other twin is similarly affected in 72% of cases. Where bipolar disorder occurs in a fraternal twin, the other twin is affected in only 14% of cases. Although it is accepted that bipolar disorder may have an heritable component, the exact mode of transmission is unclear (James *et al.*, 1975). This genetic transmission is shown by the number of adopted children whose biological parents had an affective disorder, and who subsequently develop affective disorder themselves. Although genetic factors appear to be implicated in the development of unipolar depression, these do not appear to be as important.

## Biochemistry

Two major biochemical theories, which relate depression to neurotransmitters, have been proposed. Depression may result from low levels of norepinephrine: where the level is extremely high, mania will result (Schildkraut, 1965). Another view implicates low levels of serotonin.

These theories arose from the observations that drugs that raised serotonin and norepinephrine levels in animals relieved depression in people (tricyclic antidepressants and monamine oxidase inhibitors). However, increased neurotransmitter levels occur only when the drugs are first taken; the levels then return to their earlier low levels. Given that antidepressants take seven to fourteen days to act, such temporary increases in norepinephrine or serotonin cannot explain why depression subsequently lifts. More recent research has focused upon the sensitivity of the norepinephrine and serotonin receptors. The hypothesis being tested is that the neurotransmitters are put to better use because the receptors have been made more sensitive by the action of the drugs.

A specific form of severe depression, known as **seasonal affective disorder** occurs only in the winter months. It is thought to arise from a build-up of the neurotransmitter hormone melatonin, which normally is suppressed by bright light (Rosenthal, 1985).

## Psychological theories

A wide range of psychological models have been developed to explain the origins of depression. Freud saw depression as the long-term outcome of some childhood problem. If the child's needs were not met, or were over-sufficiently gratified, the person might become stuck, with a fixation, becoming dependent on others for the maintenance of self-esteem.

Freud's celebrated piece 'Mourning and Melancholia' (Freud, 1917) became the basis for the notion that depression represented anger turned against oneself. Where actual losses are experienced in childhood, for example of a parent, the mourning child identifies strongly with the lost person in an effort to recover the loss. In overly dependent people, the mourner directs anger towards the lost person, who has deserted the mourner, criticizing and castigating her or himself for the loved one's failings, thus turning anger inwards. Where no real loss has been experienced, a symbolic loss may occur, for example, divorce may be interpreted as a loss of love due to the loss of the loved one. Freud later revised this theory, suggesting that depression resulted from discord between the super-ego and the ego: the super-ego venting its rage against the ego. Using his newly formed hypothesis of the death instinct, he stated that if aggression was not turned outward, it would be turned against the self (Freud, 1922) (Chapter 8).

Little evidence exists to support Freud's explanation of depression. Dream studies have found that loss and failure are more prevalent than anger and hostility, and projective tests show that the depressed person identifies more with the victim than with the aggressor (Beck *et al.*, 1961). More importantly, studies have shown that depressed people can express intense anger towards family and friends. Despite these findings, it is clear that Freud's original concept contains some validity, which has been developed by a number of subsequent theorists, most notably John Bowlby, who has articulated a highly sophisticated attachment-loss theory, which serves as a valuable explanation for the development of depressive disorder (Bowlby, 1981).

### Behavioural theories

A number of behavioural theories suggest that the depressed person fails to be 'reinforced' sufficiently, and subsequently becomes in-active, withdrawn, and depressed (Lewinsohn, 1974). In some cases, people who become depressed may have lost the ability to experi-ence pleasure, or have failed to acquire this skill. Empirical studies lend some support to this hypothesis.

The concept of learned helplessness is an extension of this theory (Chapter 11). Seligman *et al.* (1979) proposed that the depressed person sees himself as unable to control negative events: he expects to not be able to control what happens, to find solutions or to harness support. As a result he feels helpless. This represents a sophisticated cognitive explanation of depression: 'I think I am help-less, therefore I feel depressed'.

A compatible theory was developed by Beck *et al.* (1979) that suggests the depressed mood is associated with characteristic thinking errors, which derive from views of the world that develop in early adolescence. When the person encounters a stressful event that compares in some way with the situation in which the world view was developed, it triggers related thinking errors. Beck suggested that some people see themselves as incompetents, expecting always to fail; others take responsibilities for everything that goes wrong in their lives. There is some evidence that similar negative thinking styles and belief systems are implicated in manic depressive psychosis (Barker, 1988).

### THE PSYCHOSES

Two main groups of psychotic disorders are commonly described: **organic** or **biogenic**, and **functional psychoses**. Organic psychoses stem from degenerative changes in the brain. Here, we are concerned with disorders that cannot as yet be attributed to any distinct physical cause.

Until the mid-nineteenth century, the term 'psychosis' was used to refer to a wide range of mental disturbances. From the beginning of the twentieth century, psychosis has tended to exclude the mental consequences of physical disorders and neurotic disorders.

Psychoses generally refer to severe or major psychiatric disorders. There is a common misconception, however, that all forms of psychosis are of equal severity. In reality, some people with a psychotic disorder may be less disabled than people with, for example, certain forms of neurotic disorder. The term 'psychosis' is also often confused with insanity. By law, a person may be defined as 'incompetent' (*non compos mentis,* 'not of sound mind') due to a disabling psychosis, recognizing the need for special control or supervision of a person unable to function responsibly. The severity of the psychosis refers to the outcome of the disorder, or what results from the psychosis. In this sense, the competence of some people is so badly affected that their competence as people is called into question. Although this might apply to many, it does not apply to all people with a psychotic disorder.

A psychosis might be described as an unrealistic way of appreciating the self or the world. In very simple terms, the person with a psychosis believes that his view of himself or of the world is not defective, and he behaves accordingly. This is not to say the person is always happy or content with this world-view; simply that this view is accepted by him or her as right. People who are, for example, psychotically depressed do not complain about how they feel in the way a person with a neurotic depression might; they do not fight the disorder but accept it, and in many cases may appear to encourage it. The person may be described as having no insight, lacking awareness of the disturbing or distressing nature of his or her behaviour.

The net result is that the person who experiences a psychotic disorder appears to inhabit a different order of reality from the rest of us. He may become so enmeshed in his own world that his capacity to maintain contact with our world becomes impaired. When this happens, the behaviour and reasoning of the person becomes incomprehensible to most other people, and special care and treatment services may be essential to keep him from danger.

Three main forms of functional psychotic disorder exist: those which display major disturbances of mood – **affective psychoses**; those characterized by a disturbance of thinking – **schizophrenic disorders**; and those characterized by disturbances of belief systems – **paranoid psychoses**.

In affective and schizophrenic psychoses, several forms of disturbance of thought, feeling, and behaviour may co-exist. In paranoia, the abnormality may be limited to beliefs alone. As we have already addressed affective disorder in some detail, attention will be given to a consideration of disorders of thinking, with specific reference to people diagnosed as suffering from schizophrenia.

DISORDERED THINKING

The person considered here may exhibit one of many forms of disordered thinking: at one level this can involve specific beliefs, at another it may affect how the person processes information about himself or the world. The outstanding feature is the individual's peculiar use of language. (We shall assume that the way the person speaks is a direct reflection of his thinking; one being dependent upon the other.) This disturbance of thought has a significant knock-on effect: the disturbance of thinking influences mood, and ultimately both affect the person's relationship with the world, which is expressed through behaviour.

Although we speak generally about the person suffering from schizophrenia, the experience can be highly specific to the individual. In Arieti's (1979) words, 'schizophrenia has a thousand faces'. We should not forget, therefore, that although all of the people considered here may present some of the patterns all of the time, none of them show all of the patterns all of the time. Furthermore, some people who might be described as psychotic appear to be normal, and behave quite normally, much of the time.

The following points characterize the form of thinking for this individual:

- The way the sufferer thinks, organizes his ideas, and communicates them is unusual.
- The person may appear incoherent, as he uses fragments of thought or images that are not directly connected in an effort to communicate; words may be coined (neologisms) that are meaningless to the listener.
- He may find it difficult to stick to one topic, drifting off on a tangent, led by a train of loose associations.
- Such associations may be exaggerated further by the use of rhyming speech (clang associations), which rarely are logical or grammatically correct.
- Although the person says a lot, he may communicate little (poverty of content).
- Certain ideas or words may be used repeatedly (perseveration).
- Speech may be repeatedly interrupted by irregular silences (blocking), after which the person cannot recall what he was trying to say.

**Thinking: content**

The content of this person's thinking is grossly disordered, but he is unlikely to be aware that his thoughts, or associated patterns of behaviour, are in any way unusual (lack of insight). The person holds firmly held convictions which have no obvious basis in reality. Such delusions are evident in a wide range of disorders – including mania, severe forms of depression, organic syndromes, and drug overdose – but are commonest in people described as suffering from schizophrenia.

Delusional thoughts can take a variety of forms. For example, the person may believe that:

- others are plotting, watching, or joining in a conspiracy against him (delusion of persecution);
- some ordinary event takes on a special significance, quickly developing, for example, an elaborate message about unlikely, if not impossible, future events (delusional perception);
- his bodily sensations are being influenced by some external agency (somatic passivity);
- other people's thoughts are being inserted in his mind by some external power (thought insertion);
- other people have access to his thoughts (thought broadcasting);
- other people are suddenly and unexpectedly stealing his thoughts (thought withdrawal);
- he is suffering from some hideous disease, or bizarre affliction (hypochondriacal delusion);
- he has committed some unpardonable sin (delusional guilt);
- he does not exist, is returned from the dead, or that the world or people within it no longer exists (nihilistic delusions);
- he is famous, important, or powerful; he may even claim to be some famous person from history (delusions of grandeur).

Other delusional processes that relate to feeling and related actions were described by Mellor (1970). The person may believe that:

- his feelings are being made up and projected on to him by some external controlling agency (made feelings);
- he is a puppet, whose body is manipulated by some external force (made volitional acts);
- he is subject to inexplicable impulses, deriving from external influence (made impulses);
- loved ones, and even objects, such as houses, keys, cars, are substituted duplicates.

## PERCEPTUAL PROBLEMS

Many of the problems of thinking form or content noted above may be a function of a breakdown of selective attention. The basic problem of the psychoses – upon which all other problems of living experienced by the psychotic are built – remains unclear. There are, however, strong indications that the kind of person we are considering experiences a specific problem in co-ordinating or pro-cessing all the information that floods into his brain through his sensory channels. Kraepelin and Bleuler first suggested that people with schizophrenia were unable to select from the mass of information provided by their senses. One hundred years later, studies suggest that the individual works out strange beliefs or odd patterns of behaviour as a defence against the information overload which faces him (McGhie *et al.*, 1961; Maher *et al.*, 1979).

A further problem exists when the person perceives things that are not present in objective reality. Everyone has the capacity to imagine, often vividly, using all sensory channels. The person considered here is largely unable to distinguish whether or not his experience is real or imaginary (hallucination). In more severe examples, the person believes firmly in the reality of the hallucinatory experience. The most common hallucinatory experience involves hearing voices. These can be classified as:

- audible thoughts, whereby someone else is heard repeating the person's own thoughts;
- arguing voices, whereby two or more voices are heard disagreeing with one another;

- voices commenting, usually in a negative, critical fashion, about the person's own behaviour, attitudes or secrets. These invariably are the most distressing form of auditory hallucination.

Other forms of hallucinatory experience are reported much less frequently. Visual hallucinations are often thought to be indicative of some organic psychosis. Olfactory hallucinations occur most often in association with epilepsy.

## AFFECTIVE AND BEHAVIOURAL FEATURES

In addition to the cognitive disturbances noted above, the person with a severe psychosis such as schizophrenia is likely also to show disturbances of mood and behaviour. They may appear to show little emotion (blunted or flat affect); the voice may be monotonous, and the face show no expression. Alternatively, the person may display wholly inappropriate affect, for example, laughing while telling a sad story, or shouting angrily during an otherwise pleasant interaction.

The range of disorders of behaviour are infinite. These are most easily classified as inappropriate in their given context. The person might jump up and down, shred paper, rub parts of his body: all of these behaviours appearing incongruous in the setting in which they occur. Where the pattern is repeated for long periods it is described as **sterotypy**. Some people may also become motionless for long periods (**catatonia**).

One final class of behaviour deserves special mention. Here, the individual is likely to keep others at a distance, rarely engage in small talk, and often avoids eye contact. While this pattern of social withdrawal can be interpreted as a means of dealing with sensory overload, it may be more a function of the difficulty the person experiences in making himself understood.

## THE CLASSIFICATION OF SCHIZOPHRENIA

Although schizophrenia is often depicted as a single form of disorder, the title suggests a group of psychotic disorders in which marked thought disturbance, perceptual distortion, affective disturbance, bizarre behaviour, and withdrawal are evident. Schizophrenia is a convenient term for a range of disorders, which differ in presentation or symptoms, and also have different possible causes.

The earliest accepted description of schizophrenia was offered by Eugene Bleuler, who coined the term as an alternative to the earlier description of dementia praecox. Bleuler identified four fundamental characteristics of schizophrenia:

1.  Association – evidence of thought disorder, usually expressed through a specific language style.
2.  Affect – the emotions appear blunted or inappropriate.
3.  Ambivalence – the person is indecisive and unable to complete normal tasks.
4.  Autism – evidence of withdrawal and self-absorption.

These were supported by a list of secondary features, including hallucinations, paranoid thinking, grandiosity, and hostility and belligerence.

In the 1960s, greater emphasis was given to the importance of hallucinations and delusions as the key characteristics of the disorders. However, more recently, interest has been shown in Bleuler's 'four As': this is mainly due to the finding that anti-psychotic drugs can influence these symptoms, having little effect on the secondary characteristics.

We have noted that a wide variety of types of disorder is possible. These can, however, be classified under the following three main headings:

- **Disorganized hebephrenic type** – the person mainly shows incoherent speech and inappropriate affect.

- **Catatonic type** – the person mainly shows a behavioural disturbance, usually exaggerated activity (hyperactivity) alternating with speechless inactivity,
- **Paranoid type** – delusions of persecution or grandeur are accompanied by similar hallucinatory experience.

## EXPLAINING SCHIZOPHRENIA

### PSYCHOLOGICAL AND SOCIAL EXPLANATIONS

Research explanations of the origins of schizophrenia are diverse. It is worth noting that Freud had little to say about psychosis; in his view the person had a weak ego, which could not deal with unacceptable impulses from the id, resulting in regression. Harry Stack Sullivan devoted most of his work to people with psychosis, and developed an important interpersonal model that emphasized the damage caused by mother-child relationships, resulting in withdrawal (Sullivan, 1962). Later theorists developed models that emphasized the role of disturbance, especially anxiety and hostility, within the family (Arieti, 1974: Lidz, 1973). Fromm-Reichman (1948), who earlier had argued that mothers could induce schizophrenia in their children, formulated the idea of the double-bind, in which the mother gives the child contradictory messages, resulting in severe anxiety and confusion (Bateson, 1956). Laing (1970) suggested that schizophrenia was a special strategy that a person invents in order to live in an unliveable situation.

Little evidence has been presented for any of these viewpoints. What is clear from objective studies is that communications within families of people with schizophrenia can be muddled, vague, and fragmentary (Lewis *et al.*, 1981). Other studies show that stress within such families can be high. Where this stress is translated into family arguments and frictions (high expressed emotion), schizophrenia symptoms are more likely to recur or to be exacerbated (Leff, 1976; Miklowitz, *et al.*, 1986).

### BIOLOGICAL EXPLANATIONS

The available evidence on adopted children who developed schizophrenia suggests a strong relationship between having a schizophrenic parent and developing the disorder (Kety *et al.*, 1968). This genetic predisposition may also result in biochemical disturbance specific to the disorder. Although tentative, there are indications that excess dopamine activity may explain schizophrenia where positive symptoms (hallucinations, delusions and outlandish behaviour) are most pronounced. (Seligman *et al.*, 1985). Other brain dysfunctions, such as enlarged ventricles, cortical and cerebellar atrophy and diminished alpha rhythm, are postulated as explanations of negative symptoms (flattened emotions, poverty of speech, anhedonia and inattentiveness) (Weinberger *et al.*, 1983).

### BEHAVIOURAL PROBLEMS: PERSONALITY DISORDERS

The last group of mental health problems we shall consider focuses upon some form of behavioural disturbances. Some such people seek help, complaining of the unfairness of others or of the world in general. Others may not be aware of any problems, although friends or family may well see things from another perspective. In most of the examples considered here, the individuals may well be seen as disturbing rather than disturbed. Although the problems are clearly visible, in a behavioural or interpersonal sense they are highly complex. For this reason, this group is referred to as personality disorders.

The concept of personality disorder is a broad one. A wide range of disorders has been described, most of which are little understood. Although the term has been used for generations, the definitions of such conditions vary enormously, and often are inconsistent. This is not surprising, given that definitions of the normal personality are also wide and varied. For the purpose of the discussion here, we shall consider personality disorder within the American Diagnostic and Statistical Manual (DSM).

The American Psychiatric Association's diagnostic system requires that the person is described on five separate axes. Any of the personality disorders described here may coexist with other forms of abnormal behaviour, such as substance abuse disorder, or psychosexual disorder. This form of classification recognizes that a person may be showing a current problem, such as drug abuse, against the background of a longer-term problem, such as a personality disorder, requiring that the clinician consider more than the immediate symptoms in framing a diagnosis. The kind of people nurses might encounter can be described under four headings, discussed below.

## ODD OR ECCENTRIC BEHAVIOUR

All people display a degree of uncertainty, hesitation, and even suspicion in their dealings with others. The person we shall consider, however, is consistently suspicious of others, which may reflect an expectation that he or she will be badly treated, or offended in some way.

His means of dealing with this expectation is to become overly secretive – constantly on guard against the threat of offence or injury. Although blaming others is a common coping strategy, especially among men, this individual blames others even where he is clearly at fault. In addition, he may be overly jealous; sensitive to any criticism, whether or not intended; argumentative; or manifestly uncomfortable in the presence of others. Those who know him well may describe a dour and humourless character, showing little emotion, and especially lacking in warmth. Such an individual is likely to be described as a **paranoid personality**.

Our second person has great difficulty in establishing relationships. He has few friends, is seen as stand-offish and lacking warmth and the ability to express feelings, which are all part of friendship. This person is seen as a loner, and is largely indifferent to praise or criticism. He appears to prefer his own company and interests. Although he may appear to be lost in thought, unlike the person with schizophrenia he is in close contact with reality. This person is likely to be described as a **schizoid personality**.

Our third person also has relationship problems, but these are enhanced by the presence of specific eccentricities. He may believe he is in touch with invisible forces or with dead people – these are illusory rather than hallucinatory experiences. He may experience and describe readily perceptual disturbances, such as the feeling that either he or the world about him changes from time to time (depersonalization). He may also be unusually superstitious, believing he can foretell the future or read minds (so-called magical thinking). He may also speak in an eccentric fashion. This person, who may be mistakenly diagnosed as suffering from schizophrenia, is likely to be described as a **schizotypal personality**.

## THOSE WHO APPEAR VULNERABLE

Four kinds of people make up the vulnerable group. The first is unhappy about the absence of close, loving relationships, but he is reluctant to get involved with people, fearing rejection or humiliation. His self-esteem is so low that he expects no one will love or accept him. Even when others reassure him, he remains sceptical that their affection will last, and interprets any upset as a major sign that the relationship is failing. This person reports mixed feelings of depression with the world, and anger at himself for being a failure. He is likely to be described as an **avoidant personality**.

The second person also lacks self-confidence and, characteristically, allows others to make the important decisions that affect his life. He cannot make demands, and submits himself to the will of others rather than to risk damaging a relationship. This person might be described as suffering from an inferiority complex. This personality type is commonly used to describe women who surrender to men, who may even abuse them, rather than risk abandonment. This person is likely to be described as a **dependent personality**.

The third person is preoccupied with maintaining order in his life. He is likely to be more concerned with work than pleasure. He forms poor relationships largely because of his rigid rule-making. This pattern is more likely to be found in men, who may prize success or power over the enjoyment of loving or friendly relationships. He should not be confused with those suffering from obsessive-compulsive disorder, where more specific patterns of severe behavioural disturbance are present. This person shows a wider range of compulsive organizing and planning routines, which interfere with decision-making and general efficiency. This person is likely to be described as a **compulsive personality**.

The last person in this group experiences relationship difficulties by indirectly resisting others. This may be shown by habitual lateness, forgetfulness, dilly-dallying, or procrastination. This person rarely says no, may express the best of intentions, but appears to covertly undermine others, or sabotage their efforts. He experiences major problems at work or in confirmed relationships like marriage. Where this pattern is longstanding across a range of situations, the person is likely to be described as a **passive-aggressive personality**.

## DRAMATIC OR ERRATIC BEHAVIOUR

Three patterns of behaviour characterize the third group. The first person shows much variability in behaviour patterns involving other people. She (in this case) can be argumentative and sarcastic, showing unpredictable impulses for gambling, sex or eating – any of which may be self-damaging in the long term. She cannot bear to be alone, but enjoys only short-term, intimate relationships, expressing uncertainty over commitments, either to people or careers. She may also swing from appearing depressed and engaging in numerous suicidal attempts, to appearing psychotic, especially when under stress. Although these patterns of behaviour are more often attributed to women than men, this may represent no more than the traditional sexism of psychiatry (Chesler, 1972). This pattern of behaviour has been viewed as overlapping with a number of neurotic psychotic disorders: as a result, the person may be described as a **borderline personality**.

The second person is overly dramatic, perhaps as a means of drawing attention to herself. Again, this classification is most often attributed to women. She is seen as manipulative, trying to attract sympathy by, for example, fainting at the first sight of blood, or being overcome with emotion. She may make heavy demands on people, but easily becomes bored or upset with routine relationships. On first acquaintance, she exudes charm, warmth, and sincerity. Through time this fades, and the person is seen as shallow and lacking in sincerity. This is the stereotype of the flirtatious, sexually provocative woman, and is described in the DSM IIIR classification as the **histrionic personality**.

The third person is seen as self-absorbed and possessing an almost grandiose perception of their own uniqueness and importance. He is seen as exploiting others, showing a distinct lack of understanding of their needs, expecting to be served hand and foot, though never reciprocating. This person may be preoccupied with fantasies of success or power, and may be largely indifferent to the problems of people around him. Although this person appears to have a very unrealistic view of himself, this may hide a fragile self-esteem. This person is likely to be described as a **narcissistic personality**.

PRIMARILY ANTISOCIAL BEHAVIOUR

Our final group focuses upon people who behave badly towards others, and appear to experience no shame or guilt. Such people tend to engage in criminal behaviour; many of those in special hospitals or forensic units are representative of this group. There may, however, be an equally large group of people who display similar or even worse patterns of behaviour, but, because they have not been convicted of any offence, are assumed to be normal. The person considered here:

- has a long history of problems in sustaining relationships, with family, friends, or lovers; similar problems are met in maintaining employment; he shows little sense of obligation, and may walk out on the family, abandon a job, or ignore creditors;
- often gets into trouble before puberty by stealing, lying, and challenging authority. In adolescence such social difficulties may become exaggerated; casual sex, drug abuse, vandalism, and truancy are among the antisocial behaviours which, in adulthood, may be translated into prostitution, pimping, drug-dealing, and other criminal acts;
- is very likely to display irritable and aggressive behaviour, for example, brawling in public and abusing family members in private;
- is impulsive and reckless, pursuing an adventurous lifestyle, with little planning or forethought; sexual liaisons, petty crimes, and other forms of thrill-seeking may be undertaken whimsically: the easiest and most gratifying actions rule the day.

This person is likely to be described as an **antisocial personality** disorder. This represents an extension of the earlier diagnosis of psychopath, which assumed that the problem was of hereditary origin; later, this was changed to 'sociopath', on the assumption that the source of the problem lay in the environment. This form of personality disorder embraces a wide spectrum: at one extreme are highly unsuccessful petty criminal types, who may commit callous murders on impulse; at the other are highly successful people who build empires through the systematic manipulation of their employees (Harrington, 1972).

EXPLANATIONS OF THE PERSONALITY DISORDERS

The development of the concept of the personality disorder originates from psychodynamic theory. The idea that people can develop sustained, deeply ingrained, handicapping personality traits is most evident in the psychodynamic literature. Such disorders are attributed to frustration or over-indulgence at one of the stages of psychosexual development. For example, the obsessional personality is said to experience stresses during the anal-retentive stage of psychosocial development (Chapter 11); his holding-in being expressed in a need for order and rigidity (Fenichel, 1945). More extreme forms of antisocial personality disorder are attributed to failure on the part of the super-ego to develop control over the id's demand for instant gratification.

These explanations are highly speculative: the same could, however, be said of others. This person is more likely to come from a poor background, suffering the effects of poverty, urban deprivation, and a pervasive sub-culture. The absence of appropriate parental role models or parental discipline are also often cited (McGarvey, *et al.*, 1981). This does not explain, however, the small proportion of antisocial personalities who do not come from disadvantaged backgrounds.

Perhaps the most significant answer lies in the observations that have been made of the physiological responses of the person with antisocial personality disorder. The person is likely to:

- show abnormal amounts of slow-wave EEG activity, which may explain his lack of inhibition;
- have a low level of arousal, or is able to control his autonomic arousal, which may also explain the thrill-seeking lifestyle;
- be able to ignore or tune out aversive events, like punishment;
- lack the capacity for planning, foresight, and impulse-control, which may be connected with malfunction of the frontal lobes (Gorenstein, 1982).

The list of mental health problems reviewed here are a mixed bag in more than one sense. The patterns of behaviour described as representing this or that disorder overlap often with the descriptions of other disorders. It is not unusual for people with, for example, a neurotic illness, to show also one or other of the personality disorders described here. It is clear, also, that although we have discussed the behaviour of such people, emotional and cognitive disturbances also feature strongly in most of the disorders. We should not forget, either, that the distinction between these so-called disorders and the normal personality, is not easily made.

Nurses will meet people, from time to time, who display such behavioural characteristics: they might well be advised to remain open as to what such behaviour patterns might mean in a diagnostic sense. The mix of explanations as to the origins of such disorders is considerable. Nurses also should not forget that the classification of any disorder is not a substitute for the understanding of the person, and of her or his needs and experience, which are the focus of the nursing assessment.

## THE CHALLENGE TO NURSING

The major mental health problems described in this chapter represent a significant challenge to nursing. Nurses need to be aware of the complex nature of each of the various disorders present under the three classifications of disturbance of affect, cognition, and behaviour. What are the biological, psychological, and social factors that might play a part in an explanation of the disorder? What are the likely components of an appropriate nursing care plan? Complex problems, such as those described, require individual solutions.

Medical treatment has the specific aim of reducing the presentation of the symptoms associated with different conditions. The nursing role focuses more on life problems, which can be peculiar to specific disorders, but may be common to a variety of mental health problems.

The nurse's primary responsibility is to undertake a careful assessment of the person. This should address the three points of the bio-psychosocial pyramid (Figure 13.1). These points serve as a useful anchor for the definition of specific problems, and a format for examining possible links between one problem and another. The person who suffers a loss of appetite (biological), associated with specific thoughts and feelings (psychological), against a background of a disrupted or unsatisfactory relationship (social) may be diagnosed as severely depressed.

Nurses have long appreciated the need, for example, to help people who are anorexic to eat, or when they suffer insomnia to sleep better. The challenge facing the nurse in caring for the kinds of people described here is to develop a response which acknowledges as appropriate the interaction one problem may have with another. Such a care plan will focus more specifically upon the human needs of the person with an affective, cognitive, or behavioural 'disorder', without ignoring the features that give the disorder its characteristic stamp.

## REFERENCES

American Psychiatric Association (1987) *Diagnostic and Statistical Manual* (3rd edn. revd) APA, Washington, D.C.

Arieti, S. (1974) *Interpretation of Schizophrenia*, Basic Books, New York.

Arieti, S. (1979) *Understanding and Helping the Schizophrenic: a Guide for Family and Friends*, Basic Books, New York.

Barker, P. J. (1988) An evaluation of specific nursing interventions in the management of patients suffering from manic depressive psychosis, unpub. thesis, Instit. Tech., Dundee.

Bateson, G. Jackson, D. D., Haley, J. *et al.* (1956) Towards a theory of schizophrenia. *Behavioural Science*, 1, 251–64.

Beck, A. T. and Ward, C. H. (1961) Dreams of depressed patients: characteristic themes in manifest content. *Archives of General Psychiatry* 5, 462–7.

Beck, A. T., Rush, A. J., Shaw, B. F. *et al.* (1979) *Cognitive Therapy of Depression*, Guildford Press, New York.

Bowlby, J. (1981) *Attachment and Loss: Vol. 3 – Loss, Sadness and Depression*, Penguin, Harmondsworth.

Chesler, P. (1972) *Women and Madness*, Doubleday, New York.

Clare, J. (1991) Implications of the care programme approach. *Community Psychiatric Nursing J.* 11, 24.

Depue, R. A. and Monroe, S. M. (1978) The unipolar-bipolar distinction in the depressive disorders. *Psychological Bulletin*, 85, 1001–29.

Fenichel, O. (1945) *The Psychoanalytic Theory of Neurosis*, Norton, New York.

Freud, S. (1917) Mourning and melancholia, SE IV, Hogarth press, London, and Vol. II, Penguin, Harmondsworth.

Freud, S. (1922) Beyond the pleasure principle, in SE, Hogarth, London, and Vol. II, Penguin, Harmondsworth.

Fromm-Reichman, F. (1948) Notes on the development of treatment of schizophrenics by psychoanalytic psychotherapy. *Psychiatry* 11, 263–73.

Gorenstein, E. E. (1982) Frontal lobe function in psychopaths. *J. Abnormal Psychology*, 91, 368–79.

Harrington, A. (1972) *Psychopaths*, Simon and Schuster, New York.

Hirschfield, R. M. A. and Cross, C. K. (1982) Epidemiology of affective disorders: psychosocial risk factors. *Archives of General Psychiatry* 39, 35–46.

James, N. and Chapman, J. (1975) A genetic study of bipolar affective disorder. *British J. Psychiatry*, 126, 449–56.

Kety, S. S., Rosenthal, D., Wender, P. H. *et al.* (1968) The types and prevalence of mental illness in the biological and adoptive families of adopted schizophrenics, in *The Transmission of Schizophrenia*, (eds D. Rosenthal and S. Kety) Pergamon Press, New York.

Laing, R. D. (1967) *The Politics of Experience*, Pantheon, New York.

Leff, J. (1976) Schizophrenia and sensitivity to the family environment. *Schizophrenia Bulletin*, 2, 566–74.

Levitt, E. E., Lubin, B., and Brooks, J. M. (1983) *Depression: Concepts, Controversies and Some New Facts* (2nd edn), Lawrence Erlbaum Assoc., London.

Lewinsohn, P. M. (1974) A behavioural approach to depression, in (eds T.M. Friedman and M. M. Katz) *The Psychology of Depression: Contemporary Theory and Research*, Winston, Washington.

Lewinsohn, P. M., Mischel, W., Chaplain, W. *et al.* (1980) Social competence and depression: the role of illusory self-perceptions. *J. Abnormal Psychology* 89, 203–12.

Lewis, A. (1934) Melancholia: a historical review. *J. Mental Science*, 80, 1.

Lewis, J. M., Rodnick, E.H., and Goldstein, M.J. (1981) Intrafamilial interactive behaviour, parental communication deviance and risk for schizophrenia. *J. Abnormal Psychology*, 90, 448–57

Lidz, T. (1973) *The Origin and Treatment of Schizophrenic Disorders*, Basic Books, New York.

Maher, B. A. and Maher, W. B. (1979) Psychopathology, in *The First Century of Experimental Psychology* (ed. E. Hearst), Lawrence Erlbaum, New Jersey.

Mellor, C. S. (1970) First-rank symptoms of schizophrenia. *British J. Psychiatry*, 117, 15–23.

Miklowitz, D. J., Strachan, A.M., Goldstein, M. J. *et al.* (1986) Expressed emotion and communication deviance in the families of schizophrenics. *J. Abnormal Psychology*, 95, 60–66.

McGarvey, B., Gabrielli, W. F., Beutler, P. M. *et al.* (1981) Rearing, social class, education and criminality: multiple indicator model. *J. Abnormal Psychology* 90, 354–64.

McGhie, A. and Chapman, J. (1961) Disorders of attention and perception in early schizophrenia. *Brit J. Medical Psychology* 34, 103–16.

Rosenthal, N. E., Sack, D. A., Carpenter, C.J. *et al.* (1985) Antidepressant effects of light in seasonal affective disorder. *Amer. J. Psychiatry* 142, 163–70.

Schildkraut, J. J. (1965) The catecholamine hypothesis of affective disorders. *Amer. J. Psychiatry*, 122, 509–22

Schinnar, A. P., Rothbard, A. B., Kanter, R. *et al.* (1990) An empirical literature review of definitions of severe and persistant mental illness *Amer. J. Psychiatry*, 147, 1602–8.

Seligman, M. E. P., Abramson, L. V., Semmel A. *et al.* (1979) Depressive attributional style. *J. Abnormal Psychology* 88, 242–7.

Seligman, M. E. P. and Rosenhan, D. L. (1983) *Abnormal Psychology*, Norton, New York.

Sullivan, H. S. (1962) *Schizophrenia as a Human Process*, Norton, New York.

Weinberger, D. R.; Wagner, R. L.; and Wyatt, R. J. (1983) Neuropathological studies of schizophrenia: a selective review. *Schizophrenia Bulletin*, 9, 193–212.

Weissman, M.M., Klerman, G. L. and Paykel, E. S. (1971) Clinical evaluation of hostility in depression. *Amer. J. Psychiatry*, 128, 261–66.

## 14

# HIV AND AIDS

*This chapter is dedicated to the memory of Paul Sheen. Royalties have been donated to Body Positive Northwest, Manchester, in his name.*

## *Jean Faugier*

AIDS (acquired immune deficiency syndrome) and HIV (human immunodeficiency virus) constitute a unique challenge for nursing. Associated with sexuality, drug misuse, stigma, fear, serious illness, and death, AIDS presents a complexity and diversity of emotional and psychological problems that affect every aspect of a person's life. Such stresses can in turn diminish the immune response, creating a vicious circle of stress and illness (Bridge *et al.*, 1988). In addition to such stresses, nurses need to be aware of the impact of AIDS on lovers, families, spouses, and friends, who may require the opportunity to discuss their feelings with nursing staff in an atmosphere of confidentiality and acceptance.

HIV infection is associated with the highest incidence of neurological and neuropsychiatric morbidity of any serious common condition that is not primary to the nervous system. Estimates of neuropsychiatric dysfunction in persons with HIV infection, at 25 – 70%, vary considerably (Paine, 1988).

Many studies have shown that HIV infection has an affinity for brain tissue, and can strike the central nervous system (CNS), either in the form of degenerative neuropathological changes occurring as a result of the virus itself (primary brain infection), or as a result of non-viral, opportunistic infections such as toxoplasmosis encephalitis, a parasitic infection of the brain, or cryptococcus meningitis, a fungal infection that can cause CNS dysfunction.

As many of the opportunistic infections affecting people with HIV can be treated, it is essential that the nurse should be alert to the early signs of any neuropsychiatric symptoms, as he or she may be the first person to become aware of them. Early diagnosis, however, is complicated by the tendency of neurological infection to present symptoms that can mimic those more commonly associated with depression or anxiety (Paine, 1988). The person with HIV infection will be subject to all the cognitive, behavioural, and emotional changes that accompany a stigmatized, life-threatening disease. General nurses working in the hospital or in the community will need to expand their repertoire of skills in order to be able to deal with the whole person, and not simply his physical condition. Conversely, psychiatric nurses will have to become more familiar with the impact and consequences of HIV infection and its treatment. In this sense, HIV infection presents nursing with the challenge of breaking down arbitrary barriers, not simply between the biological and the psychological, but also between branches of the profession.

Nurses cannot provide skilled support to those affected by AIDS unless they recognize their own limitations. The effective nurse will be the one who is aware of his or her own feelings as a human being. He or she must appreciate that the stresses experienced by clients and their loved ones will inevitably be transferred on to them, either in a conscious or an unconscious form. The nurse must be able to deal with these emotions to be of value to the client. In order to avoid a build up of emotional stress, nursing staff need to develop methods of support that allow them to address these issues in a positive way, ultimately improving their knowledge and skills in dealing with the emotional and psychological problems of others.

## THE DIAGNOSIS

People who are diagnosed as having AIDS and HIV are often young and active, and may have had no previous occasion to question their longevity. Diagnosis of a life-threatening disease – potential or actual – will produce myriad emotional and psychological responses, ranging from a positive approach to despair and hopelessness.

Due to the manner in which the virus is transmitted – through unsafe sexual activity or contaminated blood, particularly through the sharing of injecting equipment – a diagnosis of AIDS or HIV can identify the affected individual as a member of a socially stigmatized minority. This may happen before they themselves, or their loved ones or families, have had time to work through their feelings. On occasion, others' reactions may cause the person extreme pain and distress. The enormous strength of the social stigma associated with the disease can lead, for example, to former lovers, family, and former friends, avoiding social and physical contact with those affected, whose deep feelings of loss and despair can be significantly increased by such rejection and withdrawal of love and approval.

Because AIDS is associated in many people's minds with death, disfigurement, and disability, including dementia, it is not surprising that a diagnosis of AIDS or HIV can produce terror and fear, to the point of seriously interfering with the individual's normal functioning, and leading to acute anxiety.

Due to the often negative media coverage given to HIV and AIDS, HIV-infected people are made to confront feelings of guilt, responsibility, self-hatred, and rejection, along with all the other emotional and psychological sequelae of HIV. For this reason, *blame should have no place whatever in the vocabulary of nursing.*

Society's preoccupation with what is currently the most important public health issue in the world results in the person with HIV being subjected to a constant barrage of media coverage. Not only distressing, this can make it almost impossible for those infected to do anything without being constantly reminded of their situation. Nurses must be aware of these constant pressures, and their potential to disrupt or undermine the confidence and self-worth of clients. The nurse should work with the client to devise strategies that will minimize the impact of distressing and inaccurate material.

## PSYCHOLOGICAL AND EMOTIONAL PROBLEMS OF HIV INFECTION

### ANXIETY AND STRESS

The anxiety and stress experienced by those with HIV infection is caused by the nature of the disease, and by the actual or anticipated reactions of others. Each one of us has at some time or other experienced anxiety; in the context of HIV infection, such anxiety is likely to be more severe and long lasting: a diagnosis of HIV infection can be devastating. Currently there is no known cure, and for many the disease has already proved fatal. For those in various stages of HIV, or who are antibody positive, the fear of HIV can become a constant source of worry and anxiety, making them scarcely able to think of anything else (Elaskerud, 1989; Green and McCreaner, 1989).

Some common anxieties experienced by those with HIV infection include:

- The risk of infection they represent, or have represented, to others.
- Rejection either by loved ones or in a social or occupational context.
- Fear of losing one's home and job.

**Table 14.1** Symptoms of HIV-related anxiety

| | | | |
|---|---|---|---|
| **Muscular** | Tension headaches<br>Pains in muscles and joints<br>Tremor<br>Tension in muscles | **Gastro intestinal** | Nausea<br>Lack of appetite<br>Diarrhoea<br>Frequent bowel movements |
| **Cardiovascular** | Increased heart rate<br>Sensation of heart pounding<br>Peripheral vasoconstriction<br>Flushing | **Frequent micturition**<br><br>**Affective symptoms** | <br><br>Fear<br>Panic<br>Feelings of being out of<br>control<br>Sudden and extreme mood<br>swings |
| **Breathing** | Feeling of tightness in chest<br>Difficulty breathing<br>Excessive yawning<br>Hyperventilation | | |
| **Sweating** | Sweating excessively in<br>axillae<br>On soles of feet or palms<br>Generalized sweating | **Cognitive symptoms** | Difficulties concentrating<br>Preoccupation with<br>problems<br>Difficulty remembering<br>things<br>Confusion |
| **Dizziness** | | | |
| **Blurred vision** | | **Behavioural<br>symptoms** | Avoidance of particular<br>situations<br>Pressure of speech<br>Jerky or sudden movements<br>Excessive use of tobacco,<br>alcohol, legal/illegal drugs<br>Overactivity, inability to<br>relax |
| **Loss of libido** | Loss of desire<br>Impotence<br>Lack of arousal<br>Lack of vaginal lubrication<br>Failure to reach orgasm | | |
| **Sleep disturbance** | Difficulty getting to sleep<br>Fitful sleep<br>Frequent wakening and<br>bad dreams | | |

Source: Miller, D. (1987) *Living with Aids and HIV*, Macmillan Press, Basingstoke.

- Fear of losing physical and financial independence.
- Having to face the physical and psychological consequences of the disease alone; ultimately, perhaps, having to die alone.
- Feelings of futility and hopelessness; being powerless to alter the situation.
- Concern about physical and neurological degeneration; a declining ability to cope in the future.
- Loss of dignity and privacy.
- Being identified as a member of a socially stigmatized group.
- Doubts about the ability of those close to them to cope with the problems.
- Possibility of future social and sexual unacceptability.

When one considers the range and importance of concerns which HIV brings, it is hardly surprising that sometimes those affected can be overwhelmed by such anxieties to the extent that they may attribute them to a worsening of their physical condition.

The physical symptoms of anxiety can easily be mistaken for the onset of a new or recurrent infection common in those who have HIV (Table 14.1). Shortness of breath, diarrhoea, headaches, and dizziness are all often seen as a result of opportunistic infections. It is important, however, that in attempting to detect signs of anxiety, the nurse should not make the mistake of missing the symptoms of physical illness. Where there is any doubt about the origins of symptoms, they must be thoroughly investigated to ensure nothing is missed.

HELPING PEOPLE TO COPE WITH ANXIETY

The general nurse is quite capable of dealing with people who are demonstrating feelings of anxiety. This will be nothing new, as many people experience such feelings when they are seriously ill, or even when admitted to hospital. Knowledge from the field of cancer nursing has provided an important baseline of useful nursing strategies to meet the needs of those with HIV infection.

### Simple explanations

The nurse can greatly assist people to better understand and cope with their feelings of fear and anxiety by explaining to them what is happening to their body. A clear explanation of the symptoms of anxiety, and the way in which the body deals with feelings of fear – by translating them into physically distressing symptoms – can be a great reassurance to those who feel they are losing control.

### Teaching positive responses

At times, the anxiety experienced will be so severe that the person may feel they could be completely overwhelmed by it.

Working with clients to identify the methods of coping they have previously found effective when under pressure is useful in identifying positive diversions. The nurse should, with the individual, identify times when feelings of anxiety are strongest; there is no doubt that an understanding of what triggers such feelings is an important step in being able to deal with them.

Simple breathing exercises or relaxation techniques can demonstrate to the client that with help they can learn to control these feelings. Clients often spend lots of time alone and unoccupied, dwelling on feelings rather than expressing them in a way that helps them and the nursing staff to understand their hopes and fears. Art therapy, music and writing are also useful tools of positive expression (Chapters 36 and 37).

### Talking about anxiety

In HIV infection, anxiety is the result of a very real and frightening situation in someone's life. It will often be sufficient for the nurse to simply be there for the client. Spending time talking about worries can put such feelings into a clearer, more manageable, perspective. By expressing fears and anxieties, clients have the opportunity to name and identify them to themselves. If this can be done in an atmosphere of acceptance and empathy, in which the client feels safe from being judged, it is possible to significantly reduce the power of such feelings to disrupt the individual's capacity to live with HIV.

### Know your limitations

It may occasionally happen that in spite of all the efforts made by the nurse to help the client to cope more effectively with feelings of anxiety, some will fail to respond to the interventions outlined above. In these cases, it is vital that nursing staff seek the help or advice of mental health nursing staff to ensure the best possible quality of life for the sufferer. Such a referral should be seen as a highly professional response, rather than a failure on the part of general nursing staff. Following short specialist intervention, or the provision of expert advice, nursing staff in the ward or community can usually continue to cope with appropriate support.

DEPRESSION

All of us have at times suffered from feelings that can be described as depression. Fortunately, most of these states of depression are self-limiting, and eventually we recover as the causes of the depression subside, or as we exercise self-determination to effect a positive change.

It is not surprising that for those with HIV infection, depression is a common reaction, particularly in the period immediately following diagnosis (Green and McCreaner, 1988). By its very nature HIV infection can involve the client in a catalogue of loss. While anxiety is often seen as the threat of loss, depression may be viewed as the consequence of it. Losses caused by HIV may include:

- Loss of acceptability, both social and personal.
- Loss of function, decline in physical health.
- Loss of status, employment, and economic security.
- Loss of home. It is not uncommon for those with HIV infection to lose their home either through ill health or intolerance.
- Loss of loved ones. In some cases, those closest to the person with HIV infection may find it impossible to accept the situation, and may reject him/her.

**Table 14.2** Symptoms of HIV-related depression

| Depressed mood | Feeling downcast, angry, miserable, sad, and despondent |
|---|---|
| Loss of interest in | Previously enjoyed activities<br>Appearance |
| Absence of feeling | |
| Feelings of worthlessness and guilt | Dismissive of past achievements<br>Self-blame<br>Deserving the disease |
| Low self-esteem | Unworthy of help<br>Incompetent<br>A 'bad' person |
| Helplessness | Incapable of action, even routine daily tasks |

- Loss of future. The absence of a cure can result in feelings of hopelessness and despair, the individual feeling powerless to do anything towards achieving longed for hopes and ambitions.

### Coping with depression

People suffering from the understandable depression associated with HIV infection can be helped most by being given back control. Serious illness reduces most of us to feelings of dependency, which seems out of our control and inappropriate to our adult status. Nursing intervention should be aimed at helping the person to express that sense of self that is unique and individual to all of us.

Working together, the nurse and client can get through the worst times by emphasizing the rewards and the good things in the client's life, which will help him towards having a less distorted view of his worth. An essential contribution in this process is the way in which clients are valued by nursing staff. If the client can genuinely be made to feel he has worth for those who are caring for them, it will be difficult for him to maintain a feeling of worthlessness. Many are able to transfer such renewed feelings of self-worth by helping others who are struggling with similar feelings. For some, medical intervention and treatment, particularly in the form of a short course of antidepressants, may also be beneficial.

### Suicidal thoughts

People whose depression is severe will often consider suicide as the only way out of what seems to be an unbearable situation. In HIV infection, as in other life-threatening conditions, suicidal thoughts are an understandable reaction. In the vast majority, such thoughts will come and go throughout the illness in the same way as depression will wax and wane. Although suicidal thoughts are transitory in most people, they are nevertheless serious; it is essential that nursing staff treat them as such. Time needs to be spent with clients and their loved ones, not to reassure, but to acknowledge the depth and reality of their feelings. Nursing staff should not leave the client isolated, with no one to share his frightening feelings with.

Nurses may find it distressing to discuss the feelings expressed by some clients that a self-determined end is preferable. For those who have previously misused illegal drugs, a painless overdose may have its attractions.

Research shows that the motivating factors behind attempted suicide are all relevant to HIV infection (Miller, 1987). These include:

- Threatened or actual loss of a loved one.
- Social isolation, living alone.
- Financial problems, recent unemployment.
- Poor physical health, incapacitating incurable illness.
- Alcohol or drug dependency.
- Recent violent quarrels with a partner.
- Organic brain syndromes.
- Previous history or threats of suicide.
- A desire not to become a burden on others.

The most effective way of helping people through such periods or despair is to provide intervention aimed at prolonging life rather than prolonging death. The client should be fully aware of all aspects of treatment, and care should be organized to provide a constructive, optimistic atmosphere in which the most important issue is the quality of life for the individual. In such an atmosphere, it will be easier for the client to permit the general nurses to call in the considerable body of expertise represented by mental health nursing staff, who can help them to talk through their feelings, and identify ways of facing the future.

## HIV INFECTION AND INJECTING DRUG MISUSERS

Injecting drug misuse with contaminated equipment has been identified as the method of transmission of HIV in 16% of known cases of injection in the UK (Bennett, 1989). Even before the onset of the psychological and emotional trauma of HIV infection there already exists an enormous number of unresolved emotional issues surrounding the user's lifestyle and his injecting drug misuse (Kennedy and Faugier, 1989). HIV infection can make the emotional burden already carried by the injecting drug misuser too much to bear, who may continue to use drugs, or even increase drug misuse, in an attempt to blot out the painful feelings. Others may alternate between attempts to gain some control of their drug misuse, and erratic, chaotic misuse when their anxiety about HIV infection is severe.

People with HIV infection who demonstrate their greatest difficulty in coping with the psychological and emotional stress of the disease are those who have poor accommodation; few or poor family ties; low peer acceptance; and guilt over past behaviour.

Many injecting drug misusers lack a network of carers in the community on whom they can depend when they need support when in hospital, and help when out of hospital. This often condemns them to spending long and lonely periods in hospital, during which time they will be dependent on nursing staff for all their support. In this situation, where the client may have to deal not only with the immense emotional consequences of HIV infection, but also with the psychological damage inflicted by a drug misusing career, it is essential that nursing staff establish ready lines of support from specialist psychiatric and drug-misuse staff.

Since HIV infection is primarily a disease of the sexually productive, many female drug misusers will be faced with the questions related to pregnancy, childbirth, and HIV infection. Such women will need extremely supportive nursing care while dealing with these questions. Most importantly, they should have access to empathetic counselling, aimed at enabling them to reach their own choice (Richardson, 1989).

## AIDS DEMENTIA COMPLEX

It is now widely accepted that HIV infection can cause changes in the brain that give rise to dementia. Initially, complaints and presenting symptoms of those with AIDS dementia complex can mimic the signs one would expect to see in cases of extreme anxiety or depression (Page 145). Early recognition and correct identification of symptoms (Table 14.3) is essential, as many persons have experienced relief when treated with AZT (Zidovudine).

Caring for people who have developed dementia as a result of HIV infection requires a particular compassionate and skilled response from nursing staff. Clients may become very distressed by their own inability to grasp things mentally, or to perform quite simple everyday tasks. Lovers, relatives, and friends will need support through the painful experience of witnessing upsetting changes in the loved one, and in dealing with their own feelings of helplessness and futility. While all nursing staff have at some time in their career nursed elderly people suffering the indignities of dementia, they will not have nursed large numbers of previously active, healthy, young people in such a condition. This is likely to impose an extra emotional burden on staff, as they adjust their expectations of these young persons' abilities.

## THE WORRIED WELL

In relation to HIV infection, the 'worried well' is something of a misnomer, as all sexually active people should be concerned about the risks of contracting the virus. However, some individuals, who do not have a history of any activity that would give rise for concern, are nevertheless wrongly convinced they have HIV infection. As a result, they may subject themselves to repeated tests, the negative results of which fail to offer any relief from their anxieties.

In addition, there are members of the at-risk population who, in the absence of testing, can fall prey to chronic, disabling anxiety. The nursing management of these people is a psychiatric and psychological issue and should be treated seriously and sympathetically, as the obsession with HIV infection may be masking far more worrying psychiatric problems. Such people may be identified by:

- Frequent contact with counselling services, often by telephone.
- No history of high-risk behaviour.
- Repeated antibody tests.
- Mistrust of test results.
- Unshakeable conviction of having HIV infection.
- Guilt related to innocuous activity in the past.
- Relationship difficulties caused by their concerns about the virus.

Management of such people should be aimed at motivating them towards understanding the psychological nature of their concerns, and attempting to engage them in therapy.

## STRESS ON FAMILY AND FRIENDS

Like all life-threatening diseases, HIV infection has a devastating effect on the lovers, spouses, family, and friends of those involved. All of the reactions that occur in the person with HIV are also experienced by the people who are close to them: shock, denial, anger, guilt, depression, and anxiety. These people may themselves be in need of skilled help and care from all branches of the nursing profession.

There may be pre-existing problems relating to the client's sexual preference or injecting drugs misuse that family members find hard to deal with, and which may have caused difficulties in the past. For some families, the knowledge that their child has HIV infection may be their first knowledge of homosexuality, drug misuse, or involvement in other relationships. Sometimes information about the lifestyle of the client has been shared with some family members and not with others, causing resentment, anger, and guilt.

Many of those so far affected by HIV infection are homosexual men. Often they have lived with a lover for years, sharing their lives in a stable relationship. HIV can often place lovers and family members in conflict, as the families of clients frequently fail to appreciate the lover's role as a spouse. The ability of nursing staff to appreciate the importance of this relationship can greatly reduce the emotional damage to lovers at this time, and result in them having fewer unresolved feelings about the process of care.

Nursing staff must also be aware of the role which is played by other services in the community, such as voluntary organizations and self-help groups, which are an important aspect of support offered to clients, their lovers, partners, and families. In order to provide a continuity of support, nursing staff should establish effective communication links with such local groups. In the interests of clients' well-being, it is important for nursing staff to be sensitive to the roles and responsibilities of all those closest to them.

## CARING FOR YOURSELF AND YOUR COLLEAGUES

Nurses caring for people with HIV face enormous personal stress. Dealing with the intense physical and emotional needs of clients and others makes huge demands on the energies of health-care staff. People can struggle with HIV for many years before dying, during which time nurses and medical staff will have become close to them, often serving as a replacement for lonely and isolated clients. The repetitive experience of grief and demoralization that occur because

of the high mortality of HIV infection inevitably has an effect on those providing care.

In order to remain at an optimum level of effectiveness, all nurses require established support that will enable them to deal with their feelings in an appropriate manner. One method might be the establishment of a staff-support group, with a skilled facilitator who can assist nurses in better understanding their own and their colleagues' feelings in these difficult situations (Chapter 25).

## CONFIDENTIALITY

One of the issues that gives rise to a great deal of anxiety in those with HIV infection is the possibility of health care workers failing to treat information relating to their conditions as confidential. The consequences of inadvertent breaches of confidentiality can seriously damage the emotional state of clients and their loved ones, and undermine the relationship of trust necessary to provide meaningful psychological support (UKCC, 1984).

All enquiries from the media regarding individual clients should be directed to a single nurse manager or unit manager, who has public relations responsibility, and nurses should not make any comments to the press or other media representatives.

It must be remembered that confidentiality is an absolute prerequisite for the establishment of a safe, trusting relationship in which people can explore their deepest emotional fears and concerns.

## A DUTY TO CARE

Nursing staff have a duty to care for all those requiring their skills. They do not have to select which clients they will care for, or those to whom they will refuse this care.

There are learning opportunities available to nurses who wish to acquire or improve the relevant knowledge, skills and attitudes needed to care effectively for those with HIV infection (below).

## MENTAL HEALTH NURSING STAFF

Increasing numbers of mental health nursing staff now work in the community either as community psychiatric nurses or as specialists in the field of drug dependency. Some of these nurses are now breaking new ground as liaison mental health nurses, whose task is to bridge the gap in care between general and mental health nursing.

Many people facing the emotional impact of HIV can benefit by contact with a skilled nurse, who can spend time helping them to talk through some of the more troubling aspects of the disease. Some of these nurses are very skilled in counselling the care of the dying, and can be of great assistance to clients and their loved ones in coming to terms with their feelings of loss and grief. In addition, such nurses are in a position to provide help to their general nursing colleagues.

## SUMMARY

HIV presents psychological and emotional dilemmas, conflicts and stresses for the clients and all those intimately involved in their care. An awareness of the manner in which these stresses may manifest themselves, and of the support required to help clients and others to cope more effectively, is essential to the delivery of optimal nursing care.

Important in this process is the ability to recognize when the problem is beyond the capabilities of the general nursing team, and to professionally refer the client to skilled psychiatric colleagues.

In addition, nurses should recognize the need to care for themselves and colleagues, and to ensure that the appropriate support mechanisms are developed so that they can continue to work sensitively on clients' behalf.

## REFERENCES

Bennett, G. (1989) *Treating Drug Abusers*, Tavistock/Routledge, London.

Bridge, T. P., Mirskey, A. F., and Goodwin F. K. (1988) Psychological, neuropsychiatric and substance abuse aspects of AIDS, in *Advances in Biochemical Psychopharmacology* (Vol. 44), Raven Press, New York.

Flaskerud, J. H. (1988) *AIDS/HIV Infection, A Reference Guide for Health Professionals*, W. B. Saunders Company, London.

Green, J. and McCreaner, A. (1989) *Counselling HIV Infection*, Blackwell Scientific, Oxford, London, Edinburgh.

Jager, H. (1988) *AIDS Phobia, Disease Patterns and Possibilities of Treatment*, Ellis Horwood Limited, Chichester.

Kennedy, J. and Faugier, J. (1989) *Drugs and Alcohol Dependency Nursing*, Heinemann Nursing, Oxford.

Miller D. (1987) *Living With AIDS and HIV*, Macmillan Press, Basingstoke.

Paine, L. (1988) *AIDS: Psychiatric and Psychosocial Perspectives*, Croom Helm, London.

Richardson, D. (1989) *Women and the AIDS Crisis*, Pandora, London.

United Kingdom Central Council for Nursing, Midwifery and Health Visiting, (1984) (2nd edn) *Code of Professional Conduct for the Nurse, Midwife and Health Visitor*, Clause 9, UKCC.

## COURSES

ENB 'AIDS: Meeting the Challenge.'
ENB Course 934: 'The Care and Management of Patients With AIDS and Related Disorders'

# SUBSTANCE MISUSE

## 15

*David B. Cooper and Jean Faugier*

This chapter covers the use and misuse of both legal and illegal drugs. Legal drugs include alcohol, prescribed drugs, tea, coffee, and tobacco; illegal drugs include cannabis, heroin and cocaine. In this chapter the word 'drug' is used in a general sense, including legal and illegal types, except when there is specific mention to the contrary.

In a recent editorial, Dunne *et al.* (1989) argued that it is, 'misleading to consider alcohol and drug misuse as separate entities'. They went on to suggest that the similarities of 'social, psychological, and medical factors' were such that a 'multi-disciplinary approach to treatment is desired for both alcohol and drugs.' It is useful to keep this in mind while reading this chapter.

We stress the importance of the well-known saying that 'prevention is better than cure', adding that early intervention is better than no intervention at all, especially in relation to treatment outcome. As nurses we act as advisors on health prevention issues, interventions, and treatments; with the expansion of the primary nursing system, we now have the ability to undertake these obligations and responsibilities with maximum effect.

## HISTORICAL OVERVIEW

Throughout the history of civilization, man has used drugs in varying forms, either by accident or design, for their mind-altering qualities. Depending on which society one belongs to, the 'legal' drug(s) of use vary. In Britain it is legal to consume alcohol, to take prescribed medication, to drink tea or coffee, and to chew or smoke tobacco products. Indeed, our society has been dependent on such drugs for some time.

Alcohol is thought to be the world's oldest drug, and is still produced widely around the world. A description of the distillation of alcohol has been traced back to an Arabic manuscript of AD 712–813; it is believed the Romans used alcohol liberally for its mind-altering qualities.

Because alcohol and tobacco products produce vast incomes for many governments, it is difficult to control their use as they depend upon the money the sale of these products create. In excess of 759 000 people work in the drinks trade in Britain, and approximately 18 000 in the tobacco trade. In addition, the government receives enormous sums of money from excise duty and VAT; in 1985 the income from alcohol sales alone exceeded £5700 millions, and tobacco brought in some £5000 millions (Plant, 1987).

It is thus an uphill struggle when we talk about altering attitudes to, and usage of, alcohol and tobacco. In 1986, 20% of all hospital admissions were alcohol related – that is some 15 800 clients per year. Smoking alone causes 100 000 premature deaths each year.

The monies invested in preventative work remain small in comparison to the income received. This discrepancy becomes especially clear if one relates it to the expenditure of alcohol- and tobacco-producing companies, which use huge amounts of cash encouraging us to drink or smoke their products. For example, in 1985 £100 millions were spent by the alcohol industries on advertisements. The tobacco companies expended £500 millions. And these figures exclude the £10 millions used for sponsorships and other indirect product promotion.

Opium and cannabis were the traditional drug of use on the Indian subcontinent as far back as the ninth century AD. In 1898 the British government in India produced a report that demonstrated the historical pattern of illegal drug use in that country. At that time the nature of opiate use was largely ceremonial, the social use of such drugs being widely accepted by the general public as a normal way of life. The report cautioned the government against prohibition because of possible public outcry. However, in 1925 Mahatma Gandhi presented a petition to the International Opium Conference favouring the worldwide restriction of trade in narcotic drugs. It is interesting that these debates continue to date, the opinions still being divided.

To put things into perspective: if a government receives no financial income from illegal drug use, then it is easy to condemn their use; but if a government gains tax revenue from so-called legal drugs, it is difficult to condemn their use.

A great deal more work needs to be undertaken into the nature of drug dependence. The development of services for this client group is slow. Those that do exist contribute considerably by undertaking local research, as well as direct client care. It is largely due to the efforts of community drug and alcohol teams over the last eight years that more positive local and national steps are being taken to provide adequate interventions for this client group. A great achievement has been made with the introduction of regional alcohol and drug co-ordinators.

## DRUGS COMMONLY USED AND MISUSED

Drugs have always been used for their ability to affect the function of the mind. The types of drugs that have the desired effect are extensive. The legal drugs include tea, coffee, tobacco, prescribed medication, and alcohol; illegal drugs include cannabis, heroin, and cocaine.

Dependence on a drug develops when an individual becomes physically and/or psychologically reliant on the substance, without which the individual feels life to be intolerable. Over time the body adapts to the introduction of the drug of choice to the system. It is then said we 'tolerate' the drug. Gradually, it takes larger amounts of the substance to achieve the required effect. When the drug is withdrawn, the body reacts to the deprivation. The duration of this withdrawal depends on the drug of use and to the extent of both physical and psychological dependence.

### DEPRESSANT DRUGS

## Alcohol

Alcohol, along with tranquillizers, solvents, glues, hypnosedatives, heroin, and opiates, directly affects the central nervous system (CNS), and depresses heart and respiratory rate and the mental and physical processes.

Although alcohol currently is the most socially misused drug, there is no evidence that in small, infrequent amounts it does more than act as a social lubricant. The Royal Colleges have collectively suggested that the limit considered to be safe is 14 standard drinks per week for women, and 21 for men. They recommend a maximum limit of six standard drinks on two to three drinking occasions for men, and no more than two to three standard drinks on two to three drinking occasions for women. What is considered safe is defined as 'the limit'; above this, one could expect to experience some physical harm.

A standard drink is said to contain approximately 15 mg of alcohol (ethanol), and can best be described in terms of pub measures. Half a pint of beer or lager; one single spirit; one glass of wine or one glass of fortified wine is each classed one standard drink. It is important to remember this refers to average-strength beers and spirits: this system does not take account of all the varying strengths of many of today's alcohol products. Equally, when we talk about safe limits per drinking occasion, we refer to an average person, of average weight, height, health, and build. The system of measurement does not make allowances for any variation.

Alcohol is believed to be one of the fastest-acting, orally administered drugs available today. It takes only approximately five minutes to pass unchanged in chemical composition from the stomach into the blood supply. There it waits for the liver to eliminate it from the body at the rate of one standard drink per hour. For example, if five pints and two single whiskies were drunk, it would take 12 hours for the liver to eliminate the alcohol.

Most harm is done when alcohol remains in the body for prolonged periods of time; each and every organ can be affected. As well, alcohol may reduce effectiveness, sometimes markedly, of prescribed medicines, such as the Pill.

The harm related to alcohol misuse can be divided into three main headings: intoxication, excessive regular drinking, and dependence. The lists in Table 15.1, while not comprehensive, illustrate the types of problems associated with each of these.

If a client has experienced withdrawal symptoms in the past, or is likely to in the future, then a properly supervised withdrawal programme will need to be discussed and agreed before commencement. Contrary to popular belief, it is possible for someone with a drink-related problem to return to social drinking or controlled drinking, in certain circumstances, at some later stage.

**Table 15.1** Harm due to alcohol misuse

**Intoxification**
Acute poisoning
Drug overdose
Head injury
Accidents
Epileptic-form seizures
Acute gastritis
Suicidal behaviour

**Excessive Drinking**
Cancer of the mouth
Cancer of the throat
Sexual impotence
Pancreatitis
Stomach haemorrhage
Peripheral neuritis
Minor brain damage
Fatty liver
Liver cancer
Liver cirrhosis
Depression
Anxiety
Phobic illnesses

**Dependence**
Anxiety
Depression
Hallucinations
Paranoid states
Delirium tremens
Multiple drug taking
Alcoholic psychosis
Withdrawal epileptic-form seizure

## Tranquillizers

Librium (chlordiazepoxide), Valium (diazepam), and Ativan (lorazepam) have all received a great deal of negative press coverage over the past few years. The right dose, properly supervised and regulated for a short period of time, is appropriate for some mental health problems. The danger is from prolonged use and/or over-use, which is sometimes accidental, sometimes deliberate, or may result from inadequate supervision.

These drugs are often prescribed as anxiety relieving agents. When taken orally on a regular basis, tolerance quickly develops, along with dependency. They are readily available on the black market.

Tranquillizers should never be stopped abruptly. Frequently, withdrawal symptoms resemble the initial presenting complaint, for example, the client may complain of palpitations, breathlessness, sweating, a feeling of shaking inside the body, nausea, and butterflies in the stomach. There is also the need to deal actively with the psychological dependence these drugs produce.

## Hypnosedatives

Barbiturates such as Tuinal, Nembutal, and Seconal Sodium are usually taken orally, but can be injected for quicker effect. Though less widely prescribed than seven years ago, they are still available on the black market.

The effect of the drug lasts 3–12 hours. Low doses induce a relaxed mood, sociability, and good humour; high doses lead to slurred speech, clumsiness, and aggression, especially if mixed with alcohol. Barbiturate overdose is very dangerous, and can quickly lead to respiratory failure; the dividing line between a normal and a fatal dose can be very close. The abuser may develop severe physical and psychological dependence. Abrupt withdrawal may be associated with convulsions and brain damage; in some cases the outcome can be fatal.

## Glue and solvents

Solvents include glue, dry-cleaning fluids, paint, anti-freeze, nail varnish remover, and Tipp-Ex; propelled gases include aerosols; and fuels include cigarette-lighter gases and petrol.

Any substance that gives off fumes can be inhaled or sniffed by the abuser; a plastic bag is sometimes used to concentrate the fumes. Absorption via the lungs enables the inhaled chemicals rapidly to reach the brain. Breathing and heart rate is lowered and oxygen intake decreases, leading to disorientation, loss of control, and eventual unconsciousness.

The toxic content of glues and gasses include acetone, chloroform, methanol, butane, and carbon. Signs to look out for in solvent abuse include adhesive marks on clothing, sores and redness around the mouth and nose, red and glazed eyes, streaming nose, and dilated pupils. In addition, the abuser may behave as if drunk, and have slurred speech. It is also useful to be aware of the distinctive smell given off by such products.

Major hazards from short-term use include injury from falls and inhalation of vomit. Suffocation, caused by the use of plastic bags, is also a potential hazard. Long-term behaviour problems result in poor performance at school, truancy, and delinquency. Increased usage can lead to medical complications, such as lung damage and kidney failure. Failure to inhale gasses correctly, for example, lighter fuel, can cause respiratory arrest and subsequent sudden death.

## Heroin

Heroin – or 'H' or 'smack' as it is sometimes called – is derived from the opium poppy. It can be sniffed, injected IV or IM – otherwise known as 'shooting' or 'mainlining' – or smoked over aluminium foil through a small tube, which is known as 'chasing the dragon'.

Because the purity of the drug is often unknown or unreliable, users can easily accidentally overdose. Heroin is usually 'cut' with other substances such as chalk or baking powder. Risks of infection are high when needles are shared, increasing the incidence of septacaemia, hepatitis, and AIDS.

Heroin induces euphoria, drowsiness, and a sense of well-being and personal worth. Tolerance develops quickly, demanding increasing doses to achieve the same effect. Physical and psychological dependence is inevitable, especially as withdrawal is unpleasant, which is often described as being like a severe dose of flu; goosebumps are also common. A gradual reduction of dose is advisable so the experience of withdrawal may be brought to a tolerable level.

Contamination of the drug with noxious substances, leading to a severe allergic reaction, is often exacerbated by poor diet and self-neglect. This degenerative process may lead to death if considerable care is not available.

## STIMULANTS

Stimulants increase alertness and concentration over a long period. Side-effects include raised breathing and heart rates; decreased sleep and poor appetite are additional complications. The main types of stimulants used are nicotine, caffeine, amphetamines, and cocaine.

### AMPHETAMINES

Amphetamines, often called 'speed' or 'whizz', have become very popular. Their effect usually lasts from three to five hours. They are usually sniffed, or 'snorted', but some users prefer to inject in order to enhance or quicken the effect. These drugs were initially introduced for the treatment of depression and as appetite suppressants, but now are readily available on the black market.

The effects of these drugs include an increase in pulse and respiratory rate and a reduction in fatigue, leading to increased muscular activity. This in turn produces restlessness and talkativeness. Users often complain they cannot sleep. Weight loss can be a complication, and should be checked frequently in order to avoid anorexia.

The user may complain of headaches, tiredness, and lack of interest in both work and self. During intoxication, there is an increased risk that the user will take inappropriate actions and 'dares', which may lead to accidental injury or death.

An overdose of amphetamines can cause fever, paranoid psychosis, respiratory failure, hallucinations, epileptic-form seizures, coma, disorientation, and cardiovascular collapse.

There are no specific withdrawal symptoms, however, the user may complain of lethargy, prolonged sleep, excessive hunger, and, with regular high usage, paranoid psychosis may develop. Another major obstacle to be overcome is that of psychological dependence.

### Cocaine

Cocaine, often referred to as 'coke', is derived from the coca plant. This white powder is a powerful stimulant, and its user-group crosses all social barriers, although it is frequently the drug of choice of the more financially affluent members of society.

The drug is usually sniffed ('snorted'), although it can be injected IV, and is occasionally mixed with heroin to maximize effect, which is known as 'speedball'. Cocaine can also be purchased mixed with heroin and LSD in pill form (white dove). Additionally, cocaine can be mixed with common baking powder and water to form 'crack'.

The effects of cocaine peaks within 15–30 minutes, then gradually decrease. During that time the user experiences a tremendous feeling of physical and mental power. Physiological arousal and euphoria lead to an indifference to pain and fatigue, with the user feeling the need for less sleep. Dietary intake is often poor. Large doses can lead to bizzare and erratic behaviour, with marked agitation, anxiety, and hallucinations.

Dependence on cocaine is usually of a psychological nature. During withdrawal the user may complain of depression, fatigue, and the inability to cope with work and life.

Chronic and frequent use may lead to restlessness, nausea, insomnia, paranoid psychosis, weight loss, hyper-excitability, and severe depression. Repeated sniffing leads to damage to the membrane lining of the nose.

# HALLUCINOGENS

## CANNABIS

When used on occasional basis, cannabis is believed to have no long-lasting effects, and is safer than alcohol. The experimental legalization of this drug in Amsterdam is claimed to have led to a reduction in the number of heroin addicts and to the sale of hard drugs. However, in this country cannabis remains illegal; the user has to purchase it from a 'pusher', and therefore access to harder drugs becomes easier.

Cannabis is available in three forms: as grass, which is a dried leaf (marijuana); as resin, which is a compact block 'hash'; and as oil, the strongest, most highly concentrated form of cannabis. It is usually smoked, though occasionally it is eaten. Commonly it is mixed with tobacco in a 'joint'.

The effect is one of induced relaxation, talkativeness, and hilarity, with an intensification in the perception of sound and colour. There is a reduction in short-term memory function, and a decrease in motor skills. Concentration becomes poor. These effects last for an hour or more after use.

High doses can lead to confusional states, but the main health hazard is from inhalation of the tobacco smoke, which is linked to lung cancer.

## LYSERGIC ACID DIETHYLAMID (LSD) AND PSILOCYBINS

### LSD

LSD, or 'acid', is a derivative of ergot, a fungus that grows wild on rye and other grasses. Initially produced for therapeutic purposes, LSD became widely abused by the hippies in the mid-1960s. It is now associated, as well as other drugs, with acid house parties (large warehouse parties, usually organized events), and more recently with rave parties.

The short-term user of LSD experiences a 'trip', a term used to describe the hallucination. This includes disturbance of perception, increased levels of awareness and disorientation, and dissociation from the body. These experiences usually commence within one-half to one hour following ingestion of the drug, and peak between two to six hours, before gradually fading after ten to twelve hours.

Long-term excessive use can cause prolonged psychological reactions and a marked re-experiencing of past trips, known as 'flashbacks'. LSD is not known to cause dependence. There is documented evidence that some users have plunged to death while deluded, believing they could fly.

### Psilocybins

Psilocybin is the active ingredient of 'magic mushrooms', commonly known as 'Liberty Cap', *Psilocybe Semilanceata*. These may be eaten or brewed as tea. The user experiences an effect similar to that of LSD, with added euphoria and hilarity. The use of this drug produces increased heart rate and blood pressure, with dilation of pupils. The drug takes effect more quickly than LSD, starting within half an hour, peaking at approximately three hours, and lasting between four to ten hours.

While dependence, withdrawal, and overdose are unlikely, the main danger to health comes from picking and eating the wrong, perhaps poisonous, mushrooms.

## RECOGNITION OF DRUG MISUSE

Because many signs and symptoms of drug misuse overlap with other physical, social, and psychological problems, it is wrong to assume that any of the factors in Table 15.2, which lists the types of complaint the client or someone close to him/her have made to health care workers over time, is a definitive

**Table 15.2** Complaints related to drug misuse

Significant behavioural changes not related to
family circumstances
Loss of appetite
Loss of weight
Change in sleeping patterns
Increase in aggression
Increase in fatigue
Decrease in motivation at work and leisure
Lack of interest in family and friends
Increased involvement in crime and police
Break-up of relationship
Financial problems
Recurrent stomach problems
Occupational changes, type of occupation
Monday-morning absenteeism
Feeling depressed
Anxiety
Blackouts
Frequent doctor visits or investigations ordered
Poor appearance
Accidents at home and work
Head injury

indication of the abuse of legal or illegal substances. In all assessments, general questions relating to prescribed, social, and illegal drug misuse need to be addressed.

**EARLY IDENTIFICATION AND INTERVENTION**

The prospect of developing drink- or drug-related problems often depends on the social resources available to the individual user. The wealthy are unlikely to suffer monetary problems as a result of substance abuse. Equally, teenagers today are far more susceptible to intensive pressures urging them to drink alcohol and take drugs than their parents are, or indeed were.

The problems raised or encountered by the drug user often go unnoticed by the caring professions, or they are misdiagnosed and treated symptomatically. For example, the abusing client who complains of heartburn

and upset stomach may be prescribed or advised to buy antacid medication. Or the mother who complains her baby will not settle, and that it cries all the time may be advised that 'some babies are like that' when the reason actually lies with a drug-misusing husband: the resulting lack of money and increased family tension is passed on to the baby by the over-anxious mum.

Many people who are admitted to hospital with the initial diagnosis of depression or anxiety on further investigations are found to have underlying drug-related problems. A survey undertaken on an acute mental health admission ward over a three-month period revealed that 38% of all patients drank more than the 'safe' weekly limits (Cooper, 1985). A three-month pilot study which covered an outpatient department and two acute admission wards of a mental health unit indicated that 17% of respondents were believed to be misusing alcohol to such an extent that it exacerbated the presenting complaint. All the individuals screened had no previous drug behaviour assessment; all had a diagnosed mental health problem. Clients with a known alcohol- or drug-related problem were excluded from this study (Cooper 1985).

**THE NURSE'S ROLE**

'It's not right her being here. It's different when people have to come in through no fault of their own.'

'He's always coming in and out; never changes.'

'They're *all* psychopaths.'

The above statements, made by nurses about substance abusers, have all been voiced in mental health and general wards. Sadly, they are commonplace, and the reader will most likely hear them too. Despite the fact that research projects regularly highlight the need to educate nurses on how to identify drug misuse problems earlier and to respond appropriately to this client group, there remains a lack of drug education targeted at all levels and groups of nurses, from RMNs, RGNs, health visitors, school nurses and CPNs, to district nurses and midwives. To illustrate the point, the following case study highlights some of the difficulties the problem drug user encounters.

CASE STUDY – THE CARING PROFESSION

Roger was a 37-year-old businessman who led a very active business and social life. Work often included long lunches, where many a good deal was clinched after not a little help from alcohol. In the evening Roger liked to unwind with a drink or two before dinner, and, of course, life would not be the same without a bottle of wine with the meal. His wife did not appreciate wine very much, so Roger would often finish off the bottle.

Most days ended with an evening at the local pub with his friends; sometimes his wife would go with him. Roger always arranged for his wife or a friend to bring him home, as he did not believe in drinking and driving, although he did not mind if the friend had had a drink. 'After all,' he would reason, 'it's a free choice, and its his licence, not mine.'

Roger found it increasingly difficult to sleep, and suffered from indigestion and heart-burn. His GP prescribed sleeping tablets and antacid medication, but these did not appear to help.

Roger could no longer cope with his business commitments; he was often late for or missed important appointments, and lost a lot of custom. The business quickly ran into financial difficulties and eventually folded. Shortly after, his wife left him.

To help him get through the day, Roger turned increasingly to drink. The problem became so great that his GP referred him to the local mental health unit for detoxification. On admission, he was prescribed Heminevrin (chlormethiazole),

which enabled him to go without alcohol. Roger could not identify with his fellow patients. 'After all,' he thought, 'you can see they are ill.' He also felt the staff did not like him. Admittedly, he felt anger and bitterness, and did not always feel like socializing – but then again he had lost a lot, and felt frightened and degraded being in this place.

The ward staff were often busy with the chap who kept running away. Roger felt the staff resented him because he needed too much time and persuasion before he would do anything. They were suspicious when he isolated himself, especially when he went out for those 'long walks'.

Some senior staff, who had seen many such detoxifications, were convinced Roger was secretly drinking – after all, why would he keep sucking those mints? They would often threaten him with discharge, just to remind him of his admission contract, whereby he had agreed to remain dry.

Finally, Roger felt unable to manage and discharged himself. The staff felt vindicated: 'After all, he must have needed a drink. They all do. People like him don't want help.'

On discharge, Roger was given a two-week supply of Heminevrin syrup. No more was heard from him for six months, when Roger was readmitted to the ward. He had not drunk alcohol since his last discharge. This time he needed detoxification from Heminevrin. It appeared that Roger had increased his usage of the drug, obtaining supplies through his GP's repeat-prescription system. Roger was taking one-half to one bottle of Heminevrin syrup a day to help him to cope with life.

Roger was reluctant to accept admission to hospital because of his past experience, however, his need for help was great and he eventually agreed, although some of his own prejudices still remained.

On this occasion, a new keyworker system was in operation on the ward. Roger felt pleased to have someone he could identify with. Lacking experience of drug problems, the nurse decided to contact the community drug team. She felt it useful to obtain their advice.

The specialist and keyworker, together with Roger, agreed on a care plan both during and following his discharge. He progressed well and participated in ward activities. He felt the keyworker understood him, and was able to confide about his past experiences and future plans.

Roger was discharged to the care of the community drug team. Two years following his discharge he no longer needs the help of prescribed drugs. He now drinks alcohol socially, after participating in a controlled-drinking programme, and teaches business studies at his local college.

It is possible to see from the above how the attitudes and interest of those professionals involved in Roger's care was important. Nurses remain in a privileged position. The client often sees us as the human face of the care system, believing we are on their side, practical, and down-to-earth. We have the ability to talk, observe, listen, support, advise and reassure when it is most needed. Because the client feels we are trustworthy and approachable, we are in an ideal position to give physical and emotional care. How many times have clients asked, 'Can you explain what he means?', as the doctor leaves.

However, we need to be as aware of the pressures on ourselves as on those we care for: it is as easy for us to misuse substances as it is for anyone. The case studies below demonstrate the consequences of drug misuse in nursing, and pose the questions: 'Should they have received help earlier?' 'If they had, would it have changed the outcome?'

CASE STUDY – THE STUDENT NURSE

Andrew, a 19-year-old student nurse, liked to unwind after the pressures of a busy day, usually in the staff social club. He often went with a group of friends; the buying of rounds was common practice. When the bar closed, many customers would take their drinks away with them and consume them in their rooms at the nurses' home. On one such occasion, Andrew was introduced to 'wacky backey', or cannabis. In time he came to enjoy the combined effect of both drugs.

Andrew found it hard to get up in the mornings, and was experiencing many bad hangovers. His concentration – especially on early shift – was poor, and his patience very low. His ability to study deteriorated quickly. He was offered some tablets by a 'friend' to help him through the mornings, and at lunch time he would have a couple of pints to 'steady him up' until the shift ended – when the process would start all over again.

After a 'good session' one night, some people Andrew had met asked for a lift. He dropped them off at their destination around three in the morning. Two miles from home on his return journey, Andrew was involved in a head-on collision with another vehicle and died instantly.

Andrew's colleagues knew of his drink and drug problem, and indeed often covered when he was late or missed lectures. They experienced first-hand his drug misuse and how this affected his work. No one wanted to discuss this with him or with the tutors for fear of losing his friendship. It is conceivable that had Andrew received advice and counselling, the outcome may have been different. His friends may also have experienced less guilt following his death.

CASE STUDY – THE TUTOR

There was always something odd about Ms Pierce: she would often arrive late for lectures, especially first thing in the morning; sometimes she did not arrive at all. There was always a weak excuse for this behaviour. The group of students began to realize that the content of some of the lectures was less than accurate. On occasions, Ms Pierce appeared confused and irritable, especially if challenged about the errors.

The students grumbled among themselves, but because of their position did not like to raise the problems they were having with a higher level of management. Many behind-the-hand comments were made between students and tutors.

Ms Pierce approached several members of the group individually, asking them to obtain a small supply of Valium (diazepam), from the ward drug cupboards. She gave the excuse that they were to be used for lectures. Each student was sworn to secrecy. She also gained access to ward drug cupboards during 'individual tutorials'. The topic was drugs and their side-effects.

The need for Valium increased to such an extent that Ms Pierce acquired a blank prescription pad, for 'lecture purposes', and presented forged prescriptions, using a rotating system of chemists.

Ms Pierce overdosed several times. Colleagues and superiors were aware of her problem, but declined to formally challenge this behaviour. She had been there many years and was a 'good tutor'. They felt her frequent 'rests' would do the trick.

The misuse of Valium became a disciplinary matter following a missing drug enquiry. At its conclusion, Ms Pierce was dismissed from service. No help or referral on to an outside agency was offered. All agreed that it was a shame to loose such a tutor. It was a sad end to her career.

In the above case study, had a student, colleague, or manager discussed their fears earlier and acted upon their concerns – for example, by involving the occupational health department or the community drug team and instigating the work place policy relating to drug and alcohol misuse – Ms Pierce may have responded to intervention and treatment. She could have continued her employment with the Health Authority, and others would have undoubtedly benefited from her experience.

PROBLEMS FOR NURSES SEEKING HELP

It is hard for an individual to approach a colleague they suspect of having a drug problem; it is equally difficult for the abuser to come forward for help. Below are some questions that illustrate the anxiety that may prevent the nurse from seeking appropriate help or advice:

- Will my colleagues find out details of my problem and treatment?
- Will I be considered responsible enough to continue in my profession if I accept help?
- If I cannot look after myself, how will others be entrusted to my care?
- Will treatment for a drug problem be noted on my record, and limit my professional development?
- How will I relate to the nurses who are caring for me?
- Will I be suspended, disciplined, or asked to leave?
- How will I convince others that I can be trusted to hold drug cupboard keys?
- How will I arrange regular time off to keep my appointments?
- How can I impress on senior administrative and nursing staff that time off from work is through a genuine illness, and not drug-related?

## PREVENTION

A great deal of headway has been made in preventing drug-related problems. Over the last few years, new health promotion initiatives at national and local level have been implemented at a rapid pace. Health-promotion campaigns targeting drug users, potential AIDS/HIV victims, and, more recently, the annual drink-wise campaign, are beginning to have some effect. Policing for drug traffickers has also enjoyed some success. Recently, three men were successfully convicted after what transpired to be the longest international surveillence exercise yet, with cocaine with a street value of some £100 millions being seized in Scotland.

Most district health promotion departments have a staff member who deals with drug-related issues, and over the past eight years community drug teams have developed. The introduction of both of these has proved useful in the early identification of drug-related problems.

Most health districts offer a needle-exchange scheme, which has developed as a result of increased awareness of AIDS, and the sharing of needles and syringes, or 'works'. At such centres, used 'works' are exchanged for clean equipment, which is usually done on a one-to-one basis.

Equally, the introduction of outreach workers working within the community and closely with community groups has lead to active involvement in the early identification of drug-related problems. The case study below demonstrates the type of work undertaken by such outreach workers, and gives some idea of their effectiveness.

## CASE STUDY – GARY

Gary was a bright 18-year-old college student in his first year of study. The college he attended was some way from his home, which meant he was independent of parental control for the first time. During the week he lived in digs, returning home for the weekends.

Like most men of his age, Gary was heavily into music. He looked forward to the college disco, when he could stay out late and have a good laugh with his mates. Gary was given his first joint by a friend. He grew to like the effect it had on him, and soon began to purchase his own. Through a pusher, Gary soon gained access to amphetamines.

Gary's college work deteriorated, failing to hand in assignments on time and missing several lectures. He became increasingly argumentative, and was involved in several fights. His parents saw the change in him, but any attempts to discuss this were spurned. As his habit grew, Gary started to experiment with other drugs. Eventually, he was given a final warning from the college. By this time his parents had refused to allow him home because of his disruptive behaviour and its effect on the family.

By chance Gary met an outreach worker at one of the college discos. They talked about drugs and Gary's problem, and as a result Gary agreed to seek help.

Although he has not kicked his habit, Gary is making good progress. The college is aware of the drug problem, and with its support his work and attendance is beginning to improve. He now feels more confident about himself, and is working towards rebuilding his relationship with his parents. Gary is beginning to enjoy life once more.

The problem drug user often comes into daily contact with members of the caring professions, and it is here that further education on how to identify and help this client group is needed.

A national multidisciplinary symposium called 'Responding to Alcohol' was held in September 1989. A statement to the UKCC and government was issued, urging them to take positive action to make drug education a priority in both basic and post-basic education for nurses.

Although the conference was on alcohol, the same should, and does, apply to all drug misuse.

## TREATMENT

The Advisory Committee on Alcoholism (1979), stated that:

> Members of the primary health care team have considerable opportunity to identify problem drinkers. The aim must be that, not only shall they do this, but, they shall also provide treatment and care.

They went on to add:

> The main task of primary level workers, in the management of problem drinkers, should be to recognize the causes and effect; to have adequate knowledge of the help required by the problem drinker, and the family; to give this help as far as it lies within their scope and, to know where and when to seek more expert help.

With these recommendations in mind, the nurse needs to know where to get specialist help and advice. Most district health authorities have a community drugs team. The senior nurse or tutor should be able to advise on how to contact this service. Equally, the Citizens' Advice office or Community Health Council may have useful phone numbers. Most teams now advertise in the Yellow Pages. Public information material is available from district health promotion departments at no cost. They can be contacted direct or via senior colleagues, as above. For technical information, including information on voluntary-sector services, a list of agencies and their addresses are given at the end of this chapter (page 163).

Treatment offered to the abuser can only be agreed upon following full assessment. It is important to gain a clear picture of the drugs misused, their affect on the client, and the client's desired treatment outcome, for example, reduction of use, change of use to a less harmful substance, controlled use, withdrawal to total abstinence.

The drug user may initially sound out the service and the help available. It is important at this stage of contact to give written and clear verbal information such as a name and future contact address, plus basic leaflets on drug misuse.

It may be helpful to arrange a joint assessment with a specialist team member, especially if the nurse wishes to continue as the key worker (she or he will be able to offer support and guidance during involvement with the client). The assessment must include detailed information about past and present use and misuse. For this purpose, it is useful to ask the client to keep a diary of his/her drug intake during the week preceding the appointment. Below are some factors to consider during assessment:

- Problematical effects of alcohol consumption.
- Psychological state.
- Work, social, and cultural factors.
- Motivation for treatment.
- Relevant personality factors.
- Family psychodynamics.
- Physical state and complications.

## DETOXIFICATION

In basic terms, this is a specific procedure designed to assist the client to a position in their life when they no longer use the drug of abuse, or require any other form of medication as a substitute.

It is not always appropriate, or necessary, to use alternative medication to assist withdrawal. Indeed, in many cases, the drug of misuse can be used in the process of gradual withdrawal.

Increasingly, detoxification is undertaken in the client's own home, inpatient treatment only being required in cases of known or identified complication. The procedure does not always need specialist supervision.

## COUNSELLING

Access to individual counselling is important. There is often a need to reassess the client's behaviour and lifestyle, and to help him or her to develop new skills and coping strategies. Awareness of relapse and its management is important. The user needs to know how and when to get help should he or she experience difficulties.

## GROUPS

Most district drug teams and voluntary agencies operate groups. These can be open or closed, single-sex or mixed, total abstinence or controlled use, client groups. Some also offer family support groups. Organized at differing levels, dependent on the identified needs of the group, they enable the user to discuss with others the problems they have experienced, and offer the chance of mutual support and advice.

## VOLUNTARY GROUPS

Drinkwatchers is organized on a similar basis to Weight-Watchers, and total abstinence is not required. It is enough to want to look at and to modify one's drinking behaviour. Alcoholics Anonymous and Narcotics Anonymous offer an individual and group support network for those wishing to stop abusing their drug of choice. Total abstinence is required. The concept is one of a disease model. It is possible to attend a meeting every night. Al-Anon and Al-Ateen are run on a similar basis to the above, but offer support to the partner or children of the abuser.

## TRANQUILIZER SUPPORT GROUPS

The withdrawal from tranquilizers can be a long process, during which time the client requires a considerable amount of support and encouragement. Many districts have a voluntary group; some community drug teams also organize such groups.

## OTHER TREATMENTS

Other treatments undertaken by drug teams may include group psychotherapy; social skills training; relaxation techniques; family therapy; education and preventative activities; medical and nursing care of physical problems; and telephone support. Most teams have access to intensive residential courses for abusers, as well as to hostel and dry-hostel care. All offer differing philosophies relating to approach. Entrance is usually following their own assessment and selection procedures.

## REFERENCES

Advisory Committee on Alcoholism (1979) The pattern and range of services for problem drinkers, HMSO, London.

Cartwright, A. K. J, Shaw, S. J, and Spratley, T. A. (1971) *Designing a Comprehensive Response to Problems of Alcohol Abuse,* London Report to the DHSS, Maudsley Pilot Project.

Cooper, D. B. (1985) The effects of a community alcohol service – the hidden 'potential' drinking problems and problem drinking (unpub.)

Dunne, F. J., Paton, A., Walker, T. (1989) Alcohol and drug services – the case for combining. *Alcohol and Alcoholism,* 2, 75–6.

Plant, M. A. (1987) *Drugs in Perspective,* Hodder and Stoughton, London.

## FURTHER READING

*AIDs and Drug Misuse* (1988, 1989) Report by the Advisory Council on the Misuse of Drugs.

*Alcohol Misuse* (1989) health notice, Department of Health.

*Drugs and British Society: Responses to a Social Problem in the 1980s* (1989) (ed. S. MacGregor), Routledge, London.

*Drug Scene* (1987), Report on drugs and drug dependence, Royal College of Psychiatrists.

Edwards, G. (1987) *The Treatment of Drinking Problems: A Guide for the Helping Profession*, Blackwell Scientific, Oxford.

Kennedy, J. and Faugier, J. (1989) *Alcohol and Drug Dependency Nursing*, Heinemann Nursing, London.

Plant M. A. (1987) *Drugs in Perspective*, Hodder and Stoughton, London.

Robinson, D. and Heather, P. (1986) *Preventing Alcohol Problems: A Guide to Local Action*, Tavistock, London.

## USEFUL ADDRESSES

Alcohol Concern
275 Gray's Inn Road
London WC1X 8QF
Tel: 071 833 3471

Alcoholics Anonymous
P O Box 1
Stonebow House
Stonebow
York YO1 2UL

Association of Nurses in Substance Abuse (ANSA)
Membership Secretary
CDTIC
Theatre Court
London Road
Northwick CW9 5HP

Health Education Authority
Hamilton House
Mableton Place
London WC1H 9TX
Tel: 071 631 0930

Narcotics Anonymous
PO Box 417
London SW10 0DP

National Campaign Against Solvent Abuse
The Enterprise Centre
444 Brixton Road
London SW9 8EJ
Tel: 071 733 7330

Standing Conference on Drug Abuse (SCODA)
1–4 Hatton Place
Hatton Garden
London, EC1N 8ND
Tel: 071 430 2341

# MIND AND BODY – THE EMOTIONS AND PHYSICAL ILLNESS 16

*Linda Rowden*

The links between emotion and physiological symptoms have been acknowledged by a number of early writers on medicine, including Hippocrates and Galen. Cartesian dualism, however, suggests that physical illness and mental illness cannot be considered in relationship to each other, either in their causation or treatment. This hypothesis is said to be responsible for the 'mind-body' divide, an expression that refers to the notion that mind and body are separate and do not interact. This attribution to Descartes has been recently challenged by Brown (1989), who has unearthed evidence of psychosomatic awareness in the seventeenth and eighteenth centuries.

In assessing health and illness, consideration of the social and psychological factors is as important as the physical assessment of the effects of disease. Any physical illness potentially has a psychological component, either in determining its existence, or in affecting the nature of its outcome: the emotional or psychological impact of the disease on the sufferer. Such manifestations that present as physical illness may have no organic evidence to support a functional diagnosis, but are able to create significant disturbance in people's lives. Thus, the mind and body interact both in health and illness. The mind may either hasten physical recovery, or contribute to the body's continued malaise. Equally, the body may have an impact on the mind.

Psychosomatic disorders are organic conditions allegedly precipitated by reactions to emotional crises, for example, peptic ulcer, irritable bowel syndrome, bronchial asthma and rheumatoid arthritis. Unemployment, job dissatisfaction, or marital discord may all result from continual episodes of irritable bowel syndrome or fibromyositis (Weiner, 1987). It is possible that these physical conditions have resulted from the emotional or social factors. Further research would inform on this. It was discovered that patients with one or more of these disorders were older and from urban backgrounds. The most common psychiatric presentation was depression. Although only 1% of the sample of 4240 adult psychiatric patients had discernible 'psychosomatic disorders', their findings determined the need for practitioners to be skilled in both physical and psychological treatments.

The division of the person into mind and body nevertheless continues to be a model some practitioners pursue, partly because of the complexity and inadequate understanding of interactions between the mental state and the physical condition. A simple example of this might be the investigation of episodes of high blood pressure and rapid pulse rate either by complete cardiovascular testing or by referral to a psychiatrist; it is in fact possible that both physical and psychological factors are involved. Specialism has its advantages, provided it exists to the same level for all aspects of care required by the person in need. Bias exists on both sides of the mind-body issue; the hope is that good communication is established to maintain the balanced view.

## QUALITY OF LIFE

Awareness of the whole person has developed particularly during the last 20 years, with consideration of a person's quality of life receiving attention especially if he or she suffers from cancer. (Although many of the subsequent examples are taken from the experiences of clients in cancer treatment centres, many of the conclusions reached are equally applicable to other forms of illness.)

A definition of 'quality of life' depends on the individual concept of what is important. For example, Bard *et al.* (1955), working psychodynamically, assessed a number of women who were treated for cancer of the breast with the surgical procedure of radical mastectomy. From extensive observation and interviews, they developed a psychological framework for the impact of this major intervention on the woman and her husband. In their interpretation, they drew on the mother-daughter relationship during puberty to explain some of the reactions of the women to mutilating surgery. For example, some women react with feelings of guilt, unconsciously experiencing the disease and its treatment as a punishment for being sexually desirable or active, which may be due to their experience of the mother's response to her own breast development.

Other appraisals measured issues such as activities of daily living in relation to cancer and/or its treatment effects. Additional aspects included date of discharge from hospital following treatment, time of returning to work, and return to participation in social activities (Eisenberg *et al.*, 1966). Such factors are key to the coping abilities of a person with cancer, but they do not necessarily describe their emotional status.

Psychiatric problems occurring in patients following breast surgery for cancer has been shown in many studies to range from 15–30%. Maguire (1978) found that 25% of women who had a mastectomy required treatment for anxiety or depression, or both, a year following surgery.

These different presentations, feelings, and behaviour reflect the variety of concepts that exist in the assessment of quality of life. In a more recent review, De Haes (1988) points out that the observer's views of a person's quality of life differ substantially from the subjective opinion of the person with cancer.

The quality of life is very dependent on individually held views. The sportsman or outdoor worker, for example, often finds confinement to bed or ward with an IV infusion in progress far more frustrating than does the person with a more leisurely lifestyle; the lonely widow or widower may derive feelings of unity with patients she or he is spending time with, while others prefer not to socialize; fellow patients' problems may offend, annoy, bore, or threaten the loner.

In their study of women undergoing radical mastectomy, Bard *et al.*, (1955) classified reactions into three phases: anticipatory, operative, and reparative. These were then extended into ten critical periods by Galbraith Thomas (1978) in order to investigate the psychosocial issues:

1. Prodromal period, when the patient is her usual self.
2. Prediagnostic period.
3. Diagnostic period.
4. Preoperative phase.
5. Operative period.
6. Immediate postoperative period.
7. Extended postoperative period.
8. Adjuvant treatment period, when drug or radiation treatment is given.
9. Recovery period.
10. Terminal period.

Galbraith Thomas suggests the relevance of personality, coping patterns, and health beliefs and attitudes, which may be studied during the first phase.

While much of the research work done focuses on people with breast cancer – one of the most common types of cancer – it has been found that people suffering with lung cancer experience a greater amount of distress that those with breast or colonic cancers, Hodgkin's disease, or malignant melanoma (Ryan, 1987). This is possibly due to the rapid progression of the cancer, with associated debilitating effects and drastically altered lifestyle. Ryan also puts forward the idea of guilt: do people who smoked blame themselves for their illness? Further research would be interesting.

Despite the presumption that there are identified responses to specific cancers, Cella *et al.* (1989) have found that the cancer site does not determine the severity  of the reaction. Pancreatic cancers may, however, provoke a depressive syndrome which may be a physical reaction to altered enzyme levels.

Enquiry into the psychological aspects of other physical illnesses also explores the links between mind and body. For example, the relationship between the physical and psychological factors in men with severe heart disease has been explored (Bass *et al.*, 1987). In assessing men who underwent coronary artery bypass graft surgery, psychiatric morbidity and personality factors were evaluated. The only significant variable associated with atherosclerosis was the expression of fear. This finding is the reverse of earlier conclusions, but leaves some uncertainty. There can be no doubt of the existence of emotional distress in patients with heart disease.

## REACTIONS TO LIFE-THREATENING ILLNESS

Today, attention is more commonly given to the impact of the physical illness on a person's psychological state. There are hundreds of adjectives used to describe a person's reaction to a diagnosis of a life-threatening illness: 'shock', 'afraid', 'desperate', 'numb', 'disbelieving', and 'hopeless', are but a few. Psychiatric complications may be found in up to half of physically ill people (Lipowski, 1977). Although considerable work has been documented on the effects of specific cancers

on psychological state, it has been demonstrated that the diagnosis is not the significant factor: patients with diabetes, renal disease, arthritis, cancer, or dermatological disorders do not experience different levels of distress from each other. The severity of a disease or disability is a predictor of significant anxiety or depression, rather than a specific diagnosis (Cassileth *et al.*, 1983).

AIDS is receiving increasing attention, and the peak of its incidence has coincided with an enhanced awareness of the emotional consequences of life-threatening disorders. The public reaction to this condition matches that which existed towards cancer 20–30 years ago. As treatments have improved for some cancers, and prognoses are less devastating: more people with cancer are likely to live with it than to die from it, since the advent of more effective treatments.

In contrast, one study identified more distress and mood disturbance in patients with cancer than in people who had experienced a myocardial infarction. The type of concerns expressed in patients with cancer tended to be more of an existential nature, such as, 'Why me?', and, 'What is it all for?' By comparison, those suffering from cardiac problems tend to be more concerned with financial matters, employment prospects, and so on (McCorkle *et al.*, 1983).

North (1988) describes reports of affected memory, concentration, and abstract reasoning after coronary artery bypass surgery, which disappear in the majority of patients after six to eight weeks; the life-threatening aspect cannot be denied. In another study, the psychiatric morbidity in people with multiple sclerosis, a chronic debilitating disorder, was significantly greater than in people who were equally physically disabled by rheumatic or non-brain-involving neurological disorders. (Ron *et al.*, 1989).

The diagnosis of a life-threatening illness can have a multitude of reactions. Ask yourself how would you feel if you were told you have cancer? For some, it means a minimal inconvenience; for others, a devastating affirmation of their greatest fear. There are many shades of feeling experienced at times like this: disbelief, despair, and denial may alternate with fear, fortitude, and fatalism. The initial crisis encompasses a turmoil of many feelings, which come and go with a confusing unpredictability.

The age of the sufferer makes a difference to the immediate response (Edlund *et al.*, 1989). Younger people experience more distress, but older people are less positive about the outcome. This suggests that the young feel more cheated but are better able to learn coping strategies to deal effectively with the disease and its treatment. The person's knowledge and previous experience also will inevitably affect his response and beliefs about the future.

In terms of the nurse's own beliefs about the prognosis of patients in her care, it is likely that he or she may significantly influence the client's views about cancer and its treatment. Assessment of the nurse's perspective reveals a pessimism about prognosis that exceeds reality. While the nurse's attitudes to cancer are based on experience, this outlook may be underpinned by irrational assumptions: his or her experience will not necessarily reflect the total picture of cancer, its incidence, the way it affects the body, its prognosis, and potential for cure (Ray *et al.*, 1984). The beliefs and feelings the nurse has about the effectiveness of treatment is likely to be internalized by the client, emphasizing the importance of nurse input in caring for the person with cancer.

Attitudes to cancer have been evaluated in relation to both the quality of life and the outcome of the disease (Greer *et al.*, 1979), and it has been suggested that the way a person reacts to the disease may influence its course. Women with breast cancer were assessed three months postoperatively, and outcome evaluated at five years. People without recurrence were more likely to have been assessed as having a 'fighting spirit' or exhibiting denial than being fatalistic or hopeless. Nelson

*et al.* (1989) has attempted to analyze these attitudes, and determined that a 'fighting spirit' and information-seeking are linked to the ability to fight back, conquer, and recover from cancer.

Some people with cancer are demonstrating their lack of fatalism and passivity by seeking treatment not generally available through the NHS, for example, healing therapy, hypnotherapy, drastic dietary changes, aromatherapy, and reflex zone therapy. For some these are viewed as alternative to orthodox treatment, for others an addition.

The controversy recently was fuelled by an address given by the Prince of Wales, which challenged the medical profession to examine in more detail the claims made by alternative therapy (BMA, 1986). One of the comments made in the report, which summarized their findings, is that, 'only properly designed clinical trials will justify the choice of alternative treatments'. The effects of many of the alternative therapies were assessed as being equivalent to the sort of good medical practice that takes the whole of the person into consideration.

The possibility of stress as a provocateur of disease arises frequently in clients who seek alternative or complementary therapies in their fight for control. In their search for the reason 'why', recent traumas in their life are often cited as the 'cause' of the cancer. Greer (1983) reported there was no evidence to support the idea that stress can cause cancer in the work he reviewed. Nevertheless, the search continues to demonstrate a link between emotions, defence mechanisms, and oncogenesis, the cause of cancer.

The reactions outlined above are the expected and common responses encountered in people with life-threatening diseases. For a proportion of those, the adjustment to their disease is not effective; they may be unable to cope adequately either with the fact of the disease or with its treatments. Although the presentation of anxiety states and depressive illnesses is still relatively uncommon in people with cancer, there is still a large group of people whose emotional state is not adaptive. If these people were assessed in a psychiatric setting, they may not necessarily be evaluated as mentally ill; in the physical-illness setting, degrees of adjustment are defined differently.

## ASSESSMENT

Determining the psychological state of people following a diagnosis of a life-threatening illness is part of the nursing role. Methods of assessment include interviews with the person and the family, observation of affect and behaviour, and psychometric testing. In a physical-illness setting, it is easy to take the client at face value: 'How are you, Mrs Smith?' 'Fine, thank you.' The person in the client role still tends to believe the doctor knows best: 'The nurses and doctors are much too busy to listen to my worries.'

Channels of communication between the client and the helper are frequently the source of distress. Many patients wait to be given information, while the doctor may at the same time be waiting for the client to ask the questions. The nurse wishing to assess the psychological state of the client is more likely to get the information he or she seeks if they are prepared to set aside time to ask the right questions and to wait for the full answers to be given. The interview, therefore, is one of the first methods to use when attempting to evaluate a person's emotional state. Observation of the person's demeanour may give some indication, but in this setting, where serious physical disorder predominates, it may be wrongly assumed that 'this is the way Mrs Smith has always behaved'.

People admitted for physical care do not automatically give a full social and psychological history. It is unsafe to assume, for example, that Mrs Smith's husband will be supportive and care for the children, and that their relationship is sound and stable. Their sexual relationship may not be satisfactory; the practicalities of coming into hospital, leaving a full-time job, rearranging family commitments, and so on, may have a major impact on Mrs Smith's reactions to this event. It is therefore relevant routinely to discover the social history of people with physical disease.

Evaluation of psychological status with the use of psychometry, measurement with standard tests, has increased, along with the concern for the quality of life. Structured interviews with predetermined questions or self-report questionnaires may be used to assess certain aspects of a person's coping style.

Tests that are well recognized in the field of psychiatry, however, have been found less useful when applied to physical-illness settings. Many people with cancer or other disabling illnesses experience physical symptoms that may be identical to those of depression and/or anxiety. This prompted the development of the Hospital Anxiety and Depression Scale (Snaith, 1976), a self-report questionnaire focusing on some non-physical attributes that feature in anxiety and depression. It helps to identify the seriously distressed person more effectively than the observations and enquiries of a physically oriented doctor.

The following case study highlights the need for routine psychosocial assessments of patients with physical illness.

CASE STUDY – MRS CASTLE

Mrs Castle attended a treatment department regularly for a brief time each day for cancer-related therapy. No one appeared to notice her depressed state. During part of a research enquiry, which does not include all patients, she was interviewed by a research assistant and asked to complete a number of psychometric questionnaires. During the second meeting with the researcher, a psychiatric nurse, she described a history of serious depression for which she was continuing to take antidepressant medication, a fact that had been noted without further qualification in the medical notes.

The existing prescription of an antidepressant can lead us to believe there is no need to enquire more deeply into a person's emotional state. Without the use of specific enquiry, this person's serious psychiatric morbidity would not have been detected at the beginning of her therapy, as her belief system was based on assumptions that no one and nothing could help her. She was also able to mask her depression for the brief time of interaction required for the cancer treatment. Her reaction to the cancer was just another major hurdle for her to climb. She appeared less distressed by the cancer diagnosis than by the irrational fears concerning the radiotherapy. In assessing her quality of life in one perspective, she may pass the test: she was looking after her appearance; saying the 'right' things to short, superficial questioning; and maintaining household activities as previously.

Specific questionnaires have been developed to gain further information in physical-illness settings. Greer *et al.* (1987) have developed a self-report questionnaire that aims to assess a person's attitude to cancer and beliefs about their illnesses. It is currently in use at cancer centres in many countries. In order to evaluate the effectiveness of a new treatment, adjuvant psychotherapy, so-called as it is given in tandem with any other physical therapy required, is given to patients experiencing high levels of psychiatric morbidity. Clients are assessed one to three months following their learning of a primary diagnosis or first recurrence of cancer, with a prognosis of at least a year. (Greer *et al.* 1992).

It is important to note that people do not always reflect their true feelings when answering a questionnaire. All methods of assessment used in tandem are more likely to give an accurate picture. When a person's reactions and coping style are accurately identified, it is more likely that interventions will be accurate, preventative, and educational.

A diagnosis of cancer may be given to someone suffering from other physical or emotional difficulties, with which they had been coping adequately. 'The last straw' of a cancer diagnosis may precipitate such people into a phase of acute distress, resembling perhaps an anxiety state or a depressive illness. The resolution of this reaction can be relatively quick, especially when crisis intervention is given. Unidentified maladaptive coping, however, may progress into disorders requiring longer-term therapy.

## SPECIFIC PROBLEMS

Despite investigations, it is sometimes difficult to differentiate between physical, emotional, and neurological symptoms. The most effective way to achieve the differential diagnosis is within the multidisciplinary team, whereby the members are able to use the diverse perspectives of their specialities to discuss, examine, and therefore apply a wider sphere of knowledge.

Is the bizarre behaviour the patient is displaying due to cerebral secondaries from the cancer? Perhaps it is the result of a biochemical disturbance, due to the side-effects of a drug, or an electrolyte imbalance created by the disease. Acute or chronic pain, inadequately controlled, provokes distress and irritability. Nausea and vomiting caused by the disease or its treatment can reduce a person's tolerance to his or her acquired limitations. Decreased nutritional intake with resulting malnutrition and weight loss has a major impact on a person and his relatives; altered appearance as perceived by the person may create an emotional vulnerability. Equally, physical weakness may provoke deep fatigue. It is not always immediately obvious to any of the team which problem is causative; it may be a combination of several.

Often, the resolution of a physical problem enables immediate emotional recovery. The less resolute person, however, may succumb to a depressive illness that does not resolve when relief from the physical problem is gained. Observation, investigations, and discussion will clarify the difficulties in many situations, and facilitate the most effective remedies.

The demands of attending for cancer treatment over many weeks, months or years, draw on the person's physical and psychological resources to the limits of endurance. The thought of another course of treatment may sometimes be more than seems possible to take. The cumulative effects of emotional and physical traumas may precipitate a psychological crisis. An instance of this is apparent in the following case:

CASE STUDY – NONA

Although Nona had asked for help, her emotional distress had not been identified by professionals in the clinic. She had been through a series of investigations over several months, the results of which had not been positively indicative of a particular abnormality. Eventually, a firm diagnosis was made of cancer of the kidney. Nona, however, was not given any treatment, nor was there any to be given for the time being: the disease in her case was not operable, nor was it likely to respond to conventional treatments. A drug under research was the only option.

Nona found the lack of treatment very frightening, worrying that every physical change she experienced might be the cancer spreading. A fear of death predominated her thoughts. Despite this, she felt she should be able to completely control her life, to the extent that a dramatic change in diet precipitated abdominal difficulties.

She was equally disturbed by having to come to the centre frequently for assessment of her disease. During clinical appointments she experienced such severe panic that any questions or opinions she had wished to voice vanished. She became distraught, weepy, and noticed her heart racing, hands shaking and her throat blocking. She thought she might not attend the centre again, as it felt intolerable. Psychotherapy enabled her to face more realistically the uncertainty with which she had to live, and to be able to express her viewpoint at the clinic. Her fear of death, however, only diminished a little.

Again we see an example of a person who is continuing to work, appears physically fit despite considerable disease, is participating actively in her social life, but is experiencing a major anxiety state, which has not been identified by the physically oriented professional.

There are people who regard their diagnosis with irrational pessimism: despite having no further evidence of disease following treatment, which is known effectively to control and cure some cancers, anxiety and depression may persist, preventing some people from participating actively or appropriately in life, as reflected in the next example.

CASE STUDY – WENDY

Nine years after a initial diagnosis of breast cancer, Wendy asked for help, complaining of a tight feeling in her chest, and fears of going on buses, of talking to people, and of a feeling in her stomach that the cancer had come back. Since her treatment, Wendy had been physically completely clear of any evidence of cancer, yet these feelings were interfering with her ability to continue with life as she felt she would like. For example, she had changed employment from a clerical position to a part-time domestic job in a motel because she thought she was not strong enough to stay on, and she did not drive, despite having passed her driving test some years ago.

With the help of a counsellor, Wendy was able to resume life more effectively. Her new job is more rewarding. She travels on buses without fear, and chats to her neighbours without the same nervousness. She has also taken some refresher driving lessons, with the hope of increasing her chances of visiting family living further afield. She is able to challenge any thoughts of her cancer spreading.

Wendy was able to see for herself that life was not as it should be for her, and asked for help; she had not been assessed by a researcher with regard to quality of life or emotional status.

The appearance in a cancer ward of unusual behaviour is commonly due to a drug effect, at other times it may be the effect of the disease process, which is less easily rectified. Appropriate treatment for this may not take effect immediately, giving the person and carers a troublesome period. The change in behaviour can be sudden, the actions unpredictable, and the responses emotionally laden. It may be some time before the answers are accredited to cerebral organic disease.

## CASE STUDY – ANDREW AND JULIE

Andrew shouted suddenly at Julie, his wife of five years. After a traumatic few weeks, a cancer was found to have spread to his brain. Julie was overwhelmed with despair: Andrew was her life; they had married late and were very close. There was no curative treatment available, therapy rather aiming to give relief from symptoms.

The cancer continued to spread, and Andrew died after a year of progressive pain and disability. Julie was very angry: Andrew knew Julie would find his death overwhelming, but he had been ready to face the end of life because his faith in God was strong.

Julie raged, wept, and despaired for several months after Andrew's death. He had not been well looked after; she was angry with him 'for being at peace at the thought of leaving her'; she was angry with his family for laying claim to him; she was angry with the world for being cruel; she felt no support from her sisters; she turned away from her faith.

Bereavement work over eight months on a weekly basis enabled Julie to feel there was a future for her without Andrew. She has found some peace, has looked again at her faith, and is working towards a deeper involvement in her church. She is giving limited support to a neighbour who later lost her husband, offering the name of the support service she had found useful. Julie looks now at the possibility of finding employment; she has taken driving lessons and passed her test. She can now speak about Andrew without the heart-rending sobs that used to accompany her words. Although she felt cancer destroyed her life, she was helped to find new purpose and meaning.

## SEXUAL FUNCTIONING AND ILLNESS

The impairment of sexual functioning during physical illness has been explored by health professionals. For example, North (1988) describes the existence of sexual problems in a large percentage of patients following bypass operations, and Bard *et al.*, (1953) reported a fear of sexual relations following breast surgery. Such anxiety may be experienced by both partners, which may then lead to an absence of physical closeness, especially when individual fears are not discussed. In patients with lung cancer, sexual problems were rated as a significant difficulty (Ryan, 1987); and patients with testicular cancer reported a deterioration in their sexual lives following diagnosis (Moynihan, 1988).

Cancer and its treatment may affect fertility and/or libido, the causative agent being physical or psychological; it may also, however, be based on faulty assumptions. The woman with breast cancer who has had surgery, radiotherapy, and medication to block hormone function will commonly experience a loss of libido. The traumatic experience of a cancer diagnosis, and the subsequent physical assault on her body drives physical desire to a lower level of priority. Following the initial period of treatment, many women recover libido, and are able to resume physical relations.

## ANTICIPATORY FACTORS

A significant problem encountered in the care of the person with cancer is anticipatory nausea and vomiting. The person who is required to attend a cancer centre for frequent drug treatment that induces nausea and vomiting may develop such symptoms before the administration of the drugs. The timing of the appearance of the symptom depends on the pairing of stimulus and response, which may take place as in classical conditioning. Some clients may experience symptoms the day before they are scheduled for admission; others will vomit when they see, smell, or taste something associated with the feelings. Pratt (1984) cites anti-emetic chemotherapy, and behavioural techniques such as relaxation, biofeedback, and desensitization as ways of alleviating the problems.

## INTERVENTIONS

The mental health nurse has a more significant part to play in treating physical illnesses than is generally realized. Though helping people to face the problems caused by illness and the physical problems, the negative effects are diminished. Skills that are practised in a psychiatric setting are equally valid in the care of the physically ill person (Chapter 19). Adaptation to caring for the physically ill person is within the range of abilities of the mental health nurse.

While short episodes of emotional distress may be anticipated and accepted as reaction to bad news, if the person does not adjust and resume adaptive coping styles, psychological morbidity ensues. By using active listening, the more psychologically distressed person can be identified and referred on to a psychotherapist. The need for referral depends on the skills and the time available of the professional in daily contact with the person. Appropriate help, with support and advice, can be given to the nurse by the mental health nurse. Any member of the caring team may be the key person for the distressed client. A physiotherapist, for example, spends frequent and long periods of time encouraging and facilitating a disabled person towards rehabilitation. There are, however, inevitably times when more specialized psychotherapy is required.

The style of therapy deemed to be appropriate depends on the skills of the therapist and on the reaction of the person in distress. In a physical-illness setting, where the promptness of physical treatment may be of life-saving importance, speedy relief from psychological distress is valued because such relief has a positive effect on recovery; and effectiveness of physical treatment is often dependent on active co-operation from the patient. A therapist with the ability to use different strategies is therefore appreciated. Alternatively, access to a number of psychological practitioners with differing skills may be preferable. Behaviour therapy techniques can be most effective with patients experiencing anxiety, anticipatory nausea and vomiting. Cognitive therapy is an effective technique for people able to give regular time to sessions, and who are committed to improving their coping ability.

Moorey *et al.,* (1989) describe a combination of helping skills that may be given at the same time as any cancer treatments. Allowing the person to express his feelings, so as to clarify the problem areas, is the first stage of this therapy. Collaboration is an essential component, with the client being given control over which problems are to be tackled. Behavioural strategies and cognitive techniques are a major component of the sessions.

The following case study shows the value of using more than one model of therapy.

## CASE STUDY – MARGERY

Margery was referred for help following a bilateral mastectomy. She was a 55-year-old unmarried woman, who had recently moved to a rural location with an old friend following their retirement. On initial assessment, Margery appeared to be mildly depressed, and so supportive counselling was begun. An unfortunate break in counselling saw a severe change in Margery's emotional state, resulting in her admission to a psychiatric hospital near her home.

On her return to the cancer centre, Margery was prescribed antidepressant medication, and a programme of therapy was planned. Behavioural strategies were discussed, and explained to her friend, who agreed to help Margery to initiate the programme at home, with review and assessment on a twice-weekly basis with the therapist. After several weeks, it was possible to introduce with effect some cognitive techniques.

Depression was a new experience for Margery, who never failed to question the reasons for its existence. With some exploration of her earlier life, it was discovered that Margery had abandoned an important relationship with a man to whom she had planned to become engaged in order to look after ailing parents. The removal of both breasts may

well have triggered feelings she had repressed for many years.

Margery recovered over a period of nine months sufficiently to support her friend through surgery for a cancer which she subsequently developed.

In this instance it was appropriate and helpful to use a number of therapeutic techniques to assist one person towards a better adjustment. There are times too when long-term psychodynamic psychotherapy has its place, for example in the following:

## CASE STUDY – JANE

Jane and her mother went to visit her father in a ward in the cancer centre. Jane appeared to be very distressed, and on one occasion was seen to lose control, taking hold of her mother by the wrists and shouting at her. The registrar identified this event as the tip of an emotional iceberg.

Jane was interviewed by the hospital psychiatrist and referred for psychotherapy. An appropriately trained psychiatric nurse was therapist to Jane for 18 months. At 40, Jane had a long history of emotional turmoil associated with the disturbed relationship she had with her mother. Facilitating an understanding of her perceptions of this turmoil, and how they impinged on her other relationships, allowed Jane to grow out of many of the maternal chains that bound her.

A major change in a person's life, which strongly effects his perspective and priorities, may precipitate a wish to change his lifestyle. For some, a sense of determination combined with joy is apparent. If, however, the physical therapy takes over the routine completely, it is sometimes difficult for the person with the disorder and those close to them to reorganize their lives with a sense of purpose. Relatives may feel isolated from their loved one, and helpless in the face of suffering. Even a good relationship may shake during long-term treatment regimes, threatening its stability.

Ill people are not exempt from domestic upheavals. The professional may find that the distress a person is experiencing appears to bear little relation to his physical problems: it may, for example, be a son or daughter with drug problems, or a spouse who abuses alcohol. There is a place for help with such difficulties, which may at the diagnosis of the illness be acknowledged. Seeking help outside the treatment centre is often the appropriate answer, although sometimes the skills of caring for the physical needs of the person need to be carried out in tandem with psychological help.

Specific basic knowledge of physical treatments and their effects will assist the nurse and other professionals in distinguishing the multitude of symptoms that combine to confuse the investigator. It is usual for those who accept help for emotional problems to be outpatients, therefore time may elapse between physical clinical appointments. There are occasions when speedy physical treatment may be the more appropriate action for an apparent psychological problem. Unsuspected secondary disease may be precipitating symptoms that mimic a depression. At other times, they may cause a behaviour change that is only noticeable to the close relatives.

### A NEW APPROACH

The most important facet in establishing new approaches is to advertise the reasons for their development, and to inform and educate.

It is likely there will be many professionals who are able to help, very competently, the distressed people with whom they work. There are, however, a proportion of staff who are unable or unwilling to delve into the emotional depths of the lives of others. Equally, there are people who cannot be helped with kindness and patience alone.

Education on the relationship between mind and body is an essential component if we are to develop a new approach. The very nature of the time and privacy required to carry out therapy, highlights the input a psychiatric nurse therapist may have. The psychiatric nurse builds a working service by maintaining a high profile with other carers, along with regular personal education to keep abreast of developments. The service is most effective when focused on the concerns the nurses meet in their work; the identification of psychological problems is the key issue; without this, nurses may fail to provide the best possible care.

Supervision and support for the psychiatric nurse is an essential component of both professional personal education and growth. Links with others in similar working environments allow a network to develop, and skills and knowledge to be shared.

### CONCLUSION

The recovery of people living with physical disorders is enhanced by a number of factors. Nurses have a direct impact: empathic support from both professional and lay carers is paramount for positive change in the sufferer. Such support is most effective when the psychological needs of the ill person are identified and met. Involvement of and discussion with the friends or relatives in the day-to-day treatments enlarges the working knowledge of the professional team. In many situations, key input is provided by someone from among this group who has a close affinity with the sufferer. Effective teamwork requires two-way communication that is both positive and constructive. Individuals who choose to work autonomously may find themselves without important information, which could influence their treatment approach.

Improved psychological status inevitably hastens the recovery from the physical condition, and may enhance the prognosis of the person with a life-threatening physical disorder; constant monitoring of the whole health status is vital to this end.

The attitudes of the people in close contact with the sufferer are likely to influence the expectations and mode of coping within the immediate circle. It is therefore of paramount importance that nurses have up-to-date facts, and check their own outlook continually. Consequently, the nurses' educational and emotional needs should be met through regular support and clinical supervision (Chapter 25).

Adapting psychiatric skills to help the physically ill is a rewarding activity, and is beginning to be accepted and viewed as an integral part of the care a person is offered. However, there are still many treatment centres with staff members to whom the person is just a body. Attitudes are slow to change. Innovation requires commitment, understanding, skills, and energy. The financial constraints which changes in NHS structure have produced, specifically in the psychological care available, provide an equally demanding challenge. Research-based clinical practice and education, developed together, provide the individual with the best chance of acceptable recovery and rehabilitation.

## REFERENCES

Bard, M. and Sutherland, A. (1955) Psychological impact of cancer and its treatment. *Cancer*, 8:4, 656–72.

Bass, C. and Akhras, F (1987) Physical and psychological correlates of severe heart disease in men. *Psychological Medicine*, 17, 695–703.

BMA Alternative Therapy (1986) Report of the Board of Science and Education, BMA, London.

Brown, T. (1989) Cartesian dualism and psychosomatics. *Psychosomatics*, 30, 3:322–31.

Cassileth, B.; Lusk, S.; Strouse, T. *et al.*, (1984) Psychosocial status in chronic illness. *New England J. Medicine*, 311, 506–11.

Cella, D.; Tross, S.; Orav, E. J. *et al.*, (1989) Mood states of patients after the diagnosis of cancer. *J. Psychosocial Oncology*, 7:1/2, 45–53.

De Haes, J. C. J. M. (1988) Quality of life: conceptual and theoretical considerations, in *Psychosocial Oncology* (M. Watson, H. S. Greer, Pergamon Press, London.)

Edlund, B. and Sneed, N. (1989) Emotional responses to the diagnosis of cancer: age-related comparisons. *Oncology Nursing Forum*, 16:5, 691–7.

Eisenberg, H. S. and Goldenberg, I. S. (1966) A measurement of quality of survival of breast cancer patients, in *Clinical Evaluation in Breast Cancer* (Hayward and Bulbrook), Academic.

Galbraith, Thomas S. (1978) Breast cancer: the psychosocial issues. *Cancer Nursing*. Feb., 53–60.

Greer, S., Morris, T. and Pettingale, K. W. (1979) Psychological response to breast cancer: effect on outcome. *The Lancet*, Oct. 785–87.

Greer, S. (1983) Cancer and the mind. *Brit. J. Psychiatry*, 143, 553–43.

Greer, S. and Watson, M. (1987) Mental adjustment to cancer: its measurement and prognostic importance. *Cancer Surveys*, 6, 439–53.

Greer, S., Moorey, S., Baruch, J. D. *et al.*, (1992) Adjuvant psychological therapy for patients with cancer: a prospective randomized trial. *British Medical J.* 304, 675–80.

Lipowski, Z. J. (1977) Psychomatic medicine in the seventies: an overview. *Amer. J. Psychiatry*, 134:3, 233–44.

Lugton, J. (1989) Relatives: identifying anxieties. *Nursing Times*, 85:17, 50–1.

Maguire, G. P., Lee, E. G.; Bevington D. J. *et al.* (1978) Psychiatric problems in the first year after mastectomy. *British Medical J.*, 15 April, 963–5.

McCorkle, R. and Quint-Benoliel, J. (1983) Symptom distress, current concerns and mood disturbance after diagnosis of life threatening disease. *Social Science and Medicine*, 17:7, 431–8.

Moorey, S. and Greer, S. (1989) *Psychological Therapy for Patients with Cancer: A New Approach*, Heinemann, London.

Monynihan, C. (1988) The psychosocial effects of the diagnosis and treatment of testicular cancer: a retrospective study, 7:2, 18–20.

Nelson, D.; Friedman, L. C.; Baer, P. E. *et al.* (1989) Attitudes to cancer: psychometric properties of fighting spirit and denial. *J. Behavioural Medicine*. 12:4, 341–55.

North, N. (1988) Psychosocial aspects of coronary artery by-pass surgery. *Nursing Times*, 84:1, 26–9.

Pratt, A., Lazar, R. M., Penman, D. *et al.* (1984) Psychological parameters of chemotherapy-induced conditioned nausea and vomiting: a review. *Cancer Nursing*, Dec. 483–90.

Ray, C., Grover, J. and Wisniewski, T. (1984) Nurses' perceptions of early breast cancer and mastectomy, and their psychological implications, and of the role of health professionals in proving support. *Inter. J. Nursing Studies*, 21:2, 101–11.

Ron, M. and Logsdail, S. (1989) Psychiatric morbidity in multiple sclerosis: a clinical and MRI study. *Psychological Medicine*, 19, 887–95.

Snaith, R. P.; Bridge, G.W.K. and Hamilton, M. (1976) The Leeds Scales for the self-assessment of anxiety and depression. *Brit. J. Psychiatry*, 128, 156–65.

Specht Ryan, L. (1987) Lung cancer: psychosocial implications. *Seminars in Oncology Nursing*, 3:3, 222–7.

Weiner, H. (1987) Some unexplored regions of psychosomatic medicine. *Psychother. Psychosom.* 47, 153–9.

# MENTAL HEALTH AND THE ELDERLY

## 17

*Mic Rafferty*

To understand the issues involved in working with and caring for elderly people with brain failure, one has to understand something of the position of the aged person in our society.

Ageing could be seen as a preoccupation of the 1990s. This is due to demographic realities: as census data and projections show (Table 17.1), we are a greying society (OPCS, 1981, 1988).

Although there is emerging evidence of changing attitudes to elderly people – as a result of the increasing awareness of the contribution older people make to the social good, because of child and sick-care services (Jeffries, 1987), and the growing economic power of the 'young old' (Abrams, 1989), – there is still a fair measure of ambivalent and frankly negative feelings towards elderly people. This is no more blatantly obvious than in cartoons. Sheppard (1981) identified four categories of cartoons about the elderly: disparagement, ineffectuality, obsolescence, and isolation. He also noted the frequent appearance of stereotyped characters, such as the 'dirty old man' and the 'little old lady'. This may be because there is a negative, or ageist, reaction to the physical changes, and the increased potential for death and dependency on others, which is an inevitable result of the biological ageing process (Robb, 1984).

Decisions about retirement age, which has led to the dependence of elderly people on a paternalistic state and restrictions on earning potential, play a part in producing a complex social norm (Blaikie *et al.* 1989). This has later life portrayed as a time for a forced well-earned rest, with expectations of incompetence and a marginal guarantee of life quality. This is demonstrated, for example, by a 'cold-weather allowance', which does not prevent the UK from having the highest death rate among elderly people from the cold among member states of the European Common Market (Verstbeeg, 1990).

Such biological and social realities must interrelate with and be shaped and shape psychological development in later life. Erikson (1965) suggests that a task of old age is the summative synthesis of one's experience; pushed together are past experiences, present realities, and anticipated futures, which potentially contain the origins of extreme perspectives about the self and one's social congruence, best characterized by integrity on one hand and despair on the other.

The issues of later life are complex and vibrant, and can begin to be conceptualized as a bio-psychosocial experience.

**Table 17.1** Size of population aged 65 and over (in 100s, England and Wales)

| Total aged | 65+ | | 65–74 | | 75–84 | | 85+ | |
|---|---|---|---|---|---|---|---|---|
| | No. | % | No. | % | No. | % | No. | % |
| 1981* | 7274 | 100 | 4488 | 61.7 | 2279 | 31.8 | 507 | 7.0 |
| 1991** | 7939 | 100 | 4446 | 56.0 | 2719 | 34.2 | 774 | 9.8 |
| 2000** | 7808 | 100 | 4131 | 52.9 | 2726 | 34.9 | 951 | 12.2 |

Source: *1981 Census (OPCS, 1981); **OPCS Projections (OPCS, 1988).

## DEMENTIA

Chronic brain failure is not an uncommon event of later life; research estimates suggest a rate of 1–7% of those aged 65 and over. Prevalence rises markedly with age, and may affect as many as 20% of people over the age of 80 (Askham *et al.*, 1990). This also is a bio-psychosocial experience, although one that often seems savage rather than vibrant.

Little is known of the subjective experience of severe brain failure; what is often proposed is inferred from behaviour. With cognitive decline, it is assumed that higher-order experiences, for instance the ability to have a range of emotions, ceases. This, coupled with the loss of the ability to move one's body in a co-ordinated way, and to have or control reflexes or sphincters, and to use verbal avenues to be understood and understand, leads severe dementia to be described as a 'vegetative state' (Huppert *et al.*, 1986). This has been described as a living death: 'What you have to all intents and purposes is an uncollected corpse, the living dead. It is a bereavement (for the carer) which is constantly stressed and irritated by the fact that the body has not departed.' (Miller, 1988).

It is important to try to counter such a bleak and harrowing reality by remembering that the real person is not submerged by dementia until late in the process. The tragic climax has to be seen as an end-stage picture of a syndrome that may span ten years or more, and which may begin innocuously with headaches and visual disturbances.

## CASE STUDY – MR IDRIS

"Six months after Mr Idris retired, he began to complain of headaches and visual disturbances. Shortly after he suffered a cerebral vascular accident (CVA), but made good recovery, even regaining his driving license a year later.

However, Mr Idris's interest in his former activities gradually declined, for example, he would not go to the pub any more, almost as if attributing all the blame for his CVA on drink. In fact, the only things he would drink now were tea and water. As time passed, he found it increasingly difficult to make decisions, and he reluctantly gave up driving after his car handling became erratic.

Six years later, Mr Idris suffered an acute confusional state brought about by viral pneumonia and a urinary tract infection (UTI), and was admitted to hospital. Deterioration in his mental function was rapid. Behavioural difficulties manifested themselves in the form of being unable to hold a conversation, to concentrate, or to dress himself. There were bizzare episodes of persecution during which he would believe the people on television were after him, so he would hide in the cellar for hours at a time. He continued to take his daily walks, but in the middle of the road. He would shout at the neighbours, and pull up newly planted shrubs in the garden.

Mrs Idris found it increasingly difficult to cope with her husband's forgetfulness, aggression, and anti-social behaviour, and her husband was admitted to hospital for respite care. It was then suggested by the geriatrician that his needs would be better met in a long-term care ward, and he was admitted informally."

R. Johns, 1989

Such a process of transformation has to be understood in terms of identifiable neuro-psychological deficits and medical conditions, which together produce the brain failure. But if we accept that, like ageing, brain failure has social and psychological dimensions, then dementia must be understood with reference to the psychological and social process.

Dementia, like ageing, is a negatively valued experience. This statement, however, does not do justice to the dread and stigma associated with this condition. One only has to acknowledge that such individuals have been described as the 'living dead', or that the integration of elderly people with psychogeriatric conditions and those with geriatric conditions is extremely difficult – the 'geriatrics' (and often their staff) finding the presence of psychogeriatrics disturbing – to realize that the person with brain failure quickly becomes a non-person. A common response to anticipating this state is 'shoot me first.'

The psychological consequences of insight about cognitive changes, coupled with the experience of others changing their ways of relating, can easily result in catastrophic reactions: that is, terror and panic. This can provoke further bio-psychosocial crises, leading to a cycle that may have significance in the way the dementia career unfolds for the individual with brain failure.

## THE AGEING EXPERIENCE

That a bio-psychosocial process is central to understanding dementia suggests that effective work with people who have dementia will be based upon an understanding of the process of ageing.

There are many different explanations for the process of ageing. One, supported by research, has demonstrated an aged-related decline in the efficiency of homeostatic systems necessary to enable the cells that make up the major organs to cope with and repair damage caused by physical, chemical, and biological adversaries (Hipkiss *et al.*, 1989). This is demonstrated in clinical practice when a fragile, if competent, homeostatic balance is stressed to breakdown. For example, in ageing there is a tendency for the large bones to become increasingly brittle. This is usually not problematic until the aged person falls, when the critical homeostatic balance in the bone can be overwhelmed, and a fracture occurs.

That 'life invariably leads to death' is no better illustrated than by the recognition that the fall might have occurred because of a number of biological changes found in later life that can influence balance and mobility. This may be followed by reactions in other homeostatic systems, for instance those concerned with the protection or repair of soft tissue, or the oxygenation and circulation of the blood, demonstrating the aged body's inability to maintain the *status quo* when faced by a stressor outside a certain range.

Biological trauma has been demonstrated to have psychosocial consequences, for instance, the older person experiencing negative changes in self-concept as a result of falls (Downton, 1990); or becoming more dependent upon their partner or concerned others to manage communication with the wider community, as a result of unwillingness to venture outside the home because of fears of falling.

It is important, however, not to overemphasize homeostatic fragility. It helps if old age is viewed as a time period that can cover two generations. There is then the likelihood of markedly different health status, psychological attitudes, and social expectations of people at different ends of the two generational continua. Two such age bands describe as the 'young old' people who are aged 65–74, and 'the older old' as aged 75 or more (Abrams, 1989). Homeostatic frailty should be viewed as something that has a tendency to increase with age in a graduated way, and which is linked to individual genetic dispositions.

That the ageing process is an individual experience is further illustrated by attention to the psychological aspect. A current understanding of the psychological process of later life suggests inevitable mourning for what one has not achieved. This is a normal experience, as no one can achieve perfection, where individual deficiencies, difficulties, and losses are taken up, reworked, and grieved for, hopefully with the outcome of successful adjustment to old age.

When this is not the case, as, for example, when the loss of a partner results in a pathological grief reaction, the implication for homeostatic systems balance may not just be confined to psychological aspects of the self. Physiological aspects can be undermined as a result of failure to maintain competence in activities of daily living, for example, as a result of an inadequate diet. Physiological disturbance can also result from the mal-adaptive strategies the individual employs to help him deaden the feelings of despair, for example as a result of alcohol abuse. That physiological changes result from life trau-mas is most powerfully illustrated by re-search showing that immunological systems are suppressed by psychological stressors (Wilson-Barnett, 1979).

The tightness of the interaction between the biological, psychological, and the social aspects of the aged person is reinforced by studies that explore the social context of the person, and show that the formation and maintenance of relationships are necessary aspects of well-being and health. In one study, 'among those in their 60s at the start of a nine-year follow-up period, the risk of dying among the most socially isolated females was three times that of those with most connections.' (Grundy, 1979).

An emphasis in turn upon three aspects of the aged person demonstrates that each has the potential to produce a transformation in all three aspects, and provides a foundation for understanding the dementias.

## DEMENTIA

We will now explore the condition of dementia, focusing in turn upon biological, psychological, and social dimensions.

ORGANIC EMPHASIS

The Royal College of Physicians (1981) define the condition as:

Global impairment of higher mental function including memory, the capacity to solve the problems of day-to-day living, the performance of learned skills, the correct use of social skills, and control of emotional reactions without clouding of consciousness.

What this means in terms of the devastation of the individual's sense of self may be appreciated by reference to a three-stage model of severity for Alzheimer's disease (Huppert *et al.*, 1986).

In the first stage, decline in memory of more recent events is the most pronounced feature. Ability to recall and use mental ground plans and judge distance deteriorates, and disorientation, particularly in a time sense and the ability to locate the self accur-ately, becomes frequent. The person begins to have problems focusing for any length of time upon a task. A general tiredness may become self-evident, coupled with a gener-alized agitation and state of hyper-alertness. The individual's usual way of expressing himself through idiosyncratic habits and ways may become exaggerated or altered, and there may be disturbances of mood.

In the second stage of Alzheimer's disease, all aspects of memory are seen to fail. The person has difficulty speaking, carrying out actions, and identifying objects. Evidence of neurological damage is shown by the occur-rence of fits in 5–10% of those diagnosed as having the disorder. The range of emotional expression available to the person begins to be lost. He is experienced as lacking in in-terest and indifferent to events around him. Abilities to decide between alternatives, and to exercise problem-solving and numeracy skills have gone.

In the final, third, stage:

...there is gross disturbance of all intellectual functions. There are marked focal neurological deficits, and increase in muscle tone appears with accom-panying slow, wide-based and unsteady gait. There is gross emotional dis-inhibition, and the former personality becomes submerged. Patients cannot recognize relatives or even their own face in the mirror. They are bedfast and increasingly incapacitated through spasticity and myoclonus. Double incontinence is almost invariable at this stage. There is progressive wasting despite a voracious appetite, but life may continue for one or more years in an almost vegetative state.

Huppert *et al.*, 1986

This picture of a relatively short life expectancy for the person who is severely demented is supported by the identification of an epidemiological relationship between poor cognition and increased mortality. Death often results from pneumonia or some other intercurrent infection (Brayne *et al.*, 1988).

Caution, though, needs to be exercised in assumptions made about the early demise of the 'chronic dement'. The studies reviewed determined the duration of the disease ranged from 2.5 to 20 years, although the majority of cases did fall within a narrower band of approximately 5–10 years (Hart, 1990).

It is important to emphasize again that the clinical picture will be unique to the individual, and diagnostic generalizations may actually be unhelpful, leading to assumptions and unfounded expectations about presentation and progression. What is presently agreed is that memory disturbance is an early presenting feature, but considerable disagreement exists because of individual variation as to the point of occurrence of other symptoms. Such disagreement about symptomatology explains something about why it is difficult to make a definitive diagnosis. For example, Alzheimer's disease cannot be diagnosed with certainty during life; and even at death there is apparently no tight definition of what are the criteria to indicate brain failure pathology at post-mortem.

Particular attention has been paid to a diagnostic stereotype for Alzheimer's disease because it is the most prevalent diagnostic type identified, and a patient career model is helpful to illustrate a general progression. The intention is to focus on general models and cautions that are relevant because they may assist the understanding of what can be a very painful family event. It is important to realize that each dementia type, such as Huntington's chorea or Parkinson's disease, may have unique characteristics that will have important significance for management and nursing care.

This approach is appropriate, for although the early symptoms and course of the most common dementias – Alzheimer's and multi-infarct – may differ slightly, by the time the patient has a moderate degree of impairment, one preliminary study found few behavioural differences, and no overall difference in impact on the family (Zarit, 1990).

Scepticism about diagnostic views of disease progression is important in challenging the assumptions of inevitable decline that are evoked by the concept or label of dementia. There are problems with accepting without question that a diagnosis of dementia means progressive and irreversible decline. For example, when those who are diagnosed as mildly demented are followed over time, it is usually found that a substantial proportion become clearly demented, another group stays much the same, and another group is better, i.e., were misclassified (Brayne *et al.*, 1988).

Clearly, the problems with establishing sharp borderlines between cognitive changes associated with normal ageing and those found with dementia make it imperative that we strive to keep them as distinct entities. That dementia is in some way an acceleration of normal ageing is unhelpful, and supports the unfounded notion that it is an inevitable terminal stage of life, in the absence of death due to other causes. This readily supports ageist expectations that cognitive and behavioural decline are an inevitable part of later life, which can promote a passive response to such changes in elderly people themselves, and, unfortunately, often in the health care professionals working with them (Hart, 1990).

It is better to regard dementia as a syndrome with an individual mode of presentation, which is revealed in disturbances of cognition, daily living, and social behaviours. Disturbances vary according to the true cause, the source of a problem, and the area of the brain affected.

Such an open perspective facilitates the identification of other causes of confusion, which in this case result from an altered level of consciousness, misdiagnosed in the past as dementia. Acute brain failure or toxic confusional states, which present with a rapid onset and fluctuation in the level of consciousness, can be the result of many causes other than organic damage to the brain. For example, 'psychiatric, medical, and neurological disorders can cause acute confusion or delirium, and emotional stress, excesses of drugs or alcohol, toxic gases, even environmental changes can affect a person's state of mind' (Holden, 1988). Holden suggests that careful screening for these alternatives to the dementia diagnosis has undoubtably contributed to the fall in the reported cases of dementia. The ability to be able to identify and then to respond appropriately to non-organic causes of confusion must be seen as central to the care of elderly people.

## PSYCHOLOGICAL EXPLANATIONS

Psychological explanations for dementia involve two separate themes. One is concerned with studying and understanding behaviour and how it relates to nervous system function and structure. This is **neuropsychology**. The other theme is more difficult to label tightly and to describe. It involves the psychological responses to the familiar and routine becoming increasingly unfamiliar and unique.

This is a psychological consequence of the social world providing less and less support and more and more stressors; managing such stressors must become a universal concern of people with dementia.

Kitwood's paradigm (Froggatt, 1988) for the syndrome of dementia, or loss of self, explains it as a response to the interrelationship of significant life events and losses. What should be considered is the personality style of the individual, which is the result of his life experience and more recent social and psychological events. The downward spiral towards the loss of self, for example, precipitated by life stressors the individual cannot manage, leads to anxiety, and then withdrawal or confusion.

Neuropsychological changes also bring about a changed relationship with self and the taken-for-granted world. One can only imagine the experience and consequences of not being able to turn a door handle the way you want it to go; or forgetting your train of thought in mid-sentence; or failing to recognize the face of your partner.

A neuropsychological approach enables identification of the ways brain failure impacts on how the person perceives, communicates, and behaves. The person who has word-finding problems is going to value a care giver who is able to identify such a phenomenon in their presentation, and institute compensatory strategies.

Dementia is still shrouded in mystery and myth. Neuropsychology is one way of mapping into this uncharted territory to find how to understand and explain the individual dementia experience. Not understanding can readily lead to misidentification of the meanings of a behaviour, and then attribution of wrong explanations for it; for example, a wilful act, rather than a symptom of apraxia.

People's sense of self-control and image improve when they realize that those caring for them recognize their expressive aphasia, but also their retained ability to understand what is said to them. A neuropsychological approach is thus concerned with identifying retained abilities as well as disabilities, and can be a way of keeping human the individual who is in the end stage of dementia. As its focus is behaviour, it helps to identify what is there. For example, Church *et al.* (1988) suggest that the use of eye-contact, gaze-shift, turn-taking, and responsiveness to tone of voice and facial expression are skills learnt early in development, which may be thus preserved even in severe dementia.

Given that a neuropsychological approach increases understanding of the subjective world of the dementia sufferer, difficulties with achieving empathy with the inflicted rather than their caregivers may be lessened.

Tentative assertions are being made about the social consequence or stigma attached to the diagnosis, in particular the effect it has upon relationships with others. Holden (1988), for instance, suggests the consequence of inadequate diagnosis leads people who have Parkinson's and Huntington's diseases to receive inappropriate and over-compensatory care, which can lead to hopelessness and an unwillingness to try to overcome disabilities.

There is a paucity of psychological work with cognitively impaired people who are experiencing an inexorable pattern of decline. Accepting Kitwood's (1989) explanation that dementia is a collapse of accepted meanings about self and environment takes us back to the personal experience of dementia. What has to be explored are the ways in which processes might be mediated by the personality of the person inflicted with the disorder. Froggett (1988) suggests we have to 'grasp the nettle', and assume that personal experience and disposition play a part in the aetiology and progress of the disorder. Certainly the individual's ways of coping with severe life stressors, for example, denial, aggression, acceptance or despair, and so on, will have an impact on the person and those who have relationships of meaning with them.

It is increasingly recognized that a depressive response is an inevitable part of the dementia experience for many people. What research is showing is that less attention needs to be placed upon looking for other explanations for cognitive impairment, such as pseudo dementia, and more upon recognizing and treating the common problem of depression found in people with dementia (Reifler *et al.*, 1990).

A model for psychological work with people in early-stage dementia is offered by Thompson *et al.* (1990). Based on the cognitive approach developed by Beck, it works on the assumption that the root of depression lies in the cognitive set, or bias, of the patient. Patients would receive assistance to keep a check upon distortions of reality, which might lead them to over-generalize their disabilities and lead them to 'catrastrophizing' limitations.

## SOCIAL EXPLANATIONS

There is recognition of a 'therapeutic nihilism' or subjective feeling that little or nothing can be done to help surrounding the dementia experience (Hart *et al.*, 1990). Holden (1988) has recognized that this must have a psychosocial impact upon the process of the disorder, given what is understood to be the consequences of labelling upon an individual's behaviour. However, this seems to be an under-explored aspect of the dementia experience.

In their discussion of the 'patient career', Bond *et al.* (1986) suggest that the very act of labelling will affect behaviourally the person labelled and those in relationship to him: '...if we start to call elderly relatives senile and, perhaps more important, to treat them as if they were senile, it is amazing how quickly they begin to behave in somewhat bizarre ways. This process is sometimes called a "self-fulfilling prophecy".'

The social dread of the diagnostic label is perhaps illustrated well in Froggett's (1988) exploration of the experience of people in the early stage of dementia:

> "The third women, aged 78, lived with an alert but physically disabled husband. A recent hospital admission had accelerated her decline, so that she failed to recognize a son who visited her from a distance. In the interview she recognized her lack of memory, and diverted my attention by offering to make tea, and describing their domestic arrangements in detail."

Certainly this act of confabulation takes on a different level of meaning if it is understood primarily as an individual's way of hiding from others memory incapacities, and, secondarily, as a psychiatric symptom of an organic disorder. That such face-saving strategies come to be used may be an example of the way relationships with others are altered as a result of a dementia diagnosis. Changed relationships, suggestive of ageism, are most obvious in the way risk potential is assessed: 'Thus, for example, an elderly person who is living in squalour is likely to be perceived quite differently from, say, a drug-addicted young person living in similar squalour.' (Norman, 1988).

The consequence is that elderly persons with dementia will be given less consideration of their rights to liberty, choice, and self-determination than would be given to a younger person. Deprivation of the right to control major aspects of life will have psychological consequences: anger, disappointment, shame, fear, and negatively altered self-concept are all possible outcomes.

Social rationalizations are available, which, if they are not quite able to justify treating people with dementia differently, at least suggest why such treatment is of no special consequence to the dementia sufferer. For instance, the assumption that elderly confused people do not suffer or are unable to have a good time (Gilhooly, 1984).

The social expectancies for the behaviour of the person with dementia and those who have contact with him are powerful. Research has shown that there is a relationship between dementia and social isolation – even for those living with family – with inevitable consequences of a decrease in social stimulation and meaningful contact with others (Gilhooly, 1984). Whether this is a consequence of difficulties in communicating because of the apathy and disturbed communication abilities, or a manifestation of social dread associated with dementia, the consequences are often the same: social death.

## CARING RELATIONSHIPS

No consideration of the social construction of dementia would be complete without consideration of those involved in caring relationships. In the first instance, this is family; 80% of people with dementia are cared for within the community (Hart *et al.*, 1990). What this is likely to mean in terms of numbers of people in the UK can be judged by Gilhooly's (1984) extrapolation:

> Around 36 000 (46%) of males and 16 000 (10%) of females with dementia live with a spouse; 21 600 males (27%) and 52 800 females (33%) live with others; 21 600 males (27%) and 91 200 females (57%) live alone. Looking at the problem in another way, these estimates indicate that 52 800 spouses care for a dementing person and 74 400 other relatives (mainly adult children) care for a dementing person.

According to Cohler (1990), adult children provide more care and more difficult care to more parents over much longer periods of time than they did in the mythical 'good old days', when supposedly the aged were diligently cared for.

## WHY DO PEOPLE CARE?

That so many people provide care, to such an extent, for such extensive periods of time, and often at considerable costs – social, psychological, and biological – to themselves, suggests that caring is satisfying for many people. It also seems to imply that it is more than merely the reciprocal response to indebtedness incurred earlier in the family's life-line when dependency roles would be reversed (Antonucci *et al.*, 1989). Although Cohler's *et al.* (1990) review of the literature suggests that one does not particularly have to like another family member to provide care and assistance at time of need, positive regard does help mitigate some of the strains involved.

## PROBLEMS FACED BY THE CAREGIVERS

Caregivers have problems meeting the demented person's practical everyday needs concerning such things as diet, hygiene, and toilet. There are also problems caused by the demented person's behaviour: unsafe acts, wandering, incontinence, and night-time disturbance are found to be particularly difficult to cope with. Interpersonal strains, which result from the severely demented person's inability to have a memory for relationships, often are manifested in sadness, family tension, and loss of temper. Finally, the social consequences of care can lead to limited social, work, and recreational pursuits (Levin *et al.*, 1988).

## WHAT CAREGIVERS NEED

The motivation to care exists at an individual and familial level. What is required is an effective range of supports for the caregivers, in order to make care sustainable and manageable. Levin *et al.* (1988) identified ten key requirements of the supporters of people with dementia. From the problems presented, it is clear these would include financial assistance and a range of respite relief options. Practical assistance with care is usually always needed, as is information and counselling. The survey also identified needs for comprehensive medical and social assessments, which produce timely action and active medical treatment, and continue as the dementia career unfolds to provide backup and review.

Meeting caregiver needs has been shown to make a difference. Brodaty *et al.* (1990) showed by research that measures that included training in assertiveness, behaviour modification, group therapy, etc., could make a difference in coping. This was demonstrated by a reduction in the incidence of institutionalization of people with dementia when compared with a control group. This phenomenon was particularly marked when training was given early in the dementia experience.

## A MODEL FOR PRACTICE

The difficult task is to deliver the level of care that best compensates for or limits the negative consequences of dementia; is respectful and zealous to protect the demented person's rights to self-determination; while also equipping concerned others to cope as effectively as possible with the ravages that dementia brings to their relationships and lifestyle, and their ability to be autonomous.

For care to be effective, there is a need to attend to a series of interrelationships. These begin with determination of significant bio-psychosocial aspects of the person who has dementia, and extend to include interrelationships with others in concerned and caring relationships and their bio-psychosocial interrelationships.

General systems theory (Von Bertalanffy, 1968) is useful to aid the description and analysis of such interrelationships, and its principles can provide a direction to practice (Chapter 22). This suggests that the behaviour of any system – for example, cell, person, family, street – will be determined by certain principles; thus it is possible to view all the participants of a particular dementia experience as a unified whole. Systems theory allows for the inclusion of a limited number, or for an ever-widening number, of subsystem interrelationships, into the focus system in question. In clinical practice this ability to move the boundaries means interventions can be determined according to the need of the person who has dementia, and, as necessary, the needs and abilities of others sharing that particular dementia experience.

Given the usual level of need of the person with dementia and their concerned others, be they family, friends or neighbours, it is appropriate that the nurse sees all these characters as the means to understand and engage with about their dementia experience.

A principle of general systems theory is that change in one system is likely to bring about changes in systems in interrelationship. This directs attention to looking for the knock-on consequences of a normal ageing or a pathological process upon related systems. For example, cardiac failure can cause lower-order disturbances as diverse as acute confusion, abdominal pain, and insomnia (Nicklason *et al.*, 1990), or have consequences for higher-order system relationships; for example, the demented partner of a person in cardiac failure might require residential care. Therefore, a function of the nurse is to anticipate as much as possible knock-on consequences for systems in relationship.

Wilson's (1989) model of the ways caregivers cope with the dementia experience suggests that trial-and-error coping, with a consequent risk of physical and emotional exhaustion, best characterizes the early stage of the dementia process. Here, then, is an opportunity for the nurse to attempt to forestall such negative consequences by such things as education about the dementia process, and practical measures to limit physical and emotional stress.

Accepting that systems are influenced by changes and inputs from related systems helps the nurse to be mindful that a transformation will inevitably occur as a result of the involvement of professional agencies. Hopefully, some of these changes will be of benefit, but inevitably, other less-welcome consequences can occur. The dementia diagnosis has a powerful social stigma, and provides the sufferer with a limited medical identity, which can negatively determine interactions with others.

As much as possible it is important to try to contradict such a process by recognizing with the patient and care system their disadvantaged status through providing accurate and balanced information about the condition and its progression and strategies for coping with problems. The marginalization and stigmatization of the person with dementia is enhanced when they are excluded from discussions about their care. Wherever possible, attempts should be made to avoid secrets, and to keep open communication between all participants of the dementia experience.

Identified earlier were some of the therapeutic measures available to improve the functioning of the person who has dementia, and also their caregivers – be this skill-training to help the caregiver deal more effectively with the stressors caused by the dementia experience, or treatment for the seemingly inevitable depression experienced by the person with dementia by medical and cognitive therapies. Appropriate strategies to help the person cope with the forgetfulness or communication, movement, and perceptual disturbances are all part of effective work with people with dementia, and can make a dent, by showing what makes a difference, in the therapeutic nihilism surrounding dementia.

That input can be of benefit points to the general systems theory principle that a process of interchange with the environment is necessary for survival. If we think of a factory as a system, it requires the import of raw materials to convert to manufactured goods. The cell that is a system requires oxygen and sugar to function. The family that is a system will take in and convert a great range of materials (food, clothing, information) in order to maintain homeostasis, or the *status quo*. Central to effective homeostasis is the efficient management of the interface between the system and the resource environment; to carry too many parts in stock is not the sign of an efficient factory.

If the condition progresses adversely, the person with dementia and their caregivers will require over time increasing inputs from support systems to maintain a satisfactory, that is, sustainable, steady state. Like the factory, of crucial significance to the successful maintenance of such a sustainable, steady state is the effective management of the boundary interface between those experiencing dementia and the caring agencies. This is related to the human 'need for considerable influence over the people, events, and situations that have a substantial impact on our well-being and valued life pursuits' (Renshon, 1979).

As dementia is a disorder without predictability and with great uncertainty, it is appropriate that the person who has dementia and the caregiver's sense of control is enhanced, or at least not undermined in other areas. Areas of relevance in enhancing or maintaining such a sense of control would be through meeting informational, support, and respite needs in ways best understood and wanted by the person with dementia and their caregivers. As identified earlier, those caught up in the dementia experience need opportunities to be put in contact with others who are in the same predicament, or who can offer practical help, or inform them about the range of services, aids, and benefit entitlement.

This is a service determined by the client and accords with the philosophy of the government White Paper *Caring for People* (HMSO, 1989). There is little choice, given the cost to society of an institutional model of care for people with dementia, or indeed the costs of the care burdens for their caregivers.

Part of effective care is the ability to recognize when the boundary responsibilities carried by the person who has dementia, or their caregivers, needs to be reduced because they cannot be sustained in the long or short term. For example, as the dementia career unfolds, the caregiver's need to be free from the need to be vigilant might gradually increase from a couple of hours a week, so that they may visit friends or go shopping, to weeks of respite, with the person with dementia receiving institutional care so that the caregiver might take a holiday, or gain necessary medical treatment.

Similarly, at points in the career of the dementia patient, decisions will have to be made about their ability to manage independently activities that can become dangerous as a result of forgetfulness and confusion. For example, cooking, and going for a walk, commonly known as 'wandering'. The reasons for taking over the management and control of such personal domains needs to be shared with the person who has dementia, and attempts made to work them through with them.

When considering the area of risk assessment and management it is important to remember it is not an area of precision, and therefore is very much open to the subjective assessments of the individual workers and caregivers (Askham *et al.*, 1990). There is a need for the development of assessment tools, so that measured judgement can be made about the demented person's ability to decide for themselves and manage personal boundaries.

General systems theory suggests that systems are directed towards maintaining a steady state to ensure adequate functioning. Referring to the earlier analogy of a factory, without the input of material, the factory comes to a stop. Without the removal of waste products, the ability of the cell to maintain homeostasis will gradually be impeded. Without shared rules for meaning – for example, when is day and when is night –

the functioning of the family unit would gradually become unstable.

A feature of the dementia experience is that the rules of shared meaning established over a life-time break down. Often it is the failure of the dementia victim to find meaning, recall, or have the ability to follow the social conventions of hygiene, manners, or occupation, which disturb the known rules of organization, and thus the steady-state equilibrium. But failure to adhere to established rules of meaning could equally be the response of the caregivers; for example, by rejecting or abusive responses because a member has a dementing-type illness.

Ways of determining and understanding rules of organization pertinent to the dementia can be gained by examining the coping strategies employed to manage the situation. These can give some indication of the forthcoming career of those involved in that dementia experience. For instance, it is likely that the *status quo* of meaning, which is the consequence of attributing the occurrence of dementia to chance, – ('it could happen to anyone') – rather than as a result of personal or family fault, will lead to more adaptive responses and solutions to problems.

There will also be unique rules for the management of the stress symptoms that occur as part of the dementia experience. Although the stress-reduction strategies might all serve as ways of reducing the stress experience for both the person with dementia and their caregivers, some, for instance, drug and alcohol use, or aggressive outbursts, will further undermine the capacity to sustain homeostasis over time.

When understanding the rules of organization, care needs to be taken not to focus just upon the dementia experience, but also on the significance of other psychosocial events and needs that occur for all in the dementia experience.

## CONCLUSION

To be elderly in our society is to be disadvantaged; to experience dementia as well is to be doubly disadvantaged. There is some evidence, though, that the aged person is about to be redefined socially in a more positive light as a consequence of increased economic power of the 'young old'. Nurses can play an important part in this social-attitude change, and in particular use it to promote a change in the ways dementia is experienced. The way forward is to have positive care goals that lead to the early detection of dementia, increased knowledge of the subjective world of the person with dementia, and detailed accounts of care that help to identify what it is that nurses do that 'makes a difference' (Chapman, 1985).

The challenge of providing individualized care based upon an understanding of the individual needs of the elderly person is considerable. The potential reward of meeting such a challenge is to make a crucial difference to the quality of experience for the individual and his caregivers.

## REFERENCES

Abrams, M. (1989) 'Third age' lives in the next generation: changing attitudes and expectations, in *Human Ageing and Later Life*, (ed. A. N. Warnes), Edward Arnold, London.

Antonucci, T. and Jackson, J. (1989) Successful ageing and life course reciprocity in *Human Ageing and Later Life*, (ed. A. N. Warnes), Edward Arnold, London.

Askham, J and Thompson, C. (1990) *Dementia and Home Care*, Age Concern.

Blaikie, A. and Macnicol, J. (1989) Ageing and social policy: a twentieth-century dilemma, in *Human Ageing and Later Life*, (ed. A.M. Warnes), Edward Arnold, London.

Bond, J. and Bond, S. (1986) *Sociology and Health Care*. Churchill Livingstone, Edinburgh and London.

Brayne, C. and Ames, D. (1988) The epidemiology of mental disorders in old age, in *Mental Health*

*Problems in Old Age,* (eds B. Gearing, M. Johnson, T. Heller) John Wiley & Sons, Chichester.

Brodaty, H. and Greham, M. (1989) Effects of a training programme to reduce stress in carers of patients with dementia, *British Medical J.,* 299; 1375–9.

*Caring for People: Community Care in the Next Decade and Beyond* (1989), Government White Paper, HMSO.

Chapman, C. M. (1985) *Theory of Nursing, Practical Application.* Lippincott Nursing Series.

Church, M. and Wattis, J. (1989) Psychological approaches to the assessment and treatment of old people, in Wattis J. and Hindmarch I. (ed.) *Psychological Assessment of the Elderly: Behavioural and Clinical Aspects,* (eds J. Wattis and I. Hindmarch), Churchill-Livingstone, Edinburgh and London.

Cohler, B. J., Groves, L, Borden, W. *et al.* (1990) Caring for family members with Alzheimer's disease, in *Alzheimer's Disease: Treatment and Family Stress,* (eds E. Light and B. D. Lebowitz) Hemisphere Publishing Company, New York.

Downton, J. H. and Andrews, K. (1990) Postural disturbance and psychological symptoms amongst elderly people living at home. *International Journal Geriatric Psychiatry,* **5,** 93–8.

Erikson, E. (1965) *Childhood and Society,* Paladin, New York.

Froggatt, A. (1988) Self-awareness in early dementia, in *Mental Health Problems in Old Age,* (eds B. Gearing, M. Johnson and T. Heller Open Univ. Press, Milton Keynes.

Gilhooly, M. L. M. (1984) The social dimensions of senile dementia, in *Psychological Approaches to the Care of the Elderly,* (eds I. Hanley and J. Hodge) Croom Helm, London.

Grundy, E. (1989) Living arrangements and social support in later life, in *Human Ageing and Later Life,* (ed A. M. Warnes), Edward Arnold, London.

Hart, S. and Semple, J. M. (1990) *Neuropsychology and the Dementias,* Taylor and Francis, London.

Hipkiss, A. and Bittles, A. (1989) Basic biological aspects of ageing, in *Human Ageing and Later Life* (ed A. M. Warnes) Edward Arnold, London.

Holden, U. (ed) (1988) *Neuropsychology and Ageing,* Croom Helm, London.

Huppert, F. and Tym, E. (1986) Clinical and neuro-psychological assessment of dementia, in *Mental Health Problems in Old Age* (eds B. Gearing, M.

Johnson, T. Heller), John Wiley & Sons, Chichester.

Jefferies, M. (1987) An ageing Britain – what is its future?, in *Mental Health Problems in Old Age,* (eds B. Gearing, M. Johnson, T. Heller), John Wiley & Sons, Chichester.

Johns, R. (1989) Care Study (unpublished), Powys Department of Nursing Studies.

Kitwood, T. (1989) The contribution of psychology to the understanding of senile dementia, in *Mental Health Problems in Old Age,* (eds B. Gearing, M. Johnson, T. Heller), John Wiley & Sons, Chichester.

Levin, E., Sinclair, I. and Gorbach, P. (1988) The supporters of confused elderly persons at home, in *Mental Health Problems in Old Age*, (eds B. Gearing, M. Johnson, T. Heller), John Wiley & Sons, Chichester.

Miller, J. (1988) *Life File,* BBC Television (Midlands), audio transcript.

Nicklason, F., Dewar, E., Finucane, P. (1990) Heart failure, *Geriatric Medicine,* 20, 6, 63–8.

Norman, A. (1988) Risk, in *Mental Health Problems in Old Age,* (eds B. Gearing, M. Johnson, T. Heller), John Wiley & Sons, Chichester.

Office of Population Census and Surveys (1988), OPCS Monitor, mid-1987, population estimates for England and Wales, P 8811, 18.8.88, HMSO, London.

Reifler, B. V. and Larson, E. (1990) Excess disability in dementia of the Alzheimer's type, in *Alzheimer's Disease: Treatment and Family Stress* (eds E. Light, B.D. Lebowitz), Hemisphere Pub. Co., New York.

Renshon, S. A. (1979) Control in political life: origins, dynamics and implications, in *Choice and Perceived Control,* (eds L. C. Perlmuler, R. Monty ) Hillsdale; cited in Psychological paradigms for understanding caregiving, in *Alzheimer's Disease: Treatment and Family Stress* (1990) (eds E. Light, B. D. Lebowitz), Hemisphere Pub. Co., New York.

Robb, S. S. *et al.* (1984) Nursing behaviour in the environment of the aged, in *The Aged Person and The Nursing Process,* (eds A.G. Yurick, B. E. Speir, S. Robbs) Appleton and Lairg (out of print).

Royal Coll. of Physicians (1981), cited in The epidemilogy of mental disorders in old age (1988), in *Mental Health Problems in Old Age,* (eds B. Gearing, M. Johnson, T. Heller), John Wiley & Sons, Chichester.

Sheppard, A. (1981) Response to cartoons and attitudes toward aging, *J. Gerontology* 36, 122–6. Cited in Excess disability in dementia of the Alzheimer's type (1990), in *Alzheimer's Disease Treatment and Family Stress* (eds E. Light, D. Lebowitz), Hemisphere Pub. Co., New York.

Thompson, L. W., Wagner, B., Zeiss, A. *et al.* (1990) Cognitive behavioural therapy with early stage Alzheimer's patients: an exploratory view of the utility of this approach, in *Alzheimer's Disease: Treatment and Family Stress* (eds E. Light, B. D. Lebowitz), Hemisphere Pub. Co., New York.

Verstbeeg, R (1990) *Hypothermia Briefing,* Age Concern, England.

Von Bertalanffy, L. (1968) *General Systems Theory,* Penguin, Harmondsworth.

Wilson Barnett, J. (1979) *Stress in Hospital,* Churchill-Livingstone, Edinburgh, London.

Wilson, H. S. (1989) Family caregiving for a relative with Alzheimer's dementia: coping with negative choices. *Nursing Research,* 38, No 2.

Zarit, S. H. (1990) Issues and directions in family intervention research, in *Alzheimer's Disease: Treatment and Family Stress* (eds E. Light, B.D. Lebowitz), Hemisphere Pub. Co., New York.

## FURTHER READING

Hanley, I. and Hodge, J. (ed.) (1984) *Psychological Approaches to the Care of the Elderly,* Croom Helm, London.

Hanley, I. and Gilhooly, M. (eds) (1986) *Psychological Therapies for the Elderly,* Croom Helm, London.

Holden, U. (ed.) (1988) *Neuropsychology and Ageing,* Croom Helm, London.

# TRANSCULTURAL ISSUES AND APPROACHES

## 18

*David B. Cooper*

## TRANSCULTURAL ISSUES IN PERSPECTIVE

Any individual – regardless of race, culture, colour, creed, social and/or economic status – has the right to expect and receive appropriate nursing interventions in relation to the presenting health problem. Lack of thorough investigation into a presenting health problem can cause harm to the individual receiving care, and his or her family. It can also make any interventions offered a traumatic experience.

One's approach must be holistic, comprehensive, and adequate. To look at a health problem simply on the basis of presenting symptom(s) is not only to invite problems but, one could suggest, it is also unethical. To assess, plan, implement, and evaluate all interventions and procedures thoroughly will go a long way in ensuring the client receives the correct care package. This must include the physical, social, spiritual and psychological needs of the client.

Sadly, for some ethnic minority groups the lack of adequate cultural knowledge within nursing prevents proper interactions taking place in any meaningful way.

The issue of transcultural nursing is very broad. In this chapter we will look at some of the problems and difficulties encountered by this client group when seeking care from health care professionals.

One needs to look closely at all precipitating factors relating to each mental health problem.

This has been highlighted to some extent on the MIND (July 1990) information sheets *Black and Ethnic Communities and Mental Health* which stated:

> The social conditions of Black people, and of people from ethnic communities, must be considered in any assessment of the health of these communities. Housing, employment, education and a feeling of community, all contribute to mental health. Consequently their absence can result in stress and eventually mental ill health. It has been established that Black people face racial discrimination in the fields of employment, housing, and education. This means that Black people are often denied access to, or given second-rate opportunities in these fields. Positive self-image can be lacking for Black children, and they may also learn to view negatively their own Blackness. These conditions must contribute to mental ill health.
>
> Thompson, 1988; Ward, 1988

Research indicates that racism occurs within the mental-health system: Afro-Caribbean people are ten times more likely to be diagnosed as having schizophrenia than White people (Harrison *et al.*, 1988). Furthermore, Black people receive larger doses of medication and have less access to alternative treatment than do White people (Littlewood, R. *et al.* 1982, 1980).

The cultural and religious beliefs of some groups, for example, Asian women, are rarely recognized in the planning and implementation of mental-health service provision. Many Asian women are isolated in their homes without any form of support (Flockhart, 1986; Jarvis, 1986).

When looking more closely at cultural barriers as obstacles to the way in which care is provided to ethnic minorities, Renshaw (1988) said:

> Many obstacles stand in the way of ethnic minorities receiving better and more appropriate types of treatment and care. Not least of these is the tendency of mental health services and professionals to view the obvious problems as belonging to the individual or minority group, rather than looking more broadly at our own cultural limitations. Models of health and ill health which we have developed to explain unusual behaviour patterns may be wholly inappropriate when applied to people from other countries. Such assumptions are part of the unconscious set. Planners, for example, may direct their efforts towards improving access of ethnic minorities to existing services rather than to carefully considering whether those services are actually suitable.

Renshaw goes on to suggest that some barriers to the provision of better treatment for people from other cultures may stem from the system itself. People from minority ethnic backgrounds tend to find health agencies difficult to approach and trust, for example, the client is often asked for documentation that he neither has, nor understands.

It is now generally accepted that we need to increase access to the information. Taking into account individual cultural needs, services must be more accessible to the client, and the provision of care should be improved accordingly. We need to incorporate the views and wishes of this client group, and to modify any services offered in accordance with the needs identified. The employment of staff from ethnic minorities is paramount in today's multi-racial society. There is a need to identify what is necessary to improve and increase training to all within the mental health and caring professions. This will, in turn, allow for more accurate cross-cultural work to take place.

In its recent draft consultative document, *Race Relations Code of Practice* (1991) the Commission for Racial Equality (CRE) stated:

> The Mental Health Act Commission (England and Wales), has recognized the importance of ethnicity in their own code of practice, in which they state as a broad, general principal that persons to whom the 1983 Mental Health Act applies should: 'receive respect for and consideration of their individual qualities and diverse backgrounds – social, cultural, ethnic, and religions' [sic].

The CRE draft code of practice in the provision of mental heath services was circulated for discussion in July 1991. The emphasis is on the law and the providers of mental health services and others to take steps to comply with the code and to avoid racial discrimination. It also offers examples of good practices in the implementation and promotion of equal opportunities.

## OTHER FACTORS FOR CONSIDERATION

We live in a multicultural, multicoloured, and multiracial society. For mental health nurses to provide good-quality care and make necessary and appropriate nursing interventions, it is vital they have an awareness and understanding of cross-cultural values, beliefs, and attitudes.

Ethnocentricity – the tendency to judge the beliefs and behaviours of others against the standards of one's own culture – creates a barrier to understanding. In dealing with a client from an unfamiliar culture, it is important to understand the cultural context of the problems presented. The nurse enters a landscape where it is not always possible to identify important landmarks, nor to separate the uncommon features from the common ones.

There are many different minority groups in Britain today, some of whom interrelate but who also pose different issues and difficulties. They may also be at diverse stages and levels of cultural readjustment, for example:

- Those who come to Britain for better work prospects, with the hope of improving their socio-economic status.
- Refugees who flee their own country in order to escape political, and sometimes tribal, oppression; such people present with behaviours and problems that may be mistakenly perceived as a form of paranoia.
- Second-generation minority groups who arrive at a young age to join their parents, or who are born in the host country. Here, there is exposure and adaptation to Western culture, and the adoption of its values and beliefs. This often leads to conflicts and generational difficulties within the family.

The client from an ethnic minority background – in hospital or in the community – experiences a great deal of stress. There is often downward social mobility, lack of opportunity, thwarted ambition, and job dissatisfaction as some are forced to accept positions they are over-qualified for, rather than to face unemployment. There is a concomitant lowering of moral and self-esteem.

These experiences may be attributed, justifiably or unjustifiably, to racism and prejudice. The expression of these feelings by a member of an ethnic minority group, however, may lead to a diagnosis of paranoia. In consequence, social isolation may increase in the absence of structured and established methods of dealing with these stresses, which the origin culture could have provided.

## ASSESSMENT

As well as attending to the client's mental health history in the usual way, the nurse will need to make every effort to assess the issues related to the client's migration and culture. If this is ignored, the client's racial and cultural identity is rebuffed. It would be a mistake to assume that by treating an ethnic minority client as you would any other, adequate care will be provided. Also, the nurse may deal with the client as a cultural stereotype, thereby ignoring the social and interpersonal factors that are so relevant in assessment, which often results from the nurse being overwhelmed by unfamiliar racial and cultural characteristics. Another difficult area relates to differences in the presentation of emotional, psychological, and psychiatric problems.

Where there are language difficulties, an interpreter should be used. The interpreter, however, must be carefully selected. If he or she is not from any of the caring professions, they may have difficulty explaining information or asking questions in a meaningful way. Equally, if the interpreter is a member of the client's family, this can lead to embarrassment, for example, if he or she is asked for information, or is required to voice the client's complaints clearly.

Below are some examples of how references and beliefs can be misinterpreted through a lack of knowledge on cultural issues:

When a Pakistani refers to himself as being 'Royal', he is not necessarily deluded; it means simply that he comes from a wealthy family. This is not a grandiose delusion in cultural terms.

'The good lord is talking to me', is an expression often used by Afro-Caribbean people of religious background. This can mistakenly be perceived by the nurse as the client experiencing auditory hallucinations. In a study of Barbadians in Britain and Barbados that looked at beliefs about causes of mental illness, Clarke (1979) found that mental illness was attributed to:

- Too much thinking.
- People make you mad by witchcraft, Obeah, or by poisoning or tampering with food. (Obeah is a form of witchcraft associated with the poorer classes of the West Indies. The individual will often go and see the Obeah for minor illnesses. Those from a more educated background tend to think of Obeah the same as English people would view the bogey man.)
- Lack of rest after childbirth to allow the body to 'knit' together.
- High blood pressure from hot sun.
- Inheritance of bad blood.

Building a rapport requires time, patience, tolerance, and perseverance on the part of the nurse. Clients may be reluctant to allow a cultural outsider to get too close. The style of questioning adopted by western society often does not fit the conceptual models used in other cultures. The nurse who insists on using such a style of questioning may lose credibility in that he or she may be perceived as ignorant, which makes it difficult to facilitate client participation and involvement in care planning. On the other hand, members of other cultures often expect the nurse to have all answers.

There are some syndromes that in the client's view stem from particular causes, for example, auditory hallucinations are sometimes thought to be a sign of divine or supernatural intervention; somatic discomfort may be attributed to human enmity and witchcraft; and manic over-activity to astrological causes.

It is good practice to understand this, as it gives a common ground that enables the nurse to maintain a dialogue. This is not to suggest that the nurse should go along with the client's beliefs, but rather to try to understand them, and placing them within the appropriate context. Gaining the co-operation of the client in prescribed care and treatment calls for educating, advising, and supporting the client and significant others, which must be undertaken in a sensitive way.

## FOOD

This can be costly, as often immigrants choose to keep to an ethnic diet, the ingredients of which are imported. Much money, therefore, is spent on food, and very little is left to pay heating bills or for warm clothing. For the elderly and the young, there may be an increased risk of hypothermia, as heating is used in a very limited way.

## RECREATION AND ENTERTAINMENT

Second-generation ethnic minority groups appear to have better resources for recreation and entertainment. For the elderly, as well as those of refugee status, such needs, if met, are very poor and inadequate, with the result that such groups may become insular and more isolated.

## EDUCATION

Educating ethnic minority groups about Western culture, beliefs, values, and attitudes alongside health education should be encouraged. This endeavour, however, will be ineffective if ethnic cultural beliefs are not also taken into account. A focal-point might be educating the client, the family, and the community at large to recognize areas or situations that can cause stress. There also needs to be more information about what help is available, and where and how to get it.

## INFORMATION-GIVING

It is not enough to give information verbally. A number of studies suggest that messages and information might be given more successfully with the use of technical and educational aids.

One model suggests that a community is likely to be more receptive to the introduction of innovations and ideas if it is seen and believed to be simple, observable, advantageous, possible, and compatible with existing cultural practices. In this model, two key figures are identified: change agents, who act as intermediaries between experts, in this case the health services, and opinion leaders, members of the community who are well respected and may have a high social status and exposure in the media. For example, in an Asian community, an opinion leader is usually a man and a senior member of a family, or, in cases to do with childbirth, a senior woman. The 'hawkim' or 'vaid' – the traditional healer or doctor – may also be accepted as an opinion-leader. In Afro-Caribbean cultures, senior members of Obeah, the traditional healers, or pastors of churches may be positively used. In some areas where such innovation has been used it has been seen to be significantly beneficial in facilitating and promoting a healthy integration.

As professionals, we need education just as much as, if not more than, the ethnic minority groups. As a starting point, training institutions should include such important issues in the syllabus. Also, workshops, seminars and day-release courses should be established in which leaders of various ethnic minority groups would be invited to participate. Talking to clients and their neighbours and showing a genuine interest in finding out about their culture is a valuable endeavour that must not be over-looked.

There are a number of ethnic minority groups that are well organized and established as voluntary bodies in some boroughs. It would be worth the effort of the practitioner to familiarize herself with these groups and to attend their meetings. This has proven to be beneficial to health care workers who have already involved themselves in this way.

## MISTAKEN IDENTITIES

The occurrence and patterns of mental health problems vary depending on: reasons for migration, the country of origin, cultures, social situation, and the climate of the host country. It has been suggested that depressed Asian and Afro-Caribbean clients tend to present with somatic symptoms. Vague, physical symptoms are often described, such as general aches and pains, alternating hot and cold sensations in the stomach, etc., and often an accompanying denial of depressed mood. Below are some case examples, to clarify some of the points raised earlier.

### CASE STUDY ONE

A 42-year-old Pakistani woman was admitted to hospital after exhaustive and thorough investigations following complaints of various physical symptoms. The woman had been in England for eight years, arriving to join her husband following an arranged marriage, in accordance with custom. She had not received any formal education, and she spoke no English at all. She would often be left on her own at home while her husband went to work. She was isolated and led a solitary life.

After several attempts to conceive, she began to suspect that a cousin still in Pakistan, who was to have married the client's husband, had cast a spell on her. She believed this explained the hotness and coldness she experienced in her stomach, particularly during sexual intercourse. She often complained that her cousin and other relatives were plotting against her, and she admitted to hearing voices.

The diagnosis given to the client was schizophrenia, and she was prescribed neuroleptic medication. The only effect this had, besides giving her distressing side-effects, was to make her spend long periods of time on her bed, looking very bewildered, dejected, and frightened.

It was not until after her fourth admission that she confided in the only nurse she had built up some rapport with during her previous admission. Her story gradually unfolded, with the help of an interpreter. She felt she had let her husband and her family of origin down, she wanted to return to Pakistan, but felt she could not do so because of this, and yet she was so alone. The woman believed her husband must want a divorce.

The neuroleptics were discontinued, and the diagnosis was changed to depression. She was referred to a day-centre that catered for isolated Asian women, where she learned to speak English and was trained in a craft that now provides her with an income. Her self-esteem improved to the extent that she now manages without psychiatric involvement, attending the outpatient department only once a year for a follow-up appointment.

CASE STUDY TWO

A 25-year-old Ethiopian refugee was admitted informally into hospital following complaints from his neighbours of self-neglect and bizarre behaviours. He spoke very little English.

He was given oral neuroleptic medication, which he was observed to withhold, seeming reluctant to take it at times. It was decided that he could not be relied upon to take the medication, and was placed on Section 3 of the Mental Health Act (1983), and given his medication by injection, against his wishes, which was a traumatic and distressing experience for both the client and the staff. The man became mute, refused food and fluids, and was unwilling to leave his bed.

A third-year student nurse devoted a lot of time to this young man. She spent time researching the cultural and customs of the Ethiopian people, and from this found out a few interesting things about Ethiopia, especially Eritrea, the client's home region. The nurse showed genuine interest, and was

patient, tolerant, and non-judgmental in her approach to the client.

Her perseverance was eventually rewarded. The client began to trust her, and gradually his story emerged. He had refused his medication only at times when he had not yet has his meal. He reacted to the decision to be given injections with extreme panic, expressing apparently paranoid delusions towards doctors and nurses. He had taken to his bed as he had given up living; he was expecting to die as a result of the injections. The client had come to England as a refugee, having run away from a camp in Ethiopia, where he had been subjected to torture and was given noxious injections for 'experimental purposes'. Some of his friends had died as a result of this torture. This accusation against the camp officials was confirmed by other refugees with whom the student nurse had spoken during her research into her client's background. His reactions on both counts were understandable in the light of his explanation.

When dealing with this man, various health-care workers had failed to take an holistic view of his problems. Carrying out detailed research into his background added important information, which in the end supplied the key to some of his problems. There were similarities between the care he was given and his past experiences of torture, and it was simply against his custom to take medication on an empty stomach.

CASE STUDY THREE

A 30-year-old Ghanaian man had arrived in England to study accounting. He lodged with his mother and stepfather; the relationships were strained, particularly between him, his stepfather, and his half-siblings. He often felt excluded from the family gatherings. However, due to financial difficulties, he had no choice but to continue lodging with his family. He worked as warehouseman and petrol-pump attendant to finance his education. Both employers were aware that he was an illegal immigrant, and used this knowledge to exploit him financially. He was under a tremendous amount of stress from family conflict, employers' exploitation, the fear and anxiety of being discovered by immigration officers, and his studies for his accountancy examinations.

He had four admissions into hospital in two years; each time he was escorted by at least four police officers, and was detained under the Mental Health Act (1983). His behaviour has been described as wild and excitable, he was expressing grandiose delusions, threats of violence, was accusatory, irritable and generally restless and overactive. This behaviour often caused a great deal of disturbance on the ward. He was treated with large doses of Haloperidol. His behaviour improved gradually, and within two weeks he was back to his normal polite, pleasant, and unassuming self. He was diagnosed as suffering a manic illness.

Without the background information given above, the young man was assumed to be manic, with a biological frame of reference, but this diagnosis was changed to reactive mania as a stress reaction, thus recognizing that his breakdown was related to factors in the real world, over which he had no control (Chapter 11).

The client had always rejected Black nurses on the ward, and had been most suspicious of them. It would have been counter-productive if these nurses had forced a relationship on such a client. On recovery, he explained that he felt the Black nurses were in on a plot to hurt him: 'How come they are Black and yet seem to have made it in a foreign world?' he asked. This is often the case, par-ticularly in clients from other cultures who present with apparently psychotic behaviour.

## CASE STUDY FOUR

A young Asian woman was transferred from a maternity unit to a psychiatric ward after having a baby a week previously. She had become disturbed on the ward immediately prior to the birth of the child, which was delivered by Caesarean section. After the birth, she had been very fearful and rejected the baby, describing him as the devil, and refusing to have anything to do with him.

The diagnosis was of puerperal psychosis. As her mental state improved gradually, the story that unfolded was that she had been trying to have a baby for five years. She became pregnant after she visited a Davi, a religious leader, who told her that her difficulties in conceiving were due to witchcraft, instigated by her unmarried and jealous aunt in India. The Davi gave her a talisman to wear at all times (Tavees), for protection and healing.

Preoperative care included taking off prosthesis and jewellery. Her Tavees were thought to be jewellery, and despite her attempts to explain, they were removed. The client consequently thought this must be a return of the witchcraft, and that her unprotected child was possessed by the devil; all of which explained her behaviour toward the child.

The Davi came to visit her at the request of the staff, said prayers over the baby, and gave Tavees for mother and child. Her health improved and she was able to resume her sound abilities as a mother. Mother and baby were discharged home shortly after the visit from the Davi.

## SUMMARY

Nursing interventions for any client should be as free from trauma as possible. Clients from minority cultural backgrounds are often placed at a disadvantage by a system designed for White Europeans.

The UKCC Code of Professional Conduct requires that we 'Take account of the customs, values and spiritual beliefs of clients'; and that we 'Take every reasonable opportunity to maintain and improve professional knowledge and competence'. As nurses, we are always at the forefront of change.

The section on useful addresses at the end of this chapter, along with the further reading list, gives information on agencies that are willing to help that nurse overcome any problems related to minority groups and their care.

To end this chapter, there follows a list of do's and don'ts. The list is not exhaustive; it is anticipated that it will be used as a reference when one is involved in the care of clients from any ethnic minority culture.

## DO'S AND DON'TS

### NAME

**Don't** use Western titles, such as Mr, Miss, Ms, Mrs.

**Don't** ask non-Christians for a Christian name.

**Do** ask for family name or first name.

**Do** avoid repetition in clinical notes. Find out the correct family name first rather than misuse several differing names.

### LANGUAGE

**Don't** assume that all ethnic minority groups speak English.

**Don't** assume that all ethnic minority groups do not speak English.

**Do** avoid making assumptions by using accurate assessment procedures.

**Don't** use the family to interpret intimate questions.

**Don't** use a family member to break bad news. He or she may avoid the issue if it is believed to be too stressful for the client.

**Do** use an interpreter who understands medical terminology; this will avoid stress for the interpreter and client and also avoid misinterpretation.

**Do** be aware that women may only ask intimate questions of women in some cultures. This will avoid wrong information being passed, and avoid embarrassment.

### RELIGION

**Don't** generalize about a client's religion.

**Do** remember that for Buddhists, Christians, Jews, Sikhs, Hindus and Muslims, religion may be an integral part of daily life.

**Do** avoid incorrect assumptions; find out the different beliefs and approaches.

**Do** record clearly and make note of the client's wish to see or have present a representative from his/her religion.

**Do** ask the family who you should contact if the client is not able to relay this to you.

**Do** remember that many Eastern Religions fast on certain days; pray at certain times; wear religious objects or symbols.

**Don't** mistake religious objects or symbols for jewellery.

**Do** check to see if any nursing interventions will compromise any religious beliefs.

**Do** inform the client and/or family of any nursing interventions before commencing, to check religious beliefs.

**Do** check religious observations with client and family.

**Do** consult with religious advisors or teachers to gain permission and/or to obtain exemption, to allow procedures to take place. Ensure he/she explains this to the client.

## DIET

**Don't** give Jews or Muslim pork or pork products.

**Do** make sure that other meat offered to Muslims has been religiously slaughtered by the *halal* method (naturally slaughtered).

**Do** remember that not all Jewish people eat kosher food (specially prepared to make pure).

**Do** remember that not all Muslims eat *halal* meat.

**Do** consult the client regarding any diet preferences.

**Do** remember that meal times are family occasions in Eastern culture; matters relating to the family are often discussed here.

**Do** remember that being taken out of a close family environment can be frightening and cause loneliness, which may cause loss of appetite.

**Do** invite the family to bring in food and to join in meal times, if at all possible and practical.

## PERSONAL HYGIENE

**Do** remember that to Sikhs, Hindus, and Muslims washing in still water is considered unclean.

**Do** supply the client with a jug of water and bowl and/or running tap and empty wash-basin to allow hand, face and body washing.

**Do** make exceptions if the client is dependent.

**Do** remember that Muslims use the right hand for eating and food preparation, and the left hand for cleaning themselves and other procedures. Anyone unable to do this because of injury or other health reasons will need counselling and discussion relating to ways of surmounting this problem (it may be useful to supply a plastic glove).

## MODESTY

**Don't** compromise the clients dignity and modesty.

**Do** remember that exposure of the female body to a male will cause distress in certain cultures, especially if the client is in *purdah* (the duration of menstruation).

**Do** offer separate bays in mixed bedded wards, or if possible a single room, especially for those in *purdah*.

**Do** remember that hospital gowns often expose more than they cover, and are therefore unacceptable.

**Do** avoid exposure of arms or legs; for example, in the case of a fracture limb. Add additional covering to protect modesty.

## SKIN AND HAIR

**Do** remember that Afro hair may be brittle or dry; add moisturizer or oil to the scalp and comb regularly.

**Do** remember to ask the client what they use for skin moisturizer.

**Do** remember that dark-skinned people are prone to keloid scarring (hyperkeratinization); invasive treatment will cause excessive pigmented scarring.

**Do** remember to inject or undertake invasive procedures in a site that will avoid disfigurement if possible.

**Don't** assume that children of Asian, African, or Southern European decent have bruising if you see marks around the sacrum, buttocks, or hand and wrists; these may be 'Mongolian blue spots'.

**Do** avoid accusation of child abuse by undertaking full and proper assessment and advice.

## HOSPITAL PROCEDURES

**Do**     give careful thought to procedures and routines before commencing them.

**Do**     remember that discussing elimination or other intimate health issues may be culturally offensive.

**Do**     approach all patients sensitively, ensure privacy, and maintain the individuals right to self-respect.

**Do**     remember that some medications and treatments may be taboo for some religious groups.

**Don't**  give Jehovah's Witnesses blood transfusions.

**Don't**  give Muslim, Jews, and vegetarians iron injections derived from pigs.

**Don't**  give insulin of bovine origin to Hindus or Sikhs.

**Don't**  give insulin of porcine origin to Jews or Muslims.

**Do**     remember that many emollients have derivatives from animals.

**Do**     remember that some medications have an alcohol base which may be forbidden in some cultural groups: the client with a drinking problem may wish to avoid these preparations.

**Do**     be aware of all preparations likely to contain potentially taboo or offensive ingredients.

## VISITING

**Do**     remember that limiting visiting to two people may cause distress in extended family cultures.

**Do**     remember West Indian, Asian, and Middle Eastern families like to visit as a family.

**Do**     remember that the 'family' may include children, uncles, aunts, grandchildren, parents, and grandparents.

**Do**     compromise over visiting, and numbers visiting per bed.

**Do**     remember that open visiting can be more accommodating.

**Do**     allow the family to participate in the client's care.

## MYTHS

**Don't**  believe that people from different races have low-pain threshold. This is not true, for example:
   – Japanese may smile or laugh when in pain, thus avoiding loss of face;
   – Anglo-Saxons may be sullen and withdrawn, portraying the stiff-upper-lip image;
   – Eastern Europeans, Greeks, and Italians express pain vocally and freely.

**Do**     remember that every individual has a different level of pain tolerance, regardless of race, culture, country of origin, or creed.

## DEATH AND BEREAVEMENT

**Do**     involve client and family in the care.

**Do**     remember that Eastern cultures like to take an active part in the care of the dying relatives, especially last offices.

**Do**     remember that in certain cultures, custom and practice will need to be followed if the client is to proceed along the continuum of life following his/her earthly death.

**Do**     ensure that you are fully conversant with specific cultural requirements for death, bereavement, and last offices.

**Don't**  deny the family the right to participate in last offices as this will increase the pain already being experienced and may slow down the grieving process.

**Do**     negotiate to minimize anxiety and allow some participation, when the family's wishes come into conflict with hospital policies and procedures. This will assist the grieving process.

**Do**     compromise; the client and family have only one chance to say their goodbyes.

## REFERENCES

Clarke, E. (1979) Imagery of Madness, transcultural psychiatric workshop, (unpub.) London.

Flockhart, S. (1986) A community at risk: isolation and Asian Women, living with racism. *Inside Out (GAHM)* 13, 4–5.

Harrison, G. *et al.* (1988) A perspective study of severe mental disorder in Afro-Caribbean patients. *Psychological Medicine* 18, 643–57.

Jarvis, M. (1986) Female, Asian and isolated. *Openmind*, April/May, 10–12.

Littlewood, R., Cross, S. (1980) Ethnic minorities and psychiatric services, in *Sociology of Health and Illness*, (vol 2)

Littlewood, R. and Lipsedge, M. (1982) *Aliens and Alienists – Ethnic Minorities and Psychiatry*, Penguin, Harmondworth.

MIND (July 1990) Black and Ethnic Communities and Mental Health Information Sheet.

*Race Relations Code of Practice* (consultation draft 1991) Commission for Racial Equality, London.

Renshaw, J. (1988) *Mental Health Care for Ethnic Minority Groups*, Good Practices in Mental Health, London.

Thompson, C. (1988) Pain and poverty in the inner cities: Racism and its impact on social deprivation in the black community. West Indian Standing Conference, paper printed at the MIND annual conference.

Ward, L. (1988) Racism and Mental Health in Britain. *Radical Community Medicine*, Summer issue, 27–30.

## FURTHER READING

Fernando, S. (1988) *Race Culture Society*. Tavistock/Routledge, London and Mind, mail order.

Renshaw, J. (1988) *Mental Health Care for Ethnic Minority Groups*, Good Practices in Mental Health.

*Race Relations Code Practice*, (1991). The Commission for Racial Equality, London.

Rack, P. (1982) *Race, Culture Mental Disorder*. Tavistock, London MIND, mail order.

## USEFUL ADDRESSES

Transcultural Psychiatric Unit
Lynfield Mount Hospital
Heights Lane, Bradford, BD9 6DP

Transcultural Psychiatric Society UK
University Department of Psychiatry
Royal Edinburgh Hospital, Morningside,
Edinburgh EH10 5HF

Centre for Ethnic Minority Health Studies
Fieldhouse Postgraduate Centre
Bradford Royal Infirmary
Duckworth Lane, Bradford 9

Commission for Racial Equality
Elliot House
10–12 Allington Street
London SW1E 5EH

Good Practices in Mental Health
380–384 Harrow Road
London W9 2HU

MIND, National Association for Mental Health
22 Harley Street
London W1N 2ED

# PART FOUR

# NURSING INTERVENTIONS – STRUCTURE AND PROCESS

*Ralph Nichols*

Intervention is about 'doing', feeling and being aware of oneself and the needs of the client. Since it is fundamentally a humanistic endeavour, we should be interested in people. Moreover, these same principles apply when interacting with colleagues and associates. This section reflects the author's belief that the quality of mental health nursing intervention is influenced by a variety of interacting factors, including the type of professional education the nurse has received; the type of culture within which she or he works; and the attitudes that prevail within the employing organization.

The viewpoints expressed here are not written in stone; they should promote discussion and debate. More importantly, it is hoped they will create an awareness of people-centred values that influence the thinking, actions, and feelings of the reader.

As professionals we need to speak in a more ordinary way if we are to be understood. In any social system there is a predominant language; in nursing it has sadly become techno-speak rather than people-speak. This is not acceptable. We have to give something of ourselves in order to explain, learn, and discover.

This chapter explores aspects of nursing intervention. The intention is not to provide a 'how-to' of the nursing process or nursing models; there is already a considerable literature in this area (Further Reading). Rather, a descriptive and creative approach is taken to illustrate how concepts associated with nursing assessments and research methods are adapted to the real world of mental health nursing. Hence, such terms as 'openness to experience', 'self-awareness', and 'learning through evaluation and supervision' take on a more realistic meaning.

The chapter first examines therapeutic engagement, a process that lays down the foundations on which the nurse/client relationship is built. The use of the medical model as a major influence on nursing organization and structure is then considered. The nursing process itself is considered in five stages: assessment, formulation, planning, implementation, and evaluation/research. Each stage is introduced and a description of the central concept is given. Basic principles associated with each concept are identified, as well as their importance and value. Finally, the author offers a critical commentary, often from personal experience, about how the concept is utilized and interpreted in the real world. This provides an analysis of the concept at a higher level, for those readers who are familiar with it and wish to further explore its application.

## A DESCRIPTION OF THERAPEUTIC ENGAGEMENT

'Therapeutic engagement' is a term that refers to the process through which the mental health nurse in the early stages of contact builds the foundations of a positive relationship with the client. The aim is for the client to begin to feel that the nurse has a realistic and non-judgemental appreciation of her or his needs, and that she can be trusted. Central to the variety of skills involved is the establishment of rapport. Therapeutic engagement can occur before meeting clients, for example, when writing letters informing them of an appointment.

What is known as the therapeutic process is often centred upon humanistic principles, notably the work of Rogers (1965) and Maslow (1970). Therapeutic processes seem to be generally the opposite to what Menzies (1970) described as mechanisms to relieve stress associated with caring. In order to be therapeutic, nurses need to get involved with their clients, assist them to take responsibility, and create changes for themselves. This is what Barker (1991) describes as 'getting personal with our clients'. Like Menzies, he describes how nurses can use their status, uniforms, titles, and hierarchical pecking-order to protect themselves from the stressors involved with clients. The latter also imposes a form of control and a power-base from which nurses can work. Interestingly, the same principles apply to relationships between teachers and students, researchers and the researched, and managers and clinicians.

## PRINCIPLES

Barker (1989) suggests the following principles or 'rules of engagement':

Rule one: No weapons. I will try not to use my status or position, real or imagined, to control the person in my care.

Rule two: Feel the fear. I will try to appreciate why he thinks this is a problem. There is no need to explain it away.

Rule three: Climb down from the pedestal. I need to explore this life with its owner. I need to get involved; to collaborate, to work with him.

Rule four: Build a raft. I need a simple structure if I am not to be drowned in the sea of possibilities.

Rule five: Mind your p's and q's. I will try to help the person on his own personal quest. Let him be his own judge and jury.

## IMPORTANCE AND VALUE

How can we assess if a relationship is therapeutic? Guidelines for good practice will not suffice; the therapeutic process has to be discovered. It is also a process of growth and development through self-evaluation. It has, and will continue to have, different values and meanings for different people according to their past experiences, their present reality, and the kind of visions they have for the future. It will also depend upon the values they attach to their work and their relationships with clients and colleagues.

First and foremost, the practitioner – teacher, researcher, manager – needs to understand and be able to interpret what the term 'therapeutic' means to them. Next, a means of self-evaluation is required. Campbell (1980) offers a general framework for promoting self-awareness as a means to evaluate the quality of therapeutic engagement with clients. He suggests four components:

The physical component is the knowledge of personal and general physiology; body reactions, body-image, body language and the physical potential we have.

The environmental component consists of our social environment, our relationships with others, and the knowledge of the relationships between people.

The philosophical component refers to the sense that life has meaning. It may involve a belief in the world as it is, how we would like it to be, and the ethics of the behaviour that evolves from it.

The psychological component includes knowledge of self-awareness, motivations, self-concept, and personality. It means being sensitive to our feelings, and the external stressors that affect those feelings.

## CRITICAL COMMENTARY

Therapeutic engagement can be more effective if the nurse utilizes a process of self-evaluation. Such evaluation may be achieved by using a series of frameworks, starting with the simple and moving towards the sophisticated. The 'rules' associated with engagement previously listed could be useful as well as, for example, the human needs hierarchy suggested by Maslow (1970). The nurse can simply reformulate each component of the model or checklist into a question by asking, 'Have I?', 'Did I?', Could I have done better?'. Similarly, nursing models can be used as means to review the therapeutic process. This example illustrates their versatility as a means not only to think about nursing and to assess the needs of clients, but also to review the effectiveness of intervention.

The most important principle is the awareness promoted by thinking and exploration, rather than the components of the models used to guide the process. Rowan (1981), for example, provides us with what is a sophisticated and detailed framework for self-evaluation, which may have been undervalued in the past. He describes an approach to self-questioning, orginally utilized to promote and demonstrate the change in thinking between researchers and the researched, that can be used at any point during a person-centred relationship. The framework consists of the following sections: being, thinking, project, encounter, making sense, and communication.

### BEING

Being is about existence. It asks: What are you trying to do? Is the problem relevant to your life, your career, a client, the organization, your unconscious? Is the client involved? If so, is there honesty, or deception, or lack of communication? Who provides the problem? Who defines what the problem is? Who owns the problem? Who is the client? Who is the real client? Why do you do your job? Is it for competition, recognition, power or acclaim? Are you sexist, racist, classist, or ageist? Are you aware of the social, organizational, hierarchical, moral, and professional pressures that influence your actions? Do you listen to others? Are you aware of the motives of others? Are you intellectually tough enough for real, in-depth, self-evaluation and awareness? Can you handle the stressors involved?

### THINKING

This is the creative process of invention and testing. It continually poses the question: Will this do? It is an inward movement, gathering in information about unfamiliar relationships and trying it against a template of what would be acceptable. It is the time for organization, using criteria for an assessment of nursing needs and the principles of people-centred work.

### PROJECT

This is an outward movement, where you take a risk and form an intention. Rowan (1981) suggests that this will involve some form of bridging distances to another person, to a new situation, to a new idea. Hence, we can ask, 'How is the client to be involved with the planning of his care?', or, 'How is a team of nursing staff to be involved with your project?' It is at this stage of self-awareness, through evaluation, that the nurse can contradict the present reality and bring into being a new situation. This stage involves plans and decisions.

### ENCOUNTER

Action is the most important thing. In action you are fully present; here and now. Plans are merely guides that reflect past reality and influence future action. Encounter means 'doing' and actually meeting the client; it involves engagement. It is at this point that we can compare what was expected with what actually happens; it is potentially revealing. It is the place for involvement and spontaneity. The question is, 'Are you really open to experience?' If the nurse is not genuinely encountering reality she or he is not likely to learn.

MAKING SENSE

Action is not enough. The nurse needs to withdraw and find out what her or his engagement with a client means. The question is, 'How can I understand what I have been through, and what the client and my colleagues have been through?' Perhaps there is more than one message, more than one way of viewing the situation and taking action. What are the contradictions, and how can they be resolved?

It is at this point that information, feelings, and biases have to be acknowledged and formulated into something that is understandable. It is at this stage that the fears, the self-esteem, the caring, and the learning of both the client and the nurse have to be contemplated honestly. Moreover, this may be the time for confrontation, risk-taking, and the upholding of the beliefs, values, and rights of the client and the nurse. Hence, supervision, support, and assertiveness skills become important because there are always consequences when such an awareness of individual need is realized.

COMMUNICATION

An analysis of thoughts and actions is not enough. The nurse needs to tell people, including the client, what it means and how she or he has understood what they have been through. What was actually accomplished or achieved? Can others learn from our mistakes and successes? It is at this point that

the nurse goes back into the field and practices nursing, only now on a higher level. Rowan (1981) suggests that the contradiction here is between 'everything is [now] all right as it is' versus 'everything is not all right as it is'. He further suggests that one's daily work is essentially a resting place, a place for contentment. It always hurts to leave it and explore what is happening.

Self-awareness can commence at any point. It may start with encounter, being, or thinking. One category should lead to another. The important thing is not to get hooked on just one category.

EXERCISE

Describe an initial encounter with a client (student, subject(s) of research) using the headings described above. Consider how your feelings influenced your understanding of therapeutic engagement.

THE MEDICAL MODEL AND TRADITIONAL APPROACHES TO CARE

Prior to a discussion of the nursing process and nursing assessment, the nature of traditional approaches to nursing needs to be addressed. This is compared with the nursing process as a means of individualizing care. We shall examine the origins of the nursing process, its purported influence on the quality of care, and its limitations.

The intention of the 'process' philosophy was to challenge traditional approaches to care that centred upon the medical model. The history of nursing, like all social history, reflects the values of society in the past. In the nineteenth century, industrial production was controlled by task division. The allocation of a series of tasks to members of a team created a hierarchy of jobs. Nursing developed at that time, and employed similar approaches to the organization of work. When the care of people is managed in this way the individual may be lost within the system.

Goffman (1968) in his book *Asylums* shows how institutions militate against individualism. He found that institutions depersonalized both staff and patients, and as Tedman (1985) and Walsh *et al.* (1989) confirm, the resulting loss of identity led people to carry out procedures without asking why they were done, or how the recipients felt; many nursing actions become rituals. Goffman (1968) describes vividly the effects of living one's whole life – eating, sleeping, working, playing – in one institution; the result is uniform and predictable behaviour by patients and staff. Tedman (1985) further comments that depersonalizing situations can intensify conformist tendencies to obey without reflection.

## THE MEDICAL MODEL

Traditionally, much of nursing work and thinking has been determined by the medical model; nursing practice has been determined by the patient's medical diagnosis. According to the medical model, a person is a complex set of anatomical parts and physiological systems. Within the medical model, much of the person's social bahaviour and many of their psychological processes are thought to originate from physiological and biochemical activity. This view is now considered inadequate, not only by many social scientists, but also by many nurses, since it encourages an understanding of people as 'passive hosts of disease and machines'. The medical approach to care emphasizes the existence of biological needs within people, and stressses the structure and function of the body, rather than the uniqueness of the individual or their position within society.

The medical model focuses on signs and symptoms that are usually identified by taking a medical history, and by physically examining the person in an attempt to identify physiological systems that are disturbed in their functioning. This leads to a diagnosis being made, which is usually recognized as a medical condition and classified as such. Intervention then centres on putting things right. Hence, the focus is not upon the whole person, but upon the particular physiological system that is perceived to be malfunctioning.

Wright (1986) argues that nurses working with the medical model may find themselves subservient to the orders of doctors. This may lead nurses to ignore symptoms or aspects of the client that do not fit neatly into the medical label. The medical influence upon the management of care has also reinforced the practice of dividing jobs into a series of tasks, such as bed-making, washing patients, and giving out meals. Often student nurses were assigned the task of taking 'patients' to the occupational therapy department. Similarly, clothing for long-stay patients was allocated from the ward stockroom. Each nurse has historically been responsible for the completion of certain tasks during a working shift.

Binnie *et al.* (1984) notes that when task allocation is used in a hospital setting, a fairly rigid ward routine prevails. A nurse working within the task-allocation system frequently has brief contact with a large number of clients; each client typically encounters many different nurses. This traditional approach to nursing means that tasks are carried out by nurses according to their skill and status within the hierarchy. Low-status skills usually involve helping clients with their daily living activities and other jobs concerned with physical care.

Tasks associated with basic nursing care are usually allocated to untrained or junior members of the nursing team. Paradoxically, it is such tasks associated with nursing care that involve most patient contact and require interpersonal skills. Although such skills may determine the quality of care, they continue to be associated with low-status work. The nurse/patient relationship has been identified as the most important single factor to influence the quality of care (Royal Commission on the Health Service, 1979).

Tasks accorded high status are usually those considered to be technical, or those of a clerical or organizational nature that tend to involve less client contact. These tasks are generally allocated to senior learners or qualified staff, and involve decision-making about client care and liaison with medical staff or senior members of the nursing hierarchy. Many high-status nursing tasks are considered to be technical because they involve the operation of equipment, although the reality is often a repetitive medical procedure, such as preparing a clinic for the administration of ECT to a number of clients.

## THE NURSING PROCESS

The nursing process has been well described in the literature. Such descriptions were thought to require elaboration, in that the process was considered to be an interactional approach that promoted a philosophy of individualized client care by influencing the culture of a nursing team and the thinking and behaviour of nurses. One of the problems with the introduction of the process was its rigid interpretation, associated jargon, and its emphasis on paperwork, which was the opposite of the original intention to focus on the nurse/client relationship.

Similarly, a number of definitions of quality care have been suggested. Unfortunately, these definitions, like many others, tend to be rhetorical and difficult to operationalize. It is suggested here that quality care is determined by how well nurses interact with clients. This relationship is considered to be dynamic because it is influenced by personal and organizational values. Such values probably influence how nurses perceive the quality of the care they provide.

Dickinson (1982) argues that with the use of the nursing process, basic care is redefined as an activity requiring scientific knowledge and equality with doctors. Hargreaves (1979) described the nursing process as a combina-tion of thought processes and nursing actions. These involve assessing client needs or problems; formulating the nursing needs of the client; drawing up a plan of nursing care on the basis of those needs or problems; implementing the plan of care; and evaluating the effectiveness of the care given.

In summary, the nursing process is a model in five stages, which should direct the thinking and behaviour of nurses towards individualized care. The approach requires support by service managers to allow for nursing autonomy and development of positive attitudes towards changing practice.

The past decade has seen increasing emphasis on the process as the core activity of nursing practice, and the foundation-stone of nurse education. Crow (1977) notes that the World Health Organization proposed an eight-year plan to familarize European coun-tries with the nursing process. She further identifies the process as simply a kind of prescription of how nurses do, or ought to do, their work. Improving patient care, she argues, will ultimately be achieved 'by nurses themselves with the "process" to help them'.

From the mid-1970s onwards the educational implications of the process were recognized in curriculum designs for nurse education; it was seen as 'a unifying thread for the study of patient care and a helpful framework for nursing practice'. For the preparation of nurse educators, the teacher was expected to 'interpret and synthesize the strands of learning which form the stages of the nursing process' and formulate training objectives for nurses (GNC, 1977, 1978, 1982). More recently, the guidelines for the clinical grading of nurses utilized the process for the operationalization of the associated pay-scales (DHSS, 1988).

## THE ORIGINS OF THE NURSING PROCESS

The nursing process evolved as a response to a need for change in the way nurses and society approached care. Its origins were probably more academic than pragmatic. The idea that nursing was a process rather than a set of separate actions emerge in the US in the 1950s. Peplau (1952) recognized nursing intervention as an interpersonal skill. Likewise, other nursing authors began to centre their attention upon the patient, rather than the completion of nursing tasks.

Strangely enough, the origin of the nursing process concept remains something of a mystery. It appears to have grown from a need for American medical insurance companies to find a way of auditing the nursing care given to patients. In addition, the process was seen as a coping mechanism for the discontent among American nurses, which coincided with a change in health-care expectation within American society. De la Cuesta (1983) writes that these changes included the expansion of education; the emergence of the Women's Liberation Movement; the growth of knowledge in the medical and social sciences; the rise of costs in health services; and an increase in other health-care occupations. These led to a movement towards the professional status of nursing, including the quest of autonomy, knowledge-based practice, and personalized services.

In the UK, the nursing process did not grow autonomously. It was not considered something completely new, but was seen to have precursors that prepared the way for its diffusion. National debates on the existing system of delivering care promoted the publication of the first British article (Crow, 1977) and the first British book (Kratz, 1979). These initial theoretical works attracted attention from nurse educators, the appeal being that they represented devices to enable the understanding and teaching of nursing.

The nursing process adopted in the UK was not a copy of the American approach. The autonomy and accountability of the nurse and the intellectual skills involved with problem-solving were not emphasized; instead the process seemed to be taught as a framework for the documentation of nursing care. The client's involvement was mentioned, but in terms of gaining their co-operation and collaboration, rather than their active participation; it was considered to be a method for improving the quality of care. However, aspects of the nurse/patient relationship as catalysts for quality were neither explained nor operationalized in the literature.

The adoption of the nursing process was very rapid, emerging around 1973. By 1977 it was included in the training syllabus for general nursing.

The medical profession was concerned following the publication of a Royal College of Nursing guideline about the nursing process (RCN, 1981), which proposed that only professional nurses could set standards, assess nursing needs, and measure the quality of care. Mitchell (1984) voiced medical doubts over the development of the nursing process, and suggested it should be properly evaluated. He further urged that the process should not be adopted blindly; rather it should be considered a catalyst to promote better health care by all professionals.

Ashworth *et al.* (1978) argue that good care within the medical model is significantly different to care under the process approach. They suggest, first, that medical plans were often based upon inadequate information and inference, rather than observation and questioning. Nurses tended to record what they assume was happening, or what was meant to happen with reference to the medical condition, rather than consider individual needs. Second, the individual aspects of care under the medical model were often not stated, therefore the care given by different members of staff was probably unco-ordinated. Furthermore, the plan of care was often not written, but communicated verbally to different members of staff causing some discontinuity. Third, planned evaluations of traditional care rarely occured.

The author's personal experiences and previous work concerning the use of the nursing process is next used to illustrate the need for a change in attitudes in the way the process and assessment are used.

The author worked in a hospital that was a prime example of an institution that demanded uniformity and conformity of behaviour from both clients and staff. The clients' physical care was seen as a measure of their well-being, and was the lowest common denominator that seemed to motivate nurses to take action; this was the goal of care. The work was dull, uninteresting, and always the same.

It did not occur to the author that at the time he was perpetuating a routine that was supported by the culture of the organization. Nurses, including myself, may not be able to identify and value good care until they have experienced and unknowingly provided poor care. This experience illustrates the power and influence that organizational values can have upon individuals and how it may affect present and future approaches towards quality care. The process philosophy purports to promote individualized nursing for patients, and autonomy for nurses to make decisions about care, but is destined to fail when imposed within organizations that insist upon conformist behaviour.

The nursing process was introduced to the hospital as a means of recording care. Managers approached the implementation of the nursing process in an autocratic way; it was seen as another management task to be completed. The emphasis was upon how to write nursing objectives, plan the appropriate care, and evaluate its effectiveness. Little mention was made of the importance of changing work organization or extending the autonomy of trained nurses.

Nurses were being encouraged to think and write about care in the same way. Like many other nationally directed initiatives, the nursing process became an imposed model of care. Some writers tend to be directive and prescriptive with regard to the correct way to write clients' problems and nursing goals. The thinking and behaviour of nurses who use the nursing process has been thus constrained towards what was called a 'systematic approach to nursing care'.

Interpretations of what the process is, how it should be implemented, and the benefits of its use for clients and staff vary. The process was intended to create a change in organizational culture by steering the thinking and behaviour of nurses away from the medical model. However, the dynamics of such a change were probably over-simplified. Moreover, the benefits of process use for the organization as a whole are barely mentioned in the literature.

Questions about the quality of care were frequently asked; at the time, quality of care was a new and popular issue within most management circles. Managers acted as nurse administrators, rather than clinical specialists. Good managers were expected to monitor the clinical situation, rather than to influence hands-on care. Evaluating care was based upon simple quantitative approaches such as numbers of staff available and the dependency of patients. Phrases associated with caring, such as 'client-centred attitudes' and 'interpersonal skills' were often quoted from the literature. However, these attitudes and skills were neither defined or operationalized.

Established quality monitoring tools were used in an attempt to measure care. However, the concepts that made up the tools did not fit the practical situation, although it was some time before it was realized that most concepts reflected the value systems of other organizations.

## NURSING ASSESSMENT

### BASIC PRINCIPLES

Assessment is the collection from any available source, particularly the client, of the information that is relevant to his or her health state and care. Assessment involves the interpretation of information gained by interviewing, systematic observation, and the review of records. Approaches to assessment are likely to vary; each health district, service or clinical team may develop its own individual stategies and methods.

## IMPORTANCE AND VALUE

Assessing a client's nursing needs will additionally reflect the beliefs the nurse holds about people, society, health and illness, and nursing itself. Assessment is thus culturally and socially specific. The assessment should lead to a description of the client's limitations and strengths, which in turn should lead to the identification of nursing goals.

To ensure that a systematic assessment is carried out, most health districts have designed a nursing process assessment form. The design is often based upon a stated nursing model.

## CRITICAL COMMENTARY

Wright (1986) warns that some universal nursing assessment formats may result in information being collected that is not always appropriate to the individual client. He further states that 'there needs to be as much flexibility in the creation of nursing notes as there is in the model used to assess patient needs.' To impose a rigid set of forms which may not be applicable to the setting within which nurses work may meet with resistance and hostility. The assessment of client need may become merely 'another form to fill and yet another task to be completed'. Similarly, De la Cuesta (1983) found that nursing histories were regarded more as reference sheets containing client information than as a base upon which to draw up care plans.

## FORMULATION

Myers (1973) suggests that the formulation stage of the nursing process, which she calls 'nursing diagnosis', occurs when the nurse considers what the information gained from the client and/or their relatives reveals. Once nursing needs are identified, the nurse then considers how best to meet them; hence, a plan of care is drawn up. Formulation also means the nurse can utilize subjective and objective feelings resulting from interacting and observing a client.

It should be noted that some writers considering the formulation of nursing needs refer, in the first instance, to the use of case notes and medical opinion rather than how a nurse interacts and/or engages with a client. Moreover, the nurse as an influencing factor upon the client's behaviour and conversation, and in turn the quality of care provided, is often omitted.

The formulation of nursing needs is based upon many factors, the most important being the client's involvement. Formulating a nursing viewpoint can be stressful; hence the importance of supervised practice. Ward (1985) argues that 'nurses must be discouraged from always seeing biological man as the most important one'. However, he goes on to suggest that the formulation stage of the process is what makes it scientific rather than innate. The author believes that the word 'scientific' in this context is taken too literally because it is generally associated with objectivity. Therefore, in order to use subjectivity and gut feeling, an element of interpretation or 'art' is necessary. There needs to be a mix of objective and subjective interpretation. This means that the objective information should be based upon what the client says and does. There needs to be caution, however, when formulating the nursing needs of the client because an over-reliance upon subjectivity could mean that nursing action is meaningless to the client; whereas to be too objective could mean that nursing intervention may be irrelevant because it ignores the nuances of the person.

Ward (1985) offers the following flow-chart to assist with the formulation of nursing needs.

- Establish which needs the client is not meeting for themselves.
- Does the client agree with your outline? If not, why not?
- Discuss alternatives; if appropriate, compromise.
- Establish which needs are to be met first.
- Convert statements into behavioural conclusions.

The author believes that statements that make up formulated nursing needs should also consider cognitive conclusions; the way that the client thinks must influence their behaviour.

## CARE PLANNING

### BASIC PRINCIPLES

This stage involves identifying goals and objectives for nursing care and writing them on a care plan. Hunt *et al.* (1980) describe the nursing care plan as a 'visible written record of care that is to be given'. The plan should make explicit the details of care to be given by the nurse and the response of the patient. Crow *et al.* (1979) suggest that without careful planning nursing care will be disorganized and less effective.

### IMPORTANCE AND VALUE

An important part of such planning is involving clients and engaging their understanding and co-operation in what the nurse is doing.

Nursing care plans are not always consistently written. Often, the nursing problems identified are concerned with physical care and centre upon the medical diagnosis.

Nursing care plans may be a major drawback to the full implementation of the nursing process if viewed as imposed formalities to be filled in when there is time; something for administrative purposes only.

Wright (1985) comments that the writing of care plans depends upon several important features, including the assessment skills of the nurse; the willingness/ability of the client to give information; the type of assessment used; the quality and content of the assessment; the nurses' knowledge and skills; the degree to which the clients' medical diagnosis affects their ability to care for themselves; and the ability of the nurse to express these things on paper. However, such influences, while having an effect upon the quality of care plans, may not affect the quality of care provided.

### CRITICAL COMMENTARY

Like nursing assessment formats, the design of nursing care plans varies from district to district, although their components may be similar. Most care plans are usually of the problem-solving type, divided into preprinted columns with headings such as 'problems and nursing needs', 'objectives and dates resolved', and 'management and nursing actions'.

Some clinical teams have interpreted the components of the nursing process by designing their own documentation according to their own values and understanding of the approach. This allows for innovation and creativity. The traditional documentation has been replaced with either multidisiplinary notes and logbooks or diaries, particularly for continued-care clients. This means that a simple checklist of components for an assessment are used for reference. Hence, this alternative to the preprinted type of document is used as a guideline for assessing and planning care, rather than as a form to fill in. This has not only influenced the effectiveness of the nursing process and its understanding, but also the quality of care.

# IMPLEMENTING CARE

## BASIC PRINCIPLES

Implementing care means that nursing action should meet the objectives identified by assessing nursing needs and planning client care. Ward (1985) considers implementing care to be an exciting prospect because it is at this stage that nurses can put their skills to the test. Without intervention and follow-up evaluation, assessing and planning care is academic and meaningless.

## IMPORTANCE AND VALUE

The implementation phase of the process is not so well illustrated in the literature. Authors are significantly less prolific in giving their views on implementation. McGilloway (1980) commented that 'although specific therapies and procedures of client management have been comprehensively described in the nursing literature, very little attention has been given to the implementation of care'. Goble (1986) considers implementation to be simply the carrying out of the prescribed nursing action, while Ward (1985) states that 'the actual delivery of care' was not an appropriate subject for his book on the nursing process in psychiatry.

Many writers simply discuss the autonomy of the nurse as a means to improve and facilitate the nursing process. Little mention is made of the interpersonal skills involved with the development of the nurse-client relationship. Duberley (1979), while discussing 'giving nursing care', merely talks about the changes in priorities for care planning, and the benefits of nurse to nurse reporting.

Given that effective and improved care provision is the reason for developing and using the nursing process, it is unfortunate that many writers seem to emphasize benefits that centre upon plans or records rather than implementation.

# INTERPERSONAL SKILLS AND ORGANIZATION OF WORK

## BASIC PRINCIPLES

The links between interpersonal skills, the organization of nursing work, and the nursing process were neglected in early descriptions of the approach. Chavasse (1981) commented, however, that the way in which the nursing work in a ward is planned and allocated among the staff available may have a considerable influence upon the continuity of care, nurse-client relationships, nurses, satisfaction with their role, and the learning experiences of students.

## IMPORTANCE AND VALUE

Many writers suggest that most, if not all, of the proposed benefits for clients which may result from the use of the process are also benefits of primary nursing, which is considered to be the organizational and behavioural interpretation of the process philosophy. Early writers described the nursing process as a cognitive approach, assuming that appropriate nursing behaviour directed at individualizing care would automatically influence the organization of nursing work.

## BENEFITS OF INDIVIDUALIZED CARE

A recent study (Nichols, 1991) allowed for a sensitive and detailed analysis of nursing process use and its effect upon the quality of care. The results illustrated that all the nursing teams identified as using a high standard of the nursing process had not only interpreted the approach in their own way, but also provided the best quality care.

The findings of this study suggest that some of the assumptions associated with nursing process use may now be better termed as predictions or implications. The assumption that nursing care would be more effective when using the process may be enhanced if the measure of effectiveness is an increased number of qualitative psychosocial interactions between the client(s) and the nurse. The study illustrated that writers who suggested across-the-board improvements were probably referring to an improved effectiveness of physical care. Second, that dignity and respect for the client(s) is increased with the use of the process. Third, decision-making, choice, control, and autonomy for the client(s) may be improved and finally, nurses were able to give more time, and were able to listen and probably elicit more cues from client(s) when working in process teams.

The results illustrate that further research is required to strengthen the assumption that client(s) gain a greater sense of individuality, self-esteem, motivation, and responsibility. Interestingly, the results suggest that such attributes may be improved for nurses when they interpret the process. Assumptions regarding improved continuity of nursing intervention, client(s) involvement, hypothesis-generation, and client(s) teaching remain speculative.

All the nursing teams identified as using a high standard of the nursing process had thought about and explored ways to improve the effectiveness of their approach to care. This could be an important factor influencing the quality of care. It may also result in a knock-on effect in that staff feel more valued because their interpretation of the process becomes the focus of attention for client(s)' needs.

However, it could be argued that documentation is only a record of this care. Unlike traditional approaches towards documentation, interpretations of the process reflect the thinking and identification of values essential for the provision of quality care. Such an approach not only allows nursing teams to identify components of an assessment and care plan, it also provides a focus for thinking about individual client(s),

and is more likely to promote a sense of responsibility for the care of clients. Nursing teams, permitted by managers and educationalists to interpret the process in their own way, are able to reflect their understanding of the approach and their ability to challenge traditional practices.

## EVALUATION AND RESEARCH

The act of evaluation is concerned with ascertaining whether nursing intervention has met the needs of the client. Some actions will be measurable and objective, while others may require subjective evaluation by the client. This final stage of the process provides the means by which the nurse may revise the plan of care. It requires a comparison of the client's physical and psychological needs before and after intervention. When expected outcomes do not take place, the client and nurse should reassess the particular area of difficulty. Stenhouse (1984) considers that evaluation is more about learning and thinking than measurement of goal achievement. He proposes that evaluation should have meaning, understanding, potential, and interest.

The processes of reviewing care are the same as those associated with research. Luker (1981) describes what she calls a continuum of evaluation. Values have to be recognized when reviewing the care of a client and assessing the quality of care provided by a nursing team. The fundamental difference is that the evaluation stage of the nursing process relies upon the nurse's personal value system, whereas evaluative research has in some ways to rely upon the organization's value system.

It is important, therefore, that the values of practitioners influence the values of the organization. The process may have been an underestimated catalyst that changed the value system of organizations and the way that the quality of care was assessed and developed. This further strengthens the need for practitioners to be involved with and decide upon the approaches used for quality assurance. It also calls into question the validity of orthodox research methods where the researcher 'does' research 'on' practitioners rather than 'with' them.

## VALIDITY OF EXPERIMENTAL RESEARCH

The author believes that studies involving human behaviour undertaken in the real world cannot be called true experiments. Extraneous variables that may also affect the quality of care include: the education of the nursing staff; their interpretation of the nursing process; management values appertaining to innovation; and risk-taking associated with bottom-up approaches. Moreover, the organizational culture that either supports or stifles approaches towards the use of the nursing process and the autonomy of the individual nurse or nursing team needs to be considered.

### THE UNIVERSALITY OF CONCEPTS

In order to construct a nursing model, an element of subjectivity has to be permitted. Objectivity cannot be achieved when evaluating human behaviour, although the process philosophy tells us it should be. The following trade-offs may have to be made.

First, to be totally objective when evaluating care, a practitioner would have to rely upon a retrospective audit of the nursing records. The trade-off is for nurses to evaluate their own practice.

Second, to evaluate the quality of care objectively, a practitioner can only record if a nursing task was completed or not. Recording the outcome of care in relation to a specific area of client functioning may be a means of recording objective data, however, total objectivity may not indicate the nuances of quality. The trade-off is to indicate quality by evaluating how care was given, thereby

acknowledging the usefulness of subjectivity.

Finally, nursing assessment checklists, models and instruments designed to identify the quality of care are limited in that they cannot capture all the social and psychological influences that are a part of the caring function of the nurse. The trade-off is the realization of such limitations in the context of social research and development, compared with the objectivity of models constructed using methods derived from the biological sciences. Such limitations enable the identification of only some of the actions that nurses perform, and likewise may only allow for the identification of some of the effects such actions could have on clients.

### CHANGE OF DIRECTION

While conducting the study to review the influence of the nursing process upon the quality of care, the thinking of the author was pulled in different directions. Originally, the traditional approach described was considered appropriate. This so-called positivistic, or traditional, methodolgy was useful as a foundation for the study in that it promoted and organized exploration. However, because this research took place in natural settings, the need emerged for more subjective interpretations of the findings. Throughout the study a logbook was kept containing not only notes appertaining to the process of the research, but also subjective descriptions of the wards involved, the type of care provided, and the consideration of other influences thought to support the findings. Therefore, the design for a follow-up study is planned that depends much more upon interpretation.

The study illustrated that the interpretation of a particular way of working (the nursing process) influences the quality of care, rather than the uptake of the modality *per se*. A hierarchy of influences affecting the quality of care were identified. The study further suggests cultural changes associated with the research. It is the comparison of the quality of care between nursing teams at different stages of development that future research will aim to address.

It could be that the conceptualization of the nursing process has evolved through three stages of development. The first stage was the original interpretation of the idea, which emphasized paperwork and centred upon the universal design and completion of care plans. The second stage was marked by nursing teams interpreting the approach according to their own values and understanding. The third stage could involve the evaluation and teaching of the process as an interactional tool. The nursing process may, therefore, be more effectively utilized where the organizational ethos is client(s)-centred, and where priority is given to exploring quality issues related to the nurse/client relationship, rather than relying upon staffing levels and aesthetic values as measures of care.

Similarly, values appertaining to the quality of care could have evolved through several stages of development. The first stage was marked by descriptive approaches that centred upon nursing tasks. The second was achieved when behavioural interpretations of quality care centred upon how well nurses interact with clients, were accepted, and utilized. The third stage will be reached when caring is explored and improved according to cognitive and emotional interpretations, without a reliance upon scientific frameworks, and hence a realistic consideration of managerial, organizational, and interpersonal influences.

The study previously described demonstrates that positivistic, or traditional, research methods can be incorporated with interpretive approaches. Reason and Rowan (1981) call positivistic or scientific frameworks for research the 'old paradigm', and approaches that involve the interpretation of events by the researcher the 'new paradigm'.

The conceptual framework used to guide the study allowed it to move only half way towards the new paradigm. This was because it utilized a research design that relied upon interpretation and explanation with the assistance of control groups. The new paradigm suggests that an over-reliance upon experimental research designs, control groups, and generalization may limit the creative aspects of research involving what Parlett (1981) calls illuminative evaluation. The author believes that conceptual frameworks for research merely enable the creation of ideas generated at the vision stage of a project.

Hence, the new-paradigm approach has evolved from its scientific counterpart. This illustrates that the achievements of the past help in the search for present continuities; they present step-by-step connections. The new approach supports the notion that researchers look at what is actually happening rather than what is a provable theory. It suggests that theory evolves from a synthesis of what people do and say. The author believes that there is a need to add some diversity to the seemingly restricted menu offered by traditional research frameworks.

Reed *et al.* (1991) suggest that gut feelings should be an acceptable part of an investigation. They argue that many research techniques used by nurses may be defence mechanisms or rituals against a stressful task. Moreover, they consider that clinical rather than statistical significance may be a more valuable way to assess the validity of research.

For these reasons risks have to be taken; there is a need to illustrate the hidden agenda that is often implicitly suggested by the findings of most traditional research. This suggests that the happenings associated with real life may yield more valuable insights than trying to categorize data associated with human behaviour according to preset frameworks. When using such frameworks, it seems that the complexities and ambiguities of the real world may get lost in the sweep of the grand plan.

Can the findings of research, using traditional approaches, reflect reality, when it is possible to fiddle with it? Like the novelist, researchers need to achieve a combination of documentary detail coupled with the ability to abstract meaningful data. Research frameworks may then emerge that accurately reflect reality. Therefore, hypotheses, theoretical frameworks, and research designs may be abstracted and constructed as a study unfolds. The author suggests that an initial research question is sufficient only as a means to organize and tentatively operationalize a study.

EXERCISE

Consider ways in which your intervention with clients may promote research questions. Use your previous work associated with self-awareness, nursing assessments, and models as a guide. Remember, your interpretation of events and feelings associated with 'doing' and the processes of change are as important as numerical data.

**COMMENT**

Like other questions, there can be no model answers. The author offers some research questions that have evolved from his own experience and exploration.

In order to allow nursing teams to evaluate the quality of their own interactions with clients, the indicator of 'quality care' could be operationalized as a self-rating scale in a similar way to the process indicator. Hence, nurses' perceptions of how well they provide care could be compared with the findings of an outside observer.

ORGANIZATIONAL INFLUENCES

Organizations which permit and acknowledge challenge from practitioners may further influence practice by acting as catalysts whereby quality care is promoted and improved. Organizations which prevent nursing teams interpreting the nursing pro-cess, by directly or indirectly coercing them into a unified approach, generally seem to follow managerial models based upon institutional, bureaucratic, and authoritarian values. Such organizations would probably dictate not only values appertaining to the nursing process, but also the quality of care and the methods employed for its evaluation.

Bureaucratic organizations rely upon the assumption that all concepts of a top-down nature associated with the process and quality care will fit reality. In the past, if a nursing team did not implement the process according to set rules, the fault was thought to lie with the staff when perfect quality was not achieved. It was never considered that the organizational interpretation of the process was incorrect and in some ways unworkable. If thinking is restricted to what is accepted by organizational culture and what is well known, little progress will be made and new knowledge will not be discovered.

The influence of the organization on quality of care is undoubtedly an important implication for further research. Yuen (1986) assumes that the nurse/client relationship has changed because it is now managed less on authoritarian lines, whereby clients and nurses are less controlled according to a system of hospital regulations. Work needs to be directed towards identifying democratic or autocratic attitudes that dictate organizational culture, and how this may effect the use and interpretation of the process and the quality care provided by nurses. Van Maanen (1980) considers, when measuring the quality of nursing care, that organizational variables should be evaluated as separate entities and not viewed as elements of the nursing process. However, Dimmock (1986) comments that organizational values do not exist but are merely a reflection of the values of individuals or dominant groups.

The introduction of general management in the NHS was expected to lead to greater autonomy for managers and clinicians. However, 'few clinicians were subsequently involved with management decisions' (Best, 1985). The NHS provides little scope for managerial and clinical initiatives involving risk, experimentation, or innovation. Furthermore, organizational strategies that encourage nursing teams to experiment and develop their practice need to be explored with regard to their effect on staff morale, and, in turn, how this influences the quality of care.

Additionally, replicated studies are required, particularly in acute areas and community settings, in order to identify influences upon the quality of care other than the nursing process and medical intervention. If nursing teams identified as using a high level of process were involved with such a study, other predominent variables associated with their team cultures could be illustrated. Such influences may include an autonomous nursing structure, an emphasis upon education and staff development, or value identification.

## TEAM LEADERSHIP

Nichols (1991) suggests that the role of the leader, as facilitator of change, has emerged as a major influence upon the attitudes and behaviour of nursing staff and the quality of care they provide. Further research is required in order to identify the leadership potential of the nursing manager and how this may influence the interpretation of the process and the quality of care provided. This should establish how valued members of a nursing team feel before and after development programmes; particularly if this incorporates a staff support mechanism such as personal supervision for nurses involved with change and the development of practice. Such studies could identify further important variables influencing the quality care provided for clients.

Current measures of quality care centre upon subordinate activity. Prior to embarking upon either developmental and evaluative approaches towards quality care, team leaders require an indication of the management support available for innovation and change. Instruments designed to assess the quality of management should be constructed using an inductive approach involving all health care personnel.

Cultural influences upon quality care are closely linked with organizational values. However, these need to be differentiated from the values appertaining to organizational and managerial support for ward-based innovation. The quality of care provided for clients may be determined by either financial, aesthetic, institutional, or client-centred values. These require comparison with care provided by nurses who have developed practice and their use of the process. Such a study could illustrate how management support and the culture of an organization influences attitudes and the type of care provided.

The process needs to be taught as an interactional approach with the associated documentation used to support and direct nursing activity. In this way, as Hale (1987) argues, terms such as task allocation, client allocation, and nursing process, which tend to identify ideal types of practice, may be avoided because they evoke stereotyped and static conceptions of nurses and nursing. She further argues that such terms may cause the image of nursing to be confused with reality.

The evolution of the process may explain why staff working within institutional settings have seemed to struggle with the first stage of development. They become satisfied that the process is operational, despite the limitations, and rely upon documentation as a measure of process use and the quality of care. McMahon (1988) suggests that the process is a developmental term. He warns that bottom-up interpretations can interfere with manager's quality assurance programmes and may cause a dichotomy between care planning as taught in a school of nursing and as practised on the wards. Bradshaw (1986) suggests that those in control should respond to change from the bottom-up and not vice-versa.

The effect of nurse education upon the quality of care also needs to be identified. An educational programme for selected nursing teams could be easily devised, and the effects upon the quality of care evaluated. It is envisaged that such programmes would involve a self-directed learning approach. This could, for example, incorporate the interpretation of the process by nursing teams, and, in the first instance, the identification of values appertaining to good care. With this information a nursing assessment could be constructed and a method of care planning designed.

The implementation of the process would take account of interpersonal skills operationalized as qualitative aspects of the nurse/client relationship. The role of the nurse as keyworker and how this may reduce the routine care provided for clients, either in the community or residential settings, would also need to be explored. Finally, the benefits of evaluating care on a regular basis would need to be stressed. A development programme could include other aspects of quality care decided by a nursing team, for example, team building, clients' rights, the effects of routine care on the client(s), and the stresses involved with challenging practice and creating change.

Like the process indicator, concepts of care and quality will require to be reviewed and altered according to changes in attitudes and values of practitioners. Replicated studies will validate the concepts identified as components of quality care.

Most instruments for quality evaluation purport to focus on care provision. It is argued that, unless quality is evaluated according to how care is given, criteria for measurement are likely to veer towards structural aspects of nursing activity. Measures based upon either documentation, what nurses do, or how much they do of it are quantitative. Therefore, inferences about the quality of care given have to be made. These approaches are limited in that the results appertain to 'quality related activities'. In contrast, approaches that identify the 'how' aspect of quality are truly process-based because care is observed as it occurs. In this way explicit qualitative nursing outcomes can be isolated.

The results may be further validated by repeat studies that utilize, in addition to the approaches used for this research, a summative analysis of nursing activity to identify the amount of nursing time spent on physical and psychosocial care. This may further indicate changes in attitudes towards the care of clients if, when nurses interpret the process and explore their practice, they spend more time on psychosocial care. In addition, staff attitudes to elicit their priorities in care and how they may change towards social aspects of the nurse/client relationship when nurses identify their own values requires further exploration.

In addition to the process and quality-care indicators, other instruments need to be developed that are sensitive to educational input; the leadership style of the clinical manager; organizational values associated with innovation; and the autonomy and organization of the nursing team. These indicators may show how such influences, because they allow for exploration and explanation of nursing action, affect the cognitive and emotional interpretations of caring, and in turn how nurses interact with clients.

The following key statements/hypotheses emerged from the study and will require further work:

- Nursing teams that develop their knowledge and skills, and interpret the nursing process according to their own values, interact with more clients and provide a better quality of psychosocial care.
- The nursing process, when interpreted by nursing teams, is more effective if supported by managers and educationalists

who promote the learning potential of the organization.

- It is the interpretation of the nursing process concept that has the greatest influence upon the quality of care. Such interpretations possibly affect how cognitive and emotional interpretations of caring influence behaviour, and therefore how well nurses interact with clients.

- The use of the nursing process will be more effective if the approach is taught according to behavioural definitions centred upon interpersonal skills.

- Nursing teams who are supported and encouraged by their leaders to interpret the nursing process may feel more valued, have positive attitudes towards the nursing process, and are more likely to provide and maintain the quality of care.

- Initiatives are more effective when a bottom-up approach is used for the construction of instruments for the evaluation of quality care.

- Nursing staff may be more responsive to the social pressures of their peer groups when their awareness of client need is heightened rather than to the incentive and control of management.

- Subjective interpretation is a useful research approach for assuring quality. It demonstrates that scientific methodology should be incorporated with interpretive approaches.

- The unexpected findings suggest that hypotheses can be abstracted as a study unfolds, and that an initial research question is sufficient only as a means to organize and tentatively operationalize a study.

- The nursing process is more effective where the organizational ethos is client-centred, and where priority is given to exploring quality issues related to the nurse/client relationship, rather than relying upon staffing levels and aesthetic values as measures of care.

- The value of caring as a contribution towards quality assurance has been established. Attitudes towards caring as a low-status, innate nursing activity may be altered. This illustrates the need for practitioners, managers, and educationalists to differentiate between caring, staff support, and service issues associated with quality assurance.

- Change does not have to be imposed upon practitioners. They will create the change themselves if allowed to interpret concepts and compare them with their own practice and experience. The author believes, therefore, that nurses can be self-actualizing when given autonomy, independence, and self-control. They are able, when facilitated within a creative culture, to use and develop their capabilities and skills because they are primarily self-motivated.

## LIMITATIONS OF THE NURSING PROCESS

The nursing process was not always considered to be a major breakthrough for nursing development or the only means by which to improve client care. The adoption of the process as a vehicle for nursing professionalism mirrors the same hierarchical attitudes that historically exist between the nursing and medical professions.

Many writers thought that the process, being similar to the scientific method, would enhance patient care, but neglected to study the limitation of the scientific method, particularly the notion that logic and objectivity reign supreme. Roper *et al.* (1983) argue that the process seems to belittle the artistic side of nursing.

The process was taught from a theoretical stance, without the realization of organizational variables, which have since shown to have greatly affected its use and interpretation.

## NURSING MODELS

A nursing model is a description of how an individual or group of professionals view nursing. Roy (1984) lists the essential elements of a model for nursing practice as being:

- a description of the person receiving care;
- a statement of the goal of nursing;
- a definition of health;
- a specified meaning of environment;
- an identification of nursing activities.

Similarly, McFarlane (1986) suggests that models have a value for practice in the following ways. They may:

- serve as a tool which links theory and practice;
- clarify our thinking about the elements of a practice situation and their relationship to each other;
- help practitioners communicate with each other more meaningfully;
- serve as a guide to practice, education, and research.

Pearson *et al.* (1984) consider that nurses need to share their ideas and thoughts about their beliefs about man, the goals or expectation of care, and the knowledge required to achieve the goals (Fig. 19.1).

The model below may be a means to explain how practitioners can influence organizational change. First, exploration of practice means that knowledge is gained

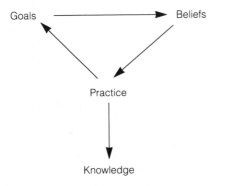

**Figure 19.1** Nursing model

from experience. This influences the value or belief system of nurses, which in turn affects their goals of care and the quality of their nursing intervention. Secondly, the expectations of practitioners with regard to what they consider to be acceptable practice within the organization may change. Hence, such beliefs may influence the expectations of the whole organization and the way in which quality of care is evaluated and improved.

McFarlane (1986) goes on to identify the following types of model: interaction models focus on the nature of nurse/client interactions; developmental models focus on the development and change to explain a nursing situation; self-care and daily living models have a common basis of human needs as the focus of intervention; and systems models centre upon how a client interacts and adapts to their environment.

The author proposes a model of caring as a means to describe and explain nursing phenomena. Most published nursing models view people according to the particular stance favoured by the model's creator. Such models may merely replace the medical approach with another imposed world view. Some nursing models, centred upon physical and psychosocial needs, may be no more than checklists for assessing clients; they barely touch upon human relationships. Rather, nursing models should provide a framework upon which nurses can base and understand their own role and self as an interacting agent with clients. The author suggests that practitioners design their own models, which can be used in part to assess the nursing needs of clients, taking the best from published works and adding to them from their own experience.

Only a few theorists have acknowledged the primacy of nurturing and caring in nursing. Leininger (1981) states that 'caring is the central and unifying domain for the body of knowledge and practices in nursing and that it is caring behaviours that distinguish nursing from other disciplines'.

Stanley *et al.* (1983) consider that a social science 'should begin with the recognition that personal direct experience underlies all behaviours and action'. They go on to state that we need to find out 'what it is that we experience'. A reliance on recognized models may insulate the nurse from other problems that are not part of the conceptual framework.

Most nursing models propose a scientific view of people. Hence, as Hagell (1989) comments 'as nurses become more and more scientific they lose what is essential to nursing ie caring itself, because science cannot conceptualize caring nor can caring be measured, only experienced'.

Botha (1989) suggests that responsible education of future nursing staff requires the exposure to as many conceptual frameworks and models as can possibly be fitted into a curriculum. She further considers that the construction of nursing models calls for a revolutionary type of activity that promotes bold, creative, and imaginative questions to be asked, and therefore provides novel ways of dealing with the needs of clients and nurses.

EXERCISE

Design a nursing model based upon your own experience. Your model could incorporate some, if not all, of the framework to assist self-awareness and assessment suggested in the first exercise (page 219), as well as how your beliefs affect your knowledge and goals of care as described above.

**COMMENT**

From the author's experience and attempt to construct a model of quality care, the following physical and psychosocial components emerged from a review of the literature and the categorization of concepts. They were: explanation for the client, allowances for speech defects, social conversation, privacy and dignity, encouragement to ask questions, client choice, nurse interest and listening, express-ive touch, and risk-taking. What follows is an explanation of why and how the author selected the above components. The method used to identify a model of quality care was similar to that employed for the construction of an indicator of nursing process use.

PHYSICAL CARE

Henderson's (1972) model of human needs may be used to organize concepts associated with physical care. The model emphasizes biological needs within people, although she recognizes that people have important psychological and social requirements that can sometimes lead to a need for nursing care. The components of the model include what have been called 'activities of living'. In addition, it is suggested that nurses should try to minimize the dependence of the client and allow responsibility for self-care. The latter philosophy is held to be a prime indicator of high-quality physical care.

CONCEPTS OF PSYCHOSOCIAL CARE

Such models include psychosocial aspects of communication, working and playing, recreation and learning. These important components, however, need to be made more explicit, particularly in the context of mental health nursing, in order to avoid the reduction of psychosocial aspects of living to mere afterthoughts in relation to physical care. The limitation of any model is that it provides definite judgements set up as classifications and categories. The further exploration of psychosocial aspects of caring is a means to break away from the narrow definitions dictated by such models. To identify the components of psychosocial care, concepts associated with aspects of the nurse/client relationship and the caring function of the nurse could be selected from the literature.

In the first instance, very broad or summative constructs may be selected; for example, the Royal College of Nursing document, *A Position Statement on Nursing* (RCN, 1987) suggests three concepts: equity, respect for persons, and caring.

Interpersonal aspects associated with quality of care, such as respect for the person, compassion, and courtesy, have been described extensively. Some consider that caring involves interpersonal skills in order to maintain the integrity and self-respect of the individual. Others suggest touch, being near the patient, distance, sharing language, speaking directly to the person, bending to get eye contact, speaking clearly and softly, using gestures and expressions, and, using reactions of approval, thanks and praise as key points to assist the caring role. They also consider that good care is centred upon nursing that promotes choice, dignity, individuality, personal space, personal possessions, risk-taking, and a sense of identity for clients.

The 'scientific analysis of social behaviour' described by Argyle (1967) may also be used to categorize and organize the various concepts described above. Argyle's analysis was selected because it was the only comprehensive list of psychosocial behaviour which included reference to all the concepts listed above. It consists of a checklist of verbal and non-verbal communication including indicators of affiliative behaviour considered by other writers to be synonymous with qualitative psychosocial nursing interactions.

## CRITICAL COMMENTARY

### COGNITIVE AND EMOTIONAL INFLUENCES UPON CARE

To identify the observable and meaningful aspects of caring, a distinction needs to be drawn between its cognitive and emotional meanings. The former are concepts that can be defined in operational terms, whereas the latter are axioms that are taken for granted because they cannot be proved; they are truths that are accepted. Like most axioms, emotional meanings are arbitrary and self-evident only to those who see things the same way. Thus organizational and educational values may influence both meanings of care.

The evaluation of practice has to be based upon some assumptions concerning these issues. Furthermore, these issues change, in that contemporary views on any subject, in this case concepts of quality care, may be simply a matter of collegial faith and ideological consensus. Caring has, therefore, to be judged according to the context and culture in which it is given. Personal values about care may be influenced by organizational culture and attitudes. These values could be reinforced or altered by education. It is proposed that such values may influence not only how nurses interpret good physical and psychosocial care but also their emotional or gut reactions to the needs of client(s) and therefore how they interact with them.

Organizations that value getting things done may have a negative influence upon cognitive and emotional interpretations of care, and ignore its potential to create change. This not only ensures the acceptance of top-down decisions, but also stifles creativity. The culture of such organizations means that top-down approaches are preferred, as are off-the-shelf instruments for quality evaluations. Such organizations can become analytically inert, and may evolve to the point where they may impede further evolution (De Bono, 1986).

Alternatively, organizations that promote bottom-up approaches, are pragmatic, value the opinion and involvement of practitioners, support experimentation, and acknowledge the influence of people. This philosophy recognizes and utilizes the subjective human aspects of quality evaluation. It may lead to practitioners identifying more realistic and meaningful concepts of quality care, leading to imaginative and creative methodologies and the dissemination of new knowledge.

## CONCLUSION

This section, like many others, raises more questions than it answers. It may have provided new insights into how the process may be more effectively used as a catalyst of quality care. It may also have suggested new ways to look at the problems associated with the approach. The section is intended to be interpretive, illuminating and evolutionary rather than problem-solving or revelatory. Moreover, the section has suggested some unorthodox approaches towards the use of the process and nursing models as well as potentially promoting new ideas for research techniques which in the long term may add to our knowledge of methodology. An additional challenge will be the interpretation and teaching of these interventions as a means to improve the quality of nurse/client relationship.

## REFERENCES

Abdellah, F. (1984) One American's view of the quality of service provided. UMIST, unpub. notes from a conference on quality.

Argyle, M. (1967) *The Psychology of Interpersonal Behaviour*, (2nd edn), Penguin, Harmondsworth.

Ashworth, P. and Castledine, G. (1978) Subject of concern. *Advanced Nursing*, 6, 503–14.

Barker, P. (1989) Rules of engagement. *Nursing Times*, 85, 51, 58–60.

Barker, P. (1991). Finding common ground. *Nursing Times*, 87, 2, 37–8.

Best, G. (1985) General management: an audit. *Senior Nurse*, 2, 4, 20–2.

Binnie, A. and Roberts, R. (1984) Module 4: The third step of the nursing process – implementation, in *A Systematic Approach to Nursing Care: An Introduction*, Open Univ. Press, Milton Keynes.

Botha, M. E. (1989) Theory development in perspective: the role of conceptual frameworks and models in theory development. *Advanced Nursing*, 14, 49–55.

Campbell, J. (1980) The relationship of nursing and self-awareness. *Advanced Nursing Science*, 2, 4, 15.

Chavase, J. (1981) From task assignment to patient allocation: a change evaluation. *J. Advanced Nursing*, 6, 137–45.

Crow, J. (1977) The nursing process: theoretical background, in *The Nursing Process*. (ed. J. Crow, and C. Kratz) Macmillan Journals, London.

De Bono, E. (1986) *Future Positive* (4th edn), Penguin, Harmondsworth.

De la Cuesta, A. C. (1983) The nursing process: from theory to implementation. *J. Advanced Nursing*, 8, 365–71.

DHSS (1988) The Nurses, Midwives, and Health Visitors Rules Approval Order, extract from statutory instrument, No. 837, Annex E 376d/20/498–6.

Dimmock, K. S. (1986) Assenting to change. *Nursing Times*, 82, 43, 38–9.

Friend, P. and Hayward, J. (1986) *Report of the Nursing Process Evaluation Working Group*, DHSS Nursing Research Liaison Group.

General Nursing Council for England and Wales (1977), *Design of Curricula*, circular 77/19/A.

General Nursing Council for England and Wales (1978) *Preparation for Teachers of Nursing*, circular 78/3.

General Nursing Council for England and Wales (1982) *Training for Nurses Responsible for General Care*, circular 82/5.

Goble, A. (1986) An approach to care, unpub. teaching package, School of Nursing, Queen Alexandra Hospital, Portsmouth.

Goffman, E. (1961) *Asylums: Essays on the Social Situation of Mental Patients and Other Inmates*, Pelican Books, London.

Greene, J. (1979) Research design-Part 2: experimental design, in *Research Methods in Education and the Social Sciences*, Open Univ. Press, Milton Keynes.

Hagell, E. I. (1989) Nursing knowledge: woman's knowledge. A sociological perspective. *J. Advanced Nursing*, 14, 226–3.

Hale, C. (1987) *Innovations in Nursing Care: Study of a Change to Patient-Centred Care*, Royal College of Nursing, London.

Hargreaves, I. (1979) Theoretical considerations, in *The Nursing Process*, (ed. Kratz, C.), Baillière Tindall, London.

Henderson, V. (1972) *Basic Principles of Nursing Care*. International Council of Nurses. Geneva.

Hunt, J. and Marks-Maran, D.J. (1980) *Nursing Care Plans: The Nursing Process at Work*. John Wiley, Chichester.

Kemp, N. (1984) The Rush-Medicus quality monitoring instrument, in *Quality and Care Measurement Conference* Notes, Wessex Regional Health Authority, Winchester.

Kratz, C. R. (ed.) (1979) *The Nursing Process*, Bailliére Tindall, London.

Leininger, M. (1978) *Transcultural Nursing: Concepts, Theories and Practices*, John Wiley, Chichester.

Luker, K. A. (1981) An overview of evaluation research in nursing. *J. Advanced Nursing*, 6, 87–93.

Maslow, A. (1970) *Motivation and Personality*, Harper and Row, New York.

McFarlane, J. K. (1970) *The Proper Study of the Nurse*, RCN Research Project, Royal College of Nursing, London.

McGilloway, F. A. (1980) The nursing process: A problem solving approach to patient care. *Inter. J. Nursing Studies*, 17: 79–90.

McMahon, R. (1988) Who's afraid of nursing care plans? *Nursing Times*, 84, 29, 39–41

Mitchell, T. The nursing process debate: is nursing any business of doctors? *Nursing Times*, 80, 19, 28–32.

Myers, N. (1973) Nursing diagnosis. *Nursing Times*: 1229–31.

Nichols, R. (1991) The quality of care for elderly people: the impact of the nursing process in the hospital setting, unpub. CNAA thesis, University of Portsmouth, Portsmouth.

Parlett, M. (1981) Illuminative evaluation, in *Human Inquiry: A Sourcebook of New Paradigm Research*. John Wiley, Chichester.

Pearson, A. and Vaughaan, B. (1984) Nursing practice and the nursing process: module 1, in *A Systematic Approach To Nursing Care – An Introduction*, Open Univ. Press, Milton Keynes.

Pepleu, H. E. (1952) The heart of nursing: interpersonal relations, *Canadian Nurse*, 62: 273–5.

Reason, P. and Rowan, J. (eds) (1981) *Human Inquiry: A Sourcebook of New Paradigm Research*, John Wiley, Chichester.

Reed, J and Robbins, I. (1991) Research rituals. *Nursing Times*, 87, 23, 50–1.

Roper, N., Logan, W., and Tierney, A. (1983) Is there a danger of processing the patients? *Nursing Mirror*, 156, 22, 32–3.

Rowan, J. (1981) A dialectical paradigm for research, in *Human Inquiry: A Sourcebook of New Paradigm Research*, John Wiley, Chichester.

Roy, C. (1984) *Introduction to Nursing: An Adaptation Model* (2nd edn) Prentice-Hall, New Jersey.

Royal College of Nursing (1981) *Towards Standards*, RCN, London.

Royal College of Nursing (1987) *A Position Statement on Nursing: In Pursuit of Excellence*, RCN, London.

Royal Commission on the National Health Service 1979 Extract from conclusions and recommendations, HMSO, London.

Stanley, L. and Wise, S. (1983) *Breaking Out*, Routledge, London.

Stenhouse, L. (1984) *An Introduction to Curriculum Research and Development*, Heinemann, London.

Tedman, D. (1985) Passing the prejudice. *Nursing Mirror*, 160, 5, 39.

VanMaanen, H. M. Th. (1981) Improvements of quality of nursing care: a goal to challenge in the eighties. *J. Advanced Nursing*, 6, 1, 3–9.

Walsh, M. and Ford, P. (1989) We always do it this way. *Nursing Times*, 85, 44, 26–32.

Ward, M. F. (1985) *The Nursing Process In Psychiatry*. Churchill-Livingstone, Edinburgh.

Wright, S. G. (1985) How one nurse was converted. *Nursing Times*, 81, 33, 24–7.

Wright, S.G. (1986) Patient-centred practice. *Nursing Times*, 83, 38, 24–7.

Yuen, F. K. H. (1986) The nurse-client relationship a mutual learning experience. *J. Advanced Nursing*, 11, 529–33.

## FURTHER READING

Adair, J. (1987) *Effective Team Building*. Pan Books, London.

Anthony, A. (1991) Mirror images. *Nursing Times*, 87, 2, 35–6.

Armitage, P. (1985) Primary care: An individual concern. *Nursing Times*, 81, 45, 35–8.

Baker, D. E. (1973) *Future Care of the Elderly*. Macmillan, London.

Barber, P. and Norman, I. (1987) Skills in supervision. *Nursing Times*, 83, 2, 56–7.

Barber, P. and Norman, I. (1989) Preparing teachers for the performance and evaluation of gaming-simulation in experiential learning climates. *J. Advanced Nursing*, 14, 146–51.

Bergman, R. (1983) Understanding the patient in all his human needs. *J. Advanced Nursing*, 8, 185–90.

Bergman, R. (1986) Nursing the aged with brain failure. *J. Advanced Nursing*, 11, 361–7.

Bond, M. (1988). Setting up NT assertiveness training groups. *Nursing Times*, 84, 5, 57–60.

Bracey, B. and Wicikowski, D. (1989) Apportioning care. *Nursing Times*, 85, 19, 49–51.

Caddow, P. (1986) Questions of quality. *Nursing Times*, 82, 29, 42–3.

Clark, J. (1982) Development of models and theories on the concept of nursing. *J. Advanced Nursing,* 7, 2, 129–34.

Clarke, L. (1988) Ideology, tradition, and choice: questions psychiatric nurses ask themselves. *Senior Nurse,* 11, 11–13.

Clarke, M. (1986) Action and reflection: practice and theory in nursing. *J. Advanced Nursing,* 11, 3–11.

Closs, J. (1988) Cost-effectiveness in the NHS. *Senior Nurse,* 8, 7–8, 24.

Cook, M. (1987) Part of the institution. *Nursing Times,* 83, 25, 24–7.

Cormack, D. (1986) Psychiatric nursing in the year 2005. *Nursing Times,* 82, 37, 39–41.

Crosby, I. and Taylor, J. (1985) *In Our care: A Handbook of Workshop Activities For Those Caring For Older People,* training workshop series, Help The Aged Educ. Dept. London.

Darbyshire, P. (1990) Making caring count: the hear of the matter. *Nursing Times,* 86, 47, 63–4.

Davidson, L. (1991) Healing the healers. *Nursing Times,* 87, 4, 21.

Dick, D. (1985) The institutional trap. *Nursing Times,* 81, 34, 47–9.

Dickinson, S. (1982) The nursing process and the professional status of nursing. *Nursing Times Occasional Paper,* 22, 61–4.

Forrest, D. (1989) The experience of caring. *J. Advanced Nursing,* 14, 815–23.

Griffin, A. P. (1980) Philosophy and nursing. *J. Advanced Nursing,* 5, 261–72.

Hale, C. (1987) *Innovations in Nursing Care: Study of a Change to Patient Centred Care,* Royal College of Nursing, London.

Heyward-Jones, I. (1988) The final straw. *Nursing Times,* 84, 9, 47–9.

Iveson-Iveson, J. (1985) Developing self-awareness. *Nursing Mirror,* 161, 5, 25.

Jones, G. (1990) All you ever wanted to know about counselling. *Nursing Times* 85, 12, 55–8.

Kappeli, S. (1986) Nurse's management of patients self-care. *Nursing Times,* 82, 11, 40–43.

Lees, G. D. Richman, J., Salavioo, M.A. and Warden, S. (1987) Quality assurance: is it professional insurance? *J. Advanced Nursing,* 12, 719–27.

Loughlin, M. (1988) Modelled, muddled, and befuddled. *Nursing Times,* 84, 5, 30–1.

McCarthy, M. M. (1981) The nursing process: application of current thinking in clinical problem solving. *J. Advanced Nursing,* 6, 173–7.

*Memory Diary: Notes for Guidance.* Winslow Press, London.

Miller, A. F. (1984) Nursing process and patient care. *Nursing Times,* 80, 13, 56–8.

Miller, A. F. (1985a) Does the process help the patient? *Nursing Times,* 81, 26, 24–38.

Miller, A. F. (1985b) Are you using the nursing process? *Nursing Times,* 81, 49, 26–38.

Milne, D. (1986) Management, motivation and monitoring. *Health and Social Service J.* 96, 4982: 78–9.

Minshull, J. and Turner, L. (1986) The human needs model of nursing. *J. Advanced Nursing,* 11, 643–9.

Moss, A. R. (1988) Determinants of patient care: nursing process or nursing attitudes. *J. Advanced Nursing,* 13: 615–20.

Nicklin, P. (1984) Innovation without change. *Senior Nurse,* 1, 3, 9–10.

O'Donovan, S. (1988) Why bother? *Nursing Times,* 84, 15, 43–4.

Parahoo, K. and Read, N. (1988) Research skills: the research process. *Nursing Times,* 84, 40, 67–70.

Pepleu, H. E. (1962) Interpersonal techniques: the crux of psychiatric nursing. *American J. Nursing,* 6, 50–4.

Raatikainen, R. (1989) Values and ethical principles in nursing. *J. Advanced Nursing,* 14, 92–6.

Raichura, L. (1987) Learning by doing. *Nursing Times,* Quest educ. supp., 7, 2, 59–61.

Rawlins, T. (1983) Do we really need the process? *Nursing Times,* 79, 9, 64.

Richards, D. A. and Lambert, P. (1987) The Nursing Process: the effect on patient's satisfaction with nursing care. *J. Advanced Nursing,* 12, 559–62.

Rosen, S. I. (1981) One researcher's self-questioning, in *Human Inquiry: A Sourcebook of New Paradigm Research,* John Wiley, Chichester.

Stuart, G. W. and Sundeen, S. J. (1987) *Principles and Practice of Psychiatric Nursing.* Mosby, Washington, D.C.

Thomas, P. (1988) Managing change. *Nursing Times,* 84, 44, 58–9.

# PART FIVE

# NURSING INTERVENTIONS IN PRACTICE

*Brendan McMahon*

As medicine has extended its range of treatment techniques, nursing has tended to encroach upon what were once strictly medical preserves. In the nineteenth century, the process worked the other way as midwifery and the care of the mentally ill, for example, were progressively medicalized.

Not long ago, the use of the sphygmomanometer was considered beyond the powers of the nurse. The apparently infinite extension of medical and surgical technique has meant that nursing has had to develop its expertise in order to fulfill a variety of roles that doctors have had to renounce. This is in part to do with increased specialization within medicine, and in part to do with changing public expectations of the medical profession.

This process has affected not only the relationship between the sister professions of nursing and medicine. Increased specialization in medicine has been reflected by increased specialization in nursing, and the move towards the creation of increasing numbers of clinical nurse specialist and nurse practitioner posts is evidence of this. In recent years, nursing has attempted to define itself in its own terms, not just as an adjunct to medicine, while in many areas, the old, class- (and gender) based tradition of medical dominance and nursing subservience persists (Derbyshire, 1987).

This will continue to have a decisive influence on the development of the psychodynamic approach in this country. Psychoanalysis is now and always has been practised mostly by a select group of medically trained personnel, even though two of the most influential early analysts, Anna Freud and Melanie Klein, were lay practitioners, and Freud himself fought strenuously to prevent analysis falling under medical domination.

Psychoanalysis has spawned many children, many of whom would be unrecognizable to their founding fathers and mothers. Psychodynamic theory has long since broken out of the confines of the analysts' consulting rooms. The breakdown in traditional moral and religious values, the near demise of the extended family, increasing expectations from personal relationships and other social changes in the fairly recent past have produced social fragmentation and individual alienation, leading to emotional and psychological problems on such an enormous scale that psychoanalysis cannot even begin to tackle them. Increased awareness of psychological methods of treatment has led to increasing demand, and people seem more prepared to talk about their problems than their forebears were. Increased demand has led to the commitment of more resources to the provision of responsible psychological treatments, just as it has led, especially in the US, to the development of alternative approaches, which range from the harmlessly silly to the sinister.

A thoroughgoing analysis involves visiting the analyst four or five times weekly for several years and can be very expensive. Clearly this is not a practical proposition for the masses of ordinary people whose lives are constrained by psychological problems.

At the other end of the spectrum are the large numbers of people who require medication, antidepressants, or tranquillizers in order to cope with the stresses of life. All too often taking drugs of this kind can become a habit that renders the client incapable of working out more effective ways of coping with his or her problems.

Of course, people who suffer from one or other of the major psychiatric disorders – manic-depressive psychosis or schizophrenia, for example – may be helped by physical treatments such as electroconvulsive therapy or phenothiazines. The 'medical' or 'disease' model of mental illness: the theory that mental disorders have their origins in physiological changes, just as physical disorders do, has in its practical application been of immense help to countless suffering human beings. None the less, it has its limitations, as do all other attempts to explain mental disorder.

In the first place, although physiological changes do occur in mental illness, the question of whether they are the cause or the effect remains unanswered. In the second place, the analogy with general medicine is somewhat misleading. For example, non-epidemic acute encephalitis is caused by the herpes simplex virus. Neurological symptoms are often preceded by respiratory difficulty, and headaches and fitting are recognizable early symptoms; fever and coma are not uncommon, spinal fluid proteins are raised, and red blood cells are often to be found. The condition is treated with steroids and anti-convulsant medication (Shafer *et al.*, 1975). This is a clear progression from identifiable causes to a rational, explicable line of treatment.

In comparison, psychiatric terms such as 'endogenous depression' – 'one in which the disease derives from an innate disposition' (Cape *et al.*, 1974) – seem less than adequate. Similarly, the term 'schizophrenic', which would seem to describe little more than the way some people behave. To describe behaviour is not the same as to explain it. To some, the medical model denies the meaning of the client's distress and confusion, just as it takes away his responsibility for understanding and changing himself.

In addition to those suffering from grave mental disorder, there is a host of unhappy people whose sense of well-being, creativity, and social confidence is impaired by an emotional conflict that leaves them confused and powerless. The lives of these unfortunate people cannot be fundamentally changed by medication, though there may be some alleviation of symptoms in the short term, and there is a considerable risk of becoming dependent on psychotropic medication. A full-length course of psychoanalysis would of course be impracticable for the vast majority of such people, even if it were thought to be appropriate.

The health services of the Western world have attempted to plug this gap in a variety of ways. Forms of therapy that are less expensive and time-consuming than classical Freudian analysis have evolved, the most notable including individual analytic psychotherapy, group analytic psychotherapy, psychodrama, Gestalt therapy, and client-centred counselling.

Many health-care professionals find themselves in the position of having to deal with problems that call for a psychotherapeutic approach, without having either the knowledge or the skills effectively to implement such an approach. While it is true that a sympathetic ear and the ability to respond to other people's problems with ordinary human sensitivity and understanding is often of considerable benefit, many problems are beyond the reach of common sense approaches.

Current models of nursing care emphasize communicational, interpersonal skills, and nursing as a profession is less confined by considerations of organic illness-orientated conceptual frameworks than is medicine. In the nature of things, nurses spend more time with their clients than other health professionals, and nursing traditionally has always emphasized the importance of the nurse-patient relationship. In recent years, more consideration has been given to the specifics of this relationship, its objectives and parameters, and the uses to which it may be put. Some models have placed the interpersonal dimension at the heart of their professional philosophy (Peplau, 1988), while others have adopted a less interpersonal approach. It is self-evident that our relationship with our clients is the most powerful therapeutic tool we possess.

In general, interactional skills are learned by example. While many nurses possess such skills to a high degree, the quality of nurse/client interactions, as well as the quantity in terms of time spent with clients, is not in general as satisfactory as it might be (Cormack, 1976). This may be particularly so in a general nursing context. In a study of nurse-patient interactions on surgical wards, McLeod (1983) found that:

> Nurse-patient interaction was limited in terms of both quantity and quality. Moreover, nurses displayed little evidence of skills which encourage communication, while demonstrating the frequent use of strategies which block or discourage further communication. These findings reinforce those of earlier, more general studies which have identified restricted patterns of nurse/patient interaction.

Clearly, interpersonal skills need to be taught more effectively than they are at present. Moreover, the skills that nurses do possess must be supported and extended by a coherent conceptual framework, which will allow them to think about what they do or do not do with clients, and why (Chapter 25). Nurses need and deserve a systematic training in the theory of the way people are, the way people develop into who they are, and the ways in which they can be helped to change. Only on

such a basis can the nurse learn to use her relationships with her clients consistently and creatively, and learn to play her part in alleviating the immeasurable psychological distress surrounding us. The psychodynamic model is flawed like all other models of the mind, and yet it offers us a rich and complex understanding of ourselves and our clients, and of what happens between us.

## THEORETICAL BACKGROUND

Although many workers in many specialities have contributed to the development of the psychodynamic approach over the years, it owes its existence primarily to the pioneering work of Sigmund Freud, the founder of psychoanalysis and one of the most influential figures in twentieth-century thought (Chapters 5 and 8). Freud's ideas are rich and complex, and repay careful study.

Freud was born in 1856 in what was then part of the Austro-Hungarian empire. After qualifying as a doctor in Vienna, he specialized in neurology, and carried out research into the use of cocaine as a local anaesthetic. He went on to work with the great neurologist Charcot at the Salpêtrière in Paris, where he became interested in the use of hypnosis as a means of treating hysterical illness. The results were patchy, and so Freud discontinued hypnotic treatment in favour of a new technique of his own, which he called **free association**. This has been defined as, 'the mode of thinking encouraged in the patient by the analysts injunction that he should obey the "basic rule", i.e. that he should report his thoughts without reservation and that he should make no attempt to concentrate while doing so.' (Rycroft, 1972).

Stated more simply, this means that the client is encouraged to talk about whatever comes into his head, on the assumption that, owing to the operation of the unconscious, preoccupations and conflicts that have been **repressed** or pushed out of consciousness because of their painful nature, will eventually emerge, often in a distorted or symbolic way. These conflicts can, through interpretation, be brought back into consciousness, and the client then can begin to work through and resolve them (Freud, 1940). The importance of free association as a technical innovation can hardly be overstated: for the first time, the client was allowed to set his own agenda, to define his own problems, and to set his own objectives.

Free association is a technique from which nurses might learn much. It entails on the nurse's part a capacity to tolerate silence – and even confusion and pain – as well as the ability to renounce the active role of 'doer', dispenser of advice, and so on. This can be painful, since it is at variance with the self-concept which many nurses have, as Buller (1990) states:

> There is nothing worse than being with a patient and not knowing what to do. However, the psychodynamic model not only makes this permissible, but also desirable. The result of the value shift is a framework for understanding relationships which allows for learning and change.

A capacity to tolerate silence, to allow the client the space to express himself in his own time and in his own words, is particularly important during the assessment process, as the following case study shows.

## CASE STUDY – MRS. SMITH

Mrs Smith, a 24-year-old woman, was referred by her GP to the community mental health team. She had been suffering from anxiety and depression over the past 18 months, and has recently given up her job as a sales manager because of her inability to cope with the pressures involved. She is happily married, and has a daughter Emily, who is two years old. She presents herself in a bright, chatty, somewhat superficial way.

Mrs Smith's home background was somewhat unhappy: her father treated her harshly, and seems never to have given her much in the way of affection; her mother, who also suffered from depression, was usually too tired and preoccupied to spend much time with her daughter. Mrs Smith was an only child.

When Mrs Smith was seven years old, her parents moved from the working-class northern city where she grew up into an affluent, rural community in the south of England. At school she was bullied and ostracized because of her different background, which persisted into the later stages of her secondary education. After school she went to university and completed her degree, and at about this time she married her present husband. Not long after the birth of Emily, her symptoms of depression and anxiety began, and have become steadily worse ever since.

The client was assessed by a community psychiatric nurse. During the assessment the nurse considered the possibility of offering Mrs Smith a number of structured therapeutic sessions. The client showed a readiness to understand her problems in terms of past experiences and personal relationships, as well as a capacity to stay in touch with and to express painful feelings. She expressed a strong determination to resolve her problems, and there was evidence – for example, her marriage, career history, and personal resources – to suggest she was strong enough to cope with the stresses that self-exploration always entails. There was no evidence that she had habitual recourse to alcohol or drugs as a way of avoiding her problems, or that she was in danger of psychotic breakdown, both of which would be negative indications suggesting unsuitability for an intensive psychotherapeutic approach.

The nurse, however, had a growing feeling that something was not being said during the interview. In the early stages, the nurse had felt some pressure to ask direct questions in response to the client's anxiety, but as time went on she allowed silences to develop, confining herself to empathic comments, clarification, and rephrasing – or putting the client's communications into other, simpler words in order to help her to understand them. This had the dual effect of deepening the **therapeutic alliance** by assuring the client of her concern and capacity to understand, while at the same time giving the client space to talk about what she wanted, and conveying the impression that it was permissible to talk about anything. From the client's point of view, the central question changed from 'What does she [the nurse] want to hear?' to 'What do I need to say?'

After some hesitation, and with considerable distress, Mrs Smith was able to tell the nurse that she had been sexually abused by her father over a period of years. This had left her with a damaged sense of herself (she now thought of herself as both 'bad' and irreparably 'spoiled'), and with severely conflicting feelings about her father, which affected her feelings towards men in general, including her husband.

Mrs Smith's disclosure not only provided a useful focus for therapeutic work, but was a therapeutic experience in itself since it was the first time she had been able to share what had happened to her with anyone. By expressing it, she came to know it herself for the first time, and so began to resolve it, a process that is of enormous importance. As Storr (1979) writes:

Putting things into words…is a means whereby we detach ourselves both from the world about us and from the inner world of our own emotions and thoughts. It is by means of words that we objectify; that we are enabled to stand back from our own experience and reflect upon it. Words about the self make possible a psychical distance from the self and, without distance, neither understanding nor control, nor willed, deliberate change is possible.

This therapeutic outcome depends upon the capacity of the nurse to tolerate both painful silence and painful self-disclosure by the client. Nurses often feel they should 'do something' to the client, rather than simply being with her or him, which can feel like doing nothing. Often the most valuable service we can perform for our clients is to stay with them in their suffering and confusion. Premature attempts to sort out the client's confusion generally reflect the nurse's unwillingness to tolerate uncertainty and anxiety, and do not allow the client the opportunity to make sense of his own confusion in his own terms. Similarly, we sometimes unconsciously deny our clients the opportunity to make painful self-disclosures because we fear the pain such disclosures may evoke in us.

The psychiatric client is not an alien being. He struggles to make sense of his history and his relationships; he fears death, madness, and the loss of love, and we share these fears with him. For this reason self-awareness is an integral part of the psychodynamic approach. Without it we will find ourselves unable to listen to what the client needs to say, as Sundeen *et al.* (1985) state:

The nurse who cares for the biological, psychological and sociological needs of her clients will be exposed to a broad range of human experiences. She must learn to deal with anxiety, anger, sadness and joy in helping clients at all intervals of the health illness continuum. Her goal is the attainment of authentic, open and personal communication. In her nursing care she must be able to examine her own feelings and reactions as a person, as well as her actions as a professional provider of care. A firm understanding and acceptance of her own self will allow the nurse to acknowledge a client's differences and uniqueness.

Allowing the client space to be and to express himself is central to all nursing practice, not only to psychotherapeutic work: the expectant mother on the labour ward; the self-mutilating teenager in accident and emergency; and the confused man living in a care-of-the-elderly ward – each has a story, and the real need to tell it.

## BEHAVIOUR AND MEANING

Central to the psychodynamic approach is the belief that behaviour – including interpersonal style, symptoms, dreams, and fantasies – has meaning. It expresses something of the person's inner world, his sense of himself, and his perceptions of others. This is true however inconsequential and apparently meaningless the behaviour may seem to be. The bizarre behaviour of the psychotic person is an expression of his torment and inner fragmentation; if we can understand this and share our understanding with him, we can go some way towards diminishing his fear and loneliness.

The person's inner world is shaped by his or her past experience, at the same time shaping and giving meaning to – and sometimes distorting – his present experience. The psychodynamic approach is not concerned with the past for its own sake, as is sometimes believed, but with the past insofar as it lives on in the present. This is true for all of us in many ways. Our social, cultural, ethnic, religious, and family background has a profound influence on the way we are now.

Sometimes in the therapeutic setting a particular symptom, depression, for example, is connected with a repressed emotional conflict or trauma, and the consequent insight

and release of emotion causes the symptom to subside. Usually, however, it is not as simple as that. A person who has been exposed to rejecting or persecutory experiences over a period of time will develop a distorted sense of self, a sense of the self as being, for instance, bad or unworthy of love, and will develop ways of coping with the experience. While these may protect the person from pain in the short term, they may have adverse effects on the capacity to form and maintain satisfactory relationships in the long term.

The way we see ourselves can profoundly affect our perceptions of others, just as our experience of others over time can profoundly affect our sense of ourselves. In the case of Mrs Smith, past trauma and the release of emotion connected with it was only a part of the story, which also included father's rejection, her relationship with her mother, feelings of guilt, shame, and rage, as well as her current lifestyle and relationships with her husband and daughter. All of these needed to be integrated into a meaningful pattern, an accommodation with her past, which would allow her to live comfortably in the present. It is this emphasis on the dynamic interaction between past and present, the self and others, the inner and outer worlds, which is characteristic of and unique to the psychodynamic approach.

## MENTAL DEFENCES

We each have a view about the kind of person we think we are, as well as of the kind of person we think we ought to be. Our knowledge of ourselves is based on our experience, and particularly our experience at ourselves in relation to others.

If we have a satisfactory experience in our earliest relationships, most importantly with our parents; if our needs are met more or less consistently, and we receive positive feedback about ourselves – if we are loved – then we are likely to grow up thinking that, while we do have faults, we are lovable, basically good people. If, as in the case of Mrs Smith our experience is the opposite, we are likely to grow up thinking we are bad and un-lovable. This will colour the way we see the world, and lead us to misinterpret the things that other people say and do in ways that confirm our own sense of 'badness'. In this way a self-defeating spiral of disastrous relationships is established. Fortunately, what is damaged by relationships can also be treated by them, which often happens naturally in the course of things: we meet someone who loves us for what we are, and our picture of ourselves changes for the better. Some people are unable to do this, and need the help of a professional nurse, therapist, or counsellor.

Our sense of ourselves as we ought to be – as distinct from the way we think we are – is also influenced by schooling, cultural norms, and unmet needs. The latter sometimes find expression in compensatory fantasies about, for instance, becoming fantastically rich, being a rock star, and so on. If there is a very wide discrepancy between our sense of ourselves as we think we ought to be and ourselves as we really are, or if our expectations of ourselves are so high we cannot possibly meet them, then a conflict is created, and we are left feeling inadequate and bad. Instead of getting on with the business of being ourselves, we remain permanently preoccupied with our failure to become something we were never intended to be, which prevents us mobilizing the potential we really do have.

Sometimes we experience desires and im-pulses, particularly of a sexual or aggressive nature, which are incompatible with the way we are or think we ought to be, for example, 'I am a respectable person; respectable people never feel like killing their fathers; have homosexual impulses; are tempted to have affairs.' To accept such impulses would mean having to let go of our familiar self-image, and begin to build a more authentic sense of self that would allow for the expression of hitherto unacceptable feelings.

This is a frightening process. We depend upon a familiar, more or less consistent sense of self to keep us in touch with reality, and a threat to our sense of self can feel like the beginning of madness. One way we deal with this threat is to **repress**, or push into uncon-sciousness, the impulses, desires, and mem-ories that threaten us. Once they have been forgotten, we can get on with being the per-son we like to think we are.

There are problems with this, however. Repressed feelings do not cease to exist just because we are no longer conscious of them. They tend to find expression in indirect ways, symbolically, for example, in dreams, through skewed relationships, or in the creation of symptoms – depression or obsessive compuls-ive neurosis. Moreover, repression is not a once-and-for-all event; it requires continued effort to keep the repressed material uncon-scious, which uses up considerable amounts of psychic energy that would otherwise be available for more creative purposes. Since the function of repression is to defend the psyche from pain, it is known as a **defence mechanism** (Chapter 8).

Many other such mechanisms have been identified. **Denial** is a refusal to accept the reality or existence of a particular impulse, desire, or experience. **Splitting** is, in Freudian terms, the separating off of some unac-ceptable aspect of the self. Splitting also is a key concept in Kleinian thought. It refers to the primitive process in which the infant phantasizes that it is possible to get rid of uncomfortable or frightening feelings and impulses by pushing them outwards, in order to protect himself from them. To do this, he must first feel that 'bad' and 'good' can be separated (page 51).

It is easy to see how such a phantasy might develop in the infant's mind: for example, when discomfited by griping pains, he will strive to expel the wind or faecal matter causing it. In so doing, he loses the pain. With the relief he feels from releasing wind, he learns that what he is left with is good by comparison. It is thus reasonable to conclude that he would imagine he could push out other forms of discomfort in the same way.

The mother is often identified with such **projections**: that is, those unwanted, threatening or threatened parts of the self that the baby imaginatively pushes out. If I am frightened of my own aggression, for instance, I will project it into others and will then be frightened by what I perceive to be their aggressive feelings towards me. **Introjection** is the process by which the external object or part of it is unconsciously incorporated into oneself, for example when a toddler sets about to do something that is forbidden, such as put his fingers into the electric socket. He may stop suddenly, saying 'No' to himself, repeating it each time he is tempted to reach out. He has taken into himself the part of his parents that guards his safety, through policing his actions. This leads to **identification**, which can be employed as a defence against loss or separation, for example, if the external person is inside me, I cannot have lost/never could lose him/her.

**Regression** is a reversion to an earlier developmental level, when we felt safer than we do at present, and is an important part of life for all of us. We all need to behave like children sometimes, however old we are; we have an abiding need to play, and, sometimes, to cry and to be comforted.

In **reaction formation**, we disguise an unacceptable impulse with an exaggerated tendency to do or feel its opposite. For example, our aggression may be masked by an over-solicitous concern for the welfare of others. Our 'concern' will, however, invariably be experienced by the other person as persecutory, and will in this way reveal its real nature.

**Sublimation** is the process by which unacceptable sexual or hostile desires are channelled into, for instance, sport, artistic or creative endeavour, or intellectual activity.

Defence mechanisms are not abnormal. We all defend ourselves against psychological and emotional pain in one or more of these ways, though some are more adaptive than others. It is worth bearing in mind that these mechanisms are more or less unconscious: we use them without being fully aware we are doing so. We all need defences at times because they help us to cope in the short term with the stresses of life. When we use them, however, we are for a time out of touch with the reality of ourselves and of the world around us. Major problems can arise when a short-term response to stress becomes a habitual response to life.

CASE STUDY – JENNY

Jenny is a 24-year-old nurse, who has been referred to the community mental health team by her GP. She has recently been suffering from depression.

Jenny has had a sad life, but feels that things are better now that she has left home and has a place of her own. Her father has suffered from depression for many years; mother seems always to have been a dominating and aggressive woman, who has consistently bullied Jenny into doing what she wants. Jenny has always found this paralyzing, and is still unable to stand up to her mother. On the positive side, Jenny enjoys her work, music, and sporting activities, such as marathon running. She has had relationships with men, and would like some day to marry and have children.

Jenny was assessed by the nurse psychotherapist in the team, who thought her well motivated to explore her central conflict, which she took to be her relationship with her mother. She offered Jenny 20 sessions of time-limited therapy, with a view to focusing on this central conflict. The first eight sessions of therapy were very sticky. The client showed little willingness to talk without prompting, and was clearly determined, on an unconscious level, to cling to her habitual defence mechanism

In particular, Jenny denied her anger towards her mother, which was perfectly evident. Her reasons for this were two-fold. Firstly, she did not see herself as the kind of person who became angry, because of the associated guilt and because of her anxiety that mother would 'take it out' on father and so, in her fantasy, destroy him. Jenny's repressed anger has thus converted into depressive symptoms, by turning her anger against herself.

It is interesting to note Jenny's involvement in running, which might be thought of as sublimation, and her career choice, which could be thought about in terms of projective identification. When we have needs, as Jenny has, which we are unable to recognize and meet, one of the things we can do is to project into another person, and fulfil those/our needs in the other person, for example, caring for others when we ourselves wish to be cared for.

The nurse therapist gave careful thought to the question of why Jenny's therapy had got stuck. In consultation with her supervisor, with whom she discussed her casework on a regular weekly basis, she came to two separate but linked conclusions: Firstly, Jenny was in some sense re-enacting her troubled relationship with her parents within the context of therapy. In part she was projecting her own sense of importance into the nurse, and in part she was attempting to defend herself against becoming dependent on the nurse, since if she did so she would, she believed, inevitably end up being hurt, as in her experience of her mother. Secondly, because of the nurse's own relationship with a psychologically fragile father, she was finding it difficult to confront Jenny with this issue.

A careful examination of the process notes, which recorded the week-to-week progress of the therapy, was of great help in reaching these conclusions, and the casework discussions with her supervisor helped the nurse to distinguish between her own preoccupations and conflicting feelings and those of the client. This freed her to comment on the way in which the relationship between Jenny and her parents was being duplicated in therapy. Over time this enabled Jenny to acknowledge and express her anger towards her mother, both within therapy and outside of it, and to acknowledge the fantasy element in her perception of father's fragility. By the last session, Jenny was able to limit her contact with mother, and to direct her energies towards the development of new, more creative relationships, and her depressive symptoms had virtually vanished.

## DEVELOPMENT

Freud saw human development in term of shifting sexual focus. He postulated the existence of a powerful psychosexual drive, which he called libido (Chapter 8). At different periods of development, the libido is associated with different parts of the body. To the young infant, the mouth is the source not only of sustenance, but also of sensual satisfaction and intimacy with the sustaining breast, and so with mother.

This **oral phase** is superceded towards the end of the first year of life by the **anal phase** (Chapter 5). In Freudian terminology, the libido becomes focused on the anus, and the child becomes increasingly interested in the pleasurable, and aggressive, activities of releasing and later controlling his anal sphincter. About the end of the third year, the genitals become the centre of interest and this is therefore known as the **genital phase**, as both boys and girls begin to derive pleasure from playing with their genitals. From about the fifth to the tenth year, sexuality becomes latent – the **latency period** – and this is succeeded by the beginnings of adult sexual interest at around 11 years of age (Freud, 1910).

Each phase of sexual development may leave marked traces on the adult personality, depending on the extent to which each is successfully negotiated. This in turn depends on early-life experiences, environmental factors, parental attitudes, and so on. Major disturbances in psychosexual development can cause serious problems later, for example, adults who, incapable of mature sexual relationships, attach their libido to inappropriate objects or persons, such as children (Freud, 1905).

We all have a tendency to regress to earlier stages of development when under stress, to revert, for example, to the oral stage by smoking, drinking, or eating too much when we feel anxious. Some individuals, however, owing to a failure to progress satisfactorily through the phases of libidinal development, become fixated at an early stage. They are unable to relate to others on an adult level, and often present themselves with psychiatric problems. For examples, the orally fixated person may be rather dependent, preoccupied with immediate gratification, and prone to mood swings from elation to depression; the anally fixated personality may be very controlled, preoccupied with orderliness and cleanliness, sometimes lapsing into a full-blown obsessive-compulsive neurosis.

Before leaving the subject of psychosexual development, it is necessary to mention the **Oedipus complex**, which Freud named after the hero of Sophocles's *Oedipus Rex*. In the story, Oedipus unwittingly kills his father and marries his mother, and is subsequently punished terribly, both by the gods and by himself. Freud used the term to refer to the '... group of largely unconscious ideas and feelings centring around the wish to possess the parent of the opposite sex an eliminate that of the same sex.' (Rycroft, 1968).

The little boy, it is postulated, desires an exclusive, intimate relationship with his mother of the kind which his father enjoys. Because he cannot displace father, he becomes possessed with impotent, homicidal rage towards him. This makes the boy feel guilty, since he also loves his father, and also fearful that his father will punish him. Because these feelings are so powerful and felt to be dangerous, they are repressed in about the fourth or fifth year of life, only to emerge at the end of the latency period, when they are usually resolved through the formation of satisfactory sexual relationships in young adult life. The female equivalent of the Oedipus complex is the **Electra complex**, in which the feelings directed towards mother and father are the reverse of the boy's.

An inability to resolve such conflicts can result in difficult or disturbed relationships in later life, and Oedipal feelings – the desire on the part of a male client for an exclusive relationship with a female nurse, for example, or competitive, hostile feelings towards a male nurse – will often surface in the nurse/client relationship, where they may provide a vital pointer to underlying developmental problems. If these feelings can be openly expressed and examined, the client may move some way towards freeing himself of their damaging influence in other areas of his life.

The Freudian model of human development is by no means immune to criticism. Melanie Klein (Chapter 5) and others made the point that it omits any consideration of the vitally important first year of life (Klein, 1935). Mrs Klein and others, especially Donald Winnicott and John Bowlby, have gone some way towards rectifying this. The Freudian model also ignores everything that takes place after the young adult phase.

The theoretical construct has been criticized on wider grounds, often with some justice. Social psychologists in the tradition of Adler, Fromm, Horney, and Sullivan have pointed out that Freud considers his hypothetical subject as though he existed in a social vacuum (Hall, 1970). In this respect it resembles learning theory, and its clinical offshoot, behaviour therapy. The behaviourists themselves have attacked the analytic model on the grounds that it is unscientific, and indeed the scientific foundations of Freud's theory of development are rather shaky. The model is perhaps best thought of as a rough map through a difficult terrain, and as a useful basis for therapeutic interventions. Psychology is an inexact science, and we need the insights of psychoanalysis, behaviourism, social psychology, and cognitive theory if we are to approach the fullest possible understanding. (For alternative developmental models see Beard [1969]; Sugarman [1986]; Lewin [1952]; and Erwin [1978]).

## TRANSFERENCE

Freud paid particular attention to the phenomenon known as transference, which has been defined by Rycroft (1968) as:

> The process by which a patient displaces on to his analyst feelings, ideas, etc., which derive from previous figures in his life, by which he relates to his analyst as though he were some former object in his life by which he endows the analyst with the significance of another, usually prior object;
>
> The state of mind produced by 1) [the above] in the patient;
>
> Loosely, the patient's emotional attitude towards his analyst.

Essentially, in the transference the client feels towards and may relate to the analyst/ therapist/nurse as though she or he were some important person in the client's past or present life, usually a parental figure. Transference is a concept some find difficult to grasp, and yet of all the important analytic concepts, it is probably the one that addresses our everyday experience most directly: what

nurse has not experienced transference feelings towards her ward sister, nurse tutor, or teacher?

Transference can include both positive and negative feelings; a degree of positive transference is probably necessary to the formation of a therapeutic relationship. In its extreme form transference can lead to the client 'falling in love' with his or her nurse or therapist.

Initially, Freud regarded transference as an impediment to therapy, but later he came to see it as a vital part of the therapeutic process: the feelings of anger, desire, conflict between love and hate, and so on which the client re-experiences with the analyst in the transference are the cause of his disturbance. By becoming conscious of and expressing these feelings, and with the help of the therapist's interpretations, he is able to connect his present feelings with past experience, and thus begin to understand himself and integrate his past and present emotional life.

This is often a lengthy and painful process. We all like to feel our emotional responses are solely based on reality, and the notion that we harbour feelings of which we may be unaware and yet which exert a powerful influence on our current relationships is a frightening one.

The emotions which the nurse or therapist experience fall under the heading of **countertransference**, which has been described by Laplanche *et al.* (1973) as 'the whole of the analyst's unconscious reactions to the individual analysand, especially to the analysand's own transference.' The therapist's emotional response to the client can be either a response to the client's own transference, or a product of the nurse's/therapist's own emotional makeup, life experience, or current problems. It is important, through supervision and self-exploration, and perhaps through personal therapy, to work out which is which (Chapter 25). Of course, not all powerful feelings are transferential by any means; people like and dislike each other for all sorts of reasons.

Every nurse has encountered a client for whom she experiences powerful feelings of dislike, without knowing why. If we do not question such feelings and attempt to trace them to their source, we may find ourselves, quite unconsciously, neglecting or punishing the client on the basis of our personal feelings, which he has been unfortunate enough to evoke. When we find ourselves experiencing such powerful emotions about a client that cannot be adequately accounted for, our first task is to work out how much of these feeling is to do with ourselves. If we can be reasonably sure that our feelings are objective, we can make use of the counter-transference. In order to do this, we need to think of the feelings we are experiencing as a communication from the client. This can take one of two forms: firstly, 'I want you, the nurse, to feel this sadness, anger, hopelessness because this is how I, the client, feel, and I want you to understand'; or secondly, 'I want you, the nurse, to feel sad, angry, hopeless because this is how I, the client, wish someone who is or once was close to me to feel.'

Interpretation of the counter-transference needs to emerge from the nurse's/therapist's wider understanding of the client, his history, and their relationship, and must be based on a therapeutic alliance, otherwise the interpretation will not be 'heard' by the client.

## CASE STUDY – JULIA

Julia is a 23-year-old young woman who has been admitted to an acute psychiatric ward, having taken an overdose of her antidepressant medication.

Julia has been suffering from depression for some time, and has also had a long-standing eating disorder that has recently become more severe. She is a teacher and, though she generally finds her work satisfying, the pressures of work have recently been getting on top of her. She binges and then fasts for prolonged periods, and has begun to take laxatives to keep her weight down. Julia herself recognizes the connection between her emotional state and her eating pattern, and says that she diets when she feels good about herself and binges when she is unhappy, to punish herself.

Julia is an only child. Her parents separated when she was five years old. Her mother brought her up unaided, and it seems there was little time or affection to spare. Although she sees her father occasionally, the relationship between them is somewhat strained, and it seems to Julia as though he too has little time for her. Over the last year she has separated from her partner because she felt her independence was threatened. This was the latest in a long line of unsatisfactory relationships.

Julia's keyworker felt she might benefit from an opportunity to explore her problems psychodynamically. It seemed to him that her difficulties were rooted in her relationship with her father, her anger at being abandoned by him, and her frustrated need to be loved by him. This had left her with a considerable degree of damage to her self-esteem, and ambivalence in her relationships with men. This was expressed through her eating disorder, which symbolizes both her neediness and her anger, which she turns against herself.

Since she showed considerable insight and strong motivation to change, the nurse offered Julia a fixed, limited number of therapy sessions which continued after her discharge from hospital.

From the outset, Julia expressed powerful transference feelings towards the nurse. Although she was quite willing to discuss her difficulties and relationships, Julia made it clear she was sceptical about the ability or willingness of any man to be helpful to her. The nurse, who genuinely wanted to be helpful, found this difficult to take, and discussion with other nurses in peer-group supervision helped him to contain and work with Julia's hostility, and to maintain a stance of non-judgmental empathy and positive regard (Rogers, 1961). His theoretical understanding helped him to understand Julia's hostility in terms of transference: that her anger towards him and mistrust of him really 'belonged' with her father. Moreover, it became clear over time that this **negative transference** was in itself a defence against a **positive transference**: Julia needed to maintain her picture of the nurse as uncaring and persecutory, otherwise she might like and become dependent on him, and would be dreadfully hurt when he abandoned her as he was bound to do, since this is what father did, and thus what men always do.

At first the nurse found it difficult to tolerate Julia's hostility, and in particular to be seen as uncaring. He tended therefore to attempt to prove his benevolence in inappropriate ways by, for instance, directly expressing his concern for her instead of helping her to understand her hostility. Discussing his work in supervision helped him to become aware of his counter-transference feelings, which gave him space to help Julia to come to terms with her feelings about him, her father, and the other man in her life. The working-through of her anger and dependence, in a supportive, structured context, helped her to set about the task of building new relationships on a more realistic basis. This outcome depended on the nurse's willingness to discuss his feelings for the client in supervision, and on his ability to acknowledge and work with his own emotional responses.

## OBJECT RELATIONS THEORY

Many developments in the theory and practice of the psychodynamic approach have taken place since Freud's day. One important concept is that of the object-relations theory, and the work of its originator Melanie Klein (Grosskurth, 1986; Meltzer, 1978) (Chapter 5).

According to Rycroft (1968), object relation theory is 'the psychoanalytical theory in which the subject's need to relate to objects occupies the central position, in contrast to instinct theory, which centres around the subject's need to reduce instinctual tension' i.e., as distinct from Freudian analytic theory, which is predominantly instinctual.

Klein developed techniques for the analysis of children's play, and this work led her to formulate new hypotheses concerning psychological development in the early years of life, a period which Freud had largely neglected (Klein, 1932; 1961).

Freud had described the psyche in terms of the **ego** – the conscious self; the **super-ego** – the critical internal voice that tells us what is right and what is wrong, and which derives ultimately from our parental models; and the **id** – the repository of our unconscious feelings, impulses and memories. Klein suggested that the child is unable to distinguish his own ego – what he knows to be himself – from the outside world. Because the dividing line between the child's ego and the external world is so weak, his internal world comes to consist of **good objects** – those that gratify him – and **bad objects** – those that cause him pain or frustrate his needs.

The first external object the child comes to know is his mother's breast, which is either a good or a bad object to him, depending on whether it is available or not, and, if available, whether it satisfies his needs or not. The child therefore alternates between loving and hating the breast. He desires to take in, or **introject**, the good breast, which becomes the foundation of his sense of selfhood and goodness, and to get rid of, or **project** the bad, withholding breast. This 'bad' object, which is in fact the child's own aggression projected outward turns back on the child in phantasy, causing him to feel persecuted.

Klein described this as the **paranoid position** (Klein, 1935). Most children pass through this phase more or less successfully, although most of us retain a susceptibility to persecutory feelings into adult life, which are apt to come to the fore at times of stress.

This phase is succeeded by the **depressive position**, in which the child realizes that the good and bad objects are in fact both aspects of the same person: his mother. Since this realization occurs when the dividing line between imagination and reality has not yet been clearly drawn, the child experiences intense guilt, because he believes his aggressive feeling towards the bad object could also destroy the good object, as they are now one and the same. He thus becomes depressed, and remains so until he comes to realize his mother has not been destroyed by his hostility. Elements of the depressive position can also linger into adult life in the form of a tendency to see other people as either wholly good or wholly bad.

For Klein, aggression is a fundamental drive. From a clinical perspective, the expression of aggression must sometimes be encouraged, and contained, along with its associated anxiety, so that it may be resolved. Paranoid and depressive feelings often emerge in our work with clients, and object-relations theory provides a useful way of understanding and working with them (Greenberg *et al.*, 1975).

## THE PROCESS OF CHANGE

Psychotherapy has been defined by Strupp (1978) as:

> ... an interpersonal process designed to bring about modifications of feelings, cognitions, attitudes, and behaviour that have proven troublesome to the person seeking help from a trained professional.

It has been described by Storr (1978) as: 'the art of alleviating personal difficulties through the agency of words and a personal professional relationship.'

Although most nurses do not practice formal psychotherapy – which requires a specialist training and specialized working conditions - in the wider sense of alleviating personal difficulties through a helpful personal and professional relationship, all nurses can and should, and many do, work in a psychotherapeutic way.

What, then, is meant by a 'helpful, personal and professional relationship'? All interaction with clients, however fleeting, have a therapeutic potential, but a relationship that has understanding and personal change as its objectives need to be structured in the sense that it requires boundaries that are both external and physical as well as internal, psychological, and emotional.

The client needs a secure place if he is going to be able to trust the nurse and express his feelings honestly. He also needs to feel that he and the therapeutic work are valued by the nurse and her colleagues. In the most obvious sense, the client needs the physical space in which to be himself in relation to the nurse. This means that a particular room must always be available over a particular period. The time spent with the client must be free from interruption, and the nurse must ensure that neither she nor the client will be called away to do something else. It is important that other members of the team understand the need for this. If, for instance, sessions are interrupted or cancelled because the nurse is required to administer medication, this may convey the impression that medication is more important than the client's self-exploration. On a deeper level, interrupted sessions may be perceived as reflecting and reinforcing the client's sense of hopelessness and inadequacy.

Time is another important boundary, so the session must have a specific starting and finishing point. If sessions do not start on time, the client may feel his needs are not being given priority, and that the nurse is not a consistent, trustworthy person with whom he can safely share his feeling. It is often tempting to go over time at the end of therapeutic activities, especially if the client is in pain or has made some new disclosure in the final minutes. It is almost always a mistake to allow this to happen, since it conveys the message that the nurse does not believe in the client's capacity to contain his own feelings between sessions. As well, by expressing himself at this point, the client may be conveying an unconscious desire to be interrupted, and the continuation of the session beyond the agreed termination point can be quite frightening. He may, of course, be unconsciously attempting to manoeuvre the nurse into breaking her boundaries in order to test her concern for him. As a general rule, the implications of last-minute disclosures should be examined in the following session.

The same principle of maintaining boundaries applies to the emotional/psychological area. The relationship with the client is personal in that the nurse cares about – but not for – him. It is important to be sufficiently involved with the client to be concerned about him, while remaining sufficiently detached to reflect upon what is happening, in order to share one's reflections with the client in useful ways. Clients, and nurses sometimes, are occasionally tempted to convert the therapeutic relationship into one that will meet their emotional needs - for instance, friendship or love or, more commonly perhaps, a parent and a child. When this happens the relationship ceases to be therapeutic. Such relations are invariably disastrous, since they are built on false expectations on both sides, that is, on transference and counter-transference. The aim is to develop the client's capacity to meet his needs by engaging in real relationships in the real world.

Since we are often not as aware of our own true feelings as we like to think, regular supervision in which transference and counter-transference can be discussed openly is the best way of avoiding such developments (Chapters 1, 25). Close attention needs also to be paid to the predominance of different issues at different stages of the relationship. At the onset, the principal issue is often one of trust versus mistrust: does the client feel safe enough to disclose himself to you? Approaching the end of the relationship, the issue for the client is frequently one of abandonment, and he may feel hurt, angry, and rejected, as he has felt before when abandoned by others in the past. Although this may be painful for the nurse, she must allow the client to express and work through such feelings.

The importance of confidentiality cannot be over-stressed. How can the individual feel safe enough to face again and again, over time, the distress that some issues cause, if the nurse therapist cannot be trusted to keep confidential what is private and intimate? It is essential to any form of treatment that confidentiality is maintained. Each team will have its own guidelines regarding this, but we should consider them against the back-cloth of our knowledge of human emotional needs and development, and against the joint measures of what is sensible and what is appropriate.

## CASE STUDY – ELAINE

Elaine is a 20-year-old student who was admitted to hospital in a depressed, withdrawn state following the breakup of a relationship and a failed end-of-term examination.

Elaine is an only child. Her parents came from two different cultures, and their relationship has always been strained. Father left home for long periods to return to his country of origin, and the client herself had an unsettled childhood, living now with her mother, and then, though less often, with her father, and with both for fairly short periods of time. This experience has left Elaine with acutely divided loyalties, and the feeling that 'she didn't know where she belonged'. It also has left her feeling ambivalent about all close relationships, especially with young men of her own age. Although in need of affection and intimacy, Elaine is terrified at the thought of being rejected, and frightened therefore to commit herself to another person. Her inability to tolerate this conflict has led her to break off her relationships at the point where they begin to be important to her, which leaves her feeling hopeless and unloved. It was one such episode that precipitated the depression, and led to Elaine's admission.

Her keyworker, a male nurse, was able to establish a helpful relationship with Elaine quite quickly. He decided his work with her needed to concentrate on helping Elaine to work through her conflicting feelings about her father, since it was this that impinged most seriously on her current relationships. This was based upon the psychodynamic hypothesis that Elaine's ambivalence towards her father (her anger and love for him, and her feeling that being close to him implied disloyalty to her mother) had damaged both her sense of her own value and her capacity to form and maintain adult heterosexual relationships.

The nurse anticipated that Elaine's ambivalence would be powerfully expressed in the transference, and from the beginning Elaine demonstrated strong mixed feelings towards her keyworker. Since she was unable to acknowledge this, she demonstrated it, or **acted it out**, by, for instance, not communicating or rejecting the nurse, while at other times behaving in a manner that suggested she did in fact want the nurse to like her.

In response to Elaine's behaviour the nurse found himself feeling angry in a 'paternal' sort of way. He was helped to understand the counter-transferential nature of this feeling in supervision, which enabled him to help Elaine to understand her behaviour as the expression of a need to recreate the relationship with her father. Although she resisted this interpretation for a time, as the hatred and love she felt for her father emerged into consciousness Elaine eventually became aware of and able to express her own sadness. This in turn helped her to reconcile the 'good' and 'bad' aspects of herself. That she was able before discharge to express her sadness at ending her relationship with the nurse suggested that much of the conflict had been worked through. Elaine went on to complete her college course, and to engage in more satisfactory relationships, and has required no further professional help.

In the psychodynamic model, personal change is brought about through insight: as the individual is able to understand his problems in terms of his emotional conflicts and their roots in past relationships, and their influence on his current relationships, behaviour, and feelings, he is able gradually to become free of their negative influence, and is able to make significant changes in his life.

However, intellectual understanding without the expression of the appropriate accompanying emotion is not enough. In their early pioneering work on hysteria, Breuer and Freud (1895) found that:

> ... each individual hysterical symptom immediately and permanently disappeared when we had succeeded in bringing clearly to light the memory of the event by which it was provoked and in arousing its accompanying effect, and when the patient had described that event in the greatest possible detail and had put the affect into words. Recollection without affect almost invariably produces no results.

This is rarely a straightforward matter, however, as usually the original experience – and its accompanying emotions – needs to be re-experienced again and again by the client in order to be 'worked through' until the feeling, or affect, can be defused.

The experience of life itself – in particular our experiences in relation to others – is the most important source of insight. Sometimes, however, our emotional conflicts constrain our capacity to engage in constructive relationships and our capacity to learn from them; for example, we may unconsciously re-enact painful relationships from the past in an attempt to resolve them in the present. Many mental health nurses will have encountered clients whose life histories are a sequence of interpersonal catastrophes. This process, which Freud called the **repetition compulsion**, seems to stem from a desire to rewrite the original story of one's life, in the hope that it will have a different ending.

Without insight the individual can only be swept along by emotional forces he does not understand, and the pattern can only be repeated endlessly. In the end, disorders that are rooted in relationships can only be put right by relationships – usually the therapeutic relationship.

Most of us have experience of helpful relationships with friends, relatives, and colleagues. Although it shares some of the same characteristics, the therapeutic relationship is fundamentally different from these. All helpful relationships require empathy – the capacity to feel 'with' the other person – as well as honesty, reliability, the ability to communicate clearly, and to accept the person on his own terms. Equally, there are important differences. Our everyday relationships have a quality of mutuality, that is, we share our hopes and fears with our friends as well as opening ourselves to their confidence; if the communication takes place in one direction only, the friendship is unlikely to last.

The therapeutic relationship is different in that the nurse makes her or himself available to the client without disclosing personal information, and without giving judgement or advice. Only thus can the client be free to say whatever he needs to say; and only thus can the nurse be free to think about what is being said and what is happening between herself and the client, and to feed her thoughts back in a way that will help the client's understanding of himself.

We are all familiar with this process. We learn about ourselves from the feedback we get from other people – through their opinions of and their responses to us. We do not always like what we hear. Insight is often painful, and we resist it when it contradicts the image we have of ourselves, or if to accept it would mean making major changes in our lives, which we are frightened to contemplate. This is as true for nurses as it is for clients.

A client's resistance to an insight or interpretation should never be thoughtlessly confronted, since for some individuals such resistance is a necessary defence against the threat of disintegration of the personality or sense of self. Formal therapeutic work should only be undertaken on the basis of a careful assessment of the client's **ego strength**, or as Bloch (1982) says, the 'integrating force which allows a person to use his adaptive resources...assessed by considering such areas as heredity, constitution, early environmental experience, developmental history, customary methods of handling stress, and general level of social maturity.'

## REFERENCES

Bloch, S. (1982) *What is Psychotherapy?* Oxford Univ. Press, Oxford.

Buller, Steve (1990) Psychodynamic models in relationships. *Nursing Standard*, 4, 18, 32 – 4.

Cape, B. and Dobson, P. (1974) *Baillière's Nurses Dictionary*, Baillière Tindall, London.

Cormack, D. (1976) *Psychiatric Nursing Observed*, Royal College of Nursing, London.

Derbyshire, P. (1987) The burden of history, *Nursing Times*, Jan./Feb. 32 – 4.

Freud, S. and Breuer, J. (1895) *Studies in Hysteria*, SE II, Hogarth, London and Vol. 3 Penguin, Harmondsworth.

Freud, S. (1905) *Three Essay on the Theory of Sexuality*, SE VII, Hogarth, and Vol.7 Penguin, Harmondsworth.

Freud, S. (1910) *Five Lectures on Psychoanalysis*, SE XI, Hogarth, London.

Freud, S. (1940) *An Outline of Psychoanalysis*, SE XIII, Hogarth, London, and Vol.15, Penguin, Harmondsworth.

Greenberg, J. R. and Mitchell, S. (1975) *Object Relations in Psychoanalytic Theory*, Harvard Univ. Press, Cambridge, Mass.

Hall, C. S, (1957) *Theories of Personality*, Gardner Lindzey and John Wiley and Sons, Chichester, London.

Laplanche, J. and Pontalis, J. B. (1973) *The Language of Psychoanalysis*, Karnac Books, London.

Macleod, Clark J. and Hockey, L. (1989) *Further Research for Nursing*, Scutari Press, Harrow.

Meltzer, D. (1978) *The Kleinian Development*, Clunie Press, London.

Peplau, H. E. (1952) *Interpersonal Relations in Nursing: a Conceptual Frame of Reference for Psychodynamic Nursing*, Macmillan Education, Basingstoke.

Rogers, C. R. (1961) *On Becoming a Person*, Houghton-Mifflin, Boston.

Rycroft, C. (1968) *A Critical Dictionary of Psychoanalysis*, Penguin, Harmondsworth.

Shafer, K., Sawyer, J. *et al.* (1975) *Medical-Surgical Nursing*, C.V. Mosby, St. Louis.

Storr, A. (1979) *The Art of Psychotherapy*, Secker and Warburg and Heinemann, London.

Strupp, H. (1978) Psychotherapy research and practice: an overview, *Handbook of Psychotherapy and Behaviour Change*, (eds S. Garfield and A. Bergin) Wiley and Sons, Chichester.

Sundeen, S.J., Stuart, G. W., Rankin, E. *et al.* (1976) *Nurse-Client Interaction: Implementing the Nursing Process*, C.V. Mosby, St. Louis.

Tyrer, P. and Steinberg, D. (1987) *Models for Mental Disorder; Conceptual Models in Psychiatry*, John Wiley and Sons, Chichester.

## FURTHSER READING

Beard, Ruth (1969) *An Outline of Piaget's Developmental Psychology*, Routledge, London.

Erwin, E. (1978) *Behaviour Therapy: Scientific, Philosophical and Moral Foundations*, Cambridge Univ. Press, Cambridge.

Gay, P. and Freud, S. (1988) *A Life For Our Time*, Macmillan Publishers Ltd, London.

Grosskurth, P. (1986) *Melanie Klein*, Karnac Books, London.

Klein, M. (1932) *The Psychoanalysis of Children*, Hogarth, London, and Virago Press, London.

Klein, M. (1937) *Love, Guilt, and Reparation, and Other Works*, Virago Press, London.

Klein, M. (1961) *Narrative of a Child Analysis*, Hogarth Press, London.

Lewin, Kurt. (1952) *Field Theory in Social Science*, Tavistock, London.

Main, T. The ailment, in *Psychosocial Nursing* (ed. E. Barnes), Tavistock, London.

Sugarman, L. (1986) *Life-Span Development: Concepts, Theories and Interventions*, Methuen and Co., London.

# BEHAVIOURAL AND COGNITIVE-BEHAVIOURAL APPROACHES

## 21

*Gordon Deakin*

Behavioural approaches to treatment and care have become more readily available in the UK since the early 1970s as increasing numbers of clinical psychologists, psychiatrists, and mental health nurses have developed skills in applying the now wide range of research-based therapeutic methods to mental illness and psychological distress. Behaviourism's long history in the research laboratory led to the development from the late 1950s onwards of increasingly effective therapeutic techniques. Originally these excluded the mind-orientated examination of human difficulties, but with the growth of cognitive therapies during the 1970s, a merging of strategies occurred.

Both cognitive and behavioural approaches to mental health difficulty emphasize research-based, structured, participative, and time-limited orientations. They are cost-effective, and in many areas of clinical difficulty can be viewed as the first choice for treatment intervention, for example, anxiety states, fear, phobias, obsessions, and compulsions.

Central to behavioural and cognitive-behavioural theories of human functioning and dysfunction is the recognition that learning is the basis for the development of both adaptive and life-enhancing, and maladaptive and life-restricting, ways of living with the self, others, and the environment. The more behaviourally-orientated will emphasize learning embedded in activity, while the more cognitively-orientated will emphasize perception, reflection, and thinking in the learning process.

Both behavioural and cognitive-behavioural approaches emphasize the active participation of the client in the change process. Clients will learn how their problems are hypothesized to have developed, how they are maintained by environmental reinforcers and unhelpful thinking patterns; and how by entering planned programmes of graded activity (as in the treatment of escape and avoidance behaviour), together with monitoring, challenging, and modification of thinking styles they can regain control of their lives to make lasting change in their behaviour and feelings. The aim is to develop new learning to replace older, unhelpful learning.

Therapeutic interventions are available for learning difficulties among the intellectually impaired, the chronically affected and institutionalized mentally ill, community-based individuals with schizophrenia, as well as for individuals with depression, anxiety-based disorders, and sexual and relationship difficulties. Behavioural medicine has extended the field of intervention to provide strategies to manage chronic pain, ameliorate problems with hypertension, and assist people to cope with life-threatening malignant disease, and the side effects of other treatment.

## STRATEGIC ISSUES IN ASSESSMENT AND CASE MANAGEMENT

Skills in assessment are critical for nurses developing expertise in cognitive-behavioural approaches to clinical practice. Adequate educational preparation and high-quality supervision from an experienced cognitive-behavioural worker is an essential prerequisite for ethically sound, safe, and professional clinical practice. Many of the methods available within this field can be distressing and harmful if used improperly. Inadequate or incomplete assessment leads to defective formulations, inappropriate care planning, and the strong likelihood of treatment failure or client non-compliance.

Cognitive-behavioural assessment is based largely on the clinical interview, supported by observation and data collection. Directive styles of interviewing are favoured. Richards *et al.* (1990) describe such a goal-oriented method as a 'pragmatic' model of interviewing, enabling the nurse to acquire extensive amounts of client and problem-relevant material in a short period of time.

The interview style is focused, moving from general to specific open questions in an onion-peeling fashion, and on to highly specific open and closed questions. Interview questions using the '5WH-formula' – who? when? where? what? why? and how? – are particularly useful (Priestley *et al.* 1983).

A cognitive-behavioural assessment of an individual's difficulties should produce descriptive information, in an objective form, covering the following areas:

- Description of the current problem, detailing the frequency, intensity, duration, and variability of the problem behaviour or emotion. The environmental situation should be included, and the client's difficulties examined in relation to the antecedent, the behaviour itself, and the consequences that follow. Emotional responses such as anxiety, fear, and anger need to be described using a three-systems analysis (Lang, 1969), which divides emotions into their component elements for assessment and treatment planning purposes: physiological symptoms; cognitive responses; and behavioural activity.

- The development of the problem and the hypothesized maintenance factors should describe the problem history in relationship to relevant life events, how learning might have produced the current problem, and which cognitive, behavioural, and physiological factors are operating alongside reinforcers to maintain the problem.

- Social and environmental factors, including current family relationships, social networks, interests, occupational, housing, and financial information relevant to the problem and its anticipated management.

- Personal assets, emphasizing the individual's strengths as a person, and the non-problem aspects of his life.

- A detailed listing of the person's cognitive and behavioural excesses, and, separately, a list of the cognitive and behavioural deficits.

- The individual's use of prescribed and unprescribed medication, alcohol intake, and use of stimulants such as drinks containing caffeine that produce symptoms similar to anxiety (Lee *et al.*, 1985). Physical ill health and disability should be described, and the presence of health problems that will be exacerbated by high levels of autonomic arousal should be highlighted (coronary artery disease, angina, hypertension, asthma, emphysema, peptic ulcer, colitis and epilepsy contraindicate rapid behavioural exposure methods such as flooding [Marks, 1981]).

- The client's motivation for treatment and evidence of self-control. Why has s/he sought help at this time? Did s/he seek help, or did a family member pressure them to seek a referral? How does s/he currently manage the problem? What efforts does s/he make, or has made, to treat themselves? (Many individuals already use coping strategies that can be shaped into self-treatment methods.)

- Supporting data collected to confirm the above descriptive information. This may be in the form of data diaries containing frequency, intensity, and duration information (e.g., anxiety/panic attacks, episodes of handwashing) collected by the client and/or a family member. Questionnaire measures, tested for validity and reliability, are regularly used to demonstrate the range and extent of a person's problem. Fear questionnaires (Marks *et al.*, 1977), mood measures, such as the Beck Depression Inventory (Beck *et al.*, 1961), and other problem-specific questionnaires such as the Maudsley Obsessional-Compulsive Inventory (Rachman *et al.*, 1980), or the Rathus Assertiveness Schedule (Rathus, 1973) are valuable aids in the assessment process. Standardized rating scales are routinely used to measure impact of the person's difficulties on lifestyle, e.g., the life-adjustment scale (Marks, 1986), and to demonstrate problem severity, on 0-8 rating scales.

- Outcome objectives are negotiated with the client as a series of targets or goals to be achieved by the end of the treatment programme. These usually consist of a series of objectively testable outcome statements that can be rated before and after treatment on 0–8 rating scales of distress and successful completion (Marks *et al.*, 1977; 1986).

This assessment information provides the material evidence available to the nurse that will enable her to carry out a functional analysis of the individual's difficulties and make a

formulation of the problems. Such a functional analysis summarizes evidence, gives hypotheses to test, and relates the assessment information into a structure that helps to identify intervention points, and enables planning decisions and predictions to be made.

The clinical team described here usually use a standard battery of assessment questionnaires and problem-rating forms with each client; to these are added other problem-specific questionnaires as and when required to elicit more detailed data on particular clinical syndromes.

The standard questionnaire battery consists of: a life history questionnaire (Lazarus, 1976); a fear questionnaire, using a 0–8 rating scale of avoidance of 17 situations, and a 6-item general symptoms questionnaire; and a Beck Depression Inventory.

Having carried out an assessment by interview, observation, and data collection, the nurse makes a functional analysis of the person's difficulties and presents this as a formulation to the client in order that treatment plans can be discussed. Just as outcome objectives are negotiated between nurse and client, so are the intervention plans. The nurse needs to be familiar with cognitive and behavioural principles, and to be up to date on the research evidence for the various therapeutic methods available. The treatment options are discussed so that the nurse can recommend a preferred option, and the client can discuss treatment implications and make a choice from the available options. Motivation and compliance will be higher where the client fully participates in treatment planning.

Nurses using cognitive-behavioural methods aim for short-term interventions in order to maximize cost-effectiveness and minimize the risks of the client developing an unhelpful dependence upon the nurse. Treatment interventions are based upon maximum client participation.

If the client is able to undertake treatment without the nurse being present, they are encouraged to do so. The nurse then acts as an educator and treatment facilitator, who aims the client in the right direction; teaches him how to treat himself; receives feedback from the client's homework practice; gives social reinforcement for the client's gains; and fine-tunes or problem-solves any difficulties he might have in the self-management programme.

Such self-treatment is becoming increasing popular, but how many clients can benefit with low levels of nurse/therapist inputs is as yet unclear (Richards *et al.*, 1990).

Where the nurse needs to be more closely involved in treatment exercises – for example, exposure within phobic situations, or using a flooding and response prevention approach on a domiciliary basis with an individual's obsessional contamination fears – the same principle holds: the client should be moved towards maximum involvement and participation as rapidly as possible, enabling the nurse to withdraw as early as possible from the close direction and therapeutic modelling. Clinical progress is then more clearly 'owned' by the client, while the nurse can steer him more efficiently towards his treatment goals.

Outpatient treatments are appropriate for all but the most severely affected clients. Therapy sessions are usually best carried out from an outpatient clinic or health centre (Marks, 1985). Domiciliary sessions for assessment or treatment should be based on assessed need, as they tend to be time-consuming, e.g., travel, without necessarily benefiting the client more than clinic sessions. Even people with severe levels of agoraphobia can often visit outpatient clinics. On the other hand, people with obsessional-compulsive disorders affecting home or work life are often best treated at home for at least the initial sessions.

Nurses using cognitive-behavioural approaches tend to view assessment as a continuing process throughout treatment. Clients will often be expected to keep daily data diaries reporting on their progress through therapy. Periodically nurses will repeat key measures, e.g., target ratings or Beck Depression Inventory, to evaluate the clients state or progress.

Therapeutic sessions tend to work best when closely spaced, for example, weekly, with frequent homework exercises negotiated to take place between clinic appointments; these might be daily or more frequent.

Each therapeutic session needs to be structured, with an agenda that enables the nurse to effectively address her client's needs without wasting time or moving on to irrelevancies. For most cognitive and behavioural therapists, the following agenda works well:

1. Greetings and orientation.
2. Review of homework programme and significant events in the week.
3. Discussion and problem-solving of homework difficulties.
4. Cognitive-behavioural treatment exercises.
5. Reviewing and summarizing in-session learning.
6. Negotiating new homework programme and data requirements.
7. Closure and new appointment.

Unsuccessful interventions become evident very rapidly. People with problems involving phobic and obsessional-compulsive difficulties usually show improvement on at least one of the three systems model of emotion within each session. Adequate homework produces rapid generalization.

As a supervisor, reviews of progress after every fifth session should be sufficient when appointments are weekly. If appointments are less frequent, reviews ought to be programmed for a similar calender regularity. Where clinical anxiety states are the presenting problem, progress may take six to eight sessions to appear, but should be progressive thereafter. When individuals receive cognitive-behavioural interventions for depression, as many as 15–20 sessions or more will be needed, with twice weekly sessions required in the first few weeks. Progress should become evident by improvements in activity levels and mood within four sessions.

When co-operative and compliant clients fail to make the expected progress, the nurse is strongly advised to reassess the individual's problem and closely review how treatment was implemented. This will usually reveal errors in the original assessment, incomplete or inappropriately managed treatment sessions, or problems in the individual's compliance that have not been revealed in homework reviews previously. Negotiation of a modified programme is then usually possible, enabling progress to occur.

Clients who are hostile to cognitive-behavioural approaches and are not amenable to educational change should of course be transferred to a professional using other clinical strategies. A proportion of clients will drop out of treatment after a small number of sessions. Reassessment often reveals previously undisclosed hostility to the nurse or their intervention methods; or, not infrequently, clients who feel the nurse's treatment demands are higher than they feel they can cope with. For the latter, closer support and some rescheduling of homework will usually provide a solution.

While not all clients will achieve all their negotiated outcome objectives or reach a point where they view themselves as problem-free, the majority of individuals do make significant progress within a relatively short period of time. Expected success rates can be reviewed within cognitive and behavioural journals, and within some reviews of therapy (Rachman *et al.*, 1980; Foa *et al.*, 1983).

The decision to end a programme of therapy is best negotiated between the client and the nurse as a part of their regular review of progress in each session. Treatment need not be complete for discharge from the nurse's active caseload to take place; what is necessary is for the client to be confidently making progress and aware of each step he needs to make. Further monitoring can then be made with less frequent appointments as a planned programme of follow-up. Many nurses using cognitive-behavioural approaches routinely offer follow-up appointments at one, three, six, and twelve months following the date of discharge.

Discharge and follow-up points are important evaluation episodes. The nurse should collect data that demonstrates the degree of success. Where questionnaires of problem severity, life-adjustment ratings, problem ratings, and outcome-objective (target) ratings have been made during the assessment phase of the nurse's intervention, they should be repeated at discharge and at each follow-up point to provide a database confirmation of clinical change, contributing to the nurse's range of quality indicators.

## CLINICAL MEASUREMENT

Behavioural therapists in particular, and cognitive-behavioural workers to a great extent, place a high value on collecting data to supplement the client's self-report. There is an emphasis on identifying and measuring as objectively as possible otherwise subjective phenomena, for example, the intensity of anger or anxiety. There is a corresponding emphasis on collecting valid and reliable information on when things happen, how long for, and with what frequency.

Rating scales of various types have been devised to examine subjective experiences, and a wealth of questionnaire measures exist to measure difficulties and symptoms as diverse as mood, assertiveness, fear (fear survey schedules), and anxiety (Thyer's Clinical Anxiety Scale). Some of these are highly specific, for example, the mobility inventory for agoraphobia (Chambless *et al.*, 1985). Validity and reliability are critical issues in developing, testing, and choosing such measures.

The diary method of collecting data is a particularly useful means of gathering in-

**Table 21.1**  Client/patient problem-rating scales

Therapist and client define the mutually agreed problems that require treatment during assessment, and rate each one separately on two scales. The first scale examines the clients current feelings of distress, and the second the impact of the problem on their usual activities or behaviour. These ratings can then be repeated at the discharge and follow-up points in order to evaluate the effects of treatment and their persistence. The intervening odd numbers (1, 3, 5, and 7) are gradations that allow the client to give a finer discrimination between their feelings of distress and impact on lifestyle than the defined even numbers on the scale. Some workers in the field utilize 0–10 and 0–100 point scales in a similar manner. An example problem description might be 'tension headaches'.

Feelings scale for problem ratings

| 0 | 1 | 2 | 3 | 4 | 5 | 6 | 7 | 8 |
|---|---|---|---|---|---|---|---|---|
| I never feel at all upset about this problem. | | I sometimes feel a bit upset about this problem. | | I often feel quite upset about this problem. | | I very often feel seriously upset about this problem. | | I continuously feel extremely upset about this problem. |

Behaviour scale for problem ratings

| 0 | 1 | 2 | 3 | 4 | 5 | 6 | 7 | 8 |
|---|---|---|---|---|---|---|---|---|
| The problem does not interfere with my usual activities. | | It occasionally interferes with my usual activities. | | It quite often interferes with my usual activities. | | It very often interferes with my usual activities. | | It continually and seriously interferes with my usual activities. |

**Table 21.2**  Target/outcome objective ratings

During assessment, the therapist and client negotiate outcomes they wish to achieve by the end of treatment. These are described concretely as observable and repeatable activities that will reflect improvements in distress and activity. The ratings are used at discharge and follow-up, as well as during the course of treatment in order to evaluate progress. All target descriptions need careful selection and wording to facilitate this measurement activity. At assessment, the client gives pretreatment ratings on how well they would be able to carry out the activity now, and how distressed they would expect to feel on the 'Feeling' and 'Behaviour' scales. Verification can be sought using a behavioural avoidance test. Variations on these scales are used to examine the impact of problems on work, home management, private and social leisure (life-adjustment scales) and on other aspects of difficulty. They can be modified easily to evaluate satisfaction with the treatment process (Deakin, 1989).

Feelings scale for target ratings ('Carrying out this activity now will make me feel…')

| 0 | 1 | 2 | 3 | 4 | 5 | 6 | 7 | 8 |
|---|---|---|---|---|---|---|---|---|
| No distress at all. | | Some uneasiness. | | Definite distress. | | Strong distress. | | Extreme distress. |

Behaviour scale for target ratings ('I could complete this activity now with…')

| 0 | 1 | 2 | 3 | 4 | 5 | 6 | 7 | 8 |
|---|---|---|---|---|---|---|---|---|
| Complete success. | | 75% success. | | 50% success. | | 25% success. | | I would be completely unable to carry out this activity. |

formation. Clients, and/or family members, are often asked to complete data-collection sheets, recording the frequency of particular symptoms, the environmental context in which they occur, their duration, and their effects on the individual. Providing they are designed for ease of use, and given a trial-run in order to problem-solve any difficulty the client experiences in their use, they can provide extremely valuable information that the client might not otherwise be able to recall or report in detail. For example, a person with difficulties around anger might be asked to record their variable levels of irritability at set times each day, with notes on where they were and what they were doing. They might also be asked to record all episodes where anger rose above a certain threshold on a 0–8 subjective rating scale, attending to issues such as environment, activity, anger duration, expression, and the use of coping strategies.

At clinic sessions such homework diaries provide the therapist with the information on which to focus therapeutic activity. They can also be used to provide pretreatment baselines against which comparisons can be made during treatment, at discharge, and in follow-up.

## NURSING INTERVENTION FOR CLINICAL ANXIETY STATES AND PANIC EXPERIENCES

### CASE STUDY – DAVID

David, a 38-year-old married man working for the last three years as a traffic warden, sought help from his GP for frequent episodes of anxiety and tension, which occurred unpredictably on most days. The anxiety had been present for six months, and led to mild feelings of depression. Twice in the previous month David had experienced panic attacks when driving, and feared more occurring. Although his GP had prescribed diazepam 5 mgm to be taken at night two months previously, these had had no

effect on David's anxiety or panic, but there had been some improvement in his ability to fall asleep.

David lived in a small country town in his own house and worked in the busy nearby city. His marriage to Mary was happy. His two children – both boys, aged 19 and 18 – lived at home but were expecting to move out in the coming year; the eldest to marry and move into his own home, the younger to join the Royal Navy.

Seen initially by a nurse behaviour therapist in his GP's health centre for a preliminary screening interview, David asked to be seen for further sessions in the outpatient clinic of the city in which he worked, as this would fit conveniently into his working day.

David – well-groomed but with a taciturn, preoccupied appearance – gave a clear and succinct description of his difficulties over two assessment appointments, two weeks apart. As was the usual department policy, first names were used throughout treatment, with sessions taking place in a clinic office arranged with informal lounge chairs.

### The assessment

Assessment interviews lasted a total of two-and-one-half hours. David completed the department's standard battery of questionnaires and rating-scale measures, as well as a Thyer Anxiety Scale (Thyer, 1987) consisting of 25 items rated on a 1–5 scale (Figure 21.5).

David described his current problem as being attacks of anxiety occurring between two and four times a day, each lasting 5–20 minutes. The episodes were not situation-specific, and occurred at any time without warning. Physical symptoms included rapid heart rate, sweating, tingling sensations in hands, and abdominal discomfort. High levels

**Table 21.3** David's pretreatment data summary

|  | **Score** |  |
|---|---|---|
| Fear questionnaire | 26 | Not significant. |
| General symptoms | 14 | Not significant. |
| Beck Depression Inventory | 22 | Suggesting mild depression of mood. |
| Thyer Anxiety Scale | 28 | Clinically significant score. |

Life-adjustment scale:
| | | |
|---|---|---|
| **1.** Work (0–8) | 0 | No problem. |
| **2.** Home management | 2 | Slight problem. |
| **3.** Social leisure | 2 | Slight problem. |
| **4.** Private leisure | 0 | No problem. |

Problem-severity scale
**1.** Anxiety
| | | |
|---|---|---|
| a) Feelings | 8 | Severe problem. |
| b) Behaviour | 6 | Major interference. |

**2.** Panic
| | | |
|---|---|---|
| Feelings | 8 | Severe problem. |
| Behaviour | 4 | Moderate interference. |

Target-rating scale
**1.** Cope with general anxiety symptoms as they arise.
| | | |
|---|---|---|
| a) Feelings | 6 | Marked problem. |
| b) Behaviour | 6 | 25% effective. |

**2.** Manage panic episodes as they arise.
| | | |
|---|---|---|
| a) Feelings | 8 | Severe problem. |
| b) Behaviour | 8 | Ineffective. |

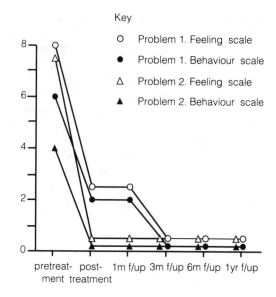

Key

○   Problem 1. Feeling scale
●   Problem 1. Behaviour scale
△   Problem 2. Feeling scale
▲   Problem 2. Behaviour scale

**Figure 21.1** David's problem severity ratings

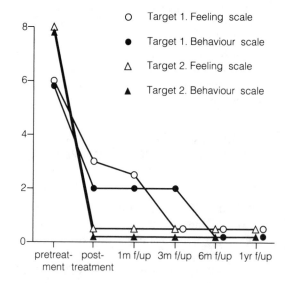

○   Target 1. Feeling scale
●   Target 1. Behaviour scale
△   Target 2. Feeling scale
▲   Target 2. Behaviour scale

**Figure 21.2** David's target-rating scales

of muscle tension were present in the neck, arms, and shoulders, leading to aching stiffness. Cognitively, David would notice negative self-statements during the attacks, such as 'Oh, no, not again.'; 'How long this time?'; 'This is bloody awful. I can't stand much more of this.' His behavioural activity would change, and he would set off walking vigorously with two aims in mind, first, avoidance of any conversation, and, second, to 'burn-off' the heightened level of arousal. David feared other people, apart from his wife, noticing his anxiety, and experienced relief when the anxiety passed. David was socially skilled and usually felt confident, but he had found

he was generally more tense than in his previous job as a dockyard fitter.

Three months before the onset of his anxiety symptoms, Mary had had a hysterectomy; she had made a full

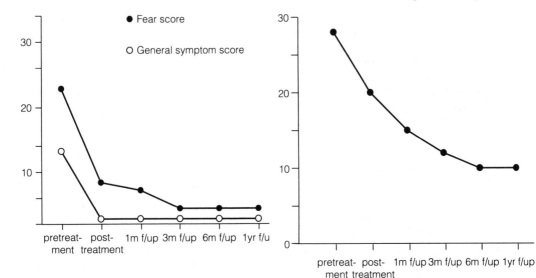

Figure 21.3 David's fear questionnaire

Figure 21.5 David's Thyer anxiety scale

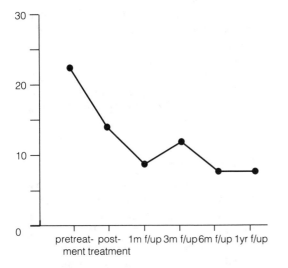

**Figure 21.4** David's Beck depression inventory

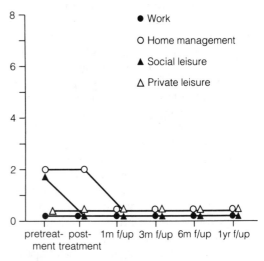

**Figure 21.6** David's life-adjustment scale

recovery, and their sexual and emotional relationship was good. The two panic experiences had both occurred while David was returning home from work. On both occasions he was delayed in traffic-jams, a regular occurrence on his one route out of the city. The panics involved high heart rates, marked shortness of breath, and a fear of losing control and fainting. Neither attack lasted more than five minutes, and had ended when the traffic flow had improved. Although he anticipated further attacks, they had not occurred in other traffic-jams.

While David's mood was described as usually good, he had felt miserable or slightly depressed for most of the preceding six months. Since his wife's surgery they had reduced their social activities markedly, only having been out together twice to local pubs, which they had previously frequented at least once each week.

## The case formulation

After analyzing David's questionnaires, reviewing his interview material and a daily diary recording his anxiety experiences over a two-week period, a formulation was made by the nurse and discussed with him.

In summary, it appeared that following his redundancy three-and-one-half years before, and a six-month period of unemployment, David had taken his current job as a traffic warden without great enthusiasm. Although competent at his job, he did not enjoy it and felt uncomfortable in a 'policing' role with parking offenders who did not welcome his attentions. David consequently felt generally more tense, restless, and dissatisfied. This heightened level of autonomic arousal was exacerbated by his wife's hysterectomy, which led to increased worries about her health. The impending departure of their two sons left him aware of further life changes as middle-age approached.

The increased levels of general physical tension produced physical symptoms that worried him, leading to negative thinking, which produced further increases in arousal that David experienced as anxiety. The mild depressive mood was seen as secondary to, but exacerbated, the anxiety. Relief associated with vigorous exercise and social avoidance led to inappropriate cognitions about coping. It was further suggested to David

that his reduced social life had increased general tension, and contributed to his lowered mood.

The two panic attacks were viewed as a progressive consequence of the frequent anxiety episodes occurring in situations where David felt less control than usual. In particular, his negative 'awfulizing' thinking produced a catastrophic sequence of thinking, which involved unwarranted health concerns that increased his anxiety, which exacerbated his negative cognitions, in an upward spiral producing hyperventilation, fear, and a sense of losing control (hyperventilation temporarily alters the acid blood base values, which further increase symptoms of distress [Salkovskis, 1988]). Relief from these panics was also outside David's sense of control, being perceived as due to the lessening of the traffic-jam. His fearful anticipation of further panics, which did not occur as regularly as the traffic-jams, increased his level of autonomic arousal and added to his general level of anxiety and tension, making further episodes of anxiety and panic – through self-fulfilling prophecies – more likely.

## The treatment plan

David found this formulation made sense to him, and with his nurse he negotiated a treatment plan based on an educational programme of treatment that he felt made sense, was problem-focused, and which could, with some compromises, fit into his current lifestyle. The nurse was able to take David straight into treatment. Problem ratings, life-adjustment rating and target descriptions with ratings were made (Table 21.3). The treatment plan was designed to use a one-to-one teaching format with prescribed homework exercises. Six clinical sessions over approximately ten weeks were estimated to provide an adequate trial of treatment.

At the last assessment session the nurse asked David to continue his daily diary of data, and explained how anxiety, as a normal human process, operates within the individual. David was given a brief role-played and modelled-teaching session on a modified version of Jacobsen's (1938) relaxation training method. This required him to set aside two 30-minute periods every day for relaxation practice, accompanied by four relaxation fantasies. This he started immediately, and with only a small number of errors practised regularly throughout the treatment programme, recording each practice in his daily diary.

In the following weekly appointments, the nurse taught David a technique to control his hyperventilation-induced panic attacks, initially using role-played hyperventilation to reproduce similar symptoms in the clinic (Clark, 1986). This improved David's sense of self-control, and effectively reduced his fear of further panic attacks; he experienced no further panic attacks.

Other elements of David's programme included discussion and teaching – supported by handouts – on the role of cognition in producing increases in anxiety. He was taught how to 'catch' automatic negative thoughts, acknowledge their presence, and then to reframe them in a more positive and adaptive manner (Beck *et al.*, 1985). This was a major element in David's homework programme.

**Table 21.4** David's post-treatment data summary

|  | Discharge | 1m f/u | 3m f/u | 6m f/u | 1yr f/u |
|---|---|---|---|---|---|
| Fear questionnaire | 8 | 6 | 2 | 2 | 2 |
| General symptoms | 0 | 0 | 0 | 0 | 0 |
| Beck Depression Inventory | 14 | 8 | 10 | 6 | 6 |
| Thyer Anxiety Scale | 22 | 15 | 12 | 8 | 8 |
| Life-adjustment scale |  |  |  |  |  |
| 1. Work | 0 | 0 | 0 | 0 | 0 |
| 2. Home management | 2 | 0 | 0 | 0 | 0 |
| 3. Social leisure | 0 | 0 | 0 | 0 | 0 |
| 4. Private leisure | 0 | 0 | 0 | 0 | 0 |
| Problem-severity scale |  |  |  |  |  |
| 1. Anxiety |  |  |  |  |  |
| a) Feelings | 2 | 2 | 0 | 0 | 0 |
| b) Behaviour | 2 | 2 | 0 | 0 | 0 |
| 2. Panic |  |  |  |  |  |
| a) Feelings | 0 | 0 | 0 | 0 | 0 |
| b) Behaviour | 0 | 0 | 0 | 0 | 0 |
| Target-rating scale |  |  |  |  |  |
| 1. Cope with General anxiety |  |  |  |  |  |
| a) Feelings | 3 | 2 | 0 | 0 | 0 |
| b) Behaviour | 2 | 2 | 2 | 0 | 0 |
| 2. Manage panic episodes |  |  |  |  |  |
| a) Feelings | 0 | 0 | 0 | 0 | 0 |
| b) Behaviour | 0 | 0 | 0 | 0 | 0 |

(m = month; f/u = follow up)

Other sessions included discussion and practice of problem-solving strategies, teaching about the effect of escape and avoidance behaviours on anxiety and fear. This was coupled with advice to change his response style when experiencing an anxiety episode so that he no longer avoided other people or indulged in vigorous walks. David replaced these where feasible with quiet episodes of relaxation and conversation with other people (Powell *et al.*, 1990).

David was asked to cease his diazepam medication with GP approval, and did so with only minimal effects on his sleep pattern. He was advised to discuss his difficulties with his wife, and asked her to re-establish their social life together, which they did with pleasure, and widening of their social network.

## Conclusion

David's treatment programme was largely self-directed homework. Nurse-led sessions occurred on seven occasions over ten weeks, totalling six-and-one-half hours of the nurse's available time. Discharge with major improvement took place 12 weeks after first contact. Further improvement continued in the follow-up period, this being maintained up to the 12-month point, when the client agreed that no further follow up appeared to be necessary (Table 21.4). David showed major improvement in anxiety, panic, and mood. No job change appeared necessary as he felt increasingly able to cope, and able to expand his and his wife's social life in a beneficial manner.

Generalized anxiety disorders are often chronic difficulties, showing 50% improvement rates with or without treatment. Our experience suggests that skilful cognitive-behavioural interventions can produce 60% improvements within three to six months of first contact, whether as individuals or as group members; little controlled research is yet available beyond this clinical impression.

## NURSING INTERVENTION FOR AGORAPHOBIA

### CASE STUDY – CHARLOTTE

Charlotte is a 27-year-old woman, married for three years to John, a 28-year-old civil servant. They have lived for four years in a rented flat. Charlotte, previously a civil service clerical officer, is a housewife who spends much of her time looking after their three-year-old daughter, Rachel. She would like to return to work in order to buy a house, but has developed agoraphobic fears over the last two-and-one-half years, following a series of panic attacks while shopping. She has been able to continue shopping alone in two shops, which are five minutes away, and can visit some friends without escort. However, she is unable to travel to or shop in the city centre alone, nor in the large superstores on the city outskirts without her husband and the family car.

Although Charlotte is an experienced driver, she now only drives when John is with her, but he uses the car to travel to work. The area they live in is 20 minutes' walk from the city centre, served by a regular bus which Charlotte cannot use. Two parks are within five minutes' walk. The local infants' school where Rachel is due to start half a day per week in six weeks is just over 10 minutes' walk, but Charlotte is unable to make this trip alone.

Charlotte experiences mild to moderately severe premenstrual symptoms (PMS) of increased anxiety, irritability, backache, bloating, and sensitive nipples eight days prior to her periods, which are regular on a 28-day cycle. The PMS symptoms are relieved on the first day of each period. Pregnancy and childbirth were uncomplicated.

John's parents live in a small town 60 miles away, and Charlotte's live 40 miles away in a county town. The couple visit both sets of parents by car about every four to six weeks; unless the parents visit them

Charlotte sought help from her GP three months previously when she realized Rachel's nursery was due to start soon. She had not previously discussed her fears with the GP, who is described as impatient with mental health difficulties; he prescribed no medication, but made an immediate referral to the behaviour therapy nursing service.

**Table 21.5** Charlotte's data summary

| | Pretreatment | Post treatment | 1m f/u | 3m f/u | 6m f/u | 1yr f/u |
|---|---|---|---|---|---|---|
| Modified fear questionnaire | | | | | | |
| 1. Fear | 34 | 25 | 17 | 17 | 18 | 12 |
| 2. Avoidance | 34 | 9 | 10 | 8 | 6 | 6 |
| General symptoms | 10 | 4 | 2 | 2 | 1 | 1 |
| Agoraphobia questionnaire | 71 | 42 | 39 | 36 | 27 | 28 |
| Mobility inventory | | | | | | |
| 1. Accompanied | 8 | 8 | 10 | 0 | | |
| 2. Unaccompanied | 55 | 55 | 31 | 14 | | |
| Beck Depression Inventory | 9 | 6 | 0 | 2 | 3 | 0 |
| Life-adjustment scale | | | | | | |
| 1. Work | 6 | 3 | 2 | 2 | 1 | 1 |
| 2. Home management | 4 | 0 | 0 | 0 | 0 | 0 |
| 3. Social leisure | 6 | 2 | 2 | 1 | 1 | 1 |
| 4. Private leisure | 4 | 0 | 0 | 0 | 0 | 0 |
| Problem-severity scale | | | | | | |
| 1. Fear of panic | | | | | | |
| a) Feelings | 6 | 2 | 2 | 1 | 0 | 0 |
| b) Behaviour | 6 | 3 | 2 | 0 | 0 | 0 |
| 2. Fear walking alone | | | | | | |
| a) Feelings | 7 | 3 | 2 | 1 | 1 | 1 |
| b) Behaviour | 7 | 2 | 2 | 0 | 1 | 0 |
| Target-rating scale | | | | | | |
| 1. Walk to city centre alone | | | | | | |
| a) Feelings | 8 | 2 | 2 | 0 | 0 | 0 |
| b) Behaviour | 8 | 2 | 2 | 0 | 0 | 0 |
| 2. Travel by crowded bus alone | | | | | | |
| a) Feelings | 8 | 3 | 2 | 2 | 0 | 0 |
| b) Behaviour | 8 | 2 | 2 | 1 | 0 | 0 |
| 3. Shop in crowded stores alone | | | | | | |
| a) Feelings | 8 | 2 | 2 | 0 | 0 | 0 |
| b) Behaviour | 8 | 2 | 2 | 1 | 0 | 0 |
| 4. Take daughter to school/home alone | | | | | | |
| a) Feelings | 6 | 4 | 2 | 1 | 1 | 0 |
| b) Behaviour | 8 | 6 | 2 | 0 | 0 | 0 |

(m = months; f/u = follow up)

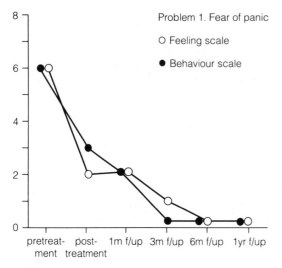

**Figure 21.7** Charlotte's problem-severity scale ratings

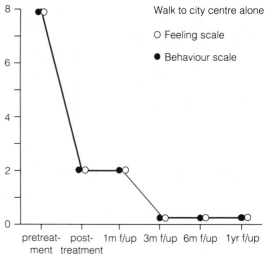

**Figure 21.9** Charlotte's target-rating scale 1.

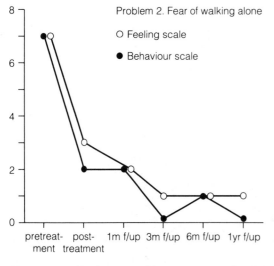

**Figure 21.8** Charlotte's problem-severity scale ratings

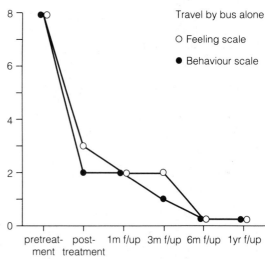

**Figure 21.10** Charlotte's target-rating scale 2.

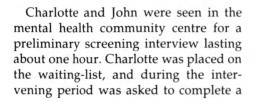

Charlotte and John were seen in the mental health community centre for a preliminary screening interview lasting about one hour. Charlotte was placed on the waiting-list, and during the intervening period was asked to complete a battery of questionnaires (Table 21.5; Figures 21.7–21.16) and to keep a daily data diary of her activities and anxiety/fear experiences. She was also asked to read a self-help manual (Marks, 1978).

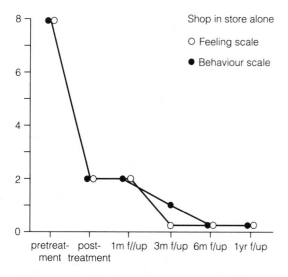

**Figure 21.11** Charlotte's target-rating scale 3.

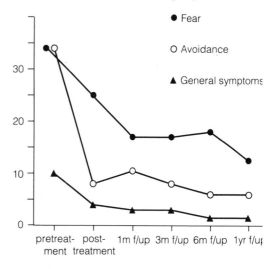

**Figure 21.13** Charlotte's modified -fear questionnaire

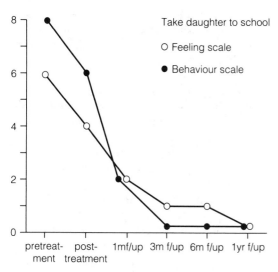

**Figure 21.12** Charlotte's target-rating scale 4.

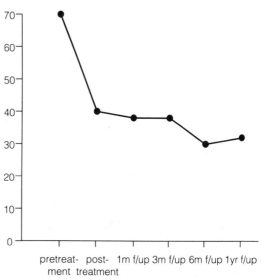

**Figure 21.14** Charlotte's agoraphobia questionnaire

## The assessment

Two one-hour interviews at the clinic over a two-week period completed the assessment. The department's standard battery of measures were completed (Table 21.5). To these were added an agoraphobic questionnaire (Burns, 1977) of 25 items rated on a 1–5 scale of fear and avoidance, and the mobility inventory for agoraphobia (Chambless *et al.*, 1985), a 26-item questionnaire that rates

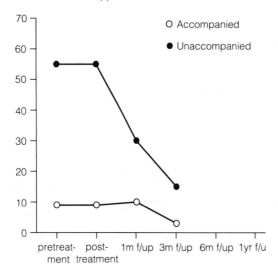

**Figure 21.15** Charlotte's mobility inventory

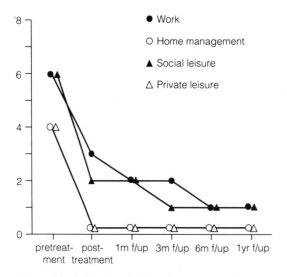

**Figure 21.16** Charlotte's life-adjustment scale

each item on a 1–5 scale of avoidance, differentiating between the client accompanied and alone.

Charlotte's description of her fear and panic experiences were examined within the three-systems context.

Although she has not experienced a panic attack for two years, Charlotte fears she will panic and lose control whenever she goes out, even locally. She feels safer when close to home, knowing she can return home or drop in on a friend. When needing to go out, her anticipation of fear and panic is vivid. She has made no attempts to travel into the city unaccompanied for two years. Although friends have offered to accompany her, she has declined, fearing they will be less effective safety signals than John.

When with John, Charlotte is able to walk into the city centre, drive or travel as a car passenger, and is able to shop in all but the most crowded stores, including queueing, providing John remains within sight. She is not free of fear, however, as she is aware of hot skin sensations, sweating, slight breathlessness, increased heart rate, 'bufferflies' in the stomach, and wobbly legs at times. Charlotte feels able to cope with this, provided John is present, but she is aware of being hypervigilant, repeatedly looking around to check John's position. When in densely crowded areas, she fears being swept apart from John, so avoids entering such situations, often seeking out his hand to hold.

Thinking is characterized by a mixture of coping phrases repeated to herself, such as, 'I'm doing OK; it's not too bad. John's just over there with the baby buggy.'; and negative, fear-inducing thoughts and images, such as, 'Oh dear, I can't manage that queue.'; 'Why is she looking at me? Everyone must think I'm mad.'; 'Where's John got to? No, this is terrible! John, where are you?' About 20% of her thoughts are negative disaster images such as fainting, being laughed at, or arrested on suspicion of shoplifting.

## The case formulation

A formulation was discussed with Charlotte and John that suggested her fears had developed as a consequence of a series of stressful life events within a 12-month period: she had become pregnant (wanted), given up her job, married, given birth to Rachel, suffered a marked drop in income, and had experienced the disruption of sleep and lifestyle a new baby brings. Premenstrual symptoms, although usually mild, were an additional stressor.

The initial fears and panics occurred when shopping alone with the baby (feeling responsible for Rachel as well as herself). Escape and later avoidance produced profound feelings of relief, which together with negative cognitive rehearsals and self-instructions (Meichenbaum, 1977) led to a strengthening of fear responses in public places and when away from a safety signal stimulus, e.g., home, husband, and friends' homes. Charlotte's fear of panic was maintained by her anticipation of its return, which was prevented from returning by her carefully structured escape and avoidance patterns.

## The treatment plan

Charlotte and John, both having read the suggested self-help manual, found the formulation made sense, but expressed concern that Charlotte would need a lot of help in facing the exposure treatment.

The nurse therapist spent an hour discussing anxiety, panic, and fear, the role of escape and avoidance in fear development, and how thinking styles can strengthen or weaken fear responses. Target descriptions for Charlotte's end-of-treatment objectives were drawn up, and a plan of treatment was devised that she and John found acceptable.

The plan was to include one session of respiratory-control training, and a hyper-ventilation-induced panic in the clinic, to be followed by breathing exercises as homework (Clark *et al.*, 1990). The nurse agreed to spend one exposure session (see below) with Charlotte, starting from her home; Charlotte and John agreed to follow a homework exposure plan following that session.

The treatment of choice for people with agoraphobia is prolonged exposure *in vivo* (Chambless *et al.*, 1982; Foa *et al.*, 1983) in sessions of two hours or more, taking place several times each week either under a therapist's direction or as homework. Exposure should take place without escape, but controlled avoidance is allowed when it prevents a disruptive panic attack in 'self-controlled exposure' (Emmelkamp, 1982). There are several ways that exposure treatment can be delivered with various adjunctive treatment methods (Deakin, 1989).

The nurse therapist decided that teaching Charlotte how to use cognitive rehearsal and cognitive self-guidance would be helpful and compatible with the present cognitive coping strategies (Meichenbaum *et al.*, 1980).

Treatment started with one session of respiratory control training, which Charlotte found helpful in defusing her fear of panic. Two days later, the nurse therapist met Charlotte at home and spent three hours in graded exposure, which involved the nurse and client walking together to the city centre and shopping throughout the pedestrianized centre, initially side by side but progressively separating, and within one hour leaving Charlotte alone while the nurse waited at an agreed rendezvous.

During exposure sessions it is usual to ask clients to give periodic ratings of the level of distress they experience on the same 0–8 scale used in assessment in order to determine fear severity. The ratings are described as subjective units of distress or disturbances (SUDs), where 8 indicates maximum distress and 0 indicates calm.

Charlotte's fear ratings initially were high (6), but rapidly fell to manageable levels (3). Practice in the crowded market, and in a range of long queues followed with time devoted to lifts in city-centre stores. To end the session, the nurse and Charlotte travelled by bus to two small suburban shopping areas, before returning to end the session over tea in Charlotte's house. By this time, Charlotte's fear ratings were 2 for walking and 3–4 for bus travel.

Coaching in cognitive rehearsal and self-talk followed, with the drafting of a homework plan to cover the next week, which required a daily walk or bus trip to the centre, with shopping to last at least one hour. Charlotte's optimism was high, and the following week she put in nine hours of unaccompanied homework practice. Two further sessions took place, with Charlotte attending the clinic unaccompanied before discharge into follow up.

Successful resolution of Charlotte's agoraphobia required three treatment sessions, following two assessment sessions and two teaching sessions. Total nurse therapist time involved 11 hours, of which three were spent in one exposure session. Charlotte's high level of motivation and strong compliance with homework instructions produced rapid treatment results; during the follow-up period, she extended her practice range, and made further gains.

Charlotte also taught herself a relaxation technique to help cope with the mild PMS symptoms. When last seen, Charlotte remained largely problem-free (one year follow-up), and was experi-

menting with dietary changes to modify her PMS. Post-treatment and follow-up results appear in Table 21.5.

## NURSING INTERVENTION FOR AN OBSESSIONAL-COMPULSIVE DISORDER

### CASE STUDY – JANINE

Janine, a 52-year-old married woman, was referred to the behaviour therapy nursing service by a consultant psychiatrist, who had been asked to see her by the family GP, and who felt a cognitive-behavioural approach was appropriate.

Janine's difficulties consisted of handicapping cleansing rituals related to a fear of contaminating others, and a series of checking rituals related to her fear of being responsible for a fire or flood in the family home. Further rituals had generalized from these involving self-doubt.

### The assessment

An assessment of five hours total occupied three sessions in the clinic and one in Janine's home. Janine described fear of dirt and germs that she felt would harm her family (husband, married daughters, grandchildren). She would wash her hands excessively following the use of the toilet (30 minutes after defaecation; 15 minutes after micturition); avoided cleaning the toilet, which her husband had to do; and spent excessive time cleaning the bath, kitchen, work surfaces, stove, waste-bins, and other rooms and household furnishings. She felt compelled to check bedlinen and laundry for 'dirt'. Cleaning and washing occupied many hours each day. On a wash day, for example, Janine spent up to five hours checking clean laundry for specks of dirt. Lowered mood would exacerbate her distress and increase the duration of her riuals.

On leaving the house and each night on retiring to bed Janine would spend between one and three hours checking the security of window and door locks, checking that water and gas taps were off, that electrical appliances and sockets were off, and that no cigarette ends could lead to a fire.

Janine's marital relationship was strained, particularly by her great need of reassurance that things were clean and the home safe. Rituals were less severe

**Table 21.6** Janine's data summary

| | Pretreatment | Post-treatment | 1m f/u | 6m f/u | 1yr f/u |
|---|---|---|---|---|---|
| Fear questionnaire | 30 | 30 | 28 | 25 | 22 |
| General symptoms | 24 | 7 | 8 | 6 | 8 |
| Beck Depression Inventory | 18 | 7 | 8 | 7 | 6 |
| Maudsley Obsessional-Compulsive Inventory | 19 | 8 | 12 | 7 | 7 |
| Obsessional-compulsive checklist | 48 | 26 | 24 | 19 | 12 |
| Life-adjustment scales | | | | | |
| 1. Work | 8 | 4 | 3 | 2 | 2 |
| 2. Home management | 6 | 2 | 2 | 3 | 2 |
| 3. Social leisure | 6 | 2 | 1 | 1 | 1 |
| 4. Private leisure | 8 | 2 | 1 | 0 | 1 |
| Target-rating scales | | | | | |
| 1. Resist checking laundry | | | | | |
| a) Feelings | 8 | 3 | 0 | 0 | 0 |
| b) Behaviour | 4 | 2 | 0 | 0 | 0 |
| 2. Resist washing hands | | | | | |
| a) Feelings | 8 | 2 | 0 | 0 | 0 |
| b) Behaviour | 8 | 0 | 0 | 0 | 0 |
| 3. Resist checking front room at night | | | | | |
| a) Feelings | 4 | 2 | 2 | 0 | 0 |
| b) Behaviour | 6 | 2 | 2 | 2 | 0 |
| 4. Resist checks leaving house | | | | | |
| a) Feelings | 3 | 0 | 0 | 0 | 0 |
| b) Behaviour | 8 | 1 | 0 | 0 | 0 |
| Obsessional-compulsive problem-rating forms | | | | | |
| 1. Checking laundry | | | | | |
| a) Discomfort | 8 | 0 | 0 | 0 | 0 |
| b) Time | 5 | 0 | 0 | 0 | 0 |
| c) Handicap | 6 | 1 | 0 | 0 | 0 |
| 2. Washing hands | | | | | |
| a) Discomfort | 8 | 1 | 0 | 0 | 0 |
| b) Time | 5 | 1 | 2 | 2 | 1 |
| c) Handicap | 8 | 2 | 2 | 1 | 1 |
| 3. Security of plugs/taps | | | | | |
| a) Discomfort | 8 | 3 | 2 | 2 | 2 |
| b) Time | 5 | 1 | 1 | 1 | 1 |
| c) Handicap | 8 | 2 | 2 | 2 | 2 |

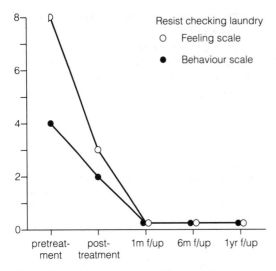

**Figure 21.17** Janine's target-rating scale 1.

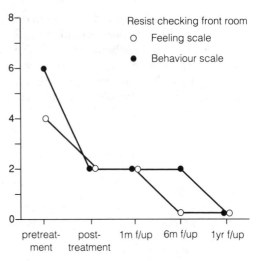

**Figure 21.19** Janine's target-rating scale 3.

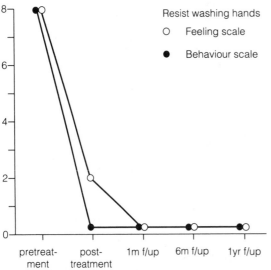

**Figure 21.18** Janine's target-rating scale 2.

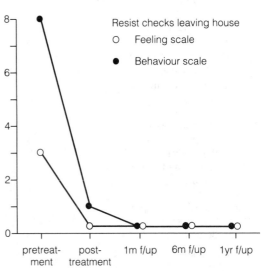

**Figure 21.20** Janine's target-rating scale 4.

when her husband was at home, but he worked long, rotating shifts in the dockyard.

Janine described her parents as meticulous, and herself as always fussy and houseproud. She recalled developing repetitive cleaning rituals at about 20 years old when her oldest daughter, now 32, was born; these had progressively worsened as the years had passed.

The department's standard battery of questionnaires were completed, including the life-history questionnaire, fear questionnaire, and Beck Depression Inventory. In addition, Janine completed a Maudsley Obsessional-Compulsive

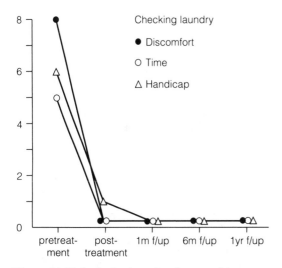

**Figure 21.21** Janine's obsessional-compulsive disorder rating scales 1.

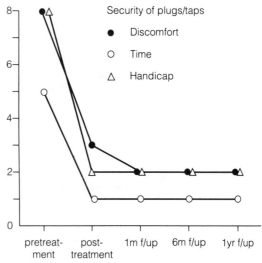

**Figure 21.23** Janine's obsessional-compulsive disorder rating scales 3.

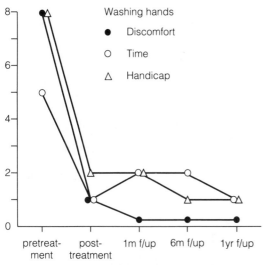

**Figure 21.22** Janine's obsessional-compulsive disorder rating scales 2.

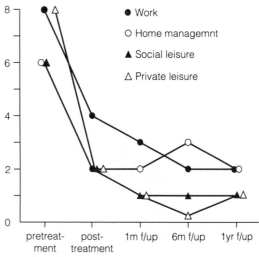

**Figure 21.24** Janine's obsessional-compulsive disorder rating scales 4.

Inventory (Rachman *et al.*, 1980), an obsessional-compulsive checklist (Marks, 1986), and separate problem-rating forms rating rituals on 0–8 scales of 'Discomfort', 'Time', and 'Handicap' (Marks, 1986), in addition to life-adjustment ratings, and outcome target with ratings (Table 21.6; Figures 21.17–21.28).

A three-systems analysis of Janine's emotional reactions showed that in addition to her rituals and avoidance behaviours she had distressing anxiety symptoms including marked muscle tension in arms, legs, abdomen, neck and shoulders, frequent headaches, shallow rapid breathing, and a persistent feeling

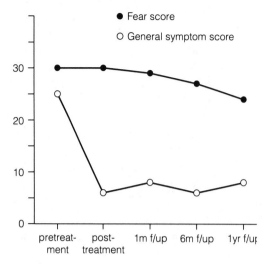

Figure 21.25 Janine's fear questionnaire

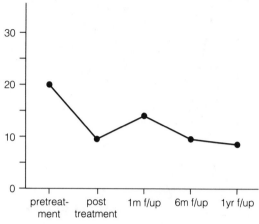

**Figure 21.27** Janine's Maudsley obsessional - compulsive inventory

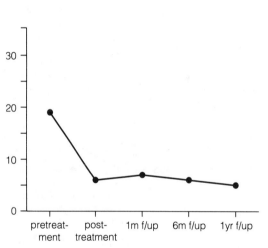

**Figure 21.26** Janine's Beck depression inventory

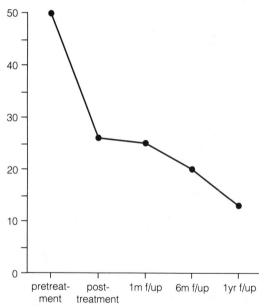

**Figure 21.28** Janine's obsessional compulsive checklist

of shakiness. Her thinking was full of negative self-evaluations and irrational patterns, for example, labelling ('I'm silly, stupid, dirty'); moralistic should's and must's ('I must not pass on dirt', 'Everything should be clean'); dichotomous thoughts ('If the house is not clean, I'm useless').

**The case formulation**

Conducting a behavioural analysis led to a formulation which the nurse discussed with Janine. It appeared that Janine's meticulous parents had been inappropriate role models, leading her to adopt excessively high personal standards of hygiene and cleanliness; her marriage and homemaking led to this being reinforced by approving husband and parents. Fears of contamination developed with the birth of her first child, negatively reinforcing further rituals over cleanliness. At about the same time, fears for the family safety led to security checks that gradually worsened over many years.

Only when Janine was in full-time employment were her obsessional problems under control, in that far less time was available for her to indulge in them. Since giving up her job, for the last five years they had returned to occupy the available time. Fears for her regularly visiting grandchildren also fuelled the need to continue to decontaminate.

It was explained to Janine that much of her thinking was self-derogatory, and that this had reduced her self-confidence and self-esteem, enabling her to slip into regular periods of mild to moderate depression that exacerbated the obsessional difficulties.

### The treatment plan

Janine was willing to accept treatment, and, like many people with obsessional difficulties, followed the nurse's instructions to the letter and kept meticulously detailed data diaries. The treatment plan that was proposed and accepted had four main components: first, relaxation training, with a modified and abbreviated version of Jacobsen's (1938) method as a means of managing anxiety; second, response-prevention methods to curtail checking behaviours for dirt and security, and to limit cleaning and hand-washing; third, exposure to contamination fears by purposeful contamination with traces of human, bird, and dog faeces on the house, its furnishings, and

all linen; fourth, Michael (her husband) agreed grudgingly to act as a co-therapist under the nurse's direction to monitor achievements, refuse requests for re-assurance, and support Janine with reinforcing feedback. In addition, Janine was asked to explore means of rescheduling her daily activities so that time freed from obsessional rituals could be used for other purposes.

The first three treatment sessions, each of one-and-one-half hours, took place in the client's home, with the husband present to be coached in the exposure and response-prevention methods with his wife.

Janine's initial reluctance to contaminate her surroundings weakened as she, the nurse, and Michael covered more and more of the house with faecal material, which was collected daily from the toilet and nearby park. Contamination involved touching the faecal material with a wooden spatula, and then touching the widest array of household items and each other with the spatula. No visible contaminant was apparent; Janine, however, felt as contaminated as if there had been a visible smear.

Janine's distress increased and then subsided over two to three hours in the first few treatment days as she followed the nurse's instructions not to do any cleaning of the house for one week, when it would be recontaminated, and no washing except immediately before the preparation of food. Cutlery and kitchen work-surfaces were contaminated along with everything else twice each day as homework. Distress levels rapidly decreased, and Janine and Michael started to do more socially as a way of using free time. This gradually brought them closer, particularly as Janine's frequent requests for reassurance that all was safe and well diminished over the next six to eight weeks.

After six weeks' exposure and response-prevention to dirt and germs, Janine carried out a similar response-prevention programme for security and safety on leaving the house and when retiring to bed. With Michael's assistance she had to leave the house repeatedly with a brief visual check of appliances, windows, and doors (maximum time allowed, five minutes), and repeat this each evening on retiring to bed, with the added refinement that various electrical appliances had to be left plugged in with the socket switch on.

## Conclusion

Treatment for Janine occupied a total of 17 sessions and 19 hours of the nurse's time over a period of four months. Major improvements occurred that had been maintained up to the one-year follow-up point. Janine was aware, however, that she was daily needing to recognize her limitations and view herself in some respects like a diabetic who requires a daily insulin dose to remain well. Each day she needed to ensure that things were left uncleaned and unchecked, and that every few days she needed to purposely contaminate herself, Michael and/or part of the house to maintain her gains and confidence. Table 21.6 shows outcome measures.

## NURSING INTERVENTIONS FOR INTERPERSONAL DIFFICULTIES

### CASE STUDY – SOCIAL ANXIETY AND SOCIAL-SKILLS DEFICIT

After seeing a television documentary on assertion skills, Bruce, a 37-year-old married man with two children aged 10 and 8, sought help for his lifelong social anxiety via his GP. He recognized that although he possessed a range of appropriate social skills, some, particularly those related to the expression of positive and negative feelings, were weak. Bruce never really felt comfortable in groups of people, either socially or at work, and at times his fear caused him to leave social situations early, and to avoid those he felt he would not be able to tolerate.

### The assessment

Assessment took place over a three-week period in two clinic-based interviews lasting two-and-one-half hours. Within a three-systems analysis of emotion, Bruce's fear responses showed the pattern usual for a socially phobic person, with physical symptoms of blushing, rapid heart rate, sweating, and a shaky sensation in his hands, arms, and legs. His thinking when anticipating a social encounter was uniformly negative, with images of social failure and humiliation. When in a social situation, strong urges to leave would surface as more people arrived or paid Bruce any attention. He would compare himself negatively with others, worry about having nothing to say, and imagine that others could see his fear and also would evaluate him in a negative manner.

Susan and Bruce had grown up in the same small city suburb, had known each other since early childhood, went to the same school, and even worked in the same insurance company offices. Their marriage was happy, but Susan did miss a more active social life, as she felt they were getting very much into a rut as 'homebirds'.

In addition to the department's standard battery of questionnaires and rating-scale measures were added a Rathus Assertion Scale, confirming Bruce's low level of self-assertion, and a social anxiety scale of 53 items rated on a 0–8 scale of fear and avoidance, which showed that a wide range of situations evoked unease and anxiety, while others produced fear with escape or avoidance.

## The case formulation

Bruce participated fully in drawing together his own case formulation with his nurse therapist. A shy and embarrassed child, he had avoided the limelight, staying with his own small group of friends. He had little interest in competitive sports or girls and parties until his late teens, when it seemed only natural to pair off with the shy girl who lived in the next street. Bruce had no difficulty expressing emotion with Susan, providing no audience was involved, and their relationship remained close and sensitive. Early shyness and embarrassment restricted Bruce from participating in the social life of adolescence, which is for most of us a rich learning environment for the development of a wide range of social skills, social confidence, and self-esteem. Low-practice frequency, together with avoidance contributed to the development of a wide range of social anxieties, confirmed for him by his self-critical negative evaluations of himself.

## The treatment plan

Bruce agreed to a treatment plan with four elements: firstly, he was to purchase and read two self-help manuals on assertion (Smith, 1975; Fensterheim *et al.*, 1975). Another therapist was due to start a time-limited series of social skills training groups one evening each week

Table 21.7 Bruce's data summary

| | Pretreatment | Post-treatment | 1m f/u | 6m f/u | 1yr f/u |
|---|---|---|---|---|---|
| Fear questionnaire | 52 | 24 | 20 | 12 | 15 |
| General symptoms | 5 | 2 | 3 | 2 | 2 |
| Beck Depression Inventory | 18 | 10 | 8 | 6 | 6 |
| Rathus Assertiveness Scale | −16 | 0 | +4 | +4 | +10 |
| Social-anxiety scale | 178 | 102 | 80 | 42 | 40 |
| Life-adjustment scales | | | | | |
| 1. Work | 6 | 3 | 2 | 2 | 2 |
| 2. Home management | 3 | 2 | 0 | 0 | 0 |
| 3. Social leisure | 7 | 3 | 2 | 1 | 1 |
| 4. Private leisure | 3 | 2 | 2 | 0 | 1 |
| Problem-rating scales | | | | | |
| 1. Social anxiety | | | | | |
| a) Feelings | 7 | 3 | 3 | 1 | 1 |
| b) Behaviour | 6 | 2 | 2 | 0 | 0 |
| Target-rating scales | | | | | |
| 1. Hold conversation with 4 people for 30 mins | | | | | |
| a) Feelings | 7 | 3 | 3 | 2 | 1 |
| b) Behaviour | 8 | 2 | 3 | 0 | 0 |
| 2. Attend busy party with wife for 3 hours | | | | | |
| a) Feelings | 8 | 2 | 2 | 0 | 0 |
| b) Behaviour | 8 | 2 | 2 | 0 | 0 |

over an eight-week period, and a place was reserved for Bruce. In addition, the nurse offered individual sessions on a fortnightly basis to coach him in cognitive strategies and to monitor a homework programme of re-socialization and exposure to socially threatening environments.

Treatment covered a 14-week period. The group operated along lines similar to a personal effectiveness group (Liberman *et al.*, 1975) and provided both exposure opportunities as well as didactic teaching and social skill role-play practice, with group feedback and reinforcement of progress. The reading focused on assertiveness skills and goal-setting, with problem-solving strategies that Bruce was able to utilize both in the group setting and homework practice. The individual sessions led to a tailored homework programme, which encouraged graded exposure to a wide range of social situations. Individual coaching in cognitive self-guidance strategies led to further

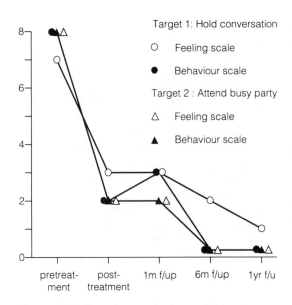

Figure 21.30 Bruce's target-rating scales

behavioural experiments wherein Bruce could test and disprove his negative cognitive thinking styles and negative evaluations, replacing them with more positive and appropriate evaluations (Beck *et al.*, 1985).

The treatment programme ended at Christmas, which proved fortuitous as work parties and many social events provided Bruce with many exposure and practice opportunities, enabling major reductions in social fear, and giving him frequent practice in social interaction, which improved his social skills and self-confidence. Bruce and Susan described this as their busiest and most enjoyable Christmas ever, and many new friendships were established.

### Conclusion

In all, seven individual sessions and eight group sessions – totalling eight and twelve hours, respectively – were used, with a major improvement in the client's social-fears skills and confidence. These

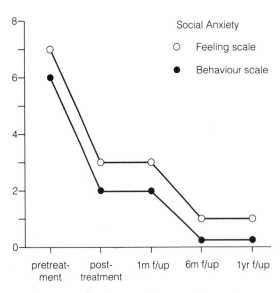

Figure 21.29 Bruce's problem-severity scale ratings

were maintained at one year follow-up (Table 21.7; Figures 21.29, 21.30).

## CASE STUDY – MARITAL AND SEXUAL DYSFUNCTIONS

Ian, a 24-year-old man, was referred to the behaviour therapy nursing service by his GP with a three-year history of difficulty in gaining and maintaining an erection during sexual intercourse. His current sexual partner, Lisa, had lived with Ian for 18 months, and had discussed sexual therapy with him several times during their relationship.

A preliminary screening appointment with Ian outlined that optimal results would best be achieved if his partner would attend sessions jointly with him, to which Lisa readily agreed. Ian and Lisa attended two assessment sessions of three-hours duration, over a two-week period. They were seen by one male nurse therapist, who interviewed them together and individually.

### The assessment

The assessment revealed that Ian's erectile difficulties had developed over a two-month period three years earlier when his worries about sexual performance with a regular girlfriend had led to self-consciousness during sexual intercourse, accompanied by negative evaluative thinking ('I'm not satisfying her'; 'I'm useless at this'). Negative self-fulfilling prophecies occurred frequently ('It's all going to fail; I can't keep this going') and a high frequency of must/ should thinking added to his stress ('I should be able to satisfy her'; I must keep this erection – she'll storm out if I lose it again').

Ian's sexual confidence had never been high since his first intercourse with a regular girlfriend at the age of 18. Apart

**Table 21.8** Ian's data summary

|  | Pretreatment | Post-treatment | 1m f/u | 3m f/u | 6m f/u |
|---|---|---|---|---|---|
| Fear questionnaire | 12 | 8 | 8 | 6 | 8 |
| General symptoms | 5 | 3 | 0 | 0 | 0 |
| Beck Depression Inventory | 15 | 10 | 6 | 4 | 4 |
| Life-adjustment scales |  |  |  |  |  |
| 1. Work | 1 | 0 | 0 | 0 | 0 |
| 2. Home management | 3 | 0 | 0 | 0 | 0 |
| 3. Social leisure | 3 | 0 | 0 | 0 | 0 |
| 4. Private leisure | 1 | 0 | 0 | 0 | 0 |
| Problem-rating scale |  |  |  |  |  |
| 1. Difficulty maintaining erection during vaginal intercourse |  |  |  |  |  |
| a) Feelings | 6 | 2 | 1 | 0 | 0 |
| b) Behaviour | 8 | 0 | 0 | 0 | 0 |
| Target-rating scale |  |  |  |  |  |
| 1. Gain and maintain erect penis during intravaginal intercourse |  |  |  |  |  |
| a) Feelings | 6 | 2 | 1 | 0 | 0 |
| b) Behaviour | 8 | 0 | 0 | 0 | 0 |

from occasional episodes of premature ejaculation within seconds of commencing vaginal intercourse, Ian had not previously experienced erectile difficulties. Questioning revealed that for several weeks before the onset of his erectile difficulties, Ian had been having a stressful time at work in his job as a salesman, and felt the relationship with the then girlfriend was fading.

Lisa was the first woman Ian had lived with, and was the longest lasting of all his emotional and sexual attachments. Although Ian's erectile difficulties frustrated him, they continued an active sex life, with mutually enjoyable masturbation and oral sex three or four evenings a week. No erectile difficulties occurred during mutual masturbation or oral sex – only during attempts at vaginal intercourse. Lisa was relaxed with sexual relationships, enjoyed intercourse, and usually experienced an orgasm with manual or intravaginal stimulation. She wanted to establish a long-term relationship with Ian, and wanted them to be able to have full sexual intercourse.

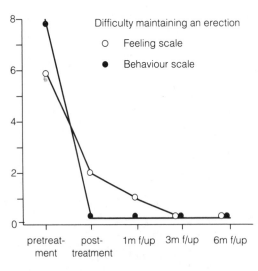

**Figure 21.31** Ian's problem severity scale ratings

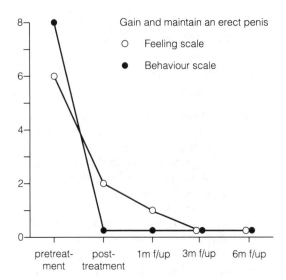

**Figure 21.32** Ian's target-rating scales

Ian completed the department's standard battery of assessment measures, and in addition completed a series of measures specific to his sexual difficulties. Lisa was asked to complete these as well, in order to identify any factors concerning her own sexuality that might need addressing. These measures included a questionnaire on sexual attitudes, based on a semantic differential examining six concepts, and a sexual-activity rating form examining activity, frequency, pleasure, and distress. Treatment targets were negotiated and rated (Table 21.8; Figures 21.31, 21.32).

As a means of monitoring sexual activity and the effects of the treatment programme, Ian and Lisa were asked to complete a standard daily diary of their sexual life, and to bring these to each treatment session.

### The case formulation

At the end of assessment, a case formulation was discussed with Ian, and shared with Lisa, which highlighted how Ian's performance anxiety had led to a distancing of himself from sex with Lisa. The role of his cognitions in both anticipating failure – producing self-fulfilling prophecies – and criticizing his own performance was discussed in relation to the autonomic arousal this produced, and its functional result in loss of erection when vaginal intercourse was attempted. Ian and Lisa were able to understand this description, found it matched their experience together, and discussed possible solutions with the therapist.

## The treatment plan

At the end of assessent, the nurse asked the couple to agree to a temporary ban on all attempts to engage in sexual activity while the treatment plan was implemented. A programme based on Masters and Johnsons (1970) model of sex therapy was described and accepted. This involved a series of clinic-based sessions, in which ongoing education would be carried out with psychotherapeutic problem-solving and communication enhancement, based on the results of a prescribed homework programme. The homework programme would require Ian and Lisa to set aside three evenings each week, during which they would use sensate-focus exercises for exploration, mutual pleasuring by touch and massage, arousal enhancement, and anxiety reduction (Hawton, 1985; Deakin, 1987). In addition, Ian was asked to purchase and read a particularly useful self-help manual on male sexuality (Zilbergeld, 1978) and to let Lisa read and discuss this with him.

Ian and Lisa agreed to the programme, and to attend the clinic every two weeks. They expressed doubts about the ban on sex, but accepted the rationale after further discussion.

Over the next two months, Ian and Lisa attended the clinic for eight treat-ment sessions while continuing their homework programme as requested.

The sensate-focus programme follows six stages, beginning with sessions of touch without genital contact, with each partner caressing and gently stroking and massaging the other – avoiding breasts and genitals – for 15–20 minutes each. The aim is to maximize sensory awareness, involvement, and pleasure, while improving verbal and non-verbal communication. The effect is to increase arousal and reduce anxiety, thereby facilitating new learning, and the unlearning of unhelpful anxiety performance and self-conscious responses. The ban on intercourse is a means of building trust, and, particularly, of preventing failure.

Ian and Lisa progressed rapidly through the first three sensate-focus stages. At week four, the fourth stage, they continued the touch-and-caressing process simultaneously and together with genital contact. Of particular importance was for Ian to gain, purposely lose, and then gain his erection again as a confidence-building exercise.

The sexual ban continued until stage five, which was reached by week six. At this point the couple were allowed to insert Ian's erect penis into Lisa's vagina, but with no movement and no attempt at ejaculation. Again, practice focused on gaining, losing, and regaining Ian's erection, both with his penis inside and outside Lisa's vagina. Communication improvements paralleling the physical exercises enabled these homework sessions to be fun, with much ribaldry and shared laughter.

The nurse now felt progress was sufficient to move on to the final stage, allowing vaginal intercourse with movement to ejaculation, which followed without any difficulty. Ian was now able to maintain his erection during active penile thrusting for up to 10 minutes, pleasuring both himself and Lisa with no sense of anxiety or self-consciousness. Lisa was pleased to report achieving orgasm on two out of three episodes of intravaginal intercourse.

## Conclusion

At the eighth session, ratings and questionnaire measures were repeated (Table 21.8; Figure 21.31). The couple were asked to continue elements of the sensate-focus programme into the follow-up phase to reinforce their mutual gains. One month later, the couple were discharged and seen subsequently for follow-up at one month, three months, and six months. Telephone follow-up at one year showed all their gains maintained, and a marriage planned for the following spring. The clinical programme required 15 hours of the nurse's clinic time, over a total period of three months.

CASE STUDY – UNCONVENTIONAL SEXUAL BEHAVIOUR

Alec, a 29-year-old man, married for three years to Sharon, 30, sought help through the Psychiatric Advisory Service (PAS) (the District's crisis intervention service) on the advice of his solicitor. He had been arrested and charged one week previously when the police staked-out a local park following complaints from several young women that a man had been seen exposing himself from a parked car. The local magistrates court fined Alec, and placed him on one-year's probation, with a recommendation that he seek psychiatric help. The community psychiatric nurse and social worker who interviewed him for the PAS found him to be only mildly depressed, and referred him to the behaviour therapy nursing service for assessment.

## The assessment

Alec attended a preliminary screening appointment with his wife two weeks later at an outpatient clinic. He presented as a smartly dressed man, who appeared anxious and distressed. Sharon, his wife, showed him warm support, but expressed distress and confusion about what appeared to her to be most untypical behaviour. Alec was interviewed alone by a nurse therapist for one hour, Sharon for 30 minutes, and then the couple were seen together for a further 30 minutes. The nurse decided to take Alec straight on to his caseload, and arranged two further assessment sessions involving both partners over the next two weeks. Assessment required a total of seven hours.

Alec's probation officer requested a report, but having worked with the department previously he was content for the nurse therapist to manage treatment without any direct involvement beyond periodic updates on progress.

Alec described how for the last 18 months he had felt an increasingly strong urge to expose himself to young attractive women while masturbating, which he had done on at least 12 occasions, usually at the end of his working day while driving home. Two venues were used, both local parks near housing estates where buses dropped passengers off.

Alec worked as a clerk in a firm of accountants, who knew nothing of his court appearance, and Sharon worked for a small estate agency as a typist. They had no children, but had plans to start a family when mortgage interest rates enabled Sharon to leave her job.

On exploring Alec's psychosexual history, he described how from the age of 15 to 18 he had infrequently exposed himself to young women in parks in another town. Then, as now, he would expose himself with an erect penis, and masturbate to ejaculation before rapidly leaving the scene. When exposing himself, Alec sought a look of shock or horror from his witnesses, but described how he half hoped they would be impressed. He had never been apprehended, and ceased that form of sexual exhibitionism when he established his first long-term sexual relationship with an older woman at the age of 18.

He described himself as a shy young man, who had only gained self-confidence slowly in his late teens and early 20's when he found himself to be attractive to women. He reported having seven medium-to-long-term sexual relationships between the age of 18 and 25, when he met Sharon. They had married within a year of meeting, and led a happy but conventional life together, which Alec felt had lost some of its original sexual sparkle. In the last 12 months sexual intercourse had dropped to about once a month, usually at a weekend after an evening out. They had not discussed this, and gradually Alec had found his old urges re-emerging.

At the time of assessment, Alec was mildly depressed, frequently felt anxious in case his employers or neighbours found out, and experienced strong guilt feelings. He no longer felt any urges to expose himself, but was beginning to feel sexually frustrated. Sharon reported they had not had sex for at least six weeks. She too felt that sex had become stale and predictable, not meeting her needs either, over at least the past year. Both Alec and Sharon reported they masturbated privately, at approximately twice-weekly intervals, without knowing the other part-

**Table 21.9** Alec's data summary

|  | Pretreatment | Post-treatment | 3m f/u | 6m f/u | 1yr f/u |
|---|---|---|---|---|---|
| Fear questionnaire | 20 | 12 | 6 | 6 | 6 |
| General symptoms | 8 | 6 | 3 | 0 | 0 |
| Beck Depression Inventory | 20 | 15 | 8 | 6 | 6 |
| Rathus Assertiveness Scale | −8 | −2 | +6 | +6 | +4 |
| Life-adjustment scales |  |  |  |  |  |
| 1. Work | 6 | 2 | 0 | 0 | 0 |
| 2. Home management | 5 | 1 | 0 | 0 | 0 |
| 3. Social leisure | 8 | 3 | 2 | 0 | 0 |
| 4. Private leisure | 4 | 2 | 0 | 0 | 0 |
| Problem-rating scale |  |  |  |  |  |
| 1. Exhibitionism |  |  |  |  |  |
| a) Feelings | 6 | 2 | 0 | 0 | 0 |
| b) Behaviour | 0 | 0 | 0 | 0 | 0 |
| Target-rating scales |  |  |  |  |  |
| 1. Control, or eliminate, urges to expose |  |  |  |  |  |
| a) Feelings | 4 | 2 | 0 | 0 | 0 |
| b) Behaviour | 0 | 0 | 0 | 0 | 0 |
| 2. Enjoy mutually active sex life with partner |  |  |  |  |  |
| a) Feelings | 7 | 2 | 0 | 0 | 0 |
| b) Behaviour | 8 | 2 | 0 | 0 | 0 |

ner was doing so. Alec's solitary masturbation usually involved fantasies that
recalled his exhibitionist episodes, further
increasing both his worries about doing it
again, and strengthening his guilt feelings.

Sexual and emotional communication
was lacking, but both partners strongly
wished to change this and re-establish

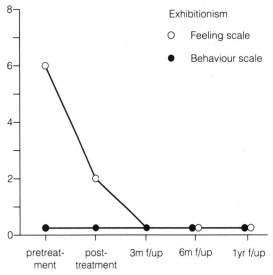

**Figure 21.33** Alec's problem-severity scale ratings

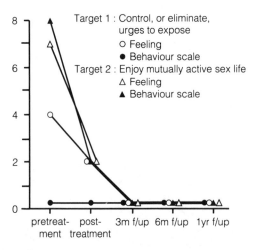

**Figure 21.34** Alec's target-rating scales

the active and enjoyable sex life they had
enjoyed previously.

After completing the department's
standard battery of assessment measures,
Alec completed sexual attitude scales
and a rating of unconventional sexual
behaviour (Table 21.9; Figures 21.33,
21.34). Alec and Sharon completed problem and target description forms for their
shared lowering of conventional sexual
interest. Sexual diaries were started.

### The case formulation

The nurse therapist analyzed the data
results in conjunction with the psychosexual histories of both partners, and
shared his formulation with them. Generally, the poor sexual communication
skills and sensitivities about sex and
sexuality they shared had led to a gradual but profound reduction in their sexual activity and mutual pleasure when
both of them had been leading busy
working lives. Their shared social life
had similarly diminished during the
same period. It was striking that neither
partner knew what the other partner
liked or wanted in a sexual encounter,
nor what either disliked. Their sex life
had gradually moved towards the lowest
common denominator, and was infrequent, brief, and unexciting.

This had led to increased solitary masturbation by Alec, to fantasies embedded
in his exhibitionist sexual past, providing
a reinforcement by orgasm, which the
nurse hypothesized had produced a re-
awakening of urges to expose himself.
Actual episodes of genital exposure were
further reinforced by orgasm, the
witness' look of shock or disgust and by
a sense of risk. The hypothesis outlined
in the formulation was accepted by both
Alec and Sharon, and was actively discussed with the nurse therapist as to how
they could eliminate Alec's unwanted

conventional urges and re-establish an active sex life together.

## The treatment plan

With the couple's high motivation for change, planning an intervention programme proved a speedy process. Both Alec and Sharon recognized a need to improve their knowledge of each other and to enhance their skill in their communication of emotional and sexual feelings. They agreed to start 'dating' each other several times each week so they could re-establish a social life. With the nurse's guidance, they agreed to the introduction of a regular programme of sexual experimentation into their evenings and weekend mornings together, which would utilize ideas from sensate focus, the sharing of fantasies and story-lines from books and erotic magazines, and experimentation on chapters from various books (Comfort, 1987 a,b).

Though this would be largely their own programme, the nurse therapist suggested they use their sessions with him as neutral ground to feedback their feelings, successes, and failures in order to ensure that neither partner felt pressured into activity they might dislike, or that might produce feelings that could prove harmful to the relationship.

In addition, Alec agreed to follow an individual programme of masturbatory retraining, based on establishing an appropriate sexual fantasy life, and to follow a programme of covert sensitization in order to reduce the probability of responding to exhibitionist urges (covert sensitization [Cautela, 1976] is a method that pairs in imagination a previously desired sequence of behaviour with a new series of unpleasant consequences).

The couple's joint programme took place over the following 14 weeks. They met with their nurse therapist once a fortnight to discuss the constructional programme, in order to enhance their communication and mutual sex lives. This showed a rapid and sustained improvement, expanding their sexual repertoire, and re-injecting a sense of fun and pleasure.

Alec met with the nurse therapist alone once a fortnight for six sessions to be coached in and monitored for his masturbatory and covert sensitization programmes. This progressed smoothly after some initial difficulties imagining negative consequences. For example, Alec was requested to set aside two 20-minute periods a day to imagine, in as vivid detail as possible, the sequence of activities that led to exposure. At the point of imagining himself exposing his penis, he was to immediately switch to an unpleasant set of imagery from a jointly prepared list.

By week 14 Alec reported no further interest in exhibitionism, either as fantasy or potential reality. Both Sharon and Alec reported a good-quality, enjoyable social and sex life. Sexual activity was occurring on average four times each week. This involved mutual masturbation, oral sex, and penetrative vaginal intercourse in a variety of positions and in a variety of places.

## Conclusion

At this point Alec was discharged into follow-up. Alec and Sharon were subsequently seen up to two years in follow-up, during which time sex remained frequent and enjoyable. No further unconventional incidents were reported, but as Sharon was now pregnant, they were advised to contact their nurse therapist should this lead to any re-occurrence of unconventional urges. The treatment programme involved a total of 13 sessions (7 jointly), and 21 hours of therapist clinical time.

CASE STUDY – COMPULSIVE GAMBLING

Graham, a 20-year-old inshore fisherman was referred for assessment by his probation officer, who reported that one year previously Graham had been fined for the theft of a motorcycle, which he had subsequently sold. Three months previously Graham had been fined and placed on probation for theft from a residential house and a lock-up shop. On both occasions he had taken money and easily saleable electrical equipment. Although it had not been evident at the time of his social enquiry report, Graham had revealed to the probation officer a long-standing problem with fruit-machine gambling, which was still a major difficulty, and had been instrumental in leading to the thefts in order to finance his gambling.

**The assessment**

Graham was seen for assessment in the outpatient facilities of a community mental health centre on three occasions over a two-week period. This involved four hours of interviews, and a one-hour period of observation in an amusement arcade and several public houses, using money provided by the nurse for assessment purposes. Although initially reluctant to discuss his gambling in any detail, Graham became more forthcoming when it was clear the nurse therapist was familiar with compulsive gambling, and was not adopting a judgmental stance.

Interviewing revealed that Graham had gambled on fruit-machines regularly since the age of 14. At first he played machines in amusement arcades, but from the age of 17 played them in pubs and clubs more often. He recalled many early wins, which supplemented his earnings on a newspaper round, but felt his luck had become fickle and unreliable over time. For the last three years, most of his

wages were spent on gambling machines. Living at home with his parents and younger sister, he owed the family several hundred pounds in unpaid lodgings and loans. He had received ultimatums on several occasions that if he did not mend his ways he would be thrown out of the family home.

After leaving school at 16, Graham had gone to sea as a deckhand on a local fishing boat. He liked the work, and was appreciated as a crew member. His skipper was aware of Graham's record, and had made it plain that he would lose his job if any future charges were brought. Neither his family or crewmates were aware of his compulsive gambling.

Graham was in many ways a loner, with few friends outside the fishing business. He was socially anxious, but apparently had good social skills. He had a regular girlfriend, Wendy, the same age as he, who he had known from his schooldays. She was the daughter of a local fisherman. Wendy knew of Graham's problem, and had said she wanted to help him in any way she could. Their social life was very limited due to lack of money, but appeared close. Wendy attended the third assessment session with Graham, and clearly was a more assertive individual. What money Wendy earned as a cashier in a local supermarket she saved; she had not, and would not, lend him any money.

Graham had no bank account or credit cards. He was paid weekly in cash. At the time of his assessment, Graham had not gambled for six weeks, due to lack of money. His pay was now given directly to Wendy at the end of the week, who passed most of it on to his parents, keeping the rest in the bank, out of which she gave Graham a daily allowance for cigarettes and food. The relationship with Wendy, and her no-nonsense handling of Graham and his money, was a major advantage from the outset of treatment.

Urges to gamble were present frequently when Graham was ashore, and were strongest when in a local pub or club. He described being drawn to the flashing lights and sounds of the fruit-machines, closely watching others play. When playing, he described a high level of excitement, a feeling of strength and optimism, and a lack of awareness of things around him or the passage of time. On such occasions he would play the machines until his money ran out or until closing time. Graham's gambling was compulsive and uncontrolled. He attempted to chase his losses, and if he could, he would borrow or steal money to continue playing. Over one weekend he spent £300 on the fruit-machines. He seemed to have little or no idea of the expected probabilities of winning. No other form of gambling appealed to him.

## The case formulation

With Graham's agreement, Wendy sat in on the nurse therapist's discussion of the case formulation. The nurse described the process by which variable ratio schedules of reinforcement – as operate in fruit machines – can produce the rapid learning of compulsive behaviour, particularly when individuals have early experiences of winning as Graham had. This, coupled with Graham's social anxiety and loner temperament, helped give him, at least temporarily, a sense of strength, of being in control, and of confidence. The consequences of playing and winning were immediate and perceived as positive, while the consequences of losing were delayed and attributed to bad luck; tomorrow would show a change for the better, and provide opportunities for big wins to recoup the losses.

Although Wendy felt this formulation was accurate, Graham was reluctant to accept it on face value as he felt that fruit-machines did require skill. As Dickerson (1984) highlights, treatment for compulsive gambling is far from straightforward; the nurse therapist therefore made it clear to Graham that with his history, he was only prepared to work with Graham towards complete abstinence. The risks of lying, distrust, and further episodes of theft, and the consequences to Graham personally, occupationally, and criminally were discussed, together with the effects on his family relationships, and any future development of his relationship with Wendy. Graham agreed to proceed with a programme of treatment, and Wendy agreed to attend clinic appointments with him and to act as a co-therapist in monitoring homework exercises.

## The treatment plan

A treatment programme based on cue avoidance, followed by cue exposure (Dickerson, 1984) and covert sensitization (Cautela, 1976) was described. Graham would continue to avoid any form of gambling and any gambling environment for several more weeks. During this time he would be taught how to use covert sensitization, a self-control technique using imagined aversion images as a means of, first, progressively weakening his compulsive urges to gamble, and, second, providing himself with a self-control technique when confronting the fruit-machines. Graham and Wendy agreed to develop a plan to establish an appropriate social and recreational life, in order to replace the many hours Graham had previously spent gambling. They further agreed to let Wendy control all his income, and, by negotiation, dispensing it to pay his ongoing living expenses, and to start paying his debts.

The treatment programme was rapid, occupying ten clinic sessions and two community sessions over a 12-week period. During the first month, Graham spent four sessions learning how to develop and utilize vivid fantasy images of himself attempting to play fruit-machines, but with a mixture of realistic and fantastic, but nevertheless distressing, imagined consequences occurring, instead of the pleasurable ones he associated with playing. As homework he had to use these covert sensitization exercises for three thirty-minute practice sessions each day. With only minor difficulties, and Wendy's prompting, he complied, and was able to maintain his avoidance of gambling machines and their usual venues.

There followed two *in vivo* clinical sessions where the nurse therapist accompanied Graham on an extensive trip around the local pubs, clubs, and amusement arcades he had used for fruit-machine gambling. Wendy joined one of these sessions. With money in his pocket, Graham had to enter each venue, initially with the therapist by his side, and sit with a drink and newspaper, alternating his attention between the machines and other activities. As urges to gamble arose, he was coached in cognitive self-guidance tactics, distraction methods, and asked to use the covert sensitization technique in the real-life environment. At each venue the therapist progressively withdrew, as Graham's confidence in resisting urges improved. Thereafter, as a homework programme, Graham alone and with Wendy re-exposed himself to the wide range of gambling venues without the therapist. Weekly clinic sessions monitored progress and troubleshot the small number of slips that occurred.

## Conclusion

After six weeks of re-exposure with no reported slips, Graham was discharged into close follow-up, with instructions to

**Table 21.10** Graham's data summary

|  | Pretreatment | Post-treatment | 3m f/u | 6m f/u | 1yr f/u | 18m f/u |
|---|---|---|---|---|---|---|
| Beck Depression Inventory | 20 | 14 | 16 | 10 | 10 | 8 |
| Thyer Anxiety Scale | 23 | 20 | 19 | 14 | 8 | 9 |
| Life-adjustment scale |  |  |  |  |  |  |
| 1. Work | 3 | 1 | 0 | 0 | 0 | 0 |
| 2. Home management | 4 | 4 | 2 | 0 | 0 | 0 |
| 3. Social leisure | 7 | 5 | 4 | 2 | 1 | 1 |
| 4. Private leisure | 7 | 5 | 4 | 1 | 1 | 0 |
| Problem-severity scale |  |  |  |  |  |  |
| 1. Compulsive gambling |  |  |  |  |  |  |
|    a) Feelings | 8 | 6 | 6 | 3 | 3 | 2 |
|    b) Behaviour | 8 | 6 | 5 | 1 | 0 | 1 |
| Target-rating scale |  |  |  |  |  |  |
| 1. To resist the urge to play |  |  |  |  |  |  |
|    a) Feelings | 8 | 4 | 4 | 2 | 2 | 0 |
|    b) Behaviour | 8 | 2 | 3 | 1 | 0 | 1 |

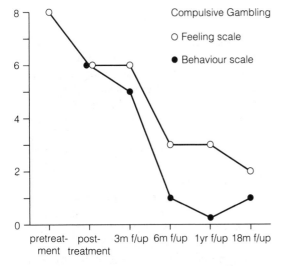

**Figure 21.35** Graham's problem-severity scale ratings

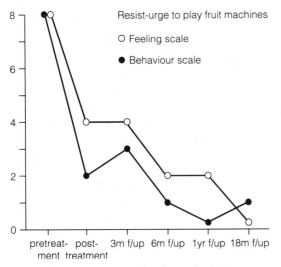

**Figure 21.36** Graham's target-rating scales

phone for an immediate appointment should any more slips occur. He and Wendy attended regular follow-up sessions on a monthly basis for three months, then three monthly appointments up to the yearly follow-up point. Further follow-up sessions were offered at 18 and 24 months to provide continuing sup-

port. Both Wendy and Graham were advised to seek immediate help should any serious slips occur in future. At the 18-month follow-up, progress was maintained, although a small number of slips had occurred involving the expenditure of less than £5 on fruit-machines. Although Graham still had debts, these were shrinking fast. As a couple, they were proposing to get engaged within a few months (Table 21.10; Figures 21.35, 21.36 for data summary).

## CASE STUDY – NURSING INTERVENTIONS FOR DEPRESSION OF MOOD

Bill, a 38-year-old manager of a busy floor in a large department store, was referred to the behaviour therapy nursing service by his GP with a depressive problem of ten months' duration. A screening appointment in a local mental health centre was followed by two assessment interviews within a two-week period.

### The assessment

Bill described how his wife, Janet, had left him a year previously to set up home with another man. They had no children. Bill blamed himself for what he saw as the irretrievable breakdown of their relationship. He felt that over the last three years of their ten-year marriage they had ceased to be a couple, principally because he worked long hours, and was so tired when at home that all he could do was sit and watch TV.

A picture emerged of Bill progressively working longer and longer hours over several years, bringing paperwork home every evening, and their social lives diminishing drastically. Occupational stress in a highly competitive business produced frequent anxiety symptoms and a feeling of exhaustion that proved destructive to their relationship. By the time Janet moved out, Bill was showing clear signs of burn-out stress syndrome (Maslach, 1976; 1982), which developed into a depressive disorder when the relationship ended.

Despite this, Bill had continued working, attempting to throw all his remaining energy into the job, with only a three-week sick leave immediately after Janet's departure. At that time, the GP prescribed a tricyclic antidepressant medication, which had been helpful in relieving the most distressing symptoms of tearfulness, sleep loss, and concentration difficulties. Bill's mood had remained depressed, however, and required a major effort on his part to continue working. A change to another tricyclic drug four months before this referral had produced no further improvement.

Anxiety symptoms (without panic attacks) continued, involving frequent worry about work, feelings of tension and persistent unease, tachycardia, and sweating and gastric symptoms that occasionally led to nausea and vomiting. Bill described how he felt profoundly sad for much of the day, and how this was worse when alone at home. He still brought paperwork home, had no social life, and often went to bed when not catching up on paperwork. Although he experienced suicidal thoughts, his religious upbringing prevented him from seriously considering this.

In addition to the department's standard clinical measures, Bill was asked to keep a detailed diary of his daily activity and mood. At the first assessment session, Bill's Beck Depression Inventory Score registered severely depressed. He was asked to complete a hopelessness scale (Beck *et al.*, 1974), which placed him at moderate risk of suicide, requiring regular monitoring.

## The case formulation

A formulation was discussed with Bill based on a cognitive-behavioural analysis of his problem description and data collection. It was hypothesized that inappropriate beliefs about his sense of self-worth being dependent on success and the appreciation by others had led to him over-investing his efforts in his work environment. This highly competitive and stressful business demanded more and more, without recognition of efforts, only of results. Bill's perfectionist need to be in control and to get things right were not achievable, but in his drive to make them so he had lost sight of his marital relationship, and a shared social and emotional life with Janet.

Burn-out stress syndrome had resulted. Janet found the emotional and social reinforcers she needed outside of their relationship. Janet's leaving provided Bill with the impetus to turn the syndrome into a reactive form of depression, whereby a sense of loss and guilt (self-blame) further reinforced and maintained his depression of mood. Although Bill continued working hard, it was with a lower level of efficiency and effectiveness and with no sense of pleasure or mastery. Bill's withdrawal from the previously reinforcing and pleasurable activities in his lifestyle further exacerbated his depressive mood.

It was suggested that the antidepressive medication could only relieve a proportion of Bill's symptoms, and could not in itself effectively treat the multiple causative and maintaining factors. Improvement depended on Bill becoming a personal scientist, developing a self-awareness of how his inappropriate belief systems (schema) generated cognitive distortions in his thinking. He would need to learn how to redesign his occupational and social lifestyle, and to develop more adaptive thinking styles, in order to challenge and progressively change the inappropriate belief systems that underlay his depressive thinking style.

Bill found this acceptable. The therapist asked that he purchase and read a particularly useful self-help manual (Burns, 1980), which would provide one element of a homework programme.

## The treatment plan

The therapist planned an outpatient treatment programme with both cognitive and behavioural elements, requiring a minimum of 25 sessions on a weekly basis over the forthcoming six months. Progress would be reviewed every six weeks formally, but the pace of treatment would be based on the results Bill was able to achieve, rather than on rigidly time-tabled plan.

A central element to a cognitive-behavioural approach to depression is the use of daily diaries for the collection of data, and as a means to identify and change both activity and thinking patterns (Williams, 1984). The first stage of treatment involved Bill extending his daily activities into a planned schedule of activities that would increase socializing and recreation for evenings and weekends. Several sessions included work with his nurse therapist on stress and anxiety management strategies to be incorporated into his homework plan. Problem-solving strategies were used to examine realistically how Bill could reduce and delegate the over-management of his department.

In his activity diary, as a self-monitoring exercise, Bill was asked to use a 0-10 scale to rate each activity for (P) 'pleasure' and (M) 'mastery'. To assist him, he used a client handout similar to that developed by Melanie Fennell (1990). In addition, Bill was asked to keep a dysfunctional thoughts record each day wherein he could identify his varying

**Table 21.11** Bill's data summary*

|  | Pretreatment | Post-treatment | 3m f/u | 6m f/u | 1yr f/u |
|---|---|---|---|---|---|
| Thyer Anxiety Scale | 26 | 12 | 12 | 8 | 7 |
| Beck Depression Inventory | 35 | 14 | 8 | 8 | 6 |
| Hopelessness scale | 12 | 7 | 4 | 2 | 2 |
| Life-adjustment scales |  |  |  |  |  |
| 1. Work | 6 | 3 | 2 | 2 | 2 |
| 2. Home management | 7 | 4 | 2 | 2 | 1 |
| 3. Social leisure | 8 | 4 | 2 | 1 | 1 |
| 4. Private leisure | 8 | 4 | 3 | 2 | 2 |
| Problem-rating scale |  |  |  |  |  |
| 1. Depression of mood |  |  |  |  |  |
| a) Feelings | 8 | 3 | 3 | 2 | 1 |
| b) Behaviour | 8 | 2 | 2 | 2 | 0 |
| 1. Stress/anxiety symptoms |  |  |  |  |  |
| a) Feelings | 7 | 3 | 3 | 2 | 1 |
| b) Behaviour | 7 | 2 | 2 | 1 | 0 |

* Although a range of short-term and interim targets were devised and utilized, the principal outcome measure with this client was to achieve and maintain a consistently low score on the Beck Depression Inventory, verified by observation and self-report.

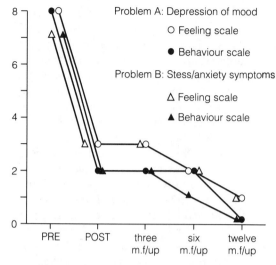

**Figure 21.37** Bill's problem-severity scale ratings

emotional responses, rate their intensity, and identify the negative automatic thoughts associated with them.

These diary records provided the working documents for each clinic session, and presented the therapist with the content of Bill's depressive thinking – the focus for his learning how to challenge and reduce their frequency and counter them by learning how to develop more appropriate and rational cognitive responses. These enabled Bill to test out in real-life his negative self-statements and expectations, while simultaneously developing a new repertoire of more positive cognitions that could be tested and confirmed with behavioural homework tasks.

Over the next eight months Bill co-operated with his programme, introducing a more satisfying social and recreational range of activities into his lifestyle, while effectively reducing a large proportion of his work-induced stress. The cognitive therapy elements of the programme led to initially slow, but later more rapid, changes in his day-to-day experience of depressive negative

thinking. This enabled Bill to examine and challenge the inappropriate belief systems that generated much of the negative cognitions, and to start to learn more appropriate ways of viewing the world, himself, and the future. Bill's mood progressively improved, his sense of loss and hopelessness diminished, and his anxiety experiences similarly reduced in frequency and intensity.

## Conclusion

At the time of discharge, Bill had received 34 sessions of cognitive-behavioural therapy for his depressive difficulty. He stopped taking antidepressant medication by his own decision four months into his programme, with no adverse effects. Follow-up appointments at one, three, and twelve months showed maintenance of clinical gains, with only moderate difficulties arising when divorce proceedings and the sale of the house occurred (Table 21.11; Figures 21.37, 21.38 for data summary).

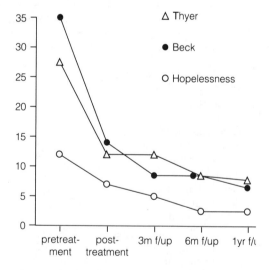

**Figure 21.38** Bill's Thyer anxiety scale/ Beck depression inventory/ hopelessness scale

# REFERENCES

Beck, A. T., Ward, C. H., Mendelson, M. *et al.* (1961) An inventory for measuring depression. *Arch. Gen. Psych.*, 4, 561–71.

Beck, A. T., Weissman, A.W., Lester, D. *et al.* (1974) The assessment of pessimism: the hopelessness scale?. *J. Consult. Clin. Psychol.*, 42, 861–5.

Beck, A. T. and Emery, G. (1985) *Anxiety Disorders and Phobias: A Cognitive Perspective*, Basic Books, New York.

Burns, D. (1980) *Feeling Good: The New Mood Therapy*, Morrow Press, New York.

Burns, L. E. (1977) An investigation into the additive effects of behavioural techniques in the treatment of agoraphobia. Unpub. dissertation, Univ. Leeds.

Cautela, J. R. (1976) Treatment of compulsive behaviour by covert sensitization. *Psychol. Review*, 16, 33–41.

Chambless, D. L. and Goldstein, A. J. (eds) (1982) *Agoraphobia: Multiple Perspectives on Theory and Treatment*, John Wiley & Sons, Chichester.

Chambless, D. L., Caputo, G. C., Jasin, S. E. *et al.* (1985) The mobility inventory for agoraphobia. *Behaviour Research and Therapy*, 23, 35–44.

Clark. D. M. (1986) A cognitive approach to panic. *Behaviour Research and Therapy* 24, 451–70.

Clark, D. M. and Salkovskis, P. M. (1990) *Cognitive Therapy for Panic and Hypochondriasis*, Pergamon Press, New York.

Comfort, A. (1987a) *The Joy of Sex*, Mitchell Beazley, London.

Comfort A. (1987b) *More Joy of Sex*, Mitchell Beazley, London.

Deakin, H. G. (1989) The treatment of agoraphobia by nurse therapists: practice and training, in K. Gournay (ed.), *Agoraphobia: Current Perspectives on Theory and Treatment*, Routledge, London.

Deakin, H. G. and Kirkpatrick, E. (1987) Sexual problems and their treatment. *Nursing*, 19, 709–14.

Dickerson, M. G. (1984) *Compulsive Gamblers*, Longman, London.

Emmelkamp, P. M. G. (1982) *In vivo* treatment of agoraphobia, in *Agoraphobia: Multiple Perspectives on Theory and Treatment* (eds D. L. Chambless and E. J. Goldstein) New York. J. Wiley & Sons, Chichester.

Fennell, M. J. V. (1990) Depression, in *Cognitive-Behavioural Approaches to Adult Psychiatric Disorders: A Practical Guide* (K. Hawton, P. M. Salkovskis, D. M. Clark), Oxford Univ. Press, London, New York.

Fensterheim, H. and Baer, J. (1975) *Don't Say Yes When You Want to Say No*, Futura, London.

Foa, E. B. and Emmelkamp, P. M. G. (eds) (1983) *Failures in Behaviour Therapy*, J. Wiley & Sons, Chichester

Hawton, K. (1985) *Sex Therapy: A Practical Guide*, Oxford Univ. Press, Oxford.

Hawton, K., Salkovskis, P. M. and Clark, D. M. (eds) (1990) *Cognitive-Behavioural Approaches to Adult Psychiatric Disorders: A Practical Guide*. Oxford Univ. Press, Oxford.

Hersen, M. and Bellack, A. S. (eds) (1981) *Behavioural Assessment: A Practical Handbook* (2nd edn), Pergamon Press, New York.

Jacobson, E. (1938) *Progressive Relaxation*, Univ. Chicago Press, Chicago.

Kanfer, F. H. and Saslow, G. (1969) Behavioural diagnosis in behaviour therapy, in *Behaviour Therapy: Appraisal and Status* (ed. C. M. Franks), McGraw-Hill, New York.

Lang, P. J. (1969) The mechanics of desensitization and the laboratory study of fear, in *Behaviour Therapy: Appraisal and Status* (ed. C. M. Franks), McGraw-Hill, New York.

Lazarus, A. A. (ed.) (1976) *Multimodal Behaviour Therapy*, Springer, New York.

Lee, W. A., Cameron, O. G. and Greden, J. F. (1985) Anxiety and caffeine consumption in people with anxiety disorders. *Psychiatry Research*, 15, 211–17.

Liberman, R. P., King, L. W., DeRisi, W. J. *et al.* (1975) *Personal Effectiveness: Guiding People to Assert Themselves and Improve Their Social Skills*, Research Press, Illinois.

Marks, I. M. (1978) *Living with Fear*, McGraw-Hill, New York.

Marks, I. M. (1981) *Cure and Care of Neuroses: Theory and Practice of Behavioural Psychotherapy*, John Wiley & Sons, Chichester.

Marks, I. M. (1985) *Psychiatric Nurse Therapists in Primary Care*, Roy. Coll. Nursing, London.

Marks, I. M. (1986) *Behavioural Psychotherapy: The Maudsley Pocket Book of Clinical Management*, Wright, Bristol.

Marks, I. M., Hallam, R. S., Connolly, J. *et al.* (1977) *Nursing in Behavioural Psychotherapy*, Roy. Coll. Nursing, London.

Maslach, C. (1976) Burned out. *Human Behaviour*, 5(9) 16–22.

Maslach, C. (1982) Understanding burnout: definitional issues in analyzing a complex phenomenon, in *Job Stress and Burnout: Research, Theory and Intervention Perspective* (ed. W. S. Paine) Sage Pubs, London, Beverly Hills.

Masters, W. H. and Johnson, V. E. (1970) *Human Sexual Inadequacy*, Little, Brown, Boston.

Meichenbaum, D. (1977) *Cognitive-Behaviour Modification: An Integrative Approach*, Plenum Press, New York.

Meichenbaum, D. and Genest M. (1980) Cognitive-behaviour modification: an integration of cognitive and behavioural methods, in *Helping People Change: A Textbook of Methods* (eds F. H. Kanfer, A. P. Goldstein) (2nd edn), Pergamon Press, New York.

Powell, T. J. and Enright, S. J. (1990) *Anxiety and Stress Management*, Routledge, London.

Priestley, P. and Maguire, J. (1983) *Learning to Help: Basic Skills Exercises*, Tavistock Publications, London.

Rachman, S. J. and Hodgson, R. J. (1980) *Obsessions and Compulsions*. Prentice-Hall, New Jersey.

Rachman, S. J. and Wilson, G. T. (1980) *The Effects of Psychological Therapy*, (2nd. edn) Pergamon Press, Oxford.

Rathus, S. A. (1973) A 30-item schedule for assessing assertive behaviour. *Behaviour Therapy*, 4, 398–406.

Richards, D. A. and MacDonald, R. (1990) *Behavioural Psychotherapy: A Handbook for Nurses*, Heinemann, London.

Salkovskis, P. M. (1988) Hyperventilation and anxiety. *Current Opinion in Psychiatry*, 1, 76–82.

Smith, M. J. (1975) *When I Say No, I Feel Guilty: How to Cope Using the Skills of Systematic Assertive Therapy*, Bantam Books, New York.

Thyer, B. A. (1987) *Treating Anxiety Disorders: A Guide for Human Service Professionals*, Sage Publications, Newbury Park, California.

Upper, D. and Cautela, J. R. (1979) *Covert Conditioning*, Pergamon Press, New York.

Williams, J. M. G. (1984) *The Psychological Treatment of Depression: A Guide to the Theory and Practice of Cognitive Behaviour Therapy*, Croom Helm, London.

Zilbergeld, B. (1978) *Men and Sex: A Guide to Sexual Fulfillment*, Little, Brown, Boston.

# NURSING INTERVENTIONS: INDIVIDUAL, FAMILY AND GROUP SYSTEMS

22

*Christine Halek*

Systems theory was developed in relation to biological (living) and cybernetic (computerized) systems. What these systems have in common is that their functioning is regulated by feedback mechanisms, which are determined by genetic predisposition or by interaction with the environment. Thus, many animals hibernate when food is scarce and temperatures drop. When warmer weather comes and food supplies increase, they wake and return to active life. If the weather remains warm, or the food supply is plentiful, the hibernation pattern changes. This behaviour is innate, but only displayed when triggered by environmental conditions. In system terms, therefore, an animal changes its system functioning according to its perceptions of its environment.

Thinking in system terms can help the mental health nurse to make sense of what is happening in therapeutic relationships. It is a very flexible concept, and can be applied just as well to individual and intrapsychic relationships as to groups and organizations.

## DEFINING SYSTEMS THEORY

Firstly, let us recap on some of the basic concepts of systems theory, and how we can apply them to human relationships. In this context, a single system is a discrete entity, which is defined by a **boundary**. The boundary is important, because it controls contact with other systems. A **closed system** is one in which the boundary is not permeable, and all the activity takes place within the system; an **open system** is one in which the boundary is permeable, like a filter, and allows things to pass in and out of the system. To work well, the boundary of an open system must be strong enough to retain the system's discrete identity, but permeable enough to allow the necessary interchanges with other systems.

A simple example of an open system is a single cell, like an amoeba, or any of the cells in our bodies. Its boundary is the cell wall. Through this cell wall the system receives input from the outside world – maybe food, or a sensory message. With throughput the cell can process this information or material, and in turn pass its own message across the wall in the form of output. What the cell does with its input, and what it produces as output will depend on its basic nature, which it will seek to maintain so that it can revert to the state it was in before the input crossed the cell wall. This state, called **homeostasis**, which means uniformity or balance, regulates the system's throughput.

Larger systems are made up of many single systems or **subsystems,** for example the many cells that make up a single organ, which is a system in itself, and the body, which is made up of many organs. The bigger systems function in the same way as the subsystems, for example, we maintain a stable level of hydration or blood gases in precisely the same way

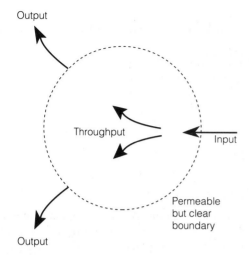

**Figure 22.1** A 'healthy' single system

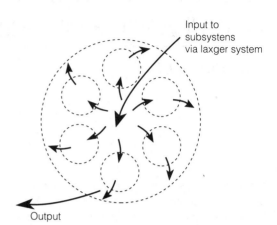

**Figure 22.2** A larger system composed of individual subsystems

that the cell maintains its essential identity or homeostasis (Figure 22.1).

In applying systems thinking to relationships and psychological processes, the same concepts are used. The individual is seen as a system, with a conceptual boundary, which we might call identity, or sense of self. Input comes in the form of sensory perceptions – things we see, smell, hear, touch, or taste. We respond to these according to our genetic makeup, together with what we have learnt about ourselves and the world. Again, the person's output into the world – what he says and does – will depend on how this input has been processed. Two people having a conversation therefore could be seen as two interacting systems: what they say to each other will depend on what they receive from each other and what they do with it according to the rules of their own particular systems.

Several systems can make larger systems, such as a family, a social club, a multinational organization, or a hospital. These larger systems will also have their own homeostases, which comes from that of individual systems, but are not the same as them. The larger system will have rules that reflect the functioning of the many subsystems it contains, but these will only be a rough average of the diverse ways in which the other systems regulate themselves (Figure 22.2).

## THE INDIVIDUAL AS A SYSTEM

One way of understanding psychological problems and mental illness is to think of them as systems in which the boundary regulation is faulty. Thus, someone who is very depressed could be thought of as a closed system, where the boundary is almost impermeable and there is little or no contact with other systems. This is one way of maintaining homeostasis, but it leaves the person isolated and cut off from others, with no hope of anything coming into the system that might improve things.

The depressed person's boundary might have become like this for several reasons: maybe some input they received was too upsetting to the system and could not be dealt with; maybe this unprocessed input is still in the system and it is not possible for the system to take in any more – one might think of unresolved grief as being like this. Alternatively, something may have gone wrong with the output to another system, such that it is felt to be too dangerous to let anything more out. Anger, or upset, or loving feelings may have been too much for another system to cope with, or may have been ignored or unwanted, forcing the system to 'clam up' and reduce its output. Or the depressed person may never have learnt how to establish open boundaries and has only narrow chinks through which communication with other people is possible. Thus, he only receives a small amount of the input directed at him, and can only respond in a similarly limited way.

Of course, it is likely that more than one dysfunction comes into play in maintaining what we think of as pathological states, but framing them in these terms can often help to make them more understandable, and also gives us a clue as to how to help.

FAMILIES AND LARGER SYSTEMS

Similarly, family and group systems may also run into problems. Families may become closed and resistant to change when the boundaries between individuals are not strong enough or clear enough to provide safety for the systems within the system. A group may be threatened by the prospect of input from another system that is due to join it. Sometimes the boundary will be too fragile, and the group will break up; sometimes the boundary around the existing group will cement, and the new person will be kept at a distance, or even forced to leave.

You can observe these sorts of processes quite easily in a school playground or at a party – anywhere where boundary maintenance, or sense of self, depends on unwritten rules. In workplaces, these rules may be enforced in a very concrete way, and a person will be expected to adapt and confirm his system's boundary and throughput to that of the workplace. If he is unsuccessful, his difficulty in conforming may be reflected in sickness, absenteeism, excessive anxiety, etc. – or he may even leave or be fired.

Healthy psychological and social functioning depends on being able to maintain the integrity of one's own system while being able to adapt to that of others. People succeed in this to a greater or lesser extent, either by having a flexible but firm system, or by finding an environment that supports their system's functioning. Successful relationships depend on finding systems that fit in with one's own without inhibiting it too much.

Any change in one subsystem will affect the others, and in larger systems this can cause problems. When we work with families or groups we have to deal with this, because working towards change in one person may well upset the system functioning of the other members of the system. It can of course also be very productive for the others, and certainly both family and group therapy rely heavily on this phenomenon.

The following examples look more closely at the clinical applications of systems theory in individual relationships, families, groups, and in our work as nurses.

CASE STUDY – AN INDIVIDUAL SYSTEM

Mrs B is a 40-year-old housewife. Although she has been depressed in the past, she has never been treated for this. Mrs B has been separated from her husband for two years, and has two teenage children. Her mother died recently, and although initially she appeared quite able to cope with this loss, more recently she has been getting into financial difficulties, having problems sleeping, and spending hours cleaning out the house rather chaotically. Mrs B's daughters say their mother cannot seem to organize things anymore, and they are worried by her over-activity and the money problems. They have never seen her like this before. If they try to sort things out, Mrs B gets very agitated, or even angry with them.

When she is assessed by the nurse, the nurse notices that Mrs B's thinking is rather jumbled, and that her ideas are rather loosely connected to one another. If the nurse tries to pin Mrs B down, even with a simple question, her answers become less coherent and angry; sometimes she just repeats what the nurse is asking her. It seems to be easier to the nurse to try and piece together what is happening by letting Mrs B talk freely, although it is very confusing. Similarly, if the nurse tries to get Mrs B to sit down or sit still during the assessment, Mrs B tries to leave the room or to do something like make tea, almost as though she is trying to distract the nurse.

If we were to represent Mrs B as a system, she might look like what we see in Figure 22.3. The boundary between Mrs B and the world has broken down rather drastically, so there is no adequate filter for input and output, nor is there any clear space in which to contain and process the input. If we look at this in terms of Mrs B's situation, we could say that her sense of security and identity has been seriously affected by the loss of her husband and her mother. We could also infer that perhaps Mrs B's boundary was dependent on a relationship with her husband and/or her mother in such a way that prevents her functioning adequately without them. Of course, in losing them she has also lost the supportive boundary around the relationships she had with them.

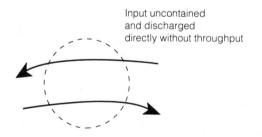

Input uncontained and discharged directly without throughput

**Figure 22.3** Mrs B's system

There is also some suggestion that before this episode, Mrs B was someone who maintained fairly rigid boundary control (the past depression), at least when under threat. Her boundary may have broken down under too much stress, and her current state is an exact expression of what she feels, without her actually feeling it directly or having to make sense of it. Thus any attempts to help Mrs B to make sense of her situation at the moment are likely to be discharged into activity or dissociated ideas (her output).

Looking at Mrs B's situation in this way can have implications for clinical management, and for understanding difficulties that may arise in trying to relate to her in a therapeutic way. One of the tasks of successful clinical management is to provide Mrs B with an adequately safe and secure boundary. This will help her to regain her sense of self, without which she cannot work through her difficulties.

Several things may be done to achieve this: she may be admitted to hospital as a place of asylum where she has less pressure from the outside world; she may be given medication, which can reduce vulnerability to stimulation from outside and help to clarify her thinking; she may be helped by a dependable relationship with someone – a system that will have its own boundaries and of which she will be a part; similarly, she could be helped by a group with clear boundaries. By successful management of boundaries to support Mrs B, it is likely she will regain her own boundary and be able to function more normally again.

Our understanding of how systems work suggests that re-establishing a clear boundary will meet with resistance, since at present Mrs B is working to maintain a homeostasis that prevents her taking in and coming to terms with the losses she has suffered. We can see how the nurse's initial attempts to put ideas or questions into Mrs B's system were unsuccessful – they were simply ejected, either directly, by being repeated, or indirectly, by being translated into another idea or a distracting behaviour. Similarly, the attempts to keep Mrs B in a boundary by being still or remaining sitting seemed threatening to her. Either the nurse will have to manage the consequence of trying to get Mrs B to take things in and keep them – (which threatens Mrs B's homeostasis) – or she will have to judge her interventions very carefully to minimize the stress caused Mrs B. This means being aware of how helping Mrs B might actually make her more disturbed, at least initially, and then being very careful as to how this disturbance is managed.

One way for the nurse to do this might be to ask one question of Mrs B, work hard to get the necessary information, and then allow her to discharge the stress caused, either in disjointed thinking or through some activity, until this is reduced and another question can be attempted. In this way, the nurse can build up Mrs B's boundary by closing the gaps slightly. This is time-consuming and difficult for the nurse, but gradually she will be able to extend the time she can make contact with Mrs B, in talking and through activity. A care plan should allow for such progress.

Another way the nurse can help Mrs B is by using her own system to do some of the work that Mrs B's system cannot manage at present. This might involve trying to make sense of what Mrs B is trying to communicate, or tolerating her distress and holding on to it until she is more able to deal with it.

In doing this, the nurse's system will be put under sometimes considerable strain. To allow Mrs B's output into the nurse's system will threaten her own homeostasis, making her feel uncomfortable, angry, frustrated and so on. While it is important for the nurse to tolerate some of this discomfort, it is equally important for her to recognize her own limits and how much strain her system can deal with. That is why the nurse talking to Mrs B for, say, five minutes at a time initially might be important not only for Mrs B but also to support the nurse's ability to help her.

Equally important is the nurse's place within a larger system – the team, or the nursing staff, or her student group; if these systems function well, they can help to take some of the strain. Particularly important is the role of clinical supervision, where work with patients can be discussed, and the nurse helped to understand how, for example, her own system is being threatened by output from her patients. Good supervision will help the nurse to untangle complex interactions and feelings, and to maintain her own system boundary in the face of such threats (Chapter 25).

To establish a therapeutic relationship with clear boundaries, the nurse must make clear who she is, when she can see Mrs B, how long for, and what the nurse expects of her. It may also mean letting Mrs B know when she is not going to be around – off-duty, on a study day, or on holiday.

The nurse's aim might be to help Mrs B establish a safe relationship within which her difficulties can be talked about. An initial objective might be to try to have a five-minute conversation with Mrs B. Strategies to achieve this might be, for example, setting a time to see Mrs B during the nurse's shift; letting Mrs B know when she will see her, and for how long at a time (five minutes); prompting Mrs B at intervals before the appointment; limiting the talking initially and just spending time with her; limiting the number of questions asked during the time, thereby limiting the pressure on her to respond; keeping instructions and information short and simple, no more than one sentence.

In this way, although the nurse's work will not be directly about systems, her knowledge of her own and of Mrs B's system, and how the two can interact to form another therapeutic system can help the nurse not only to understand Mrs B's situation, but to assess her psychological needs, and plan her psychological care accordingly; it can also help the nurse to understand and manage her own responses to Mrs B.

## CASE STUDY – A FAMILY SYSTEM

A family can be considered a system with its members being subsystems in their own right, as well as forming other subsystems. If we were to consider how an 'ideal' family system might look, we would expect to see something like what is shown in Figure 22.4. There is a clear boundary around the family as a whole; the individual family members are subsystems within the whole, and the parents (as a couple) and the children (as a group) form subsystems too. There will of course be other subsystems within the family, such as mother-children, or male-female.

> Mr and Mrs D have been separated for three years and are now divorced. Mr D lives some distance away from the rest of the family, and has little contact with them. Mr and Mrs D have two teenage children: Rob, 19, who is now at university, and Catharine, 16, who is still at school. Mr and Mrs Ds' longstanding marital problems were present for most of their children's lives.
>
> A referral to family therapy has been made because Catharine is giving cause for concern. Following her parent's separation, she started going out with her first serious boyfriend. After a few months this relationship broke up, although it is not clear who instigated this. Since that time, Catharine has become more and more withdrawn, staying at home in the evenings and at weekends to do school-
>
> work rather than going out. In the last six months she has become very tearful and depressed, crying a lot and refusing to go to school. Her work has begun to suffer, and she is very demanding of her mother's time and attention. She has also cut her arms two or three times, superficially. She recently spent a few days with her father, but was very distressed and withdrawn throughout her stay, and demanded to come home early. Over the past year, Rob has largely been absent from the family home, just coming back occasionally in the holidays. Catharine claims to hate Rob being around, saying he takes no notice of her and causes a lot of trouble to her mother.

If we look at this family in system terms, we might represent them as shown in Figure 22.5. The family boundary is extremely fragile, incomplete and unclear, and the subsystem boundary is now between Mrs D and Catharine. Mr D is completely cut off, and Rob is excluded. Catharine's system has become closed, even within her relationship to her mother.

We can see that Mr D's absence has led to a weakening of the family boundary and the breakdown of the parental subsystem. In its

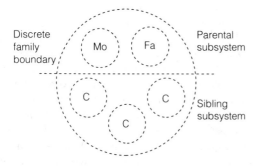

**Figure 22.4** A family system

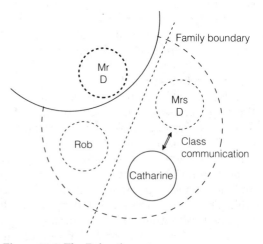

**Figure 22.5** The D family system

place, the female (mother-daughter) sub-system seems to have become dominant, with the men being more or less excluded. Catharine's withdrawal within the female subsystem would indicate that she is not happy with this arrangement. Her relation-ship with her boyfriend could be understood as an attempt to restore a male-female sub-system in her life, which failed. After this she became more and more unhappy. Catharine can also be seen as having problems with her own boundary control and sense of self, shown by the cutting behaviour – skin is a person's physical boundary – and the increas-ing dependence on her mother. Looking at the family system in this way not only helps to structure a treatment approach, but also gives clues to some of the issues that may be causing problems.

Any nurse therapist coming into this setting will first have to be accepted by the existing system. Let us assume that the nurse is male. This will mean that probably he will initially feel excluded, and pick up an air of hostility towards himself from other family members, especially from Mrs D and Catharine. If initially Mr D is not present at the sessions, then the nurse's first task might be to strengthen the boundary around the part-family, which he can do through the setting in which the therapy occurs, and by not excluding any member from the sessions. The system might look like Figure 22.6.

Once the nurse has established himself within the system, he then has several options that might promote better functioning, remem-bering that change in any part of the system will have repercussions throughout the whole system. Some possibilities might be: firstly, challenging the female subsystem by allying himself with Rob. This would give the male subsystem equal weight, and bring the male-female conflict out into the open. For example:

Mrs D is explaining to the nurse her problems with Catharine. The nurse asks Rob how he feels when Mrs D is so

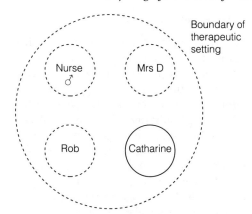

**Figure 22.6** Restoration of boundary in therapy

preoccupied with Catharine. Rob says he sometimes feels left out and angry. Catharine starts arguing with Rob, saying that things are much worse when he is at home, that he should help their mother more, and be more considerate (Figure 22.7).

Secondly, strengthening the adult subsystem by aligning himself with Mrs D, thus poten-tially freeing Catharine but possibly isolating her. Catharine would be likely to resist this intervention and its potential for returning her to a male-female child subsystem with

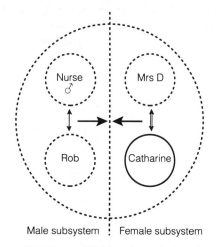

**Figure 22.7** Re-establishing the male-female subsystems

Rob. For example:

> Mrs D is explaining her problems with
> Catharine to the nurse. The nurse
> empathizes with her, discusses with her
> how difficult it is to be a parent, and
> thinks over with her how the two of them
> might help Catharine. Catharine looks at
> her mother and says she does not feel
> well and wants to go home. Mrs D looks
> helpless again, but the nurse continues
> talking to her about how they should deal
> with such 'messages' from Catharine.
> Catharine looks away from her mother
> and towards Rob. (Figure 22.8)

Thirdly, helping Catharine to open her boundary a little and be less shut off by aligning
himself with her. We could expect Mrs D and
Rob might be less comfortable with this. For
example:

> Mrs D is explaining her problems with
> Catharine to the nurse. The nurse asks
> Catharine how she feels when her
> mother talks about the problems to him.
> Catharine huddles into her chair and
> looks at her mother. The nurse says
> maybe it is difficult to talk about her
> mother to someone else, especially when
> her mother is there. Catharine nods, and
> says she helps her mother a lot. Rod
> disagrees, and starts arguing with Mrs D
> about how she treats Catharine like a

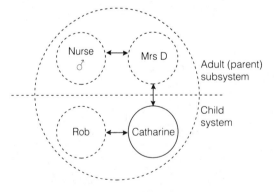

**Figure 22.8** Re-establishing the adult-child
subsystems

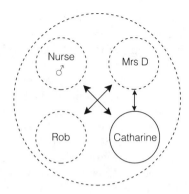

**Figure 22.9** Therapist-'patient' alignment

> baby. Catharine starts crying. The nurse
> says he thinks Catharine is worried about
> her mother being hurt. Catharine looks at
> him and nods (Figure 22.9).

Fourthly, reconstructing the family system
and strengthening the male and parental subsystems by bringing father back in and helping him to take on some of the above
interventions. This would have the effect of
enabling the nurse to move more freely within the system, observing and forming alleg-
iances as necessary to support the family
towards better functioning, even though the
parents are divorced. For example:

> Mrs D is explaining her problems with
> Catharine to the nurse. The nurse asks
> whether she misses her husband's sup-
> port in dealing with the children. She says
> she does. The nurse then asks Mr D how
> he has felt about Catharine's difficulties.
> He says he has felt powerless to help his
> family. Catharine starts to complain to her
> mother about feeling ill and wanting to go
> home. The nurse asks Mr D how he thinks
> his wife should respond to such a request.
> Mr D says he thinks she should tell
> Catharine to wait. Mrs D says there must
> be something wrong and Catharine is ill.
> The nurse says it is difficult for them as
> parents to work out how best to help their
> daughter. The parents start arguing with
> each other. The nurse says he thinks it is

hard for Rob and Catharine to see their parents argue. All the family look surprised. Mr and Mrs D say they thought the children were used to it by now. Catharine says she thinks no one understood how she felt. Rob says he feels no one saw he was upset too. (Figure 22.10)

When working with family systems in this way it is not necessary to work directly with the identified sufferer in order to bring about change for that person. Because the family functions as a discrete system, change in one part of the system can result from interventions in another. The interventions the nurse-therapist ‧ makes will be based on his understanding of the family system, and will involve the use of his own system added to that of the family to bring about change. This will appear to destabilize the stuck or skewed family system, and may throw up problems in other parts of the system, not just in one person. For instance, Mrs D's insecurities, which she dealt with since the divorce by allying herself with her daughter, may become more pronounced. Similarly, Rob's distress, and his and his father's sense of powerlessness within the family, coupled with a fear of destructive anger, can come into the open and be talked about. Catharine may become correspondingly less powerful and less 'neces-

sary' to her mother, and able to see what her particular difficulties are. She may also be able to let Rob and her father help her, rather than relying exclusively on her mother. The male-female polarization should correspondingly become less pronounced.

In this example, the nurse-therapist's gender was important; a female nurse would have had a different position in the family, although she may have seen her tasks as similar. In many cases it is possible to work with two therapists, one male and one female. In such circumstances a further range of options is available, in that there is a therapist subsystem that can model and illustrate existing problems, as well as new ways of functioning. The therapists are also able to work in a complementary way; for example, one may confront while the other empathizes, or one may be active while the other observes.

## GROUP SYSTEMS

A family is a particular form of group, one in which the members are well known to one another, and the rules by which the system functions are well established. This means that even though the boundary around the family system may be impaired in some way, the identity of the family is not usually in doubt. In groups where people are less well known to each other, even complete strangers, the question of identity is less clear. Boundary issues therefore are often at the forefront of group work, both as regards the group system, and the subsystems within it.

Groups may function either as closed or open systems, depending on the circumstances and the purpose of the group. Here we are looking at therapeutic groups, but it is worth remembering that we all spend much of our lives as members of a number of different types of groups. In most of these we are connected to other people in the group by a common goal or purpose, or by a liking for one another. It is this that establishes the boundary of the group.

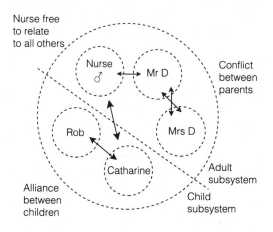

**Figure 22.10** Bringing father back into the system

Within this framework there may be many discrepancies and areas of potential conflict between the subsystems. These need to be successfully managed if they are not to damage the group or deflect it from its purpose. The tensions set up within a group by these differences between people are exploited in a therapeutic group to achieve change in its members, but this can only happen if the boundary around the group system is resilient enough to withstand the internal tensions. A group system thus can function in a similar way to an individual one, with the subsystem providing input and output to one another within the group boundary. The extent to which the group system as a whole also relates to systems outside it will depend on the nature of the group.

WARD GROUPS

Looking first at the central issue of establishing a group system, we will consider a ward group, meaning a therapeutic group that is held in an inpatient setting, and which is potentially open to all staff and patients on the ward. One of the biggest problems in running such a group is establishing a clear boundary that will give the group its identity. This is not only because the individuals in the group are only loosely connected to one another by virtue of being in the same place at the same time, but also because many of the individual systems within the group may not be functioning well for a time. There also may be frequent changes of membership, caused by staff deployment, as well as admissions and discharges.

It is clear that establishing any sort of consistent boundaries in a group like this is a major problem, but also of major importance if the group is to function successfully as a system. The fragmented nature of the boundary of a ward group is evident in lateness, absenteeism, dropping out, wandering in and out of the group, and difficulties in ending the group. Such boundary weakness is a reflection of the boundary problems of the individuals in the group (the resulting chaos can be seen as a way of maintaining homeostasis for the individuals). Strengthening the group boundary can be seen as a way of helping individuals to change.

In system terms, without a boundary the group cannot function properly. Despite the limitations of the setting, however, ward groups can work if attention is paid to making the boundary as clear and as secure as possible. This can be done both physically – in terms of time, place, and setting – and psychologically – by acknowledging and defending the importance of the group within the ward system. Most of this will depend on the staff's understanding of and commitment to the role of the group, for it is they who will be responsible for maintaining the group's boundary in the face of constant change and uncertainty on the ward, just as the nurse in the first case study (page 295) would be responsible for maintaining the boundary around a therapeutic nurse-patient relationship.

Physically, the group boundary can be established by setting aside a room for the group and a time to meet. The room should be prepared by setting out chairs for all those who are likely to attend. It is important that the staff are punctual, and firm in encouraging attendance, particularly from each other. As well, starting and finishing the group punctually are key elements in maintaining the group boundary. Ideally, the same staff should attend each group. It is also preferable to have one or two groups a week at set times with the same staff attending, than a group every day with unpredictable staff attendance. Although the latter is closer to the reality of life on an inpatient ward, the aim is to use the group as a therapeutic tool, and not only as a reflection of the ward as a whole, important as that may be.

Psychologically, the commitment of the staff to the group is of the utmost importance. If the group is regarded as a chore, or if it occurs haphazardly or sloppily, then it is unlikely to be of value to those who need it (the staffs' homeostasis will prevail). If, however, it is seen as, for example, a forum for welcoming and taking leave of others, imparting information, settling minor disputes, supporting those in distress, and establishing a group identity, then it is possible to work towards these aims and feel the group has a place among the treatment approaches used on the ward.

There will always be boundary problems in open groups like ward groups where membership changes frequently, but if the basic guidelines for establishing and maintaining a group boundary can be observed – time, place, setting, core staff membership – then ward groups can help individuals to establish clearer boundaries for themselves in their life on the ward. If boundary maintenance can be extended to the physical ward environment, so that the space which the ward occupies is clearly different from others, and those who belong to the ward have a different status from visitors (whether staff or not), then this will strengthen the identity of the ward and of the individuals there.

Ward groups are particularly difficult to run successfully, but they are likely to be the first and most common therapeutic group nurses come across in their training and subsequent practice. They are unusual and difficult in that they can be large and generally quite unstable. Smaller groups with closed boundaries or slowly changing membership (slow open) are better suited to more individualized therapeutic work, which may often be of a personal and intimate nature. Again, the nature of the group boundary is a crucial factor in enabling work to be done within the system. Indeed, everything that has been said about ward groups is true of other groups, although they will tend to be less obviously disturbed.

## CLOSED GROUPS

A closed group has a set number of members and is usually time limited, for example 20 sessions or one year's duration. The same members meet with the same therapist or facilitator, for the same length of time and on a regular basis, maybe once a week or once a month. The groups may be semistructured, as in art or drama therapy, or unstructured, as in psychotherapy.

Although the group is closed, it is not strictly speaking a closed system, in that the members have contact with other systems when they are not in the group. Therapeutically, however, it works not unlike a closed system, because the boundary is very clear and rigid, often reinforced by a strict rule of confidentiality regarding what happens in the groups. The existence of this closed boundary encourages the members to relax their individual boundary control, and facilitates disclosure, sharing, and exchange between individuals in the group, often at a very personal and intimate level. The closed boundary also make it safe to do this, as there is less risk of the group process being interrupted. (Figure 22.11)

Closed groups can become very intense, and individuals may seem to function without boundaries for the duration of the group. At first this can result in chaos in the group,

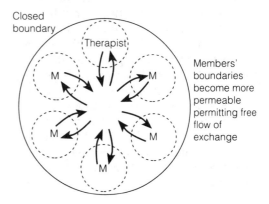

**Figure 22.11** A closed group

but gradually individuals will adjust their boundaries to contain their feelings in a more healthy way, as well as to permit interaction with other systems. A time boundary in the form of a limited number of sessions can intensify the process.

Leading or facilitating such a group requires a good sense of one's own boundaries, plus a willingness to be invaded by and process material from other systems within the group. The nature of closed groups means they may not be suitable for people whose boundary control is too fragile or fragmented, although this does depend on the skill and experience of the person running the group. However, the security offered by the closed boundary makes closed groups suitable for time-limited treatment of intimate emotional difficulties. Groups that may successfully use this format include projective art and drama groups; groups for people who have been sexually abused; groups for bereaved people; and training groups.

The role of the boundary in closed groups can be illustrated by the following example taken from a group for sexually abused women. This is an example of a homogenous group, that is, a group where members all have a similar problem, or have a similar reason for attending.

The group is to run for 15 sessions. It is being held in a health centre. In the fourth session, ten minutes into the group, a man comes into the room, thinking the meeting he is to attend is being held there. He immediately recognizes his mistake, and leaves the room without speaking. The members of the group are angry in a way that is inappropriate to the actual event; in particular they complain that they cannot be expected to talk about their traumatic experiences when they might be interrupted at any time.

The therapist recognizes that the hitherto safe boundary of the group has been infringed by the man's mistake, and thinks perhaps this intrusion and breaking of the group's boundary echoes the more serious boundary infraction of the abuse. Until now, the group members have spoken about their abuse in a fairly factual, matter-of-fact way. When the therapist puts her idea to the group that the man's intrusion has brought up feelings of the loss of safety and anger about being abused, one of the members bursts into tears and is inconsolable for some time. This leads the group members to speak with emotion about their experiences, sharing some very painful feelings with each other. Paradoxically, it is as though the group has become safer.

As well as the loss and need for boundaries, this example also illustrates how what happens in a group system may mirror what has happened in an individual system. In a group where the individual systems are similar – in this case, sexual abuse – the effect of such mirroring can be very intense in that it can affect all the group members more or less equally.

SLOW OPEN GROUPS

Slow open groups are the most common form of longer-term therapy group. The term **slow open** refers to the fact that the group membership is stable for periods of time, although people do leave and new ones join in their place. Although the boundary of a slow open group is clear, and similar to that of a closed group for much of the time, from time to time the group is subject to boundary change that can be very disruptive, but also potentially very useful. As in a closed group, personal sharing and disclosure is encouraged, but this may develop more slowly, and at a different pace for each individual depending on their stage of development within the group. The open-ended nature of the group releases some of the pressure to disclose, which can be a feature of closed groups.

When a new person joins a slow open group, they can feel at a disadvantage, usually they are joining an established system that is going to have to adjust to them, as well as having to learn the ropes of the group system. This is a tense time for the group as its homeostasis is threatened. If the group's system boundary is too rigid, the new person will not be successfully incorporated; if it is too weak, it may give under the strain and the group may fragment.

Usually the processes of adaptation happens in a muted form – for instance, existing members may be late or miss some groups, or they may band together and interrogate the new person or make him the focus of attention. Usually this dies down fairly quickly and the changed group boundary establishes itself. By implication, the nature of the group system has changed. For certain individuals, however, the adjustment may be more traumatic because of their individual system and their previous experience of being a member of a larger system. This individual resistance to change may serve to conceal or disguise the struggle of the group to resist movement and its half-seen, half-hidden consequences. The group may appear to change while continuing to seek its original homeostasis.

Because joining a group that is already established is a difficult task, the new individual may feel his identity to be threatened. For a while he may maintain quite a rigid boundary around himself, which can take the form of withdrawing or of making statements that do not seem to take into account the needs of other group members. After a while this may subside, and the person will appear to function more freely.

Before the group and the new member get to know one another, their interactions will be based on assumptions. This will mean that the existing members will afford the new person a place in the group according to the rules of their systems. Similarly, the new member will process the group as though the members were part of a pre-existing system of which he is or has been a member – one in which he knows his place. Usually this will be his family system, although it may be replicated in other personal and working relationships.

For example, a new man in a group may invite continuous critical comments from another man in the group. It may become clear that the new man was always criticized by his father. It may also emerge that the other man was very jealous of his younger brother. However, because the man who criticizes is like the father but is not the father, the new man does not have to continue to accept his criticisms and be defeated by them. Another member may be able to incorporate the new member into a system where men have a positive role, so that the new person has the chance to alter the way in which he perceives himself (input), and thereby responds to others (output). (Figures 22.12 and 22.13)

The interaction of systems and subsystems make groups a rich source of therapeutic potential, and make it possible through the interaction of relationships from the external world with relationships within the group, for relationships in the inner world of remembered experience and phantasy to be experienced in a modified form. Groups enable both the repair, to the individual, and reparation, by the individual. The injury caused by damaging systems is repaired by participation in a healthy system, which becomes incorporated by the individual.

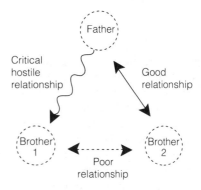

**Figure 22.12** Original pattern of family relationships

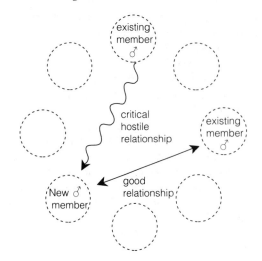

**Figure 22.13** Replication and change of family patterning in the group

Aspects of the group process that affect individuals may also be seen as having a function in the group system as a whole. So, for example, the conflict between the two men in the group may also represent conflict between the group members and the group therapist (the person in authority), or intergenerational conflict (younger versus older). All of these aspects can coexist in the group, and because change in one part of the group will occasion change in another, it may not be necessary to deal with every aspect of a situation in order for it to affect the systems on an individual, subsystem, and group level.

## NURSING SYSTEMS

As bigger systems made up of subsystems – both subgroups and individuals – groups have the potential to affect many levels of interaction. Groups such as the ones described are similar to those we live in and work in every day. The system processes and boundaries we have described are not confined to therapeutic groups.

This is particularly important to us as nurses, as we work very much in groups: as part of a team, within larger groups, units, hospitals, and the nursing profession as a whole. The organizational and institutional systems within which we work have a very specific identity, and have a profound impact on us as individuals. Such systems are sometimes called **social systems**, in order to distinguish them from naturally occurring or therapeutic systems. Individuals within social systems come together because of some common task, purpose, or role. They do not have much control over the people they work with, nor do they necessarily share common experiences or lifestyles.

As with any group, social systems are made up of many individual subsystems, and provide a framework within which these many diverse individuals can work together to achieve their goals. In order to make this possible, the larger system appears to function on behalf of the smaller ones, and takes on an identity of its own. It lays down rules that cover many aspects of institutional and organizational life.

When new people join the system, a degree of conformity is expected of them because the larger system is too unwieldy to adapt to every individual. After a while, the new person will have learnt how to conform, and will have taken on the modus operandi of the system. The boundary of the larger system may become more rigid in order to contain the many forces at work within it, which threaten its homeostasis. It may also become diffuse; a denial of anxieties regarding intimacy. This affects the systems within the system, which correspondingly reduce or increase their boundary permeability in order to fit in with the larger system.

As nurses, we experience this directly when we first begin working in the clinical area with other nurses. At first we may be surprised at the way other nurses deal with things. We may also notice that they see their way of coping as natural and do not question it. Their responses to our questions as students may seem unsatisfactory: the implication is often that this is the way things are done, and you will learn with time:

> Jane is an 18-year-old student nurse on her first day on a surgical ward. She is assigned to work with a staff nurse, who seems very nice and very keen to have Jane work with her. During the morning's work, the staff nurse has to change a dressing on an advanced fungating carcinoma of the breast. Jane is very distressed at seeing the wound, and imagines what it would be like to be the patient and to 'disintegrate' like that. The staff nurse explains to Jane what she is doing in a factual way. The patient also seems detached from what is happening to her. Jane begins to think she should not be so upset by what she is seeing. She later goes to talk to her tutor, who is sympathetic, but explains she will get used to it.

This example illustrates some of the problems of working within a large institutional organization that has as its aim the relief of illness, distress, and suffering. As Menzies-Lyth (1988) explains, the day-to-day exposure to the suffering of patients is extremely burdensome and anxiety-provoking for nurses, as we considered in the first case study (page 295). As in any situation, we need to use boundary control to regulate our input and output. As nurses, however, we are expected to respond to patients in ways which may prevent us from using our normal input-throughput-output process. For example, if a woman in the street made a threatening remark to us, we might ignore her, say something back, get angry, or upset. As nurses we may not be able to respond in our normal way because of the consequences, which puts a considerable strain on our systems and may mean, for example, that we are left with feelings we can not discharge. In this way our individual homeostasis may be seriously threatened.

One of the functions of the social system within which nurses work is to ensure that we are able to carry on doing our jobs. It therefore has somehow to deal with the stress which the job entails. The system does this largely by defending us from stress, for example, by preventing us from experiencing the full impact of the feelings that 'go with the job'.

In the clinical example above, the staff nurse – and incidentally, the patient – was able to do this, whereas Jane was not, and was left feeling as though she were the odd one out. One of the ways the staff nurse might have learnt to detach herself was by concentrating on the fungating carcinoma, rather than on the person whose body it was a part of. Or she might have been focusing on the niceties of her aseptic technique, or the fact that she was teaching a student – in other words, the task in hand. Either way, the staff nurse's boundary control had adapted to the fact that she would not be able to express her feelings about the patient's illness. Jane, however, had not achieved this, and was left feeling stressed. Here is a further example:

> Rob is a student on his first placement in a psychiatric ward. One of the things he has noticed that he finds upsetting is that the patients are always kept waiting whenever they make small requests, particularly for cigarettes or money, which are held by the nurses. When Rob talks to the nurse who is his mentor at the end of the week, he mentions this. The nurse explains that the patients have to learn that they cannot always have things just when they want them, that they have to learn to deal with frustration. Rob does not think this is a good enough response, but does not like to say so.

What is noticeable about both examples is that Jane and Rob see the patients as individuals with problems, and identify with their experiences: their systems are open to receive input from patients and to be affected by that. They bring their feelings to the situation, and presumably would care for the patients in accordance with that. The trained nurses, however, identify a 'problem' to which they can apply their nursing skills or judgment. The patients are not seen as individuals, and the nurses do not respond to them as such, but as 'bodies' or according to some prescribed ritual (the aseptic technique).

This process of depersonalization, whereby the trained staff have stopped working as though they were 'Jane' or 'Rob', but instead have become 'a nurse', responding to those in their care as 'patients' rather than as individual people, can be understood as an adaptive process. The nurse's system has changed to defend itself against having to contain too many feelings that cannot be expressed, but which would threaten its homeostasis if they remained in the system. This is one of the main ways in which the system of nursing protects those who work in it – and those who are treated by it – from experiencing the full impact of the distress and suffering caused by illness and other problems.

During their training, Jane and Rob will be expected to shed much of their personalized approach to nursing and to adopt the system defences used by other nurses. In order to be seen as a 'good' nurse, this is often required. However, although this may work in that it enables Jane and Rob to fit into the system and carry on working as nurses, it ignores the demands of their own individual systems, which they bring to their work as nurses, and which adapt at a cost. Rob, for example, feels that patients' requests should be dealt with promptly and courteously, in a way that respects each person's dignity and makes dependency more tolerable for him or her. Every time he sees someone denied this courtesy, especially if he is expected to behave like the other nurses, this causes him extra distress, because he does not think he and the other nurses are giving good care to those they are looking after. The same would hold true for Jane, if she were to approach the lady with the fungating carcinoma as the staff nurse did.

Not only do nurses sometimes do their work at great personal cost, but they can end up giving what they see as bad care at equally great personal cost by adapting to the nursing system. Jane and Rob illustrate how as nurses we may give up our individual perceptions and ways of coping to the system. These parts of ourselves then get separated, or split off, and feel as though they are no longer ours or under our control. The feelings, however, remain in the larger system as a whole and the threat is now no longer personal but institutional, and so it becomes essential to work as the larger system dictates, otherwise this threat will become reality. This explains in part why nurses can become afraid to trust their own judgement about what constitutes good nursing care and instead follow so many rules, even down to how to make beds or wash someone. Nurses often seem to have become unable to care for people in an individualized way because they have lost faith in their own abilities to work out what to do in different situations.

We can see that this creates huge problems both for nurses and for those they are looking after. To some extent, lack of individuality is a problem in all large systems (suprasystems) where it is feared that too much diversity will cause the boundary to break and the system to fragment. When we consider that as mental health nurses we often have to work with extremely disturbing feelings and thoughts, we can understand why it seems preferable to hold these at bay, rather than to be exposed to them as individuals, and to have to deal with them in terms of our own systems. This might bring up the whole issue of why we chose this profession at all, which we might not otherwise consider.

In very large systems it therefore becomes important to aim for uniformity. In nursing it is even more important, because the system acts like floodgates, holding back a deluge of anxieties and painful or chaotic feelings; any chink or crack seems terribly threatening.

In general nursing settings such uniformity is well expressed in the clothing nurses wear, usually rationalized as being 'necessary for the job'. While there is obviously an element of truth in this, it does not explain the degree of uniformity required, even down to the number of pleats in a starched cap! In psychiatry, one way in which this drive towards uniformity is expressed is through the fear of giving some patients more attention than others, regardless of the fact that each has vastly differing needs, and regardless of the reality that some patients get more attention than others anyway. There is a real anxiety about doing anything differently because one might get punished for revealing a flaw in the system and thus threaten the existing order.

Although many nurses are not satisfied with this state of affairs, changing a system as large and unwieldy – and as frightened – as the one in which we work is a daunting prospect. There is a hidden belief that the system needs to stay as closed as it is, and so attempts to change are often resisted. Consider this example:

> Sally, a staff nurse, has a new job on a ward which uses a keyworker system, and she is made keyworker for a number of patients. When Sally is on the ward, she will be expected to work with those patients. On her first day on the ward, Sally reads the care plans on her allocated patients and goes to find them, but other nurses are already working with some of them. After a few days, Sally realizes that the nurses go to the patients they prefer or are used to, and that being allocated a patient means you write up the notes at the end of the shift and talk about the patient at handover. A lot of that information is secondhand and inaccurate, and Sally feels useless and unimportant.

This example shows how an attempt to allocate individual nurses to individual patients systematically has been sabotaged by working in an *ad hoc* way. Individuals will tend to match themselves to others who do not threaten their own systems too much, but in an environment where change in a system may be necessary and desirable, that means that nothing changes, neither for the nurses nor for those in their care. Things stagnate, and institutionalized attitudes and practices quickly become the norm.

These examples from individual clinical settings can be extended to nursing as a profession – a large system with a very fixed, rigid boundary. This system is made up of a huge number of individual systems, which tend to group together to form large subsystems, particularly hierarchical ones. The complex characteristics of this large system may be distributed around the subsystems, so that senior nurses, for example, hold the power and responsibility, and junior ones the anxiety and stress. The balance of the system as a whole is very fragile, and permits very little flexibility. Individuals who want to work with their whole selves, and to deal with the stresses and difficulties of the job in their own way may find they are poorly tolerated by the system and feel they have no choice but to leave. This is one reason for the problems nursing has in retaining staff, particularly those who might be able to bring about change. Alternatively, such nurses go into areas where they have more freedom to work as individuals, for instance in the community, in teaching, or in a specialism where they can work autonomously.

Understanding the way systems function and how this thinking can be applied to interpersonal and organizational relationships can be very helpful to us in our clinical work as nurses, whether in our work with individuals, families and groups, or in our dealings with colleagues, both nurses and non-nurses. Such understanding helps us to tolerate the problems and difficulties we encounter in our work, and to devise appropriate ways of dealing with them. Systems thinking also allows us to take into account what we bring to our work as nurses, and how we are affected by contact with others. It is a simple and clear way of describing to others what we think might be happening in relationships and within the ward and institutional environment, and lends itself to be used as a tool to promote change in these areas.

## FURTHER READING

Barker, P. (1986) *Basic Family Therapy*, Collins, London.

Beckett, J.A. (1973) General systems theory, psychiatry and psychotherapy. *Inter. J. Group Psychotherapy*, 23; 292–305.

Douglas, T. (1983) *Groups: Understanding People Gathered Together*, Tavistock Publications, London.

Jacques, E. (1955) Social systems as a defence against persecutory and depressive anxiety, in *New Directions in Psychoanalysis*, Tavistock Publications, London.

Menzies-Lyth, I. (1988) *Containing Anxiety in Institutions*, Free Association Books, London.

Menzies-Lyth, I. (1988) *The Dynamics of the Social*, Free Association Books, London.

Minuchin, S. (1977) *Families and Family Therapy*, Tavistock Publications, London.

Skynner, A.R.C. (1976) *One Flesh: Separate Persons*, Constable, London.

Von Bertalanffy, L. (1968) *General Systems Theory*, Penguin, Harmondsworth.

Wright, H. (1989) *Groupwork: Perspectives and Practice*, Scutari, London.

# PART SIX

# THE PROVISION AND MANAGEMENT OF CARE: SELF-MANAGEMENT BY THE NURSE

*David Carpenter*

What motivates a person to enter mental health nursing? It is not the sort of career a person will have wanted to pursue for as long as she or he can remember. To a person with no experience, it is not even clear what such an occupation might entail. Yet people apply to train as mental health nurses with virtually no previous experience of the mental health services.

Perhaps the most obvious motivating factor is that of curiosity; not just about the mental health services and the mentally ill, but curiosity about oneself. Many potential mental health nurses claim they want to find out about people, what makes them tick and what contributes to them becoming mentally ill. Many applicants talk as though they are some other life form interested in learning more about this group called 'people'. On closer questioning, most happily admit they are really interested in learning more about themselves. In many respects this is not a bad reason for wishing to become a mental health nurse, given that a fundamental prerequisite of successful practice is self-awareness.

Many applicants have had some previous experience of the mental health services, which, given the high incidence of mental illness, is perhaps not surprising. Such experience might include that of a mentally ill relative or friend, or, sometimes, their own mental illness. The latter used to preclude any possibility of training, but more recently those responsible for selection appear to be becoming more enlightened. After all, it is often the experience of being nursed as a child that motivates a person to consider general nursing as a career; why should there not be similar considerations in the mental health field? Since those engaged in mental health nursing are usually keen to destigmatize mental illness, it seems strange to show prejudice towards people with a history of mental illness who are applying to train as nurses.

Of course, no one can train as a nurse if they are victim of some chronic and debilitating mental illness, but a recovered person will almost certainly have experience that will be invaluable in caring for others. The applicant must have resolved personal mental health problems; nursing is essentially a selfless occupation, and there will be dangers for all if an applicant is aiming to be nursed rather than to be a nurse.

There is one further large group who seek careers in mental health nursing. These are the people who find it impossible to state why they wish to undertake training. For such applicants, this is a source of great embarrassment: why should anyone aim to enter a profession without knowing what attracts them, or what they might be able to offer? It does seem that mental health nursing is an ideal career for people who are not sure what they want, other than a wish to help people. Many people have undertaken training with an apparent absence of positive motives; perhaps they are simply not accessible, or perhaps they develop as the person moves through training. Whatever the case, such people often go on to be successful practitioners.

One of the main reasons why applicants find it difficult to state their motives is the fact that mental health nursing lacks a clear image. Most people are easily able to conceptualize general nursing – even small children are able to portray at least a stereotypical image of a nurse – but mental health nursing is far more elusive. While the historical image of the 'men in white coats' has now more or less passed, nothing has developed to replace it.

It is interesting to note, however, that men are more likely than women to choose mental health nursing than other branches of the profession. Precise reasons for this are not entirely clear, but it may be because historically men were employed as lunatic attendants. Men are readily able to function as nurses, and many seek careers in nursing. Perhaps mental health nursing provided, and provides, an opportunity for men to enter a caring profession without any compromise to their sense of masculinity.

In this country, entry to training is governed by statute, in that minimum educational qualifications are specified. The current requirement is five GCSE passes, though equivalent alternatives are acceptable. One such alternative is the entrance test offered through the UKCC, which has been developed as a validated equivalent to the standard qualifications. The test has been particularly valued by mature candidates, who might not have benefited from the opportunities currently available to most younger people. In addition, various access courses have been created, which have enabled candidates who have not had recent experience of study to attain the requisite standard for entry to training.

While educational qualifications are important, there are other qualities that are equally significant in determining suitability to train as a mental health nurse. Potential candidates will typically have a caring concern for other people – a concern that will probably verge on what might uncharitably be called nosiness. A fairer description might be genuine interest in others, though that interest should never be detached or merely academic; it will involve some personal investment.

Caring in a strongly interested way entails caring **about** another person as opposed to merely caring **for** them. In the case of the former, the level of involvement is high; there is a risk of being hurt emotionally, which can be managed through facilitative supervision (Chapter 25). Generally, this interest will be driven by curiosity, a further essential attribute of the effective mental health nurse. Another important personal quality is that of being prepared to take carefully calculated risks. The over-cautious nurse will tend to stifle the client's independence, and will do little to help him to manage his own life. The enabling role of the mental health nurse is fundamental.

When students are being selected, it is usual to assess personal qualities, or at least the potential for their development. For this reason, selection procedure may well include group exercises involving the use of communication skills, as well as individual or group interviews.

Acceptance as a student nurse marks the beginning of a life-long commitment to education and further training, not the beginning of a three-year course. Continuing registration as a nurse is contingent upon the maintenance and development of professional knowledge and skill. All nurses are required to 'take every opportunity to maintain and improve professional knowledge and competence' (UKCC, 1984). While professional obligations are clear, it is fair to say that the majority of mental health nurses require little persuasion to take advantage of the increasing pool of educational opportunities that are becoming available.

## PRE-REGISTRATION TRAINING

Increasingly, nurse training is being structured according to the principles stated in Project

2000 (UKCC, 1986). In practical terms, this has resulted in student nurses becoming largely supernumerary as far as the nursing work force is concerned. They are students like other students in many respects, particularly in so far as they are equally studying to gain a higher education qualification, usually at diploma level. Nursing students, however, have the additional work entailed in achieving the statutorily specified outcomes, enabling them to register as nurses. These skills are gained in practice settings – not just wards in hospitals, but community settings as well. A significant requirement of Project 2000 is that nurses should be prepared for practice in both institutional and community settings. As nursing curricula develop, students find themselves being educated in a range of settings, both academic and clinical. While this undoubtedly broadens the focus of training, it adds to the stresses experienced by many student nurses.

Curricula designed to prepare nurses for registration as professional practitioners are subject to statutory regulation. Whilst training institutions have some scope in determining the shape and emphasis of a course of pre-registration preparation, it is recognized that all nurses registered on a particular part of the professional register must possess a common range of skills and knowledge. This range is stated in the form of outcomes, or competencies, which can be found in the Nurses, Midwives and Health Visitors Rules (1983) (Nurses Midwives and Health Visitors Act, 1979). The competencies apply to pre-Project 2000 courses, and can be found in Rule 18. They must be achieved in order to register in Part Three of the professional register (RMN). Rule 18 has been amended to take account of Project 2000 courses, and states the necessary outcomes of courses designed to lead to registration in, *inter alia*, Part 13 of the register (Registered Nurse – Mental Health Branch). The professional register is maintained by the UKCC, and training courses are monitored by the National Boards.

Project 2000 is having an increasing impact on nursing education. Most significantly, Project 2000 courses require schools or colleges of nursing to form explicit links with institutions of higher education in order to offer courses of training including qualifications to a minimum of diploma level. These new relationships have brought nursing into line with many other professions where training leads to academic qualifications as well as professional registration. Courses of training have widened to include all relevant academic disciplines, reflecting the broad knowledge-base of nursing.

Critics of Project 2000 argue that the academic emphasis detracts from the fundamental practical nature of nursing. It should be immediately emphasized, however, that the Project does not entail any reduction in clinical experience; 50 percent of all curricular time must be devoted to clinical experience (ENB, 1990). It is still too early to offer any informed evaluation of the effects of Project 2000, but if it achieves its broad aim of producing nurses who are 'knowledgeable doers', it should be welcomed.

## POST-REGISTRATION TRAINING

Changes in pre-registration training, along with other significant developments, are having a considerable influence upon the nature and structure of post-registration training. In the future, nurses will complete basic training with diploma-level qualifications, and the necessary knowledge and skill to practice in both institutional and community settings at a basic level.

It is clear that post-registration training should aim to consolidate and build upon skills and knowledge gained during training through the provision of continuing professional and academic development. In addition, the majority of practitioners who trained before the introduction of Project 2000, are looking for opportunities to build upon their existing qualifications and experience.

The personal benefits of post-registered training to individual nurses are obvious, but there are wider considerations: continuing education and training of nurses is intended to primarily benefit clients who will be cared for by nurses who have developed skills and knowledge in relation to changing patterns of health-care need. In serving its duty to the public, the UKCC is obliged to ensure that all currently registered nurses maintain and, preferably, improve upon the knowledge and skill gained during basic training.

The need for the education of nurses following initial registration has long been recognized. A range of clinical courses has been offered through the National Boards, reflecting increasing levels of specialization within nursing practice and changing trends in the nature of health-care provision. In mental health nursing, courses have been developed to prepare nurses to offer particular forms of therapeutic intervention, including behavioural and psychodynamic approaches to care. Courses are equally available to prepare qualified nurses to work in particular settings or with particular groups of clients, for example, community nursing and nursing children and families.

While specific courses are important, they do not necessarily meet all the needs of all practitioners. Clinical courses are not organized into any comprehensive framework, nor were they until recently recognized from an academic perspective. Innovations on the part of the Council for National Academic Awards (CNAA) in conjunction with professional bodies have done much to ensure academic recognition of clinical courses. The Credit Accumulation and Transfer Scheme (CATS) has been utilized in awarding pointage to clinical qualifications at both pre- and post-registration levels, such that nurses are currently able to gain credit towards higher education qualifications. In many cases, nurses pursuing undergraduate studies have been credited with up to half of a relevant degree.

Similarly, CATS can help to identify the academic level of professional courses, thus facilitating the development of structured programmes of study.

While CATS has helped to ensure appropriate accreditation of formal courses of study, other schemes have been developed to accredit learning gained through experience. Assessment of previous experiential learning (APEL) has enabled practitioners to gain formal academic recognition for learning gained through experience and, again, credit can be given against programmes of study in higher education.

In 1990, the UKCC launched Post-Registration Education and Practice Project (PREPP), with the aim of establishing a comprehensive framework of education for nurses beyond registration level. PREPP is concerned with three key areas: practice, education and standards. The Project has identified broad proposals that are currently the subject of a consultation process. It is likely, however, that the principles embodied within the proposals will be adopted. The Council envisages a future professional structure including three spheres of practice: practice following initial registration, specialist, and advanced practice. These spheres of practice are likely to be linked to a comprehensive educational framework, attracting both academic accreditation and professional approval, thus taking full advantage of CATS and APEL.

In the future, it is envisaged that continuing registration will be contingent upon the nurse maintaining professional education, thus ensuring maintenance of basic professional standards. Continuing education will not necessarily require nurses to attend formal courses, but they will be required to maintain a written personal profile of professional development. This profile will include evidence of further learning activities, as well as evidence of attempts to innovate and achieve excellence within practice. The profile will be subject to review processes, in order to establish competence to practice. The precise mechanisms for these review processes are yet to be established.

The ENB (1990) has also produced a framework for the continuing professional education of nurses, which can be viewed as being complementary to PREPP. It identifies a professional portfolio as the ongoing record of professional and academic development. The portfolio is likely to contribute to the personal profile required by the UKCC. Future requirements for maintaining professional portfolios/profiles are yet to be finally determined, but it is important to note that they are already considered by many higher education institutions in the cases of nurses seeking accreditation of experiential learning.

The future organization and structure of post-registration training is currently unclear, but it is likely that it will include a comprehensive framework of education, taking full advantage of developments such as CATS and APEL. Any vision of the future should include the idea of qualified nurses with a range of professional and academic qualifications, offering levels of practice commensurate with those qualifications.

## REFERENCES

ENB (1990) *Regulations and Guidelines for the Approval of Institutions and Courses 1990*, ENB, London.

ENB (1990) *Framework For Continuing Professional Education and Training for Nurses, Midwives and Health Visitors*, ENB, London.

*Nurses Midwives and Health Visitors Act* (1979), HMSO, London.

*Nurses Midwives and Health Visitors Rules* (1983), HMSO, London.

*Nurses, Midwives and Health Visitors (registered Fever Nurses) Amendment Rules* (1989) SI No. 145.

UKCC (1984) *Code of Professional Conduct for the Nurse, Midwife and Health Visitor*, UKCC, London.

UKCC (1986) *Project 2000 – A New Preparation for Practice*, UKCC London.

UKCC (1990) *Discussion Paper on Post-Registration Education and Practice*, UKCC, London.

*Jean Simms*

Although nurses work in organizations where caring is paramount, it is often the nurses themselves who become casualties of the system. Paradoxically, the nature of the profession itself creates much of the stress that individuals find so destructive. In this section we will look at the cost of caring, and the ways in which nurses can help to create a culture of support – one that is needed more than ever in the light of radical organizational, educational and clinical changes.

## THE STRESSES OF NURSING

According to the Royal College of Nursing (1978):

> ...the effectiveness of the individual nurse is too often judged in terms of his or her apparent ability to cope with these considerable stresses, although beneath the surface there may be concealed bitter frustration and anxiety. There has been a kind of 'destructive' stoicism which creates an atmosphere where it is difficult to meet adequately the problems of the individual or the organization, and which is partly reinforced by the nature of nursing training and discipline. In this atmosphere, nurses who cannot cope represent a threat to those who apparently manage to do so.

Chenevert (1978) takes this point further and suggests that nurses have a tendency to act like a flock of chickens: when one displays a sore spot, the rest peck at the spot until it dies. It seems that nurses who cannot conceal feelings of vulnerability often also have to cope with hostile reactions from their colleagues.

From inside the profession feelings are often expressed of being on a treadmill, with a pressure to succeed and to be all things to all people. Clinically, there is constant conflict over quality and quantity of care and, educationally, for more qualifications and higher degrees. The process of clinical grading and subsequent appeals add to these particular pressures.

The move away from institutional to community care has caused much concern, and there is much uncertainty as the major initiatives and influences become a reality. Since the Griffiths' Report (1983) on NHS management, there has been a move towards a more unitary management style. Changes include resource-management initiatives, quality and standards-of-care drives.

The government's White Papers *Working for Patients* and *Caring for People* give further emphasis to measurement of quality and efficiency, and the move towards community care leaves many nurses wondering and confused about their roles and functions. With Project 2000, changes in nurse education and the consequent effects on post-basic and continuing education also creates professional uncertainty.

What can be done to create a culture of support? Supervision, with its educational, managerial, and supportive elements is one way (Chapter 25), but potentially there are many ways to create a caring culture. First of all, it is necessary to know what people need in their personal and professional lives. Heron (1977) suggests that each person has three groups of basic emotional needs: firstly, love needs, including the need to love and be loved, and to give and to receive care, affection, warmth, appreciation, and support; secondly, understanding needs, including the need to understand and to be understood, and to communicate effectively to those around us, and to make sense of and accurately perceive the surrounding world; thirdly, the need for choice, including a need to communicate choice. Heron maintains that:

> The capacity here is the capacity to care and be cared for, to be concerned for the other's sake, and to be the conscious recipient of such concern.

and

> To be self-directing is to make autonomous choices – choices rationally made on the basis of relevant, factual considerations and in the light of one's own values.

The failure to meet these needs results in feelings of stress and vulnerability. Stress may be relieved or dealt with more effectively by either changing the demands inherent in the situation, or by changing the person's perception of them. However, it is often difficult to bring about change alone. An example of this comes from a student nurse, Graham:

> I had lots of studying and essays to write. I kept putting them off and didn't seem able to find the motivation to get on with the work. I really felt they were a waste of time and couldn't see the point in writing them. Fortunately, my supervisor helped me to look at my attitudes, and together we explored ways of making the essays meaningful and of putting academic work into practice and relating it to my work.

With help, Graham was able to change his attitude to his study, and find it more mean-ingful and relevant to his life and work. By changing his perception of the situation, his work became more enjoyable.

Nursing in a rural community setting can also be stressful. Here, Jake describes a scenario from his working day:

> It was the end of another difficult and exhausting day. I had driven many miles to see my clients, and was feeling tired and stressed. I had just seen a woman who was tearful and overwhelmed with sadness. In the course of my hour with her, I tried to help her work through her grief and anger, but knew I wasn't giving her all of my attention, and I began to get caught up in her helplessness and sadness. As I drove on, I began to get more and more confused, desperate, and sad. I tried to regain my composure and hated being unable to get my feelings under control. I turned my thoughts to home and sleep, but that night I couldn't sleep and kept restlessly and frantically turning, unable to find some peace of mind. I knew the next day would be equally demanding, and I promised myself I'd try to get out of this whirlpool of anxiety.

Jake kept the promise he had made to himself to try to make some sense of his situation and to search for ways of coping with this distress. One of the first steps he took was to understand cognitively the nature of stress as a general response of the human body to any kind of demand made on it, regardless of whether that demand was pleasant or unpleasant, emotional or physical.

The stressful effects of accidents, bereavement, or just trying to keep up, like Jake, with the often unremitting pressures of day-to-day tasks are obvious. Unless action is taken to alter the causes of the stress factors, or the body's reaction to them, exhaustion sets in. Jake was at this stage when he decided to do something positive and look for ways of reducing his high level of stress. If action is not taken, the body is no longer able to cope, and might collapse into disease; or a person may become helpless and retreat into passive resignation, failing utterly to cope with the physical and psychological demands of day-to-day living.

The first reaction of the body to any potentially harmful demand made on it is to prepare itself for action, either to face the danger (fight), or to run away (flight). Priority areas are the muscles, to make the body ready for physical action, and the heart, so it can pump more blood into those muscles. The lungs, too, need to provide more oxygen to the muscles for energy, and to the brain for alertness. High-energy foods, such as sugars and fats, are released into the blood; because of the overriding need of the muscles, the blood flow to organs, such as those of the digestive system, is cut off.

When the immediate danger passes, this gearing-up process is almost exactly reversed. The act of fighting and running away actually helps this reversal process. In our everyday lives, however, because many of the threatening situations we encounter we cannot fight or flee from, there is no physical action; the reversal process does not occur, and we remain 'wound up'.

When the body is exposed to stress over a long period of time, its biochemical state – constantly prepared for flight or fight – becomes chronic. Blood pressure is permanently raised and digestive problems arise; tension in the muscles leads to aches and pains, and disease or allergic responses may occur. This adaptation stage can last for many years without major mental or physical breakdown. Whether it will depends on many factors like the physical constitution, and the flexibility and motivation of the person to change.

Two important strategies for dealing with stress are relaxation and modifying behaviour to alleviate distress. Relaxation helps to lessen stress by distracting the mind away from stress-provoking thoughts. It also brings into play those parts of the nervous system that counter the effects of the flight-or-fight reaction. Whether clients or nurses, stress takes its toll. Many people search for deep psychophysical relaxation. Some of these, like meditation, stress the importance of manipulating the body in order to relax the mind.

The word 'therapy' originates from the Greek *therapeuein*, meaning to attend or to treat. If mental health nurses are aware of the variety of approaches to coping with distress, they can be used to increase both their own and their clients' sense of well-being.

There are many ways to cope with stress or distress. Taoism, an ancient Chinese philosophy, is about living and interacting with the environment. Jake, for example, was experiencing his 'busy syndrome', something that is familiar to many people, particularly those in the caring professions. Key words to begin to live less frenetically, adapted from Taoism, are 'acceptance' and 'going with the flow'.

Disciples of Tao do not clutter up their minds with worries, but simply adjust to what is happening around them. In the *Tao Te Ching*, the sage Lao Tzu returns again and again to the theme of letting go, exhorting, 'Stillness and tranquillity set things in order in the universe.' Non-action does not mean inactivity, but an absence of tension and strain, whatever we happen to be doing. The way we breathe, for example, signals the way we are feeling – agitated activity causes the breath to be uneven and rapid, but breathing slowly and evenly helps to calm, balance, and eventually change our mental and physical states towards a more harmonious way of being.

## CO-COUNSELLING

Co-counselling is a form of counselling that was introduced to Britain from the US in the 1970s. In the practice of co-counselling, each person takes it in turn to be counsellor and client, with the client choosing areas on which he/she wishes to work. The counsellor facilitates, listens and provides support in the form of a trusting, absolutely confidential, relationship. Co-counselling is usually done outside of the work situation, and there is a strong element of self-help to it. It is an essentially non-competitive form of therapy where two people meet on equal terms, and negotiate the time and agenda they wish to share within the context of this supportive relationship.

One crucial consideration of this type of counselling is confidentiality, and the assurance that what a client reveals in a session will never be repeated outside. Co-counsellors are more than friends; advice-giving, criticizing, judging, and making suggestions are taboo. The emphasis is on giving the best possible time, attention, space, and support to the person in the role of client.

Evison *et al.* (1988) describe the goals of co-counselling as helping individuals to:

- become more aware of their strengths and abilities, which are consequently more readily available when needed, and so can be built on and developed further;
- focus their attention where they choose, without being unwillingly or unwittingly distracted by distress;
- experience less distress from the negative events in their lives, both past and present, which continue to take up time and attention;
- break the destructive patterns that inhibit their intelligence, hinder new learning, and impede creative action.

Co-counselling is one avenue that the mental health nurse could utilize to take time out on a regular basis to explore feelings, and patterns of distress. The British Army use a buddy system, whereby soldiers are paired together as a source of support, assurance, and redirection. Nurses may adapt this as a way of formally building a relationship slightly different from the dimension of their friendships into their working life.

## FRIENDSHIP

Friendship helps to avoid emotional isolation and the symptoms associated with this, such as anxiety, emptiness, a sense of loss, and abandonment. Rogers (1959) believed that if people do not feel they are liked, they may suspect something is wrong with them and spend much time trying to earn social approval from others. Rogers called this need for social approval 'positive regard'. Friendships supply this, and meet many human needs, the basis of which is trust, survival, and mutual protection.

## STAFF-SUPPORT GROUPS

There are a bewildering number of conflicting definitions of what a group is. There are, however, attributes that theorists agree are important features of groups. The key concepts include:

- A set of people who identify with one another and who agree to meet and engage in frequent interaction;
- they define themselves and are defined with others as a group;
- they share beliefs, values, and norms about areas of common interest;
- they come together to work on common tasks and for agreed purposes.

Groups are organic and intentional, and not just a random experience. People come together to satisfy some common need or interest. Groups are about developing a sense of identity and belonging, and establishing cohesion and trust. Probably the most famous work on groups and their 'curative factors' was carried out by Yalom (1970), who identified them as : self-understanding; interaction; universality (the realization that his/her problems are not unique); instillation of hope (belief that participation in the group will be beneficial); altruism (benefit derived from the recognition that group members can help each other); guidance; identification;

cohesiveness; being authentic and taking responsibility for oneself.

There is value in nurses meeting together and supporting each other, both in daily contact and in structured support groups. Staff support groups can be useful in three dimensions. First, at a personal developmental level, they offer ways of increasing self-awareness, perception of others and understanding the therapeutic use of self. Second, for personal growth, support groups supply opportunities to seek help with personal problems, and perhaps differentiate one's own problems from those of clients; and of sharing, giving, and getting help and support. Third, managerially they are useful in enabling and ensuring team co-operation; in the formulations of policies; and in fostering effective team practices and relationships.

Through staff support groups there are opportunities for like-minded people to meet together and negotiate the agenda and areas on which they would like the group to focus. Even if there are only a few members, it is a valuable way of creating and increasing a sense of belonging, especially for people who, like Jake, feel isolated and separated from colleagues. The contact and exchange of ideas, thoughts, and feelings are all ways of enabling the mental health nurse to feel energized and creative. This type of group could be a life and sanity saver.

An alternative is to join, or be instrumental in setting up, a support group that has a facilitator or group leader. It is important that the group leader is experienced, qualified, and not motivated from self-interest, especially the pursuit of power. An effectively led group can offer insight and perception into interpersonal dynamics.

Benson (1987) gives 'survival' procedures for group workers, which are worth noting:

- Avoid crucifixions.

He sounds a warning note:

You are not a messiah nor are group members your disciples. So do not try to save, protect, rescue, or work it out for everyone all of the time. It is difficult to watch another person in pain or see them make what appears to be an unavoidable error, but often this is an essential part of their growth and you can best help by allowing it to happen.

- Do not push the river upstream. This is summarized as 'going with the flow' of the group; it is not about forcing encounters or telling people what to do.
- Learn to wait, listen, keep quiet, and remain attentive.
- Learn to forgive yourself; in the course of working with groups, mistakes are made.
- Cultivate goodwill; keep in mind why you thought the group was a good idea originally, and maintain this attitude towards group members.
- Make up your own rules; be creative and use imagination in deciding the best course of action or thing to do: 'The important thing to remember is that you do the best you can and let it go at that.'

Constructive feedback must be done in a way that is clear, specific, supportive, and about behaviour that can be changed. Feedback can be destructive if it is badly and insensitively expressed.

It is also important to avoid taking up so much time helping others that there is no time for self-care.

## ORGANIZATIONAL SUPPORT STRUCTURES

Most organizations have a formal support structure that delineates formal responsibilities and the lines of authority of individuals and organizational units. Aside from this formal structure, informal relationships frequently evolve. The organizational structure should be one in which people can perform most effectively; have information made available to them; feel valued and acknowledged; have good enough support; and appropriate ways of letting off steam. Examples of formal support are given below.

## COUNSELLING SERVICES

Many organizations have counselling and guidance services to try to meet the developmental needs of staff. These may vary, but overall the aim of such counselling is to help develop self-understanding, awareness of potentialities, and knowledge of how to best use one's capabilities.

## INDIVIDUAL COUNSELLING

I went to the counsellor because I just couldn't cope with the work. Both my parents died within months of each other, and I was trying to meet the commitment of working on a busy medical ward. I kept experiencing feelings of fear and 'butterflies' in my stomach – the grief and fear kept getting mixed up. Then I woke up in the night and kept going over my day's work and checking that I had done everything correctly.

The counsellor explored with Catherine her unrealistic expectations of herself, and the importance of allowing the expression of her feelings and giving herself time and space to grieve.

## GROUP COUNSELLING

Some counsellors arrange group sessions that can give a unique opportunity for members to compare and contrast attitudes, values, and feelings. One such group, for example, was organized after staff had been involved in counselling survivors of the Lockerbie air disaster. Pamela, one group member, reflected:

We were working individually in a very intense way with grieving relatives. The impact of the sudden and violent death

on survivors was often too horrific for words. We didn't seem to have time to take care of ourselves. I began to have dreams about being involved in the air crash myself. I thought everybody else was coping, and it was a relief to know I wasn't the only one suffering in this way. We decided to set up a group – it saved my sanity.

## ETHOS

For any form of counselling to be effective, it is vital that the counselling itself is not identified with education, service, or the administration – that is, it occupies a neutral place within the organization. It is important that it is not a disciplinary agency, and should provide a unique atmosphere where staff can explore anxieties, needs and problems in an atmosphere of trust.

If confidentiality within this relationship is ever likely to be broken, they need to know when and if this should arise. If areas of vulnerability and weaknesses are in danger of being disclosed outside of the relationship, staff will not relax their defences.

Additionally, the counsellor may have to set limits imposed upon by him/her by the organization, and these need to be made known to clients.

## STUDENT PROBLEMS

Many student nurses are living away from home for the first time and may experience difficulties in having to cope with this transition. They may experience difficulties in defining themselves, and being accepted by their contemporaries. Writing of student casualties, Ryle (1969) describes the first problems they may encounter:

The lack of dependable sources of acceptance, the uncertainty of role and the possible conflict between roles, and the exposure to the challenge of an unstructured environment in which debate about values and an absence of imposed ideologies are prized, can all combine with a sense of fragmentation and unreality in the student – the state of identity diffusion.

Other researchers have found that problems affecting students may be categorized into four main groups: academic, vocational, personal relationships, and finances. Depression was one of the most commonly presenting factors, which frequently stemmed from deteriorating relationships, parental breakdown, and remarriage. Bereavement and loss were also a major problem. Academically, students seeking help had problems in meeting deadlines and coping with their own, often unrealistic, deadlines, or trying to live up to unrealistic parental expectations.

Staff who make complaints about malpractice may need support while doing so and after. Beardshaw (1981) reports on nurses who make such complaints, and their fears. As one student nurse explained:

I have no confidence in any complaints procedures as it has been clear to me on more than one occasion that people who complain are not popular. In most hospitals the union is informally integrated into the management. People 'look after' one another to make sure no problems arise. Unions are quite likely to persuade one to be reasonable.

Being an advocate for clients is not always easy, and Beardshaw warns against concentrating just on the abuse of clients, rather than on what to do to avoid it: 'Ideally "complaining" in mental hospitals would lose all its stigma, and become integrated into a mutual support system for staff. People who work in mental hospitals do a difficult and stressful job – and one that isn't valued enough to be given the best possible conditions and facilities.' She believes, in keeping with many mental health nurses and educationalists, that understanding of basic human frailty could be the foundation for a system where open, constructive questioning and criticism would make formal complaining unnecessary.

There are outside sources of counselling, like the Royal College of Nursing, which has a counselling service for people who are going through crises and want one way counselling or help. Counsellors hold sessions in various parts of the country for its members (page 326). Personnel and occupational health departments also provide advice-giving and help, and there are also hospital chaplains who give pastoral care. Some are trained in counselling or psychotherapy, and are in the organization to help both staff and clients. Finally, the majority of schools have a system of personal tutors to help with educational and personal issues that may arise from being a student.

History has shown that conflict within organizations has brought about many changes, but when conflict gets out of hand it tends to become destructive and undesirable for all. It is therefore imperative that support systems are established that enable conflict to be confronted, and the feelings engendered to be worked through towards a healthy resolution.

At an individual level, there are many ways stress can be lessened and used creatively instead of destructively. Below is a checklist that comes from a variety of sources. People have used, added to it, acted upon it, and found the advice life-enhancing, and sometimes, life-saving. Every so often it may be read through as a reminder of the ways in which changes can realistically be made.

**Table 24.1** Take care of yourself checklist

Physical activity is a good way to work off stress, so try to take at least five minutes a day of physical exercise.

Get enough rest and sleep, and look after your own physical and mental health.

Talk to someone you can really trust, or use a telephone help-line, for example, the Samaritans.

Be gentle with yourself and learn to accept what you cannot change.

Avoid self-medication, or too many stimulants like tea and coffee.

Free yourself from your work routine at least one-and-a-half days every week.

Plan an 'away-from-it-all' holiday once a year; take time out to play and have fun.

Manage your time better; find a system that enables you to cope with the demands made on your time.

Cultivate the art of listening to drama, music, or poetry.

Plan ahead. By saying no now, you may prevent pressure piling up.

If you are ill, do not carry on as if you are not; take heed of the warning signs.

Develop a hobby – something to counterbalance your normal work or routine.

Take time to prepare food; eat it slowly and mindfully.

Use supervision or support systems regularly.

Before you go to sleep, remember and celebrate three good things that have happened to you and three things you have done really well during the day.

If you are unhappy with your present relationship or your work, look at the alternatives.

Express your feelings more; smile often.

Join a yoga or meditation class.

Know when you are tired and do something about it.

Be realistic about perfection; it is about being 'good enough'.

Agree more often – life should not be a constant battleground.

Avoid the tendency to dwell on the past - concentrate on the present.

Remind yourself you are an enabler, not a magician, and cannot achieve the impossible.

Delegate responsibility.

Avoid 'shop talk' during meal breaks.

Say 'I choose' rather than 'I should/ought/have to.'

Remember, caring and being are as important as doing.

Give support to others and learn to accept it in return - try to balance giving and receiving.

**REFERENCES**

*Counselling in Nursing* (1978), The Royal College of Nursing, London.

Chenevert, M. (1978) *Special Techniques in Assertiveness Training for Women*, C.V. Mosby, St Louis.

Heron, J. (1977) *Catharsis in Human Development*, British Postgrad. Med. Fed., Univ. London.

Tzu, L. (1963) *Tao Te Ching*, Penguin, Harmondsworth.

Evison, E. and Horobin, R. (1988) Co-counselling - historical context and developments in Britain, in *Innovative Therapies in Britain* (eds J. Rowan, W. Dryden),

Rogers, C. R. (1959) A theory of therapy, personality and interpersonal relationships as developed in a client-centred framework, in *A Study of Science* (ed. S. Koch), McGraw-Hill, New York.

Yalom, I. (1970) *The Theory and Practice of Group Psychotherapy*, Basic Books, New York.

Benson, J. F. (1987) *Working Creatively With Groups*, Tavistock Publications, London.

Ryle, A. (1969) *Student Casualties*, Allen Lane, Harmondsworth.

Beardshaw, V. (1981) *Conscientious Objectors At Work, Mental Hospital Nurses – A Case Study*, Social Audit Limited, London.

## FURTHER READING

Cartwright, D. and Zander A. (eds) (1968) *Group Dynamics, Research and Theory*, Tavistock Publications, London.

## USEFUL ADDRESSES AND INFORMATION

COUNSELLING

The British Association for Counselling
37a Sheep Street
Rugby, Warwickshire
CV21 3BX
0788 578328

Open to all individuals and organizations concerned with counselling, at all levels.

Counselling Help and Advice (CHAT)
Royal College of Nursing
20 Cavendish Square
London W1M OAB

The Westminster Pastoral Foundation
23 Kensington Square
London W8 5HN
Supply a list of counselling centres all over the country.

CO-COUNSELLING

For details send a stamped addressed envelope to:

Co-counselling International
c/o Westerly
Prestwick Lance
Chiddingfold
Surrey GU8 4XW

PSYCHOTHERAPY

Psychotherapy is sometimes, although not always, available on the NHS. Your GP may also be able to refer you to a private (fee-paying) psychotherapist, alternatively contact:

The British Psychological Society
St Andrew's House
4 Princess Road East
Leicester LE1 7DR

GESTALT THERAPY

For a list of therapists contact:

Gestalt Therapy Centre
c/o 64 Warwick Road
St Alban's, Herts. AL1 4DL

GRIEF COUNSELLING

CRUSE
Cruse House
126 Sheen Road
Richmond, Surrey TW9 1UR

Stillbirth and Neonatal Death Society
28 Portland Place
London W1N 4DE

ALCOHOL-RELATED PROBLEMS

Alcohol Concern
305 Gray's Inn Road
London WC1X

Alcoholics Anonymous
PO 1
Stonebow House
Stonebow, Yorks YO1 2NJ

The Accept Clinic
200 Seagrave Road
London SW6 IRQ

Al-Anon Family Groups
61 Great Dover Street
London SE1 4YF

If you need specific advice, your local library should have the *Someone to Talk to Directory*, published by the Mental Health Foundation. The Foundation can also provide a list of counsellors with a wide range of expertise.

If your GP cannot help, the Citizens' Advice Bureau or local church may be able to.

USEFUL REFERENCES.

Action on Smoking and Health (ASH)
25-27 Mortimer Street
London W1N 7RJ

Keep Fit Association/Sports Council
70 Brompton Road
London SW3 1EX

Women's Therapy Centre
6 Manor Gardens
London N7 6LA

Ramblers' Association
1-4 Crawford Mews
York Street
London W1H 1PT

Relaxation for Living
This is a registered charity that trains relaxation teachers, and also offers information and courses. Send an SAE to:

Dunesk
29 Burwood Park Road
Walton-on-Thames
Surrey KT 12 5LH
Yoga for Health Foundation
Offers residential courses in Hatha yoga, including special courses for people with special needs:
Ickwell Bury
Northhill
Nr Biggleswade, Bedfordshire

The Wheel of Yoga
Co-ordinates teacher training, and can give information about courses:

Acacia House
Centre Avenue
Acton Vale
London W3 7JX

*Jean Simms*

Mental health nurses encounter and engage with many and varied clients in the course of their day-to-day work. These often include clients who are distressed, depressed, overwhelmed with the problems of daily living, and who are often struggling to make sense of their lives. Contemporary mental health nursing practice is an interpersonal process that seeks to help such individuals and their families as far as possible alleviate distress, and to feel empowered in taking control of their lives.

Working with clients' thoughts, feelings, and ways of behaving within the context of complex, intense, and demanding relationships can be a minefield; the abstract nature of mental health nursing often makes the work both exhilarating and exhausting. Mental illness itself challenges many of our assumptions about normality. In mental health nursing, many dilemmas and tensions exist between what is ideal and what is pragmatic; nurses often encounter conflict as they move between the roles of clinician, educator, manager, and researcher.

For all of these reasons, supervision is an integral part of mental health nursing – a way of ensuring and enabling the nurse to give the client the best possible care available. Supervisors should enable students to become highly skilled, knowledgeable, and self-aware practitioners.

## AN HISTORICAL PERSPECTIVE

Supervision of clinical practice in a mental health setting is still a contentious issue, even though it is over 40 years since formal supervision was made a prerequisite for student nurses working in this context. Although there is still no consensus about definitions, principles, and practices of mental health nursing supervision, and very little published research, there is a growing and acknowledged awareness of and commitment to the value of supervision and the supervisory relationship.

Supervision began with Freudian psychoanalytical practice around 1925. Since then, many approaches to supervision have developed, particularly in the areas of counselling, psychotherapy and social work. Mental health nurses can learn from such professionals who extensively use supervision, and consider it fundamental to their training and practice.

As far as nursing is concerned, in 1943 the Horder Committee affirmed the need for the development of supervision in mental health nursing. Opportunities for supervision to be integrated into mental health nursing education and practice were made more possible with the implementation of the 1982 Registered Mental Nurse syllabus. The holistic nature of this syllabus changed supervision from a concept into a reality, and to a more accepted way of working – not just for students, but for trained staff also.

The practice of supervision in mental health nursing has gained momentum, as its value in helping to ensure safe and competent practice, and in developing the knowledge, skills, and attitudes of mental health nurses has become increasingly recognized by the profession.

In 1985, Ruth Schrock, nurse researcher and academic, advocated that students must be 'permitted to explore areas of knowledge, and skill on an individual basis.' With its varied tasks, supervision allows this to happen. It helps the nurse by extending knowledge, developing clinical skills, and increasing the capacity for reflection and self-evaluation.

## A DEFINITION OF SUPERVISION

In the disciplines of counselling, psychotherapy, and social work, supervision has many definitions and tasks. Whatever their differing views, all agree that supervision is primarily for the protection of the client, and a way of helping practitioners to develop skills and attitudes within the context of a trusting and supportive relationship.

For some practitioners in mental health settings, the term 'supervision' is synonymous with monitoring. The dictionary defines it as 'critical watching and directing', or the 'action, process, or occupation of supervising; a critical watching and directing, e.g. of activities or a course of action', which supports these misconceptions. This often adds to the anxiety and resistance about the use of supervision in clinical practice. To try to find less contentious alternatives, some mental health divisions use words such as 'mentor', 'preceptor', and 'facilitator' instead of supervisor.

The word 'supervision' takes on an entirely different meaning when it is broken into the two syllables 'super' and 'vision'. In this context, supervision is not only seeing beyond what is immediately obvious, but also being able to use all the senses to seek to understand the same situation from many different perspectives.

The British Association for Counselling's definition of supervision, found in their Code of Ethics and Practice for the Supervision of Counsellors (1988), also lends itself to mental health practice:

The term supervision encompasses a number of functions concerned with monitoring, developing and supporting individuals in their counselling role whilst ensuring at the same time the best interest of the client are served.

BAC stress that supervision is not just for the benefit of the supervisee, but, again, to protect the client in enabling and ensuring competence.

## MODELS OF SUPERVISION

Proctor (1986) sees supervision as a working alliance between supervisor and supervisee, a relationship in which casework is presented, and feedback and guidance then given. The dimensions within this relationship are managerial, educational, and supportive. The model of supervision she endorses has elements of the normative, formative, and restorative, and is useful since it cuts across multidisciplinary roles and boundaries (Table 25.1).

**Normative**, **formative**, and **restorative** are three shorthand words that are used to denote the variety of tasks that need to be undertaken by supervisor and supervisee in the process of supervision.

### THE NORMATIVE ASPECT

This provides the quality in supervision. The focus here is on, for example, values, beliefs, evaluation of care, documentation, Health Authorities' policies and procedures, issues of accountability, and caseload management. This aspect of supervision implies the task of overseeing; when a supervisor agrees to supervise, s/he agrees to represent both organizational and professional standards of effective practice.

Understanding organizational philosophies and principles is important. Without a clear understanding of how the organization is structured, it is impossible for the mental health nurse to work effectively and creatively.

**Table 25.1** A model of supervision

| | | |
|---|---|---|
| | **Normative** | |
| | Monitoring of standards, ethical issues. | |
| | Evaluation of work. | |
| | Caseload management. | |
| | Organizational policies and procedures, record-keeping, etc. | |

| **Formative** | **Restorative** |
|---|---|
| Theoretical knowledge. | Recognition of inherent work-related |
| Identification and development of mental | stressors. |
| health nursing skill. | Enabling the mental health nurse to work |
| Integration of theory and practice. | imaginatively and creatively. |

There may, however, be conflict between the goals of the organization and the needs of people working within it. An example comes from Rosa, a 20-year-old student nurse, who was troubled by the aggressive attitudes of some of the more experienced mental health nurses towards their elderly clients. To what degree should Rosa take responsibility for such attitudes? After all, she was only a student nurse in training. Rosa turned to her supervisor for ways of assertively advocating the clients' case.

Another example comes from Emma, who confessed to Susan, the community psychiatric nurse, that she felt aggressive towards her two-year-old son. So far she had held back and contained her violent feelings, but she was frightened she might not be able to control her anger.

Susan wanted to work with Emma, and not disclose this information outside the nurse/client relationship. She believed that trust between herself and Emma would be threatened, and even destroyed, if she did. The conflict between the need to preserve confidentiality and to work with the organization's policy, that such information needed to be disclosed, was worked through in supervision. Susan's duty of care was to protect the child and to help Emma to deal with her anger without putting the child at risk. Supervision enabled her to realize that confidentiality in the nurse/client relationship is not absolute; for example, information may need to be given as evidence in court. For this reason it is important that at the outset of the relationship the client knows the conditions under which confidentiality is both maintained and broken. The normative aspects of this example were clarification of the organization's policy, and the legal perspective on confidentially.

THE FORMATIVE ASPECT

This is concerned with the identification and development of skills, and the integration of theory with practice.

In the above example, Emma's overwhelming fear was that her anger would explode. Part of Susan's care for her would be to assist Emma to recognize and label anger, and to communicate to her that angry feelings are normal. By helping Emma to learn techniques of assertiveness, Susan began to deal successfully with her problem in an assertive way. The appropriate expression of anger became a self-reinforcing process.

The parallelling process of supervision would be that by enabling Susan to help Emma to successfully assert herself, she herself could learn to be more assertive, to deal constructively with her own anger, and to experience good feelings about herself. Through supervision, Susan also became more aware of both her own and Emma's unhealthy ways of dealing with anger, such as defensiveness, retaliation, condescension, and avoidance.

Emma told Susan she was also anxious, could not sleep, and often found herself becoming increasingly agitated. In negotiating care with Emma, it was agreed that relaxation should be included in her care plan. Susan did not feel sufficiently confident to carry out relaxation techniques but, with the guidance of her supervisor, she was able to practice relaxation techniques, and to discuss the general benefits of relaxation, and ways of encouraging her client to incorporate relaxation as part of her day-to-day living.

Emma's original needs were thus met through the protection of her defences, and the discharging of her emotions and anxiety through physical activity. While developing the therapeutic relationship with Emma, Susan also monitored her own levels of anxiety and ways of dealing with anger.

## THE RESTORATIVE ASPECT

This dimension seeks to create a supervisory relationship in which the supervisee feels '... received, valued, understood on the assumption that only then will he feel safe and open enough to review and challenge himself, as well as to value himself and his own abilities.' This supportive part of supervision is especially important, since a report for the Royal College of Nursing suggested that extreme stress was one of the reasons why nurses leave the National Health Service. As a community psychiatric nurse said:

Working in a community setting, I felt very isolated and often vulnerable in my work. Travelling around a rural area meant it was often impossible to return to base on a daily basis. The intensity of some of the encounters with clients often left me exhausted. I remember driving after such an encounter and failing to see the traffic lights. This incident made me take action. I got a group of my colleagues together. Now we meet for weekly, one-hour supervision sessions. These have proved to be life-savers. I feel much less isolated, my knowledge has increased, and my client work is more creative.

In practice, the normative, formative, and restorative functions overlap, and the different categories may become blurred. Supervision provides a medium for ensuring individual, systematic client care; a continuous learning process where mental health nursing principles and practices can be explored and evaluated.

Zelda, a mental health nurse, mentions in supervision she finds it hard to work with clients who admit to child sexual abuse. With her supervisor, she acknowledges her

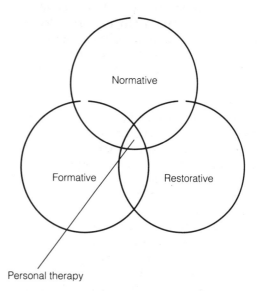

**Figure 25.1** Integration of the three aspects of supervision

prejudices and feelings when faced with this client group. She admits to her own inexperience, and discusses ways of increasing her knowledge and improving her skills. Her supervisor suggests how this conflict may be resolved, and agrees to give time in supervision to explore feelings, and to identify and work to develop the necessary skills (formative). Additionally, she will ensure that Zelda is fully conversant with the hospital's organizational policies on dealing with sexually abused clients and perpetrators of this type of abuse (normative).

This information was received by the supervisor in a non-judgmental way and Zelda felt encouraged to share her true feelings, not just pretend they did not exist. The caring attitude (restorative) of the supervisor gave Zelda the confidence that the supervisor had both time and space to reflect on Zelda's work. By really listening to Zelda, not contradicting nor blaming her for expressing her feelings, the supervisor created a relationship in which Zelda could admit to her feelings of vulnerability, without the need to defend herself. If there is a punitive, destructively critical element in the supervisory relationship, the supervisee may not feel safe to admit 'mistakes', and will be highly selective in the casework presented within the context of the supervisory relationship.

The need for supervision is based on the premise that mental health nurses want to monitor their own practice, learn from experience, and develop competence within the context of a supportive and encouraging relationship. In this way, supervision also helps to create self-aware and confident practitioners.

Three models of supervision have been described: the first is client-centred, in which the technical problems relating to the client are talked through in supervision; the second is therapist-centred, in which the focus is on the mental health nurse's psychological blindspots and counter-transference reactions;

and the third is process-centred, which emphasizes what is happening between the therapist, client, and supervisor.

Holloway *et al.* (1989), have characterized two elemental dimensions in the supervisory relationship, engagement and power, which they include in their model of supervision: Engagement and Power In Clinical Supervision (EPICS). This counselling model assumes that:

- The primary objective in supervision is to facilitate the counsellors acquisition of counselling skills, and empower him/her to utilize these skills in an appropriately professional manner.
- The supervisory relationship is the primary context for facilitating the learning of counselling skills.
- Both the content and the process of supervision are important components of supervision.
- The essential element in the supervisory relationship is power expressed through engagement.

Learning from experience is a sophisticated skill, and the relationship between the supervisor and supervisee is potentially one on which the foundations of effective practice are built.

## THE PURPOSE OF SUPERVISION

Supervision has many purposes, including the promotion of competent and accountable work, which concerns both the supervisee and the client. Another is the facilitation of personal and professional development. An example of this comes from John, a community psychiatric nurse:

John was flattered when a client he had only just met kept ringing him and telling him he was the only person who could help and understand him. The client went on to catalogue a list of grievances against past and present professionals, telling John, 'I knew instantly you would be able to sort out my problems and make things right for me. Nobody really cared about me until you came into my life.'

Without supervision, John might have begun a relationship with the client that was doomed from the outset to fail. He genuinely wanted to help his client, and the flattery made him feel powerful and important. However, if John wanted to help the client use his potential for growth, then he had to acknowledge his own feelings and be aware of issues of power and dependency within the context of his relationship with this client.

Reflecting with his supervisor on this initial contact, John was immediately alerted to possible reasons why the client responded to him in this way. First, the client's life experience had taught him to be a victim, someone who always – seemingly without any fault of their own – came out of situations badly. Second, since victims need rescuing, John could easily have taken on the role of rescuer. Third, the client could have become too dependent on John, looking to him to come up with all the answers, and to solve his problems for him.

Sooner or later, John would not have been able to meet this client's unrealistic expectations and would have been put on the client's 'blacklist'. John was also aware that he might have a hidden need for power in directing other peoples lives, especially people he considered worse off than himself.

As the relationship with this client progressed, John found himself becoming emotionally drained with this intense relationship, especially when the client continually communicated feelings of despair, hopelessness, and sadness. Supervision was a vehicle by which John could share and work with these feelings. In this way he became 'de-stressed' and more enabled to work in a creative and energetic way.

Stuart *et al.* (1987), have written extensively on this subject and make the following comment:

> The painful nature of these emotional responses make the practice of psychiatric nursing challenging and stressful. The therapeutic use of self involves the nurse's total personality and total involvement is not an easy task. It is essential that the nurse be aware of her feelings and responses and receive guidance and support in her work.

Supervision, then, is a way of reflecting on and making sense of the way people relate, both to themselves and others. It presupposes there are reasons why people sometimes behave irrationally. Reasons for this may not be immediately obvious, either to the person involved or others around. It also assumes there are processes that underlie feelings and behaviour that are constantly changing.

Many researchers and writers have drawn attention to how the process of supervision parallels the nurse-client relationship. Both are designed to be a learning process, a process that takes place within the context of a relationship that facilitates positive change, both at a personal and professional level.

Respect is a foundation of the supervisory relationship – respect not only for the process of supervision, but for the supervisee, the client, the relationship, the philosophy and aims of the organization, and the mental health nursing profession.

It is not only the supervisors who have responsibilities if the supervision process is to succeed. Supervisees need to be able to develop the ability to recognize what is appropriate to bring to supervision; to share what is creating difficulties or tensions in their work; and to be open and discriminating in the face of constructive feedback.

Supervision is an essentially enabling relationship, in which supervisor and supervisee should have a shared interest in and agree-

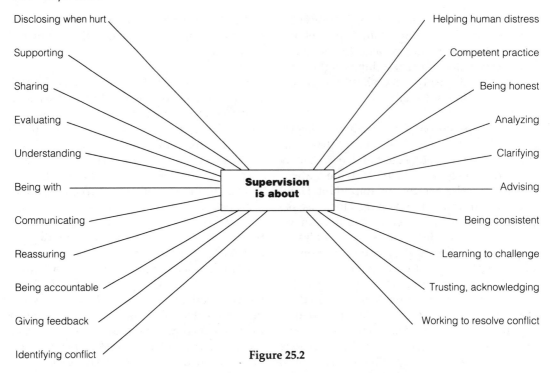

Disclosing when hurt

Supporting

Sharing

Evaluating

Understanding

Being with

Communicating

Reassuring

Being accountable

Giving feedback

Identifying conflict

**Supervision is about**

Helping human distress

Competent practice

Being honest

Analyzing

Clarifying

Advising

Being consistent

Learning to challenge

Trusting, acknowledging

Working to resolve conflict

**Figure 25.2**

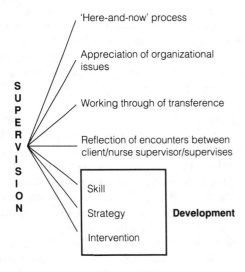

'Here-and-now' process

Appreciation of organizational issues

Working through of transference

Reflection of encounters between client/nurse supervisor/supervises

Skill

Strategy        **Development**

Intervention

**SUPERVISION**

**Figure 25.3**

ment about what is competent and effective work. Supervision involves a joint responsibility and commitment to a continuing relationship that includes challenging and confronting unwise or unethical practices, as well as teaching new skills and ways of working. As Proctor (1986) states:

> Overall the quality of the supervision depends on both parties' ability to communicate clearly and openly. The development of this ability is the foundation of accountable learning, and is the stuff of counselling and interpersonal practice. It presupposes a high degree of self-awareness, interpersonal sensitivity and political nous.

Proctor has adapted Rogers' propositions, and suggests their significance to the supervision process:

- to the extent that the supervisor can be transparently respectful, the supervisee can be self-managing;

- to the extent that the supervisor can be empathic, the supervisee can be honest;
- to the extent that the supervisor can be trustworthy, the supervisee can be confiding;
- to the extent that the supervision can be open, the supervisee can be respectful;
- to the extent that the supervisor can be straightforward, the supervisee can be self-appraising.

Here, nurses receiving supervision for their clinical practice share their own experiences:

I worked for a number of years in community settings and, although I was aware of the comparative isolation of my work, did not realize how stressed I felt. My caseload management was often chaotic, and sometimes I just responded by going from one crisis to the next. It was not until I found a supervisor and reviewed my practice on a weekly basis that I began to manage myself more effectively.

Supervision continually helps me to look at my own motivations for doing this kind of work [community mental health]. I came into the profession wanting to acquire the skills in order to help others to change. Supervision has enabled me to broaden my experience and develop both at a personal and a professional level. As a result of my supervisory relationship, I feel more confident. By dealing with my own conflicts and prejudices, for example, I now feel I can deal with those of my clients more effectively.

A mental health worker who was given a directive that he should have supervision added another perspective:

When it was suggested to me that I was to have supervision, I was very angry. I had been working for a number of years and nobody had complained about my work. It took a long time to change this attitude and to trust my supervisor, but she offered me different perspectives and taught me to identify my existing skills and build on them.

The use of clinical supervision must be a prerequisite to effective therapeutic practice. As Platt-Koch (1986) points out '...it is a disservice to both the patient and the nurse to attempt to do psychiatric treatment without adequate clinical supervision.' Supervision is a valuable tool, which the nurse should use fully to develop a professional self. However, supervision can and does fail when there is lack of appreciation and understanding of its concepts and principles and practices: for example, when there is insufficient time and attention paid to the process; where there is insufficient knowledge, skill, or negative attitudes; and where there is a culture of mistrust and suspicion.

## THE ROLE OF THE SUPERVISOR

Within the supervisory relationship there inevitably will be issues of power, which need to be spelt out at the beginning of the relationship. The responsibilities of the supervisor should be clearly set out and negotiated, and the differences between a non-managerial and a consultant supervision fully understood. Sometimes, although not always, the supervisor has clear accountability to provide written reports to the organization on the supervisee's progress. Supervisors of students in training may provide written progress reports, but with trained staff this may not be the case.

To be effective, the supervisor needs to have the same qualities and skills as an effective mental health nurse. These include the ability to listen; to create rapport; to validate; and to communicate respect, understanding, and genuineness, as well as warmth and unconditional positive regard.

If supervisors are to carry out their roles and functions, then they need not only the authority but the energy and the creativity to carry out their obligations and responsibilities to their supervisees.

Frankham (1968) has encapsulated what he considers the twelve roles of the supervisor:

1. Monitor – to ensure the maintenance of professional standards (*normative*).
2. Teacher – to impart counselling theory (*formative*).
3. Manager – to ensure the pursuit of agency policy and practice (*normative*).
4. Mentor – to provide a supportive and sustaining environment (*restorative*).
5. Trainer – to provide training in counselling skills (*formative*).
6. Therapist – to provide counselling or therapy (*restorative*).
7. Mirror – to facilitate the counsellor's explorations (*restorative*).
8. Analyst – to identify unconscious factors in the counselling relationship (*formative*).
9. Evaluator – to assess counsellor competence (*normative*).
10. Reviewer – to formulate and review counselling roles (*normative*).
11. Facilitator – to assess the counsellor's level of stress (*restorative*).
12. Union representative (*normative*).

Note: My italics

Stuart and Sundeen (1979) see the supervisor as someone who serves as a provider of theoretical knowledge and technique, and who validates an individual, systematic approach to client care.

Working with clients in often intense and demanding relationships means that nurses have to look at their relationships in more detail, and become more skilled and more creative in handling these relationships, than in other situations. Kathleen, a newly qualified mental health nurse, found it difficult to see beyond the diagnosis given to clients on her caseload:

I felt very confident when I was giving medication to clients – the effect in reducing their psychological distress was often very dramatic. While this may have been appropriate at the time, it was when I began to realize there were alternative ways of enabling clients to cope that I saw the value of supervision.

Supervision helped me to extend my knowledge of the nurse/client relationship and to identify factors that bring about client change. It also enabled me to see clients as human beings, not just as 'schizophrenics' or 'depressives'. I began

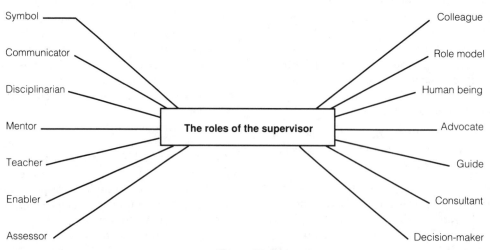

**Figure 25.4**

to feel more confident when I could identify the skills I was using, and see the relationships between myself and clients in a different light.

Negative supervision experiences have been characterized by a lack of effective teaching, inadequate role modelling, and being suddenly 'abandoned' by the supervisor. A mental health nurse shared her experience of this:

> It took time for me and my supervisor to form a working alliance, and then she suddenly announced she was leaving. We were in the middle of some difficult casework. It was several months before I got over the feeling of abandonment by her.

Supervisors who ridiculed supervisees when they disagreed with their particular way of working, or those who were either too strict or too relaxed were also disliked by supervisees. Glenda was on the receiving end of such a relationship:

> I was looking forward to working with my supervisor, but I soon began to dread seeing him. He was constantly finding fault with my work. I knew I had a lot to learn, but I soon became fearful and over-anxious about my client work. I really suffered. This supervisor had to write reports about my progress and was in a powerful position. It was only when he moved and I had another more positive experience of supervision that I realized its value and importance. I still recall those early encounters in supervision. I felt it was all my fault and felt disempowered by what was happening to me.

There are many fears and anxieties that supervisees may have as they set out to begin a supervisory relationship. Such anxieties may arise from both the relationship they have with their supervisor, and the relationships they have with their clients. For example, they may fear it is not just the skills they lack but something may be wrong with their personality. Glenda learnt the hard way, and her experiences of negative supervision made her more determined not to repeat this experience when she eventually became a supervisor herself.

## THE SUPERVISOR'S RESPONSIBILITIES

In exploring supervision research and writing, the supervisor's responsibilities seem to revolve around the following (Figure 25.4):

- Enabling supervisees to explore and clarify the thinking, feelings, behaviours, attitudes, and fantasies that underlie their mental health nursing practice.
- Sharing their knowledge, professional experiences, skills interventions, techniques, and strategies.
- Challenging practices that abuse the privileged relationships between nurse/client and are considered illegal, unethical, or incompetent.
- Identifying personal or professional difficulties that are perceived to hinder effective client care.
- Helping supervisees understand how their stereotypical thoughts, actions, and unresolved issues affect their client work.
- Awareness of the duties and responsibilities that the supervisor and the supervisee have to themselves, their clients, their organization, and their profession.

The late paediatrician and psychoanalyst Donald Winnicott (1965), introduced the concept of the 'good enough mother', pointing out that it is difficult for a mother to be good enough if she is not herself held and supported. This analogy to supervision has been used many times.

The supervisory relationship must be a place were attitudes that are racist, sexist, or ageist can be explored, modified, and positively changed. Mental health nursing needs to respect cultural differences, values, beliefs, and lifestyles with emphatic awareness and sensitive responsiveness.

## THE SUPERVISEE'S RESPONSIBILITIES AND PERCEPTIONS

Supervisees often have expectations of the supervisory relationship. As a student, who was just about to meet his supervisor for the first time, said: 'I have expectations that my supervisor will direct my work, give me instructions, demonstrate mental health nursing techniques and strategies, and provide support and security.'

Changes in attitudes and behaviour within the context of relationships can cause anxiety. The supervisor needs to manage the supervisee's level of anxiety at a point that is high enough to produce motivation for learning, and yet low enough to prevent the supervisee being overwhelmed. It is necessary to balance the supervisory relationship so that it provides challenge and support that is sufficient to avoid the relationship stagnating and becoming too predictable. This danger was spelt out by Tom:

> When I first met my supervisor, I was really impressed. He was charming and socially very skilled. He would also say very positive things about my client work, and when I asked him for feedback he would say I was doing really well. But we never moved on. I never felt my client work was considered, or my skills acknowledged.

Tom never learnt from his 'mistakes' since these were never acknowledged. The supervision degenerated into a cozy, collusive relationship. Tom never learnt from his supervisor the value of a confronting intervention that puts the spotlight on the more negative aspects of behaviour or attitudes. He could have learnt from and worked with these.

Supervisees are sometimes assumed to be and feel too inexperienced to form a relationship with an authority figure who may be critical and remind them of associations from past authority relationships. These memories of, for example, school teachers or parents are therefore likely to evoke defences that have characterized those past relationships.

Supervisees may find it difficult to admit they need help with their client work. Some mental health nurses feel the way they are working is best and will not accept the need to reflect and review their casework. Their anxiety may be denied with a defensive rejection of any advice that is extended.

Supervisees may also over-identify with their clients and become too emotionally involved, using this as an excuse for avoiding supervision. In a parallel way, they may over-identify with their supervisor and become too dependent.

Stolenberg *et al.*s' (1987) level-one supervisees are seen as commencing and continuing a long journey as they proceed through the stages of supervision. Stolenberg views them as 'dependent on the supervisor, imitative, neurosis-bound, lacking self-awareness and other-awareness, categorical thinking, with knowledge of theories and skills but with minimal experience.'

Several authors have attempted to describe how supervisee needs change over time. Researchers have all concluded that in the first stage of supervision, supervisees expect their supervision to be a highly structured experience. As they become more experienced, they move to become more autonomous, and more able to negotiate the content of the supervision sessions. In the second stage there are often feelings of hostility towards the supervisor; sometimes the supervisees express disappointment that the supervisor had in some way failed them. This stage has been likened to adolescence where there is a need for less structure but more emotional holding.

Beginning supervisees sometimes prefer 'live' supervision in which the supervisor directly observes them interacting with their clients. They also want their sessions monitored by using video/audio replays of their sessions with clients. Research has shown that supervisees perceive their supervisors as more effective when they:

- Monitor sessions, either in person or using video/audio tapes.
- Help them to understand interventions with clients.
- Provide consultations dealing with emotions and therapy styles.
- Teach practical skills, and encourage them to experiment and take risks with different strategies.

As supervisees progress on their journey, they show the ability to see the client in a much wider context, have more wisdom, and develop more depth and integration in their work.

Proctor spells out the responsibilities of the supervisee to her/himself:

- identify practice issues with which s/he needs help;
- become increasingly able to share these issues freely;
- identify what responses s/he wants;
- become more aware of organizational contracts;
- be open to others' feedback;
- monitor tendencies to justify, explain, or defend;
- develop the ability to discriminate what kind of feedback is useful.

## FINDING A SUPERVISOR

Mental health nursing traditionally has supported an apprenticeship system whereby practice has superseded theory. The varied and complex day-to-day experiences of mental health nursing make clinical supervision imperative, and generally well established. Such methods of supervision may still predominate in some nursing cultures. Ideally, supervision needs to be a mixture of both the informal and formal, the latter providing scheduled time and space on a regular basis.

There may be difficulties in seeking out a clinical supervisor. One is the lack of consensus about the word itself. Some health districts use the words 'mentor' or 'precep-

tor', to describe a person assigned the task of helping another, possibly less-experienced, practitioner to develop their skills and competences, and to practice in an ethical and effective way. Whatever the name used, the principles that underpin practice are important, especially as nurses move towards working in a more autonomous and less mechanistic, task-orientated way.

In some mental health organizations there are networks of supervisors, and as soon as newly appointed staff members take up their posts they are allocated a supervisor. Other organizations have a mixture of formal and informal supervision, so supervisor seekers are advised to be proactive and enquire about existing opportunities for supervision. If no supervision exists, the organization Standing Conference on Training of Supervisors is devoted to developing supervision systems and supporting them once they are established.

Where there are no opportunities for mental health nurses to receive supervision, every opportunity should be used to encourage the organization to develop supervision policies and practices. Other disciplines already using supervision may be useful allies.

## SUPERVISION PRACTICES

The most popular way of using supervision is for the supervisor and the supervisee to meet regularly on a one-to-one basis, although supervision can be undertaken in many ways. *In vivo* supervision is provided when the supervisor, supervisee, and the client meet together in an actual encounter. Here, the supervisor's role is mainly one of observation, followed by discussion and feedback in order to review the dynamics of the encounter.

Group supervision, mainly focusing on the presentation of particular casework, or using experiential learning techniques such as role play and structured exercises, is a useful way of receiving different perspectives. Group supervision can be carried out with peers, or by inviting an 'expert' to join the group at different times. The focus of these groups could be educational, managerial, or supportive – or perhaps a mixture of all three.

Mental health nurses may also have supervision from a member of another discipline, for example, a psychologist or social worker. This type of supervision is known as a consultancy. The consultant supervisor may work outside of the organization. This type of supervision is entered into voluntarily, and is generally concerned with professional development. Consultancy is not a substitute for supervision, but is usually reserved for qualified and more experienced practitioners, as Westheimer (1977) states:

> If the consultant does not carry administrative accountability and is therefore not responsible for the implementation of the recommended action the professional responsibility remains with the consultee, who is free to accept or reject the advice and make of it what she will.

## SUPERVISION CONTRACTS

Supervisors vary in their experience and expertise, and making a contract for supervision is a way of identifying and clarifying the conditions of the working agreement. Like any effective contract, these conditions need to be negotiated between supervisors and supervisees.

A supervision contract is a clear statement about what happens in supervision. It is essential that it includes validated statements of the organizational duties and responsibilities of the supervisor. For example, the supervisor of students in training is required to make a formal assessment of their work. The contract should answer the following questions:

- What are the place and time of supervision?
- What is the duration of the supervision sessions?
- What is a realistic agenda for the objectives of supervision?

- What are the limitations of confidentiality? For example, if the supervisee abuses the nurse/client relationship then he/she clearly needs to know whether the supervisor will take action.
- What are the supervisor's preferred methods of working. For example, is the supervisee to bring to the session nursing notes, verbatim notes, or taped or video recordings of their interactions with clients?
- Will there be a case-centred approach, where the discussion is mainly about the client?
- Or is the focus to be on the mental health nurse's feelings, behaviours, attitudes, or counter-transference?
- Is the parallel process between the nurse/client and supervisor/supervisee to be explored?
- What is likely to happen if the supervisee has personal problems?
- If the supervisee does not attend the session, how will this be explored?
- To what extent will the sessions be about training/education?
- How is the supervision to be evaluated?

The idea of a contract is not to make supervision a rigid, inflexible encounter, but to give some direction and shape to the sessions. There are dangers in working exclusively to any one approach; ideally, supervision should address any issue that prevents the supervisee working effectively and competently with his or her clients.

If the contract is negotiated between the two parties, it can be used to form the basis of a working alliance – an agreement that needs consistency and structure, and which can periodically be reviewed.

## THE SUPERVISORY RELATIONSHIP

Effective supervision can stand or fall on the supervisory relationship; this, like any other relationship, can be a minefield. The pitfalls of the supervisory relationship should be considered, particularly its limits and boundaries, for example, the division between supervision and personal therapy, which Kagan *et al.* (1977) address:

> The supervisor must work with the trainee on issues involving any of the trainee's personal attributes which hinder his development as a therapist. In this sense the task is similar to psychotherapy itself, but it has the importance of being concerned with the professional rather than the personal aspects of the trainee's life.

There has been a great deal of controversy about the counselling role of the supervisor. Potential harm can result if the supervisor is called upon to use his/her psychotherapeutic skills in the supervision of the student. For example, anxiety and guilt may be produced in the supervisee if he/she is supervised in a fashion that highlights their inadequacies. Vargus (1977) makes the point:

> The role of the therapist....encourages intrapsychic dependency. The supervisor who talks too much about the supervisee's feelings only intensifies existing personality problems. In this type of relationship, the worker fears a supervisor's criticisms and thus fears failure. Eventually the worker becomes afraid to innovate, begins to rebel against the supervisor, or, worse yet, avoids the supervisory conference.

The client's experiences may well stimulate feelings related to the nurse's own life, as the following example shows:

> Madeline was involved in working with survivors of a road traffic accident. She spent an inordinate amount of time with them, and became preoccupied and overwhelmed with intense feelings of sadness. Exploration of this in supervision revealed that Madeline's own grief

for her parents who had died in a similar way two years ago was colouring and distorting her client care. She clearly needed help in working through her own unresolved grief. Her supervisor supported Madeline in finding a counsellor with whom she could work through the grieving process.

A distinction needs to be made between personal therapy and supervision. Many of the dynamics that shape our lives are potentially borne out in the supervisory relationship, for example, issues of dependency, but if this and other dynamics are dealt with effectively, there is every possibility that supervisees will ultimately work in an independent, autonomous way (Cohen, 1987).

Over-involvement, detachment, projection, and many other forms of defensive behaviour need to be considered within the supervisory relationship. There is also the potential for abuse of power, and the possible need of the supervisor to mould the supervisee into a mirror-image of him/herself.

Supervisees are clear about the qualities they feel necessary for their supervisors to have, preferring those who are actively emphatic, genuine, warm, flexible and non-restrictive. They also want a supervisor who will value them as a person. Ultimately, their view is that supervision is about a relationship in which they are responsible for their own growth and development.

There is a consensus that the supervisor has a vital role to play in shaping and facilitating both the personal and the professional growth of the supervisee. This is asking a great deal of the supervisor and, although their needs have not been addressed here, they too need support and acknowledgement for their work.

When all the different functions of supervision are taken into account, there will be inevitable conflicts between the supervisees' perceived needs and what is realistically available in supervision. Much of this conflict will centre around the fact that often supervisors function as both mentors and consultants.

Supervision can provide support and validation; it is also often a source for evaluation and recommendations which may potentially affect the supervisees' future. Supervisees learn from supervision their skills, theories, and techniques, and move from an initial state of dependence to a more autonomous and independent way of working. Their experiences of supervision will inevitably influence and affect how they eventually function as supervisors themselves.

### GENDER ISSUES

Inevitably the context in which the supervision takes place will affect the style of supervision, and so it is one way of ensuring that non-sexist attitudes are encouraged. It is also a means of exploring and understanding the positions of women and men in society.

Often, the extent to which specific types of mental illness have been defined as pathologies of thoughts, feelings, and actions which are governed by specific gender expectations. For example, women are expected and encouraged to be sensitive to the feelings of others, to be more dependent, and to show certain types of feelings, such as sadness, fear, and anxiety. Judgments as to whether the experiences are problematic, merit medical attention, or are of a psychological nature often depend in part on the sex of the person whose actions are under consideration.

Although these observations and a history of paternalism within the medical profession, are not directly related to supervision, it is assumed that the context in which the supervision takes place influences both the supervisory process and outcomes, and the way supervisors and supervisees behave towards each other. Marked differences between male and female supervisors were found by Rubenstein (1979). Females tended

to be supportive, non-intrusive and interested in encouraging supervisees to become autonomous; male supervisors encouraged imitation and were more aware of their impact on supervisees.

There has been a constant theme that females value the supervisory relationship but struggle with issues of dependency in a system where, although they are in a greater majority, males are hierarchically in more powerful positions.

### CONCLUSION

The emphasis throughout this section has been that the foundations of supervision begin with effective supervisory relationships, in which normative, formative, and restorative dimensions are contained and balanced.

Supervision is for the professional and personal development of the supervisee; for continuation of professional standards and competent practice, but, ultimately, for the protection of the client.

Hawkins *et al.* (1989) believe that effective supervision cannot be taught:

There is so much pain and hurt in the world, that if we get caught into believing we have to make it all better heroically, we are setting ourselves to be overwhelmed and to burn out quickly.

However, if we react to this reality with professional defensiveness, we may treat the symptoms, but we fail to meet and support the human beings who are communicating through these symptoms. The middle group entails being on the path facing our own shadow, our own hurt and distress and taking responsibility for ensuring we practise what we preach.

This means managing our own support system, finding friends and colleagues who will not just reassure us but also challenge our defences, and finding a supervisor or supervision group who will not collude in trying to see who can be most potent with ways of curing the client, but will attend to how we are stuck in relating to the full truth of those with whom we work.

Effective supervision enables the sharing of ideas, feelings, perceptions – indeed, all aspects of client care. Supervision helps to increase staff morale and creates a sense of individuals and organizations working together with a unifying philosophy and shared aims.

Supervision is about the need to integrate the educative, the managerial, and the supportive aspects of experience. In the last analysis it is the quality of the relationship between supervisor and supervisee that will determine how effective it is.

Since it is vital to transmit professional knowledge, skills and attitudes, supervision has a vital part to play in shaping mental health nursing in the future. Potential difficulties will arise, however, and it would be unrealistic to ignore them. The current climate within the NHS is one of change; effective clinical supervision is a way of minimizing the more traumatic aspects of this change, a way to progressive skill mastery within a supportive climate, and a way of caring for ourselves to free us to care for others more creatively and more effectively.

## REFERENCES

British Association of Counselling (1988) *Code of Ethics and Practice for the Supervision of Counsellors*.

Carrol, M. (1987) Privately circulated paper, Roehampton Instit., Univ. Surrey.

Cohen, L. (1980) The new supervisee views supervision, in *Psychotherapy Supervision; Theory, Research and Practice* (ed. A. Hess), John Wiley & Sons, Chichester.

Frankham, H. (1987) *Aspects of Supervision, Counsellor Satisfaction, Utility and Defensiveness and Tasks in Supervision*, dissertation, Roehampton Instit. Univ. Surrey.

Hawkins, P. and Shobet, R. (1989) *Supervision in the Helping Professions*, Open Univ. Press, Milton Keynes.

Holloway, E. L. and Acker, M. (1989) The EPICS model engagement and power, in *Clinical Supervision*, Univ. Oregon.

Platt-Koch, L. M. (1986) Clinical supervision for psychiatric nurses. *J. Psycho-Social Nursing*, **26**, 17–15.

Proctor, B. (1986) Supervision: a co-operative exercise in accountability, in *Enabling and Ensuring; Supervision in Practice* (eds A. Marken and M. Payne), National Youth Bureau, Leicester.

Stoltenberg, C. D. and Delworth, U. (1987) *Supervising Counsellors and Therapists*, Jossey-Bass, San Francisco.

Stuart, G. W. and Sundeen, S. J. (1987) *Principles and Practices of Psychiatric Nursing*, 3rd edn, C V Mosby, St. Louis.

Tonnesman, M. (1979) *The Human Encounter in the Helping Professions*, London Fourth Winnicott Conference, London.

Vargus, I. D. (1977) Supervision in social work, in *Supervision of Allied Training* (eds D. J. Kurpius *et al.*) Greenwood Press, Connecticut.

Waite, R. and Hutt, R. (1978) *Attitude, Jobs and Mobility of Qualified Nurses*; a report for the Royal Coll. Nursing, IMS Report No. 130, Univ. Sussex.

Westheimer, I. J. (1977) *The Practice of Supervision in Social Work: A guide for Staff Supervisors*, Ward Lock Educational, London.

Winnicott, D. W. (1965) *Maturational Processes and the Facilitating Environment*, Hogarth Press, London.

## FURTHER READING

Bem, D. J. (1970) *Beliefs, Attitudes and Human Affairs*. Brooke/Cole.

Bernard, J. (1979) Supervisory training: A discrimination model. *Counsellor Education and Supervision*, **27**, 500–9.

British Association of Counselling (1988) *Code of Ethics and Practice of Counselling for the Supervision of Counsellors*.

Carkhuff, R.R. (1967) *Helping and Human Relations*, Vol. 2, Holt, Rinehart & Winston, New York.

Carkhuff, R.R. and Berenson, B.G. (1967) *Beyond Counselling and Psychotherapy*, Holt, Rinehart & Winston, New York.

Casement, P. (1985) *On Learning From the Patient*, Tavistock Publications, London.

Casement, P. (1990) *On Further Learning From the Patient*, Tavistock Publications, London.

Dryden, W. and Thorne, B. (1991) *Training and Supervision in Counselling*, Sage Publications, London.

Evans, D. (1986) *Supervisory Management*, Cassell Educational Limited, London.

Kipnis, D. and Gamarnikow, E. (1978) Sexual division of labour: the case in nursing, in *Feminism and Materialism* (eds. A. Kuhn, A. M. Wolpe), Routledge, London.

Eichenbaum, L. and Orbach, S. (1987) Separation and intimacy, in *Living With the Sphinx* (ed. E. S. Maguire), The Women's Press, London.

Ekstein, R. and Wallerstein, R. (1958) *The Teaching and Learning of Psychotherapy*. Basic Books, New York.

Gilligan, C. (1982) *In a Different Voice: Psychological Theory and Women's Development*. Harvard Univ. Press, Cambridge.

Greenberg, L. (1980) Supervision from the perspective of the supervisee, in *Psychotherapy Supervision: Theory, Research and Practice* (ed. A. Hess). Wiley, Chichester.

Haller, L. (1976) Clinical supervision, in *Current Perspectives in Psychiatric Nursing* (Vol. 1), (eds. C. R. Kneisl, H. S. Wilson). C. V. Mosby, St. Louis.

Hess, A. (1987) *Psychotherapy Supervision; Theory, Research and Practice*. Wiley, Chichester.

Lambert, M. (1980) Research and the supervisory process, in *Psychotherapy Supervision – Theory, Research and Practice*, Wiley, Chichester.

Marshall, W. R. and Confer, W. N. (1980) Psychotherapy supervision; supervisees' perspective, in *Psychotherapy Supervision, Theory, Research and Practice* (A. Hess), Wiley, Chichester.

Wolberg, L. R. (1954) *The Techniques of Psychotherapy*, Grune and Stratton, New York.

*David Carpenter*

Caseworking has become the dominant mode of delivery of care and treatment in mental health services; it is now far less common for mental illness and mentally ill people to be viewed as a 'collective problem' to be dealt with by some general strategy. Mental health nurses, perhaps more than any other professional group, have become increasingly orientated to caseworking.

Caseworking in nursing practice is epitomized by models such as primary nursing (Chapter 27) in which the primary nurse is identified as accountable for the provision of care to an individual client. The move towards caseworking has come about as a result of a number of related developments including increasing emphasis upon community care; increasing autonomy and accountability of mental health nurses; emphasis upon systematically planned care; and the recognition of a range of specialisms within mental health nursing. There are now several examples of specialist mental health nursing, based either on the adoption of particular forms of therapeutic intervention – for example, behavioural psychotherapy – or on working with particular client groups, such as children and families.

Caseworking has many advantages for both the client and the practitioner: the client gains from specialist expertise, and the practitioner gains professional recognition. Caseworking can, however, result in several problems; if all professional practitioners function as caseworkers, all of whom are autonomous experts, the net result can be fragmentation and duplication of care and treatment, and the client may have the bewildering experience of

encountering an ever increasing number of experts. There are also serious considerations in respect of resources: caseworking may be unduly costly if services are duplicated, and if the client is cared for by a range of experts, when in some cases a single generic practitioner might be more effective.

There are important management considerations if caseworking is to be used to maximum advantage; the main focuses include the management of:

- caseloads by individual practitioners, including mental health nurses;
- individual cases to ensure clients receive optimum comprehensive care;
- caseworkers.

A proliferation of terms and titles have tended to confuse these distinct areas of management. The term 'case manager' has been identified within the government White Paper *Caring for People* (1989); the following aspects of the role are stated:

- identification of people in need, including system for referral;
- assessment of care needs;
- planning and securing the delivery of care;
- monitoring the quality of care provided;
- review of client needs.

The Paper identifies social services authorities as having primary responsibility for case management, but does not prescribe the backgrounds of case managers. In practice, case managers are likely to be drawn from a variety of professional backgrounds, including nursing. Individual case managers are not necessarily required to undertake all the functions listed in respect of individual clients, but there is an expectation that the functions will be the designated responsibilities of named persons, thus ensuring accountability.

Case management as described within the White Paper is concerned with the second area of management identified above. Some mental health nurses will welcome opportunities to undertake case management, though there is debate as to whether it can best be viewed as a primarily clinical role or an administrative one (Bachrach, 1989). It might be argued that case management is a logical extension of primary nursing (Chapter 27) – the primary nurse acting as the nurse responsible for the provision of care, as well as taking broad responsibility for the co-ordination of the interventions of other professional practitioners (Mound, 1991). An alternative view might include the primary nurse as an example of a caseworker, to be managed by a case manager along with other practitioners involved in the same case.

Despite the confusion of terminology, a simple common goal of all models of case management can be identified, namely the achievement of a co-ordinated and comprehensive package of care and treatment, which should be developed when the client is first referred, and continue until his discharge from the service; the package of care should cross traditional inpatient/community boundaries, thus ensuring continuity (Maurin *et al.*, 1990).

The mental health nurse working as a case worker will not necessarily be a case manager, but there are other management considerations corresponding to the first point above. The nurse will need to consider the immediate management of the caseload of clients for which she is accountable.

The general idea of working with a caseload of clients has its roots in community psychiatric nursing, though examples of the approach are now far more widespread. Caseloads may be organized according to geographical considerations, diagnostic groups, or other specialist groups. The geographical approach will result in the nurse caring for a range of clients with a diversity of problems, taking a generic role. The specialist-group approach allows the nurse to operate as a specialist either in terms of caring for an homogeneous group, for example elderly people, or in terms of providing specialist therapeutic intervention, for example, behavioural psychotherapy. Both approaches tend to cut across traditional nursing hierarchies, emphasizing the individual accountability of nurses in respect of the care provided.

Both caseworking generally and primary nursing result in nurses becoming more directly accountable for the care they offer, which will require the nurse to adopt clear management strategies in respect of his or her caseload (Chapter 28).

Many nurses are concerned with such issues as the optimum size of a caseload, looking for clear numerical guidance; in practice, it is difficult, if not impossible, to determine the size of a safe caseload. As an accountable autonomous practitioner, the onus is upon the nurse to recognize her professional and personal limitations, ensuring she maintains a manageable caseload. There is little point in being willing to care for an ever increasing caseload of clients if it is not possible to provide a reasonable standard of care; indeed, to do so is an abrogation of professional duty. Many nurses gain valuable support and advice from clinical supervisors in respect of the overall management of a caseload.

Referrals to caseworking nurses can come from a range of sources. It is increasingly common for specialist nurses to receive referrals direct from GPs and other members of the primary health care team. In these circumstances, the nurse may be relatively independent, without a link with any particular team.

Some models of mental health care provision retain clear multidisciplinary team structures. Referrals are received by the team, usually at a specific meeting, and cases are passed to individual members on the basis of who is most appropriately qualified to provide the main focus of care and treatment, which might well include the direct involvement of more than one member of the team. Some teams are less egalitarian in their approach, for example, the consultant psychiatrist may be the head of such a team and the sole recipient of referrals. In this type of structure, the caseworking nurse's involvement might be little more than supervising and monitoring medication. It should be emphasized that this approach is increasingly rare, but, more importantly, teamworking should not be conceived as necessarily hierarchical. Caseworking and teamworking are compatible models, and should lead to the client benefiting from the skills of the team members, while being able to identify a practitioner who is primarily responsible for her care and treatment.

## CASE RECORDS

Part of the task of managing a caseload is the management and care of case records.

Records should include all relevant aspects of a client's history, detailed assessments, and an ongoing record of systematically planned care, including evaluation of its effectiveness. Such a record will inevitably contain personal information about clients, which should be handled with due consideration to confidentiality and general respect for the client. The UKCC (1987) has published detailed guidance on confidentiality in nursing practice, including the accessability of records. There have, however, been important changes since the publication of this document, most notably the introduction of the Access to Health Records Act (1990).

Confidentiality is primarily offered in health care to ensure that clients are free to disclose all relevant details which might, in turn, be used to their benefit in providing the most effective care and treatment. Many of these personal details are included in health records, to which relevant professionals have access. It is interesting to note, however, that the subject of a health care record previously had no right of access to their record; recent legislation has sought to remedy this situation.

In simple terms, nurses should in future remember that clients might well take advantage of their right to gain access to nursing notes. This should not inhibit the nature of the content of nursing records, but it should influence the way the record is written, avoiding the use of jargon, unnecessary technical terms, and abbreviations. The client's right of access to his records should be viewed positively. It is likely to promote trust, and ensure that care is planned on the basis of a partnership; it also has the effect of promoting the idea of a nurse's accountability to her client, which, again, is a positive development.

The Act came into force on 1 November 1991. Its main provisions include, firstly, a qualified right of access to health records by the subject of that record. The right can be overridden if it is believed that access to a part of the record could adversely affect the physical or mental health of the subject; only the relevant part can be withheld, and the subject need not be informed that the record is incomplete. Access can also be gained by parents or guardians of children. Secondly, a right to a copy of the record including explanations of unintelligible terms.

Arguably, it would seem to make good sense to continuously inform clients of the contents of nursing records, rather than leaving them to exercise statutory rights.

## REFERENCES

Bachrach, L. L. (1989) Case management: toward a shared definition. *Hospital Community Psychiatry*, 40(9), 883–4.

*Caring For People* (1989), Cm 849, HMSO, London.

Maurin, J. T. (1990) Case management: caring for psychiatric clients. *J. Psychosocial Nursing and Mental Health Services*, 28(7), 7–12.

Mound, B. *et al.* (1991) The expanded role of nurse case managers. *J. Psychosocial Nursing and Mental Health Services*, 29(6), 18–23.

UKCC (1987) *Confidentially*, UKCC, London.

*David Carpenter*

There is little doubt that the nursing profession is in the process of considerable change. While this process has been taking place over decades, there has been a recent acceleration of change, as evidenced in the proliferation of new approaches to care. Pearson (1988) states:

> For the last 20 years there has been the need to move away from the established pattern of practice based on routinization, allocation of tasks, and adherence to management and medical models to a pattern based on the individual needs of the consumer, and to focusing on professionalizing the nursing role to allow for autonomous practice.

Moves towards individualizing care and establishing professional autonomy are reflected in the new titles both of practitioners and of styles of organization, for example, 'keyworker' and 'primary nurse', but also 'nurse therapist', 'nurse specialist', 'casework/manager', and 'nurse practitioner'.

In light of this, there are fundamental questions that need to be asked:

- Has there been any change in the nature of nursing that has necessitated the new titles, or, alternatively, do the new titles describe approaches to care that practitioners are aiming to achieve?
- Do the titles refer to nursing *per se*, or merely to the organization of it?
- Do the titles reflect fundamental changes in the attitude to clients – including real attempts to become more client-centred –

or are they more concerned with the drive towards increasing professionalism?
- How meaningful are the new titles to the clients?

In answering these and other questions, the most helpful starting point is probably a consideration of the situation before the most recent changes.

Nursing has been traditionally task-orientated: it has not been unusual to organize the work of the nurse according to the 'job to be done' rather than to the 'client to be cared for'. Practising nurses can probably recollect being allocated 'the shaves' or 'the baths', or responsibility for occupying a group of patients. Although the latter example appears almost client-centred, it was equally 'a job to be done'; it was not primarily concerned with the needs of the clients either as individuals, or collectively within a group setting. This approach is not necessarily history: it is still in evidence in many institutions.

There are several factors that have spurred changes towards more client-centred approaches. Some of these factors relate to the profession as a whole, and others are more specific to mental health nursing.

The nursing profession as a whole was influenced by the introduction of the nursing process and its attendant philosophy of individualized care. In many cases, this was met with a good deal of resistance despite being enshrined in law (Nurses, Midwives, and Health Visitors Act [1979]).

While many nurses argued they had adopted the principles of the nursing process, fundamental change in the delivery of care was far from obvious. The introduction of the nursing process might have been reflected in the production of care plans and other records of care, but evidence of the basic ideology – including the systematic planned care of individuals – was often absent. Nurses became preoccupied with the completion of care plans, often struggling to get them 'just right'. While nurses were allocated groups of clients at the beginning of spans of duty, rather than lists of jobs to do, many simply identified a list of tasks, and continued in a task-orientated fashion, treating the group like a small ward. In general hospitals, for example, nurses approached the care of their groups of clients by taking all the temperatures, doing all the baths and dressings, and so on; individualized care was far from apparent.

Why did this pattern of work continue? Arguably, task orientation and routinization are inextricably part of the image of nursing. The stereotypical nurse is a person who does things to and for sick people, thus nursing is identified as a series of tasks. Task orientation was further reinforced by strongly hierarchical structures: the nature of the tasks varied according to status. Interestingly, the higher-status tasks often were those involving the least client contact, the pinnacle of achievement being seen as graduation to the ward office. Ward management was perceived as far more important than direct client contact, particularly in the context of mental health nursing.

It is reasonable to argue that a ward is no more than a group of clients, or that is all it should be conceived as from a nursing point of view; ward management therefore should be entirely compatible with direct care. In practice, however, ward management often becomes ward administration, with an emphasis upon the smooth running of the organization, as opposed to furthering the enterprise of caring. Ward administration is of course necessary, but does it require the knowledge and skill of the most senior member of the nursing team? Furthermore, if the most experienced nurses are undertaking those duties distant from direct care, the clients will be cared for by junior nurses, often students, or health care assistants.

There is some argument to suggest that nurses avoid individualizing care because they would then be forced to work as individuals. Many nurses enjoy the experience of team membership and its accompanying camaraderie. Structures – hierarchical or otherwise – bring security: if there is a pecking order, every individual knows his or her place, and who is responsible for doing what. Along with hierarchies come territories, and nurses are able to establish their own operational environments: working in the community is for community nurses; working in the hospital is for others. Working in some sort of specialist service also establishes clear territories.

Professionalization has played a part in emphasizing individualized care. The UKCC *Code of Professional Conduct* (1984) made it quite clear that nurses are individually accountable for care given to individual clients. Accountability permits autonomy (Chapter 28); autonomy is the privilege of all registered nurses in respect of the delivery of nursing care. Increasing the autonomy of nurses results in increasing the autonomy of clients, thus promoting awareness of the client as an individual, yet there is no evidence to support such an assertion. Indeed, the autonomy of a professional practitioner might well result in compromising the autonomy of the clients: an autonomous practitioner can make independent decisions, and all too often such decisions are not just made independently of other practitioners, but of clients as well. A side-effect of professional autonomy is frequently increased paternalism.

While professionalization has the potential to promote individualization of care, it can equally result in the contrary. Professionalization can be motivated either by the interests of members of the profession, or by the interests of clients.

In mental health nursing, the influence of the nursing process was accompanied by other factors that equally challenged task-orientation, routinization, and hierarchical structures. The increasing awareness of the effects of institutionalization led to more critical attitudes towards the organization of nursing care and to the environment in which it took place. Both Barton and Goffman identified the deleterious effects of rigid, ritualistic routine, authoritarianism, and lack of acknowledgement of the unique identity of individuals. Growing awareness of institutionalization was one of the many factors that influenced development towards community care. Community care is not readily organized on the basis of tasks unless of course clients are relocated to new institutions that just happen to be outside the grounds of the hospital.

Individualization of care seems to be a worthy goal to achieve, yet the organization of nursing care in many cases would appear to frustrate such an achievement. Primary nursing is one example of organization that aims to promote individualized nursing care, recognizing the autonomy of the nurse as a practitioner.

Primary nursing has been described as 'a method of organizing care that focuses on an individual nurse being responsible for a patient throughout his hospital stay' (Pearson, 1988). The approach is surprisingly simple: each client is allocated a primary nurse on admission to hospital, and that nurse takes responsibility for the assessment and care of that client throughout his or her stay. Of course, the individual primary nurse will not be able to provide all the care herself; in practice she will be supported by associate nurses and health care assistants. (Associate nurses are qualified nurses who might well be primary nurses in respect of other clients, or, in some systems, they are second-level registered nurses, whereas primary nurses hold first-level registration.)

Primary nursing might be seen as a form of keyworking whereby clients are cared for by a key person. Keyworkers, however, are not necessarily nurses. A keyworker for some clients might be a social worker or an occupational therapist. 'Keyworking' can be viewed as a generic term covering approaches such as primary nursing, though in some structures a keyworker is more concerned with the co-ordination of the interventions of other professionals, rather than being a source of direct intervention; in such structures keyworking is closely related to case management (Chapter 26).

From the client's point of view, primary nursing has clear advantages: the client is able to identify a single nurse who has primary responsibility for his care, and he is spared the difficulties of trying to understand a hierarchy and the problem of knowing to whom his questions should be addressed.

Primary nursing facilitates the development of effective therapeutic relationships; it is indeed surprising that while the value of therapeutic relationships in mental health nursing practice has been highlighted for many years, the organization of nursing care has almost militated against the development of such relationships. Before the introduction of the nursing process, there was no clear pairing of nurses and clients, though there were informal recognitions that some nurses had special relationships with some clients.

From the nurse's point of view, the advantages of primary nursing include the further development of professionalization, where the nurse is seen as an autonomous practitioner – as opposed to a member of a team responsible for little more than the satisfaction of basic needs, and ensuring that treatment prescribed by doctors is continued. There is no doubt that autonomy emphasizes accountability, which should be viewed as a distinct advantage (Chapter 28).

While the benefits of primary nursing seem clear, there remains resistance to its adoption. Reasons for this might lie in the loss of security found in team membership and task orientation, and in some cases fears of working alone. Primary nursing is a way of organizing care, and it equally requires changes in organization to be fully effective. Shift patterns, for example, do not necessarily facilitate primary nursing; in the main, shift patterns are organized to benefit staff or the organization by, for example, minimizing antisocial hours in order to maximize staff benefit and minimize employment costs. Primary nursing cannot be simply introduced into an established organization without examining other aspects of that organization.

The virtues of primary nursing as currently conceived lie in ensuring continuity of care; keeping to a minimum the number of nursing staff involved in the care of the individual client; furthering the idea of holistic care; and contributing to the establishment of professional identity of nurses.

Could primary nursing be developed in order to achieve more? It might be argued that it is still too narrow. If a nurse is identified as a primary nurse for the duration of a client's stay in hospital, why should that arrangement come to an abrupt end when the client is discharged home, and his care is continued by a community nurse? It would make good sense for the primary nurse to continue the client's care on his discharge from hospital. Although the advantages of such an approach seem self-evident, there are very few examples of it.

Many nurses will argue that ward duties do not permit the freedom to continue care in the community, while others will argue that community nursing is a specialism and should be the sole prerogative of community psychiatric nurses. While these arguments seem to be persuasive from the nursing perspective, they can readily be challenged. If primary nursing is to be valued because of its benefits to clients, there would seem to be pressing reasons to extend this value by making further organizational changes.

The only reason why nurses are unable to leave wards to continue care in the community is that duties and shift patterns are organized in such a way as to prohibit such activity. It would not be impossible to rethink this organization, with the real intention of benefiting the clients. Similarly, while it might suit professional ends to make a sharp division between community nursing and nursing in inpatient settings, it is far from obvious that this benefits clients. Presumably, in the first instance, primary nurses should be allocated on the basis of the possession of relevant skill *vis à vis* the problems of the client. If this is the case, then the primary nurse should be the most appropriate person to continue to practice this skilled intervention on the client's discharge.

The idea of community nursing as a specialism seems to be increasingly incoherent; it is vital that nurses offer planned and skilled care – perhaps the setting in which this care takes place is a secondary issue. Similarly, if it is argued that primary nursing promotes holistic approaches to care, it would be odd to limit a concept of holism to exclude the environment in which the person lives. Holistic care entails consideration of the person as a bio-psychosocial whole within the context of his environment; it requires the nurse to continue care, making appropriate adjustments according to environmental change.

Many writers argue that community nursing has always offered an example of primary nursing. In one sense this is true, assuming that primary nursing is conceived narrowly; in another sense, the very existence of community nursing as a separate specialism militates against the development of primary nursing more widely conceived.

Community nursing is increasingly the norm – it is now unusual for clients to be admitted to hospital. In the recent past, community nursing was a departure from the norm, and as such could be seen as special. The balance of hospital nursing to community nursing has changed; arguably, attitudes of nurses have not undergone corresponding changes.

It is possible that Project 2000 will result in a loss of distinction between community nursing and institutional nursing, due to its emphasis on preparation of nurses to work in both settings, but this will require accompanying changes in approaches to training. Perhaps we should no more be aiming to have a community emphasis to training than a hospital one; it is time that we had a client emphasis within training, regardless of setting. Regrettably, many current programmes of initial preparation tend to emphasize community approaches to care, which will do little towards achieving the ideals of primary nursing. If primary nursing is emphasized from the beginning of training, it is far more likely to succeed, and clients are far more likely to benefit from its deals than if there is an attempt to superimpose it on to existing structures that rely on assumptions, and in some cases frank territoriality.

Many schools of nursing are now developing new approaches to the organization of clinical experience, for example, service-allocation models are being abandoned in favour of client allocation. It is now far less common for mental health students to pursue a pattern of allocation to wards and community-based services; instead they are being allocated caseloads of clients under supervision. Students maintain contact with individual clients whether in hospital or in the community, and are prepared as primary nurses in the widest possible sense.

Primary nursing is supported and encouraged by pay-scales based on clinical grading. It is now possible to remain a committed practitioner and receive recognition in respect of both status and salary. Nurses are no longer forced to gain promotion by 'graduating' from direct care towards management or teaching roles. While these changes are welcomed by many, it should be recognized that they will increasingly impact on traditional structures and relationships.

## REFERENCES

Pearson, A. (1988) *Primary Nursing*, Chapman & Hall, London.

# ACCOUNTABILITY IN PROFESSIONAL PRACTICE

*David Carpenter*

Accountability is an issue that is often perceived with fear. The question, 'Who is accountable?' tends to be asked when something goes wrong, and has come to be understood as a polite way of asking, 'Whose head should be on the chopping block?' It is this aspect that results in nurses avoiding, or at least attempting to avoid, accountability. The hierchical structures that have prevailed in nursing have encouraged a certain amount of 'buck-passing', and many nurses seek refuge in the security they provide. As professional practitioners, however, nurses are individually accountable; it is not possible to avoid or to pass on this accountability.

It is important to note that accountable persons are not just those to be blamed when things go wrong – they are also those to be congratulated when things go well. Accountability, then, is not something to be avoided or feared; it is, however, a complex matter both conceptually and practically.

## THE CONCEPT OF ACCOUNTABILITY

Accountability is a concept that seems to have increasing application: we are told that nurses are accountable for their practice; journal articles have eye-catching titles such as, 'Are you Accountable?' (Carlisle, 1990). Moreover, we are informed that the aim of government reorganization in the public sector frequently includes higher demands for the accountability of those employed therein. In nursing practice, accountability can be said to underpin professional conduct in its entirety. The UKCC Code of Professional Conduct includes

14 clauses, all of which are qualified with the same prefix:

> Each registered nurse, midwife and health visitor shall act, at all times, in such a manner as to justify public trust and confidence, to uphold and enhance the good standing of the profession, to serve the interests of society, and, above all to safeguard the interests of individual patients and clients.

> Each registered nurse is accountable for his or her own practice, and in the exercise of professional accountability shall:...

However, despite the frequent reference to the concept of accountability, there has been little systematic attempt to define it. The UKCC (1989) in its advisory paper states that,

> Accountability is an integral part of professional practice, since, in the course of that practice, the practitioner has to make judgements in a wide variety of circumstances and be answerable for those judgements.

This description affords some idea of the part accountability plays in professional practice, but a clear analysis of the concept is lacking. Carlisle (1990) states: 'exercising accountability means using your professional judgement and being answerable for that judgement'; and Burnard *et al.* (1988) differentiate accountability from responsibility:

> While people may be held to be responsible for an action, they may not always be asked to 'account' for it. The nurse,

however, is not only responsible for the care given, but should be able to explain why it was given in the way it is [sic].

Accountability appears to have two clear but interrelated elements. Firstly, it is an entitlement to make decisions that might be properly referred to as professional judgements. Secondly, it is an obligation to explain and justify actions taken on the basis of the entitlement. It is power with an inbuilt constraint: 'You are free to decide, but be prepared to justify your decision.' There is, however, a degree of paradox, since on occasions the entitlement can be seen as an obligation, in other words, the making of a judgement can be both a right and a duty. If a nurse is accorded freedom to act or to refrain from acting, that freedom brings certain responsibilities, including the duty to exercise it in the client's interest.

Accountability can be seen as a recognition of the autonomy of the nurse – her right to make judgements based on her professional knowledge and skill; it can also be seen as a necessary concomitant of responsibility, an obligation to make decisions in the client's interest, and, moreover, an obligation to explain and justify those decisions when required to do so. Rights and duties to make professional judgements emanate from the profession, the employer, the nurse's own conscience, and the law. Such sources not only confer freedom and demand obligations, but can also demand explanations.

## PROFESSIONAL ACCOUNTABILITY

Accountability is a necessary component of professionalism. It is therefore no surprise that it should be given such weight in a professional code of conduct. A professional person provides a service to others based on knowledge and skill. The very fact that the help of a professional is sought is some indication that the recipient of the service is unlikely to make clear judgements in respect of the quality of that service. To a greater or lesser extent, the recipient puts himself in a position of trust. Given this trusting relationship, accountability can be seen as providing a necessary safety mechanism; the practitioner can be called upon to explain her actions in respect of the service offered.

Accountability is not uniquely applicable to health care professionals: it provides a safety mechanism whenever the services of an 'expert' are required. If, for example the services of a builder are required, it is not unusual to find that he is a member of some sort of guild or organization, which effectively underwrites the quality of his work. The customer will probably not be able to determine the quality of the work while it is in progress, but if he is dissatisfied with the end result, he can make an appeal to the underwriting organization. The organization will then probably provide an expert to examine the work, and if it is found to be substandard the builder may be called to account. In the absence of satisfactory explanations, the builder may be ejected from the organization, his name will be discredited, and he will lose the underwriting that previously supported his business.

Organizations of this nature often produce codes of practice that identify clear standards. Although perhaps crude, the foregoing description serves as a useful analogy to understanding the role and function of the UKCC: it is fundamentally an underwriting organization with a primary aim of protecting clients. The client has a right to expect that the practice of a nurse registered with the UKCC will conform to a reasonable standard, which will effectively apply to all nurses, since the title 'nurse' can only be applied to those people whose names appear on the UKCC register.

As stated earlier, in most cases when a person seeks the services of an expert he is obliged to a greater or lesser extent to trust that expert. This trust is particularly significant in health care, where the 'customer' by virtue of incapacity might have a limited ability to protect his own interests. In mental health care in particular many clients will suffer some impairment of autonomy to the extent they will rely on the skill of health professionals, most notably nurses. In this respect, accountability is not merely a desirable safeguard – it is a necessary requirement.

## THE CODE OF PROFESSIONAL CONDUCT

The creation of the Code of Professional Conduct represented a significant milestone in the history of nursing as a profession. It did not arise merely out of whim; it was required in law. S.2(5) of the Nurses, Midwives, and Health Visitors Act (1979) states: 'The powers of the council shall include that of providing, in such a manner as it thinks fit, advice for nurses, midwives and health visitors on standards of professional conduct.'

It should be immediately stressed that the Code of Conduct is not law, even though it is legally required. It has had a considerable impact on nursing practice, which has been highlighted by Pyne (1985), who notes its role in 'challenging practitioners to recognize their personal accountability in raising many interesting problems for managers which will not go away'. Furthermore, he states that the 'challenge to be accountable has already resulted in a 15% increase in the rate of cases reported for professional disciplinary hearings'.

The fundamental role of the Code of Professional Conduct is to clearly state required standards expected of members of the profession. It provides a clear yardstick against which the practice of a nurse can be measured, which in turn can readily serve to maintain a reasonable standard of care on the part of nurses. It is equally, if cynically, true that its purpose is to facilitate professional discipline. In other words, the purpose of the Code can be seen as an attempt to clarify the identification of misconduct just as much as it is an attempt to promote good conduct.

The Code might be seen as a guide for the direct benefit of the clients. It states the duties that should be expected of the registered nurse, and in principle there is no reason why a client should not use this list as a 'specification' against which he might assess the quality of his own care. It is a sad fact, however, that few if any clients have ever heard of the Code, let alone know of its content. Its safeguarding role therefore might be seen to be realistically limited. Professional misconduct is usually reported of professionals, by professionals, to professionals, and a real sense of public accountability may be lost.

Some nurses are currently involved in writing charters and bills of clients' rights. In part this interest has been spurred by demands to demonstrate the quality of a service which in effect is being sold in a market economy. Some of the interest has arisen from a genuine and immediate commitment to the empowerment of the clients. Often, however, locally produced charters and bills are not readily enforceable; it is one thing to make a promise, it is another to ensure that a particular promise is kept. It would undoubtedly be more beneficial to clients if they were made more aware of their existing rights, including those which are implicit within the Code of Professional Conduct. Nurses should endeavour to empower clients by making copies of the Code available. It could be displayed in prominent places, or, better still, explained to the client by the nurse. The safeguards for the client provided by the Code could usefully be included within a therapeutic contract of care. They could effectively represent promises on the part of the nurse, which might well help in facilitating relationships of trust and confidence.

## ACCOUNTABILITY OUTSIDE THE PROFESSION

The Code of Professional Conduct is not a code of ethics, although much of its content is undoubtedly ethically desirable. A code of ethics might be a list of principles based on ethical theory – it need not apply to any one person in particular, nor any specific group of persons, for example, the Ten Commandments.

Many people who have little else in common might well share a common code of ethics, whereas a code of professional conduct will apply uniquely to the profession concerned. The UKCC Code of Professional Conduct is a statement of duties that are obligatory. A breach of any of the Code's clauses could lead to the removal of the name of the nurse from the professional register; breach of a code of ethics might result in anything from mild disquiet to a crisis in conscience, but there might not be any other consequence. This is not to suggest that ethical codes should be subordinated to practical codes, but the differences do demonstrate varying types of accountability. A code of professional conduct need not state ethical principles – it need not even be ethical. It must, however, state the standards expected of members of the profession concerned.

Baher (1984) suggests a range of different types of accountability, including that the nurse is accountable to:

- society under criminal and civil law;
- his/her employer under her contract of employment;
- his/her patient under existing civil law provision;
- his/her profession under the Nurses, Midwives and Health Visitors Act (1979).

It should be stressed that each of these types of accountability are ultimately reducible to accountability to the client; each of the institutions identified can be seen as agents of the client.

It is important to add one further type of accountability, namely accountability to self. At first glance this appears to be contradictory. How can anyone demand an explanation of themselves? However, a person must be able to live with himself; a nagging conscience can be a painful thing to endure.

Many nurses, particularly more senior nurses, do not recognize primary accountability to clients. Carlisle (1990) suggests that when nurses are asked who they are accountable to,

> ...the more senior the practitioner or manager, the more likely their reply will be 'the UKCC', 'the government', 'ministers', 'general managers', or even 'doctors'. It is usually only the students and very junior nurses who reply 'my patients'.

Accountability is usually required of an individual. As an individual, the nurse might be required to explain her acts as well as her omissions, which could be demanded by any of the institutions mentioned above. The familiar childhood chant 'so-and-so made me do it' will not serve as a defence in the context of professional practice – it will be dismissed, just as it was in childhood. Accountability cannot be not delegated, a point well recognized in law: *delegatus non potest delegare* (the delegated cannot delegate). While an accountable nurse may delegate responsibilities to others, the accountability remains with her.

## CONTRACTS OF EMPLOYMENT

In terms of managerial accountability, most nurses are typically employed on the basis of a formal contract of employment, which will include statements of obligations or duties either as explicit requirements or by implication. It will also include a mechanism for calling a nurse to account. In most respects this is a fair arrangement: if an employer is offering a salary and certain conditions of service, he can reasonably expect a certain standard of work in return, and an explanation if that work falls short of the required standard.

Problems may arise, however, if an employer sets standards and expectations that differ from those of the profession. For example, a manager attempts to compel a nurse to undertake a task she feels she is not competent to achieve, such as insisting she offers a psychosexual counselling service when she has had no training in this specialist field. It would entail her breaching Clause 4 of the Code if she acceded to his request. What should the nurse do? Clause 4 states: Acknowledge any limitations of competence, and refuse in such cases to accept delegated functions without first having received instruction in regard to those functions, and having been assessed to be competent.

Clearly, the nurse should follow the requirements of her profession, and the key to this lies in the concept of accountability. Accountability in the sense of providing freedom to make a decision may require the nurses to refuse to undertake the task; it equally requires the nurse to provide an explanation for her refusal. When accountability is clearly understood as accountability to the client, few problems will arise. It is most unlikely that any manager would require a nurse to attempt an intervention that might jeopardize the well-being of a client, since he himself would be accountable for the provision of an adequate service, and called to account if that service fell below a reasonable standard.

This simple point is often overlooked by nurses protesting about shortages of staff. Many nurses become concerned when they are required to work in situations where staffing is clearly inadequate. Some nurses become aware of potential breaches of the Code of Conduct, for example, Clauses 10 and 11 state;

Have regard to the environment of care and its physical, psychological and social effects on clients/patients, and also to the adequacy of resources, and make known to appropriate persons or authorities any circumstances which could place patients/clients in jeopardy or which militate against safe standards of practice.

Have regard to the workload of and pressures on professional colleagues and subordinates, and take appropriate action if these are seen to be such as to constitute abuse of the individual practitioner and/or to jeopardize safe standards of practice.

No nurse breaches the Code merely by working in understaffed circumstances, but a breach would occur if she did not make her concerns known to those empowered to rectify the situation. Unfortunately, many nurses give 'worst case' examples when exercising accountability and making their concerns known, for example, it is generally not helpful to suggest that clients might die through neglect. This risk is unlikely to materialize, and therefore might not be taken seriously. The truly accountable nurse, aiming to protect clients through her accountability, will choose examples that will almost certainly materialize. It should be possible to produce the care plans for the clients concerned, and to demonstrate with certainty those aspects of care that will suffer as a result of staff shortage. Managers will be called to account if demonstrable shortfalls in care can be shown. In extreme cases, a manager might choose to close a service rather than risk offering substandard care and treatment.

A contract of employment that either obliged a nurse or gave scope to a manager to direct her to breach the Code of Conduct is unlikely to be legally enforceable. The employment of an individual nurse amounts to the employment of a 'package': along with the nurse is an understanding that she will be necessarily bound by professional obligations and constraints. As a manager cannot readily employ a nurse without taking account of these constraints, it is unlikely that any nurse who exercises accountability will jeopardize her employment. The obligation to provide explanations to managers when exercising professional accountability must not be lost sight of. Ultimately, successful working relationships and the effective provision of care depend on the mutual trust and understanding of employer and nurse.

## ACCOUNTABILITY TO SELF

While professional and managerial accountability are both important, other forms of accountability are often more familiar, such as accountability to self. Nurses' accountability to clients is in some ways best served by the recognition of accountability to self, which is a form of moral accountability. For example, the first test in a moment of doubt might well be the nurse's own conscience, not necessarily the 'conscience of a nurse', but the conscience of a person. The nurse might reasonably ask whether her conscience allows her to behave in certain ways. Generally, professional obligations are unlikely to conflict with personal conscience, indeed, the UKCC make special provision in the event of such a conflict: 'make known to an appropriate person or authority any conscientious objection which might be relevant to professional practice'.

The duty to make a conscientious objection known does not entail a right to have that objection respected, other than where legal provision exists, as in the case of participation in the termination of pregnancy. The most obvious way to ensure that one's own conscientious objections are respected is to choose employment carefully. A nurse is generally not free to refuse to take part in care and treatment. Any objection must clearly be grounded in some defensible moral belief, which will not include a misguided sense of self-protection or some kind of moralistic judgement of particular, or groups of, clients. A nurse is not free, for example, to refuse to care for a client who is HIV positive on the basis of an ill-conceived sense of self-protection, or a misguided judgement that the client is in some sense not worthy of care.

Can a nurse express a conscientious objection to taking part in treatment like ECT? Many nurses have attempted to express objections, but none has managed to establish a convincing argument in support of such an objection. Some nurses believe that ECT and other forms of treatment may do more harm than good. Any nurse is entitled to hold such a belief, and, reasonably, her conscience might direct her to work in areas where such interventions are not used. Other nurses might not share this belief, and argue that clients have a right to receive treatment such as ECT, which is a legitimate, though perhaps controversial, intervention.

While a nurse's objection might require her to refuse to participate in such treatment, it would not provide a licence to deprive the client, nor to undermine the beliefs of other health professionals. However, a nurse is entitled, and on occasions obliged, to withhold treatment if there is a risk of harm to the client. A drug, for example, should be withheld if the client is experiencing serious side-effects or if there is any clear contra-indication. In such circumstances the nurse would not be expressing a conscientious objection to the treatment *per se*, but would be exercising her accountability in the interests of the client.

## ACCOUNTABILITY AND THE LAW

Many qualified nurses claim that student nurses are not accountable. This is only partly true, as a student nurse cannot be held to be professionally accountable because she is simply not a member of the profession. Exercising accountability requires knowledge and skill, all of which the student cannot be expected to possess. Moreover, it would be pointless to call a student nurse to account from a professional point of view, since there would be no sanctions should she be found to be lacking in respect of determined standards; it is not possible to remove a name from a register if it has never been entered. Standards set by the profession will undoubtedly be of interest to students, who might perceive them as targets to aim for rather than yardsticks to be measured against. While a student can never be professionally accountable, she may nevertheless be given responsibilities by qualified nurses who themselves retain accountability.

Similar considerations apply in relation to managerial accountability, particularly since the adoption of Project 2000. Students undertaking courses based on Project 2000 are not employees; they hold no contract of employment, and cannot therefore be called to account as employees. Student nurses are not entirely free of managerial accountability, however. The courses they undertake impose certain duties, for example, a duty to complete 4600 hours of training. An abrogation of these duties might result in a student being a called to account, and sanctions including removal from the course could be applied.

Students, however, like any other person, are accountable to self. There is no reason to suggest that a student nurse's conscience is any less a guide to practice than that of an experienced, qualified nurse. A student nurse equally has a right to express a conscientious objection, and a duty to make this known. In a similar vein, student nurses, like any other person, are accountable in law. A student nurse is not immune from the law merely because she is a student; if she commits a crime in the course of her practice, she will be treated like any other person. Moreover, under certain circumstances, if her actions result in harm to a client, she can be sued, as any qualified nurse might be.

Like the profession, the law lays down standards of conduct, to which all citizens are obliged to conform. In some cases, the standards can be seen as a protection for society as a whole. A breach of one of these standards is likely to constitute a crime. The nurse, like any other citizen, can be formally charged and, if found guilty, punished. If a nurse intentionally kills a client, she will be called to account in law and punished. It is of course unlikely that any nurse will intentionally kill a client, but some mistakenly believe that the law makes provision for well-intentioned killings, or euthanasia. In fact, there is no place in English law for concepts such as euthanasia, and no special provision for health professionals in this respect. It would be a crime, for example, to administer prescribed strong analgesics with the intention of foreshortening a client's life, even if the quality of life by the client's own estimation was particularly poor. Although the distinction is sometimes not clear, it is not a crime to administer strong analgesics with the intention of relieving pain, while knowing that the effects might include the foreshortening of the client's life (R. *v.* Bodkin-Adams, 1957).

Some law is concerned with the protection of individuals, in the sense of providing a mechanism for redressing wrongs. This is the role of **civil law**, which provides a mechanism whereby a person can seek redress through the courts if he can establish a case that he has been wronged. Wrongs of this nature are referred to as **torts**, and should be clearly distinguished from crimes. A person cannot be accurately described as guilty of a tort as they might be in the case of a crime, nor is punishment an appropriate concept in this context.

In civil law it is recognized that a person may be liable for torts, and that the wronged person is entitled to seek damages from the wrongdoer. Damages are sums of money paid to compensate for harms done; they are not fines. Nurses, like any other person with duties towards others, can be held liable in the torts of battery or negligence if their practice falls outside of determined legal standards. If a client, for example, sues a nurse, the nurse will be called to account in law.

The law, then, rather like a professional body, offers protection to the public to whom duties are owed by others. A wronged person can sue for damages. The law sets standards, and departure from these standards might lead to a nurse being called to account. It is most unusual for an individual nurse, or for that matter any other individual health professional, to be sued.

Where a nurse is a health authority employee, it is normal practice for a wronged person to sue the authority rather than the individual practitioner. A health authority as employer is deemed to be vicariously liable for the practice of professional staff in its employ. It should be stressed that most cases are settled outside of court.

In the past, health authorities have effectively shielded many nurses from the prospect of litigation; the future, however, is not at all clear. Reorganization as a result of the NHS and Community Care Act (1990) will mean that nurses will no longer literally be health authority employees; they will be the employees of 'provider' units, whether self-governing trusts or directly managed units. In these circumstances it is possible that nurses and others might be personally liable for torts. If a nurse was to be found liable in negligence, for example, the damages could be very high, depending on the harm done. For this reason, all nurses would be well advised to ensure that they have personal indemnity, such as that offered through unions and professional organizations.

## BATTERY

The touching of another person without his consent to do so might invite a legal action in battery. In health care generally it is rare for any practitioner to be sued for battery; most clients expect to be touched, and explicit consent generally is not sought because there are sufficient grounds to suggest that implied consent has been given. It is, however, sensible to be cautious, and where there is any risk involved in a particular 'touching', for example, surgery, it is normal to record the client's consent in writing.

In mental health practice, matters are rather more complicated. By law, a person's consent is not real unless, first, he has the capacity to understand the nature of the proposed intervention, in other words he is competent to consent; second, he is sufficiently informed to

make a decision; and, third, his consent is given voluntarily, in other words, he could have chosen to decline the proposed intervention.

A client whose mental health is seriously impaired is unlikely to be able to consent to proposed treatment and care, yet it might well be in his interests to receive it; it could, for example, restore his capacity to make decisions for himself. If a nurse gives treatment and care without a client's consent, however, she risks being sued for battery. The problem has largely been solved by provisions of the Mental Health Act (1983) (page 411) and common-law powers, which enable nurses and other health professionals to give care and treatment to clients who are unable to consent if that care and treatment is necessary to save the client's life, or if it can be argued as being in his best interests.

It should be stressed that common-law power does not entitle a person to force care and treatment upon a client who has the capacity to consent; he will equally have the capacity to dissent, and his choice must be respected. It is not unusual for nurses – particular those working in mental health – to assume that because a client refuses potentially valuable treatment he must *ipso facto* be incompetent. However, competence to make a decision is the significant legal issue rather than level of competence, which might be reflected in the quality of the decision. It should also be noted that a client's agreement to, or absence of dissent from, a proposed form of care or treatment is not in itself consent. If a client is clearly incompetent as a result of mental illness, his 'agreement' will obviously not constitute consent.

## NEGLIGENCE

As mentioned earlier, it was suggested that a student nurse can be sued for negligence, just as a qualified nurse might be. In practice, many qualified nurses assume accountability can never rest with a student because he or she is a learner; there also is a popular but mistaken notion that a student nurse can offer her status as defence for practice deemed to be negligent. This can be clarified by a closer examination of the nature of the tort of negligence.

If a client is harmed as a result of the acts or omissions of any health professional, it is possible – but by no means certain – that he has been a victim of negligence. It is not certain because it is possible that the harm was a result of an unforeseeable accident, or a direct result of his own illness, or attributable to his own behaviour. Generally, an act or omission causing harm can only be negligent if that harm was reasonably foreseeable.

If a client wishes to pursue an action in negligence, the onus is upon him as plaintiff to prove that, on the balance of probabilities, he has been negligently treated. The nurse or other health care practitioner as defendant is not required to prove that she was not negligent. The plaintiff must show that a duty of care was owed to him by the defendant, and that there was a breach of the requisite duty; in other words, the care fell below a reasonable standard. The plaintiff will also have to prove that it was the particular breach of duty that caused the harm he suffered. It is clear that proving a case in negligence is no mean task, and it can be argued that the procedure favours the defendant unfairly.

Proven cases of negligence in mental health care are rare; this is partly due to the nature of psychiatry as a medical discipline, and partly due to the limited ability of many clients to take legal action. This latter point demonstrates the need for advocates of those clients who are unable to protect their own interests.

Psychiatrists are difficult to sue successfully because lack of precise medical knowledge in this area usually prevents any causal connection being established between the treatment and the deterioration of the patient. Furthermore, as psychiatry is not a science,

and so little is known by the medical profession about the workings of the human mind, it is virtually impossible to get expert evidence to prove the treatment was ill-advised (Lewis, 1988). How, then, can a client prove negligence if it is so difficult to establish norms in respect of treatment?

The principles of negligence are best understood from the perspective of a particular case. For example, many nurses working in mental health care fear being sued, especially in relation to care of suicidal clients. If a client attempts suicide, is unsuccessful, but sustains serious and permanently disabling injuries, could he sue the nurse(s) responsible for his care? Similarly, if a client commits suicide, could his relatives sue? In short, could nurses be called to account in law?

Actions in negligence such as these are rare, proven cases even rarer. Firstly, the plaintiff would have to show that a duty of care was owed to him, which his status as a client of a mental health service would establish. Secondly, the plaintiff would be required to prove there was a breach of that duty; that the nurses concerned either did, or omitted to do, something that was not consistent with the approach that a reasonably skilled nurse would have taken. As cited in Bolam *v.* Friern Hospital (1957), the legal standard of care required is 'the standard of the ordinary skilled man exercising and professing to have that special skill.'

In the case of Selfe *v.* Ilford and District Hospital Management Committee (1970), the defendants were found to be liable in negligence. The plaintiff, who was known to be suicidal, was given a bed near an unlocked window, and was in a ward where there was effectively only one nurse supervising 26 clients, three of whom were known to be suicidal. The plaintiff left the ward via the window and caused himself serious injuries by leaping from a roof. The reasonably skilled nurse would clearly not have left a client in this condition by an easily opened window, and, similarly, the hospital management committee was in breach of its duty to provide reasonable levels of supervision.

Thirdly, the plaintiff must prove that the breach of duty caused the harm that occurred; in other words, demonstrate that had it not been for the negligence of the defendants, no harm would have befallen him. In the case of Selfe *v.* Ilford, the causal link between the harm and the breach is fairly clear, but in other cases establishing this link is far more difficult. In the case of Hyde *v.* Tameside Area Health Authority (1981), for example, Lord Denning stated:

> ... the attempt at suicide here was far too remote a consequence to be the subject of damages. It is like the sequence of Benjamin Franklin: 'For want of a nail, the shoe was lost; for want of a shoe the horse was lost;... the battle was lost.' So here the sequence is, if the nurses had reported this man's depression to the doctor, then the doctors might have called in a consultant psychiatrist. If a consultant psychiatrist had been called in, he might have ordered some treatment...might have prevented him from attempting to commit suicide.

The case was lost because causation could not be established. In practice, most cases of alleged negligence *vis à vis* suicide attempts fail either because a breach of duty cannot be shown, or because the harm is too remote from the breach of duty to establish a reasonable causal connection.

A breach of duty can only be shown if care falls below the legal standard, which, as stated earlier, is the standard of the ordinary practitioner. In court this standard is identified by calling upon experts; for example, if a mental health nurse's practice is called into question, the advice of other mental health nurses is sought in order to determine whether her practice was reasonable. 'Reasonable' in this context means in accordance with current professional practice – it does not mean the highest possible standard of care, simply that there exists **a** body of professional practitioners who would have done likewise. Standards are judged according to the nature of the intervention in question, not according to the qualifications of the particular practitioner. If, for example, a nurse offers psychosexual counselling, the standard expected will be that of the reasonable psychosexual counsellor.

There is no special allowance for inexperience or under-qualification. If a service is being offered, it must be offered to a reasonable standard. This issue is particularly significant in relation to the care offered by student nurses. The care must still be of a reasonable standard, the standard of the 'reasonably skilled man', so appropriate levels of managerial supervision must be maintained. A student nurse who unquestioningly accepts a delegated task that she is not competent to perform may be liable in negligence should a client be harmed; a qualified nurse who delegates indiscriminately may equally find herself liable in negligence.

Accountability of mental health practitioners, including nurses, is clearly limited from a legal point of view. It is important, however not to allow complacency to creep in. The civil law is intended to provide protection for all members of society. The fact that it has limited effects in protecting the mentally ill is becoming increasingly well known, and more clients, and agencies advocating for them, are becoming increasingly aware of their rights. The committed nurse should undoubtedly help the client in demanding his rights, and, where necessary, seeking redress for harms that have occurred.

In the main, the law accords with common sense, and no nurse needs to have vast legal knowledge in order to protect the rights of clients, or to avoid unlawful conduct herself. Perhaps the simple test of, 'If this were me, how would I wish to be treated?' should remain the first line of approach when considering accountability.

## REFERENCES

Baker, J. (1984) Who is accountable? *Senior Nurse*, 1, 35.

Burnard, P. and Chapman, C. (1988) *Professional and Ethical Issues in Nursing*, Wiley, Chichester.

Carlisle, D. (1990) Are you accountable?. *Nursing Times*, 86, 22.

Kent, A. (1990) Protecting the public? *Nursing Times*, 86, 37.

Lewis, C. (1988) *Medical Negligence: A Plaintiff's Guide*, Cass and Co., London.

Pyne, R. (1985) Trends in accountability. *Senior Nurse*, 2, 2.

UKCC (1984) *Code of Professional Conduct for the Nurse, Midwife, and Health Visitor*, UKCC, London.

UKCC (1989) *Exercising Accountability*, UKCC, London.

## CASES

R *v.* Bodkin-Adams (1957), CLR 365.

Bolam *v.* Friern Hospital Management Committee (1957) 2, All ER 118.

Hyde *v.* Tameside Area Health Authority (1981) *The Times*, 15 April

Selfe *v.* Ilford and District Hospital Management Committe (1970), *The Times*, 26 November.

## FURTHER READING

Brazier, M. (1987) *Medicine, Patients and the Law*, Penguin, Harmondsworth.

Day, P. and Klein, R. (1987) *Accountabilities: Five Public Services*, Tavistock, London.

DOH (1990) *A Guide to Consent to Examination and Treatment*, HMSO, London.

DOH (1990) *Mental Health Act Code of Practice*, HMSO, London.

Kennedy, I. and Grubb, A. (1989) *Medical Law: Text and Materials*, Butterworths, London.

Mason, J. K. and McCall Smith, R. A. (1987) *Law and Medical Ethics* (2nd edn), Butterworths, London.

Skegg, P. D. G. (1989) *Law, Ethics and Medicine*, Clarendon Press, Oxford.

*Jean Simms*

The current literature on mental health nursing includes many references to concepts of self, self-awareness and the 'therapeutic use of self'. Beliefs central to the understanding of the self are that first, self encapsulates the whole human being, including identity, character, emotions, thoughts, feelings and sensations; and second, awareness of self in relationship to and interaction with others is essential in effective mental health nursing.

Jourard (1971) believes that during the process of socialization into nursing, nurses become estranged and detached from their true selves. The danger in this is:

> ... if a nurse is afraid or even ignorant of her own self, she is highly likely to be threatened by a patient's real self-expressions...A nurse who is more aware of the breadth and depth of her own real self is in a much better position to empathize with her patients and to encourage (or at least not block) their self-disclosures.

Self-awareness, with the verbal injunction to nurses to 'be aware' sounds easy, but life's journey towards total awareness is complex. But what are we? Shakespeare (1603) expressed praise for the human self:

> What a piece of work is man! How noble in reason! How infinite in faculty! In form, in moving, how express and admirable! In action how like an angel! In apprehension how like a god! The beauty of the world! The paragon of animals!

In writing of self-concept, the American psychologist, William James (1890), expressed his belief that people need recognition of self and that denial or indifference frustrates a deeply felt need:

> If no one turned around when we entered, answered when we spoke, or minded what we did, but if every person we met 'cut us dead' and acted as if we were non-existing things, a kind of rage and impotent despair would ere long well up in us, from which the cruellest bodily tortures would be a relief; for these would make us feel that, however bad might be our plight, we had not sunk to such a depth as to be unworthy of attention at all.

People whose selves are cut off from human contact, and who subsequently commit suicide bear out James's theory.

The concept of the self has been approached from many different perspectives. Sigmund Freud was a 'self theorist' as well as a psychodynamic theorist. Psychoanalytical theory divides the human mind into three areas: the **ego**, or self; the **super-ego**, or conscience; and the **id**, or instincts, the mental expression of instinctual needs. This theory argues that childhood experiences can profoundly affect the self and that these may be modified through life experiences.

The need to protect the self by the use of **defence mechanisms** helps us to disguise fears and anxieties, which are well documented throughout psychoanalytical literature and are succinctly described by Claxton *et al.* (1981):

> In *repression* we forbid a conflict or one of its components to conscious awareness; in *projection* we attribute a disowned portion of ourselves to another person, scapegoating them for our inadequacies. By *rationalizing*, the mind spins itself a yarn that it can accept in mitigation ('Everybody does it!' 'She did it to me first', etc., etc.,).... *Reaction formation* helps us to bury something of which we have been taught to be ashamed – sexuality and anger are the two most obvious candidates – by an exaggerated espousal of a contrary personality trait. By *regression* to behaviour of a younger age a person can hope to persuade others (and himself) to lower their expectations about his degree of responsibility and maturity. *Displacement* enables us to direct our feelings – an angry outburst – let's say – not at the real object, who may react in a threatening way (boss), but at another (spouse, children, cat) with the reaction we can cope more easily. At a more pathological level *obsessions*, *compulsions* and *phobias* may be crippling, but may also have their avoidance value.

During the first part of the twentieth century, when psychology was influenced by behaviourism, self-concept did not fit into this belief system. The notion was prevalent that only observable behaviour was an appropriate area of study, and self-concept was largely ignored.

In the 1950s, humanistic psychology revived the notion of self-concept. Carl Rogers, best known for his work in **client-centred therapy**, divided the person into the self and the organism, the former being an aspect of what individuals believe and experience as perceptions of 'I' and 'me', and the latter the real world. The 'I' is the conscious person who makes decisions and has a way of being, and there is the 'me' who elicits reactions from other people.

Gross (1987) proposes that the self-concept is a general term that refers to three major components:

- Self/image or ego identity – what sort of people we think we are.
- Self-esteem – how good we feel about ourselves.
- Ideal self – what we would really like to be.

Kelly (1955, 1969) argues that each of us has a 'theory' about ourselves, about other people, and about the nature of the world. There is a need to understand and acknowledge the past; not to repeat it, but to learn from it and to be free of its more destructive and often traumatic legacy. Kelly also believes while we are not victims of our autobiographies, we may be in danger because of the way we perceive and interpret our past.

Jourard believes that when a person has been able to disclose him/herself to another person there is increased knowledge of his/ her real self. There is no longer a need to waste energy in concealment and subterfuge:

> 'Self-disclosure, my communication of my private world to you, in language which you clearly understand, is truly an important bit of behaviour...'

It is the successful culmination of the therapeutic relationship when a client has been able to self-disclose, has been understood, accepted and valued, and can use insights to make decisions and choices in day-to-day life.

From the moment a child is born it begins an often hazardous journey to create a strong self-identity. Babies express their real selves by crying, sometimes screaming, to make their needs known; young children spontaneously self-disclose and 'tell all', but may soon learn that such honesty can sometimes be met with negative and unpleasant reactions.

The child quickly learns ways to cover up and withhold certain self-disclosures, to discriminate, to become socialized, and, to some extent to be conditioned to conform in a socially acceptable way. In Western culture, early growth and development involves training in concealment, often displaying double standards and not being 'real'. Much anxiety, anger, and confusion stems from a need to establish a self and a sense of identity.

The origins of self-awareness come from the parents, whose messages to the child can be nurturing, accepting and valuing – or cruel, brutal, or indifferent.

Children become self-aware by comparing themselves to others. Work by such people as Fantz (1961) and Bower (1971) has shown that young infants act as if they can, in advance of any experience, make sense of important visual aspects in their environment. To become self-aware, these infants need to show in their actions their place in relation to others, not just an awareness of their physical world.

The use of props, symbols, uniforms, hairstyles and fashions all help to give a sense of security, albeit sometimes a shaky one, and a feeling of belonging and mattering in the scheme of things. Youth culture abounds with subcultures that are different from mainstream society. Clothes and hairstyles are used to proclaim individuality in an attempt to be unique whilst also conforming to their peer group.

## THE TRUE AND FALSE SELF

The psychiatrist Ronald Laing (1965) wrote that in any one person there is a false system that is always very complex and contains many contradictions. The **false self** arises in compliance with the actual or imagined intentions or expectations of others – responses to what other people want or expect. This compliance is partly therefore a betrayal of one's own possibilities.

While being true to one self and dramatically disclosing can be fraught with dangers, Lake (1965) was sensitive to the effect of such honesty on the listener, sentiments with which many mental health nurses may agree:

Too bold a growth in honesty produces an irrational, claustrophobic reaction in the listener. By implication, they are being pushed by the self-disclosure to a place where unpleasant things are disclosed about themselves, whether they admit them to consciousness or not.

It is like being born forcibly into a new kind of world where you cannot be sure that anything is hideable, where nothing is reliably private...

That is the sort of catastrophe any sensible person wants to put off. So, honesty does not just tell us something about the teller. It also discloses the listener. It burdens him with the knowledge he didn't want and doesn't know what to do with, not only about the other person, but about himself.

Disclosures of intense feelings and experiences often face the listener with his or her own inner and outer reality – a hidden, inner, denied, often unknown reality, with different qualities and shades of light and darkness.

## LISTENING AND LANGUAGE

One of the most basic requirements of a therapeutic person is someone who really listens. As Fromm-Reichman (1950) writes:

...To be able to listen and to gather information from another person in this other person's own right, without reacting along the lines of one's own problems or experiences, of which one may be reminded, perhaps in a disturbing way, is an art of interpersonal exchange in which few people are able to practise without special training. To be in command of this art is by no means tantamount to actually being a good psychiatrist, but it is the prerequisite of all intensive psychotherapy.

The art of reflective listening is essential in all human encounters which purport to be therapeutic; since this book is about understanding mental health, listening cannot be emphasized too much. It is about listening in depth, with all the senses alert, listening not just to the words, but to the music of the whole person, (Perls, 1951).

In listening in depth to feelings as well as words, the mental health nurse is able to develop a fragile link between herself and the client to increase ways of breaking down barriers to communication. He or she will become more empathic and more aware of the client's subjective world.

By skilled and sensitive communication, and reflection on their practice, mental health nurses have the means to develop a strong sense of self and of therapeutic identity. This enables them to facilitate the growth of clients, and, through understanding, sharing, and the use of skilled interventions, enable clients to organize and make sense of their often confused and fragmented inner worlds.

To enable effective communication takes courage, and involves not only skills but also certain qualities. Carl Rogers (1961) believed that genuineness, respect, empathic understanding, and unconditional positive regard must be achieved in order to initiate and continue a therapeutic relationship. This is difficult for anyone to achieve, no matter how experienced, but especially so for the student mental health nurse. Techniques can be taught, but the possibility of the real self being exposed in a relationship may be frightening, especially if that self is anxious, unsure, immature, or inept.

Rogers (1961) gives some useful insights into the characteristics of a helping relationship. The first is concerned with issues of trust versus mistrust. Keeping appointments, being on time, and issues of confidentiality all serve to fulfil the considerations of trust. While Rogers believes these to be important, he adds that:

I have come to recognize that being trustworthy does not demand that I be rigidly consistent, but that I be depend-

ably real. The term 'congruent' is one I have used to describe the way I would like to be. By this I mean that whatever feeling or attitude I am experiencing would be matched by my awareness of that attitude. When this is true, then I am a unified or integrated person in that moment, and hence I can be whatever I deeply am. This is a reality which I find others experience as dependable.

Many therapists are afraid of their positive, warm feelings towards clients, fearing they may become trapped by them. One community psychiatric nurse remembers:

I always thought it was important to be detached from my clients, however, I can now allow myself to feel a genuine concern and warmth for them, which, rather than enmeshing me, makes me real, more at ease and has a more liberating effect.

Unambiguous communication is another vital ingredient of the helping relationship; again Rogers (1961) elaborates:

My words are giving one message, but I am also in subtle ways communicating the annoyance I feel and this confuses the other person and makes him distrustful, though he may be unaware of what is causing the difficulty.

How easy is it for mental health nurses to be their real selves? How is it possible to cope with work demands at so many different levels? Is it possible to meet, not just client needs, but also organizational demands that may clash with individual ones? Rob, a community psychiatric nurse, felt his true self was put in jeopardy by the high levels of staff sickness in the unit he worked from:

There was a lot of long-term sickness among the staff. I was torn between wanting to support them and trying to help cover clients on their caseload. At the same time, my wife was ill. The personal and professional stress was enormous, but it took time for me to admit to feelings of not being able to cope and to realize my limitations.

At the time, my therapeutic use of my own self was sadly lacking, however, through clinical and managerial supervision I took stock of what was happening and learnt from this experience. If I am to be therapeutic to my clients, then I need to be aware of my own limits and boundaries, and to ensure that my own mental health is maintained.

A major emphasis is on the mental health nurse's self being confronted by clients expressing intense feelings – some too much, some too little, and some just feeling numb. Such clients may be trying to cope with anxiety, depression, suicidal ideas, or phobias.

Constant exposure to such distress and trauma may result in mental health nurses becoming self-alienated by repressing or suppressing their reactions to the experience. There are also nurses who attempt to protect themselves by, for example, avoidance, and who cannot bear to work with one or another client group.

Indifference, insincerity, contempt, and impersonal mental health nursing care all undermine the sense of self and identity in clients and carers alike, and negate mutual experiences for enrichment and self-development. Reich (1948) called this protection against the acceptance and expression of real feelings 'character armour', and Moloney (1949) a 'magic cloak' donned by nurses and doctors to damp down their feelings in order to prevent self-disclosure in clients.

Self-esteem, self-image, and self-evaluation are bound up with how much we like the person we think we are, and a belief that what an individual does matters. The belief that thoughts, words, and deeds do not matter overlooks the contribution and the accumulative effects of each individual in bringing about changes.

The self can be destroyed or debased both by the individual and by others' cruelty or indifference; the ultimate level of self-destructiveness is suicidal behaviour. There are many addictions in society that take their toll on the mental, physical, social, and spiritual self. Drinking excessive amounts of alcohol, drug abuse, and smoking are usually explained by social and psychological problems, but also as potentially destructive forces unleashed on self. The anger and bitterness felt by many people in society who are often unheeded, marginalized, and oppressed serve to potentially erode the self and its full expression. The urban 'squatters' and people who live in 'cardboard city' are a few of the vast number of people whose selves are denied access to basic physical and psychological needs.

## INCREASING SELF-AWARENESS

There are many ways of exploring and expanding self-awareness. Chapman *et al.* (1982) describe two ways of exploring one's own personality. By talking in a relaxed and uninhibited way into a tape-recorder and listening to one's own free-flow thoughts, it is possible to learn something of the themes, worries, and issues that concern us. Another way is to keep a journal or diary, which can be used as a record of thoughts, feelings, behaviour, and the consequences. The journal or diary can be a combination of inner thoughts and feelings, as well as external events. Poetry, art, and music could all be included to help patterns of the self emerge, and hitherto unknown aspects of the self to be owned. Individual and group supervision (Chapter 25) can be used to review and reflect on practice, and can also be used to help develop self-awareness.

The mental health nurse aims to enable clients towards personal competence and self-empowerment. Rogers identified that the most effective therapists are those who have and demonstrate a high respect for others, who are genuine, and who display an advanced degree of empathy towards their clients.

Effective mental health nurses need to have basic qualities that include self-reliance and the motivation and commitment to continue the quest for self-knowledge and awareness. There are many complex forces and dynamics to understand and work with, both in life and within the context of the therapeutic relationship. Clients are identified as being at risk when they are referred to the mental health services, but mental health nurses are also at risk and may themselves, at times of crisis, become anxious, unsure, pessimistic, and unable to cope.

Using clinical supervision and support systems within the organization, and family and friends at a more personal level are ways of facilitating a sound concept of self, of shaping behaviour, developing perception, and refining therapeutic skills so that cues about the emotional stances in both self and others can by responded to more effectively.

Self-awareness is not a technique. It is a goal, a way of living, and is not to be confused with self-knowledge. The paradox is that knowing about self-awareness may not necessarily bring about change in either the self or in others. The journey of self-awareness is not an easy one, and there are many pitfalls along the way. There are many people who believe that the ways to self-awareness are more important than the process, that intellectualization is so powerful that experiences are never allowed to move them away from their minds into their bodies. As Rosenberg (1985) said:

As the body is the vehicle through which we express our being, it is important to include it in any process of growth that we choose to follow. The body, self and soul are all manifestations of consciousness. The body is the physical expression, the self is the individual psychological expression, and the soul is the expression of our essence as it merges with universal consciousness.

## REFERENCES

Bower, T.G.R. (1971) The object in the world of the infant. *Scientific American*, 225, 30–8.

Buber, M. (1957) Elements of the interhuman, William Alanson White Memorial Lectures, *Psychiatry*, 20, 95–129.

Chapman, A. J. and Gale, A. (1982) *Psychology and People*, Macmillan Press Ltd, in *Inquiring Man* (2nd edn) Penguin, Harmondsworth.

Claxton, G. and Ageha, S. (1981) *Wholly Human: Western and Eastern Vision of the Self and Its Perfection*, Routledge, London.

Fantz, R. L. (1961) The origin of form perception. *Scientific American*, 204, 66–72.

Fromm-Reichman, F. (1950) *Principles of Intensive Psychotherapy*, Univ. Chicago Press.

Gross, R. D. (1987) *Psychology: The Science of Mind and Behaviour*, Hodder and Stoughton, London.

James, W. (1890) *The Principles of Psychology*, Vol. 1,

Jourard, S. (1971) *The Transparent Self*, Litton Educational Publishing, Inc.,

Kelly, G. A. (1955) *The Psychology of Personal Constructs*, Vols 1 and 2, Norton, New York.

Kelly, G. A. (1969) *Clinical Psychology and Personality*, (ed. B. A. Mahe, Wiley, Chichester.

Laing, R. D. (1965) *The Divided Self*, Penguin, Harmondsworth.

Lake, F. (1965) Privately circulated papers for The Clinical Theological Association.

Mair, J. M. M. (1970) Experimenting with individuals. *British J. Medical Psychology*, 43, 245–56.

Moloney, J. C. (1949) *The Magic Cloak. A Contribution to the Psychology of Authoritarianism*. Montrose Press.

Parkes, C. M. (1972) *Bereavement: Studies of Grief in Adult Life*, Tavistock, London.

Perls, Frederick S., Hefferline, R. F. and Goodman, P. (1951) *Gestalt Therapy*, Souvenir Press.

Reich, W. (1948) *Character Analysis*, Orgone Press, New York.

Rogers S. C. R. (1961) A theory of psychotherapy with schizophrenics and a proposal for its empirical investigation, in *Psychotherapy with Schizophrenics*. Univ. Louisiana Press, Baton Rouge (eds J.6. Dawson, H.K. Stone *et al.*).

Rosenberg, J. L., Rand, M. L., Asay, D. (1985)*Body, Self and Soul-Sustaining Integration*, Humanics Ltd.

Shakespeare, W. (1603) *Hamlet* II, 2.

Stevens, J. O. (1971) *Awareness: Exploring, Experimenting, Experiencing*. Real People Press.

## FURTHER READING

Bolton, R. (1979) *People Skills*, Spectrum,

Bond, M. and Kilty, J. (1982) *Practical Ways of Dealing with Stress*, Human Potential Research Dept., Univ. Surrey.

Carkhuff, R. (1983) *The Art of Helping*, Holt, Rinehart & Winston, New York.

Dainow, S. and Bailey, C. (1988) *Developing Skills with People*, John Wiley & Sons, Chichester.

Klein, M. (1983) *Discover Your Real Self*, Hutchinson & Co, London.

Ernst, S. and Goodison, L. (1981) *In Our Own Hands*, The Women's Press, London.

# PART SEVEN

# SERVICE MANAGEMENT

*Frank Hardiman*

The purpose of this chapter is to examine, within a management context, developments in working practices within mental health. Changes in the management and structure of services, and changes in the roles of professionals, have arisen in part from legislative changes in the late 1980s and early 1990s. The immediate and longer-term impact on the provision of health care and community services is described and discussed.

The NHS is changing. Proposals set out in the government's 1989 White Paper *Working for Patients* offered hospitals, community health services, mental health services, and mental handicap services the opportunity to become more independent by applying for a new self-governing status within the NHS as NHS trusts.

NHS trusts take fuller responsibility for their own affairs, and aim to provide services to meet the local population needs and conditions. They are no longer controlled by district or regional health authorities. Instead they are managed by their own board of directors, which includes lay people as well as senior medical staff and nurses. Decisions about the day-to-day running and the long-term planning of trust services are theirs alone.

Ham (1991) states that the government expects health services to become more responsive to users through a number of reforms, including: proposals to strengthen management at all levels; measures to manage clinical activity more effectively; the introduction of a new system of contractual funding; and new arrangements for allocating resources. This change in service management and structure represents a significant challenge for health care services. There will be a continued need to bring about major shifts in attitudes and behaviour in order to embrace fully all the changes proposed in the National Health Service and Community Care Act (1990).

A key issue in the change process is the change in management culture and practice. Good leadership and management are essential to the success of any organization, as is the need for new skills to be developed. For Diskin *et al.* (1990) 'A manager is defined as a person who is held accountable for the outputs of others and for sustaining a team capable of producing these outputs.' The manager's role is to provide clear leadership to staff, with the explicit purpose of enabling staff to use their professional skills, expertise, and judgement in meeting client, family, and community service needs.

Before the NHS reforms of the late 1980s, the centralized management structure of the NHS was characterized by high complexity, high formalization, and impersonality, which restricted effective decision-making and responsiveness to a rapidly changing environment. Decisions were largely taken at the top-management level, without much consultation within and outside the organization, often resulting in duplication of services.

New management thinking in the public sector recognized the need to move towards a more decentralized structure that generate less dissatisfaction with work, increased satisfaction with supervision, and greater communication frequency among co-workers at the same level. Such a structure, it is believed, will allow for decisions to be taken at lower levels, increasing their effectiveness and giving subordinates a clearer identification with organizational goals. This in turn should lead to improved quality in the delivery of health care services to clients, and increased job satisfaction for employees.

In its White Paper *Promoting Better Health* (1987), the government has also set the agenda for reform in primary health care. Standards of health and health care are to be raised through a greater emphasis on health promotion and disease prevention. The focus is to offer more information and a wider choice to clients, with significant changes in GP contracts to facilitate the reforms. GPs will be expected to meet targets set for vaccination, immunization, and cervical cancer screening. The report encourages the development of health promotion clinics, but fails specifically to address mental health problems.

## MENTAL HEALTH CARE IN A COMPETITIVE ENVIRONMENT

There is a danger of services being developed in a competitive rather than a collaborative way.

The changes necessary to establish NHS trusts, and the new ways of financing them, are based on the concept of the internal market. This involves purchasers and providers of services where the purchaser should have a choice. The functions of the purchaser and provider are clearly separated between those with distinct responsibility for providing health care services, and those with responsibility for purchasing health care.

Ham (1991) has stated that the introduction of contractual funding will bring about managed competition between provider units. It will also mean, in some cases, that providers in the NHS will be competing with the private and voluntary sector for the resources that health authorities and GP fund-holders have to spend. It is envisaged that specifications in contracts for services will provide the incentive to ensure that resources are used more efficiently, resulting in high-quality care and best value.

It follows that most providers should be within easy reach of the market location, competing to provide just what the purchaser wants. This presents something of a dilemma for London teaching hospitals, which rely on having a national market, and whose cost of services is considerably higher. Future funding arrangements may recognize the need for continued separate funding from the Department of Health (DoH) to maintain these services, but this is by no means a certainty.

It is likely that some services presently being provided in the NHS may in the future only be available in the voluntary and private sectors. Concern is being expressed by opponents to these reforms that a move away from collaborative health care planning to one of market competition will mean the end of a national health service, funded largely by the state.

Will the survival of national health care services depend on each provider unit's ability to compete? Will services be provided on the basis of which are most economically beneficial to the organization, or will they be based on clinical need? Such questions form the basis of concern as to whether high-quality care at best value is at the expense of a reduction, or in some instances a loss, in services.

There are two types of health care provider within the NHS: NHS trusts, and directly managed units, or DMUs. DMUs remain accountable to their district health authority (DHA), but are allowed to run their affairs at arm's length from the authority. This allows DHAs to treat their DMUs as independent health care providers, and to place contracts to buy services from them.

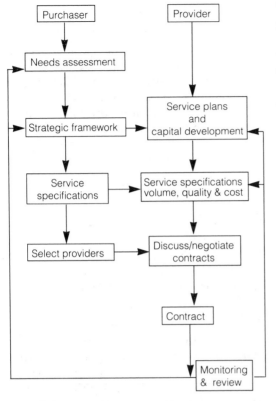

**Figure 30.1** The contracting process

The government wished to see a shift from the joint-planning system, which was designed with local authority requirements in mind, to an approach based on a national framework of planning agreements. The aim is to strengthen incentives, make responsibilities clearer, and make explicit the distinction between purchasers and providers of care.

The vital component of the contract between purchaser and provider will be that of ensuring quality. Service specifications will need to be drawn up, and specific quality measures identified for each service area.

How can health care managers work efficiently in providing services to clients if they are not clear about what resources they are using, and how they are contributing to health care outcomes embodied in care plans?

This question concerns one of sound, rational management.

For the purchaser-provider process to function effectively, it will need good information. Computer networks should enable purchasers to access data concerning the quality and availability of services and to compare costs. High-quality information should be accurate, timely, relevant, and clear.

Local authorities are to be enablers rather than sole or major providers of care, purchasing services from private and voluntary suppliers. An important concept is that the services purchased are to be determined within budget limits, by the needs of the individual client rather than by the services that are available (Millar, 1990).

There are great differences between districts providing services to the mentally ill, despite the similarity in services needed. Sadly, when resources are distributed, the needs of people with mental health problems are not often seen as a high priority. There is much rhetoric by health and local authorities about what is necessary to meet the needs of people with mental health problems, but not a lot of evidence of service provision.

In planning the statutory service provision for people with mental health problems, it should be recognized that voluntary organizations have a fine tradition in complementing service provision through the development of supported accommodation, group homes, and day-care services. Close collaboration with voluntary-sector organizations, such as MIND and MENCAP, must be further developed if duplication of services is to be avoided, and the limited financial resources are to be used effectively.

It is more important what happens to the person than where he or she lives. The purpose of developing community services for people with mental health problems should be to enrich, not to diminish, the quality and potential of their lives. In spite of expectations of extra resources following the run down of many large mental institutions in the 1980s, there nevertheless remains a dearth of community facilities. There has been growing concern about the increasing number of mentally ill people who are now homeless.

Effective community care should enable access by the mentally ill person and his or her relatives to a range of services which aim to support and enhance his or her citizenship. This will necessitate the major agents of care working in close partnership to provide and monitor standards of services in consultation with clients.

The voluntary sector has an important role in acting as an advocate, to represent the needs and wishes of individuals, or, collectively, the families of mentally ill people.

Within the present philosophy for managing health care services, it is management's responsibility to ensure that an appropriate strategy in the form of a business plan is formulated and implemented. To succeed, any strategy adopted must be able to deal with the changes taking place in the environment, and to involve clients in its formulation at all stages. It is required to be responsive – recognizing the opportunities and threats facing the organization/service and its ability to handle them by identifying the strengths and weaknesses inherent to its capabilities.

A SWOT analysis is a technique used to appraise both the present performance of the organization and the environment in which it exists. This appraisal involves analyzing internal **S**trengths and **W**eaknesses, and external **O**pportunities and **T**hreats (Cole, 1984). This analysis forms the basis for developing a business plan.

A business plan takes an overview of the whole service to be provided by:

- reviewing past years' activity and performance;
- identifying strengths and weakness of existing services;
- having an eye to future opportunities and possible threats;

- providing a clear focus for strategic planning.

Such a comprehensive strategic analysis and detailed planning is essential if providers and purchasers are to achieve their predetermined corporate objectives. The process also should be carried out in each directorate within provider units. This will ensure a continued review of service provision, assisting in determining standards of quality and costs of services provided.

BUSINESS PLAN CHECKLIST

1. Review the marketplace.
2. Analyze last year's performance.
3. Set the service objectives for next year.
4. Develop alternatives to achieve those objectives.
5. Create a first draft of the business plan.

Remember to consult and actively seek the views of staff at all stages; this will ensure more effective commitment to agreed objectives and result in better-quality services provided. Remember the formula P + I = C: Participation plus Involvement equals Commitment.

## MARKETING HEALTH CARE SERVICES

Providers of services will need to develop a marketing strategy to drive the business-planning process in order to compete effectively in the marketplace. The Chartered Institute of Marketing defines marketing as, 'the management process responsible for identifying, anticipating and satisfying customers' requirements profitably.' Applied to the NHS, this could mean using resources more effectively to ensure high-quality services at value-for-money costs. This will involve a marketing audit to review and assess the environment in which services are to be offered, identifying clearly who the customers are and what they want.

Kotler (1976) has emphasized the importance of the marketing mix: product, place, price, and promotion – the four P's – as being the ingredients to be considered when developing a marketing strategy. More recently, Kotler (1991) has described these ingredients as the seller's mix, and has suggested there is also a buyer's mix – the four C's – in the form of customer value, cost to the customer, convenience, and communication. Kotler suggests successful organizations are fully orientated to responding to the buyer's mix.

One of the aims of provider units should therefore be to highlight to potential purchasers what the differences are in the services they provide. Provider units will need clearly to communicate their competitive advantages in the form of 'differential advantage', such as the uniqueness of their service, and/or their 'distinctive competence', ability to do something well, which should stimulate market demand for their services.

## COMMUNITY CARE

Definitions of community care abound. One perspective is that the causes of mental illness lie in social deprivation, poverty, unemployment, racism, sexism, or poor education (Townsend, 1982). Here, the goal of the mental health worker is to work with the community in planning and education to help create an environment conducive to health, and thus to prevent mental illness.

For the most part, community care in the UK is provided at primary and secondary levels, with the bulk of care being provided by families, GPs, social workers, the clergy, friends, and volunteers. Secondary community care is provided by psychiatrists and a team of specialists, including nurses, CPNs and social workers.

The government's White Paper *Better Services for the Mentally Ill* (DHSS, 1975) established a blueprint for psychiatric ser-

vices into the 1990s, highlighting the need for services for patients whose needs fell between hospital care and outpatient care. This provided further impetus for the provision of day-care in day hospitals: concerned with the treatment of acute conditions, preventing more severe mental illness, and avoiding hospitalization, with day-centres providing social care rather than treatment.

Community services encompass a wide variety of services provided by the statutory, private, and voluntary sectors. These include supported accommodation, through to specialist services for adults who are mentally ill and whose behaviour causes difficulty in management.

The changes in the provision of community-based services require a greater emphasis on inter-agency working, local authority planning, social services and education, voluntary organizations, housing associations and Community Health Councils (CHC), as well as the need to develop formal links for sub-contracting and planning joint developments and new service initiatives. The government White Paper *Caring for People* (1989) represents a major shift in responsibility to local authorities, and in culture towards the purchaser/provider and mixed-contract market model.

Close co-operation between health authorities, other health care agencies, local authorities, and social services has not always been enough to remove the confusion about who is in charge, and who clients should turn to for information. Working relationships did not always exist in the best interests of people needing community care. What the White Paper does, is to give a clear point of reference for everyone in need of community care. The Paper identifies three ways in which authorities can work to improve the care offered to the mentally ill:

- All DHAs to implement a system to assess the needs of patients before discharge, ensuring effective arrangements are in place, and a named person appointed to ensure those needs are meet.

- Regions to identify sites made vacant by the closure of old long-stay hospitals that could be brought into use in partnership with the private sector to maximize value for money, and increase available options for the treatment of mentally ill people.
- From 1991–2 the government will pay a grant, through regions to the social service authorities, in order to increase the level of social care available for the mentally ill.

The principle of community care means that people where possible should be able to continue to live in their own homes rather than in institutions, and should be given every assistance by the authorities to do so. The aim of health authorities, in close co-operation with local authorities and social services, should be to develop their community services with this key objective in mind. Continuous care should, where possible, be provided in small units, offering clients their own rooms, and a home-like environment to help them to live as normally and as comfortably as possible.

Co-ordinating packages of care therefore becomes more important in the community health service than they are in an institutional service, where single accountability was the norm; in the community, the service comes from a range of different sources.

## COMMUNITY PSYCHIATRIC NURSING

A fundamental question that is still being asked is, should CPNs be primarily hospital-based, or attached to a primary health care team (PHCT)?

A review of the literature on community psychiatric nursing, suggests there is no such thing as a typical CPN service. What is clear nationally is that most CPNs have moved from being based in a psychiatric hospital, and are now based in a variety of places, increasingly as part of the PHCT. Carr, *et al.*

(1980), suggested that where the CPN is based affects the services offered.

Traditionally, the CPN was a ward-based nurse who visited discharged patients at home as part of their rehabilitation programme. The hospital-based CPN usually works as a member of the CPN team, but has close links with the ward staff and the multidisciplinary team. The CPN's caseload is indirectly controlled by the consultant psychiatrist, where he or she refers patients to the CPN, and so the caseload is subject to the psychiatrists workload and his or her contact with the GP's. Other factors include the psychiatrist's own prejudices, preferences, and his or her degree of control over the CPN.

The advantages of a hospital-based service include: close contact with the consultant psychiatrist leading to ease of access and liaison; similarly close contact with other psychiatric workers, clinical psychologists, occupational therapists, social workers, and clearer professional identity. The disadvantages of a hospital-based CPN service include: conflict of priorities of CPNs between their perception of what a client may require in terms of care and that of the psychiatrist's. Some psychiatrists may restrict the CPNs involvement with the client's whole family; lack of freedom for the CPN to be a practitioner in their own right, as most referrals have already been vetted by psychiatrists.

Being hospital-based isolates the CPN from other community services, increases the client's dependency on the hospital, and may alienate those clients not wishing to be stigmatized by contact with the mental hospital (Simmons *et al.*, 1991).

When the CPN is attached to the PHCT, he or she is usually based in a health centre or in close proximity to the team. The main difference between this type of service and the hospital service is not simply geographical, but more a shift in attitude in that the CPN is a practitioner in his or her own right and is able to accept referrals direct from all members of the team, and to terminate therapy at his or her own discretion.

The CPN's catchment area is determined by the boundaries of the GP's practice. The CPN accepts referrals from the GP for client also normally the doctor would not refer to a psychiatrist, either because he or she does not wish to bother a consultant, or because he/she fears the stigma of such a referral for the client and his/her family.

In the PHCT the CPN is able to advise on psychiatric matters for other professionals, such as the district nurse, health visitors, social workers, and other therapists.

The advantages of a PHCT-based CPN service include: GPs may prefer to talk to the CPN face-to-face, and prefer the CPN to be close by (Sharpe, 1982); early referral to the CPN leads to crisis prevention rather than crisis intervention (Leopoldt, 1979); clients prefer being seen in general practice than conventional outpatient clinics or hospital settings (Harker *et al.*, 1976; Tyler, 1984).

GPs see a need for a CPN to be based in the community, as do clients, who express high consumer satisfaction (Sugden *et al.*, 1986). It is certain that in a comprehensive psychiatric service, the CPN is essential to provide a personal nursing service. The Social Services Select Committee report on Community Care (1985) echoes this in saying 'The CPN is probably the most important single professional in the process of moving care of mental illness into the community.'

In the past, nursing has taken much of its direction for practice from the medical model, resulting in a strongly disease-orientated approach. This has played a part in preventing nursing realizing its full potential to contribution to health care If society does not perceive nursing as a discipline distinct from medicine, then little value will be attributed to nursing functions (Bridges, 1991).

The future training of community nurses in psychiatry will be influenced strongly by the location of the CPN, as will the future role of the CPN. Basic mental health nurse training is now largely linked to models of social and community care, with an emphasis on family and community skills, self-awareness, counselling, and personal skills.

The UKCC report (1991), on the future of community nursing in the context of Project 2000 and PREPP suggests a new breed of practitioner called the 'community health care nurse', who would have to have a core of knowledge, and then undertake specialist training in, for example, district nursing, health visiting, mental handicap, or community psychiatric nursing.

What is needed is research to extend the knowledge base for CPNs and to point to guidelines as to where they may develop. In particular, the client's view of the service is needed, as is some way of measuring the quality and effectiveness of the care delivered.

CPNs should continue to extend and promote their skills in health education and health promotion, emphasizing prevention of ill health and working towards empowering clients to make informed choices about the nature and type of health care services they wish to be provided. If CPNs are to make this valuable and important contribution to better health care it will be important for them often to be based in the primary care setting. It is essential therefore to develop psychiatric nurses as practitioners in their own right, to work effectively in a community setting as part of the PHCT.

## CARE MANAGEMENT

Care management, or case management as it was formerly termed, provides a process for inter-agency working, through a partnership approach focusing on the needs and wishes of the client, rather than on the individual service. The care management approach has been *in situ* for a number of years in social services, and has more recently been adopted by CPNs and others.

The purpose of care management is to work on an individual basis with the client and or family who need assistance in order to meet their particular needs. Care management also has a role in influencing service development and the provision of new services.

In practice, Richardson (1991) suggests there are two key elements of the process: firstly, it is client-led. Listening to the consumers view is central to the government's *Patient's Charter* initiative, trying to understand what is needed and consulting with the client about any decisions under consideration, and involving the client at each stage, and agreeing any necessary compromise. Care management means involving clients in the process of choice. What should not happen is the offer of a service on a take-it-or-leave-it-basis. The second key aspect of care management is that one person has responsibility for managing a client's care from beginning to end. This is to ensure that a named person is clearly accountable for obtaining the necessary services for each client, and then keeping in touch to ensure the services remain appropriate. As Richardson puts it so well, 'it involves altering the mind set of "let us see what services are available for your problem" to "let us see what can be arranged to meet your problem".'

## QUALITY CARE FOR MENTALLY ILL PEOPLE

A quality service has to satisfy client needs; quality is specific to the situation and the person. In order to achieve this the client requires information to enlarge his or her understanding and determine his or her needs.

Nurses working in the area of primary prevention in mental health may be working with any level of the social hierarchy – individuals, families, community, or even larger society. The nurse therefore needs to be highly trained and sensitive to the cultural, social, and religious needs of clients and their families, as well as providing expert nursing care. Effective communication between various service providers must be a priority, as staff in community settings can become isolated and lose their commitment to the service.

Maxwell (1984) has suggested that the overall performance of any public-sector organization needs to be considered in relation to a number of fairly discreet performance dimensions. For the health service he has suggested six dimensions, which are summarized by Best (1987) below:

- Access to services.
  Possible measures:
  - Waiting times for specific services.
  - Ambulance response times.
  - Travel times for specific services.

- Relevance to need for the whole community.
  Possible measures:
  - Percent of the budget being spent on, say, specific community services.
  - Achievement of given care group service targets, e.g., immunization rates.
  - The existence and use of follow-up assessment procedures.

- Effectiveness for individual clients.
  Possible measures:
  - Re-admission rates for the same diagnosis.
  - Infection and complication rates.
  - Existence and use of 'protocols' for given diagnoses.

- Equity.
  Possible measures:
  - Take-up and admission rates for different subgroups of the population.
  - Waiting times by population subgroup.
  - Availability of services for minority diagnoses.

- Social acceptability.
  Possible measures:
  - Annual report (statutory prepared by community representatives).
  - Complaints.

– Number of residents travelling elsewhere for services available locally.

• Efficiency and economy.
  Possible measures:
  – Unit costs.
  – Achievement of cost improvement targets.
  – Achievement of activity level targets.

These principles of measurement and standards have been incorporated in the government's *Patient's Charter* (1992) (Table 30.1).

## THE PATIENT'S CHARTER

From April 1992, the *Patient's Charter*, introduced by the government, guarantees to NHS

**Table 30.1** The Patient's Charter (1992)

| Ten Charter Rights | Nine Key Areas For Charter Stan |
|---|---|
| 1. To receive health care on the basis of clinical need, regardless of ability to pay. | 1. Patient's privacy, dignity, religious and cultural beliefs must be respected at all times. |
| 2. To be registered with a GP. | 2. Everyone, including people with special needs, must be able to use their local health services. |
| 3. To receive emergency medical care at any time, through your GP or the emergency ambulance service and hospital accident and emergency departments | 3. Health authorities must ensure there are arrangements to inform relatives and friends about progress of a patient's treatment, subject to the patient's wishes. |
| 4. To be referred to a consultant, acceptable to you, when your GP thinks it necessary, and to be referred for a second opinion if you and your GP agree this is desirable | 4. Emergency ambulance response times are 14 minutes in urban areas, and 19 minutes in rural referred for a second areas. |
| 5. To be given a clear explanation of any treatment proposed, including any risks and any alternatives, before you decide whether you will agree to the treatment. | 5. Patients arriving at an accident and emergency department should be seen immediately and their need assessed. |
| 6. To have access to your health records, and to know that those working for the NHS are under a legal duty to keep their contents confidential. | 6. No outpatient should wait longer than 30 minutes beyond his or her appointment time. |
| 7. To choose whether or not you wish to take part in any medical research or medical training. | 7. Operations should not be cancelled on the day they are due to take place; if an operation is cancelled twice, a hospital must admit within a further month. |
| 8. To be given detailed information on local health services, including quality standards and maximum waiting times. | 8. Every patient should be under the care of a named nurse, who takes responsibility for that patient throughout his or her care. |
| 9. To be guaranteed admission for treatment by a specific date no later than two years from the day when your consultant places you on a waiting list. | 9. Any decisions on continuing health/social care need to be made before discharge. Proper arrangements must be in place to make sure this happens. |
| 10. To have any complaint about NHS services – whoever provides them – investigated and to receive a full and prompt written reply from the chief executive or general manager. | |

patients ten charter rights, and introduces charter standards in nine key areas. In addition, health authorities will be required to produce local charter standards addressing other aspects of service which are of concern to local populations. The *Patient's Charter* also requires each health authority to publish annually information about performance against national standards, and also to publish an annual report of achievement against local standards.

The objectives of the *Charter* will necessarily be reflected in approaches towards commissioning developed by DHAs and FHSAs. It is hoped that DHAs and FHSAs will address the needs of people with mental health problems, as the *Patient's Charter* is more orientated to physical needs and primary health care, than to mental health needs.

There is also an emphasis on the *Charter* being hospital-centred, when in mental health there has been a shift from hospital to community-based care. It also has to be said that the *Patient's Charter* reflects largely the principles of good practice that have for many years been demonstrated throughout the health service. It is not therefore breaking new ground, for example, the named nurse has been a feature of individualized care, via the nursing process, for at least 10 years. This, however, does not detract from the importance of this initiative in setting standards of quality.

Quality is everyone's responsibility, and models of good practice will need to be developed commencing with a policy statement, relating to the pursuit of equality of access to all. Nelson (1989), suggests there is no doubt that policies are needed, are useful, and save time. The important aspect is communication; what often happens in large organizations is those propounding policy statements have not ensured that those who need to know do so, and how they should be applied.

Priorities and resources will need to be identified through extensive consultation with clients, families, and the community at large.

It has to be acknowledged also that some of the structures and practices within mental health care settings may need changing to ensure equal opportunities of access to services by all service users.

The values of a high-performing organization include quality, customer care, staff development, social responsibility, and distinctive competence. The Griffith's Report (1983) set the scene to make quality a priority for all services provided to consumers. Some initiatives have taken place in this area, with many authorities appointing staff with specific responsibility for quality assurance. Central funds have been made available by the government for medical audit, and to set up a programme of national demonstration projects, focusing on the three main areas of outpatient services; accident and emergency departments; and total quality management.

Funds were made available to regional health authorities and special health authorities to support local quality initiatives in five areas: improving information to clients; schemes to assess the quality of services provided, including consumer surveys; projects to provide a more personal service; staff training in quality issues; and improvements to the physical environment and buildings.

Quality management and service provision are central to the quality review process. Purchasers and providers will state clearly the aspects of quality to be included in the contract, which will form the basis for raising and maintaining standards.

Nurses form the largest group of health care workers, and have an important and vital contribution to make in determining and ensuring quality care. Patients with mental health problems are not the most popular in the health service, and the mental health nurse is not the most acknowledged and revered nurse in the public eye (Hardiman, 1985).

Mental health nurses not only care for acutely ill clients in institutions, but are increasing their care in the community in an attempt to prevent admissions by rehabilitating and supporting clients after discharge from hospital.

In order for quality care to be delivered to clients, mental health nurses must have a clear sense of purpose, and base their practice on research findings. At the Maudsley Hospital, London, a nursing philosophy has been written which contains the following statement:

> Psychiatric nursing practice should follow research-based principles of individualized care for clients in the hospital and community, based on a holistic approach, addressing the physical, psychological, and social needs of individual clients

A statement such as this, which was produced from extensive consultation with nurses, provides a basis upon which realistic quality nursing standards can be agreed and met.

## THE MENTAL HEALTH TEAM

Teamwork is the key to effective health care. The mental health team aims to provide a stable, well-trained, multidisciplinary team, based in a culture that fosters close, effective teamwork, with an emphasis on valuing staff as individuals, each with an important role in the delivery of services.

The Royal Commission on the National Health Service (1979) defined a multidisciplinary clinical team as 'a group of colleagues acknowledging a common involvement in the care and treatment of a particular client'. Macfarlane's (1980) description of the multidisciplinary clinical team as comprising of the client and his or her family, and all workers contributing to his or her health care, is particularly appropriate to the field of mental health nursing.

Stuart *et al.* (1991) suggest nurses may belong to three different types of teams:

- unidisciplinary, having all team members of the same discipline;

- interdisciplinary, having members of different disciplines involved in a formal arrangement to provide patient services while maximizing educational interchange; and

- multidisciplinary, having members of different disciplines who each provide services to the patient.

One might also define a multidisciplinary team as being a group of professionals with a common goal, who have the knowledge and vested authority by the discipline they represent to make the decisions for which they will be accountable.

Stuart *et al.* (1991) suggest that most organized mental health settings employ an interdisciplinary approach, which requires highly co-ordinated and frequently interdependent planning, based on separate and distinct roles for each team member.

### LEAD CONSULTANTS/TEAM LEADERS

Enabling people to work together well is the key job of every team leader and manager. The team leader in care groups may or may not be a consultant psychiatrist, particularly in the community sector, as services to clients are provided from a number of different agencies, including social services, health and local authorities, and the voluntary sector. The consultant psychiatrist is legally in charge of the cases of clients who are hospital inpatients.

The lead consultant/team leader will provide the link between management and the core professional staff working in a particular care group. Their role will include:

- negotiating with management an agreed annual contract for the clinical service to be provided;

- monitoring clinical workload against the contract and agreeing any changes;

- co-ordinating and monitoring peer review/medical audit;

- providing leadership and support to team members;

- managing financial resources.

PSYCHIATRISTS

Psychiatrists have statutory responsibilities under the Mental Health Act (1983), and carry the medical responsibility for diagnosis, medical instructions, medication, admission and discharge, and the accountability for medical treatment. They may or may not be the team leader particularly in the community setting.

NURSES

Hardiman (1985) has observed that 'the nursing service depends on the quality, skill and motivation of its staff'. Nurses are accountable and responsible for nursing care based on a primary nurse approach, whereby each client has a named nurse. This includes implementing the nursing process, and basing their practice on a nursing model of care including assessment, planning care, maintaining a safe and therapeutic environment, and evaluating nursing outcomes of care.

Nursing roles have changed with the emergence of resource management and the expanding nature of the profession. Murray *et al.* (1983) have suggested that as a mental health nurse, you may carry out a number of roles. In the UK the following key roles have emerged:

### Clinical specialist

This nurse is an expert in providing nursing care in a speciality area of work, for example child and adolescent psychiatry or HIV and AIDS counselling, based on authoritative knowledge and expert skills.

### Nurse therapist

This role was first developed at the Maudsley Hospital in London, were nurses trained in behavioural psychotherapy techniques. The nurse therapist is recognized as a trained and skilled independent practitioner, who diagnoses, prescribes and carries out treatment for clients in hospital and community settings. The nurse therapist may also be in private practice.

### Primary nurse

This is the named nurse responsible for the individual client's nursing care, throughout the period of their care programme, whether the client is in the community or in hospital.

### Nurse manager

She or he may work less directly with clients, but has the responsibility to provide nursing leadership to ensure that an appropriate therapeutic milieu is maintained. Having regard for the cultural, religious, social, and health care needs of the client, their families and friends.

A key area of responsibility is the support and development of nurses and representing nursing views to senior managers. The nurse manager is not necessarily the budget-holder for nursing resources, but plays an important role in negotiating and allocating nursing resources within clinical directorates.

### Nurse researcher

The role of the nurse has expanded with an increase in the complexity of skills required. Nurses now more than ever have an important responsibility to evaluate their practice, to develop their understanding and knowledge of nursing interventions through planned research, and to communicate their findings.

### Nurse health educator

The government's White Paper *Promoting Better Health* (1990) provides an important opportunity for nurses to promote health and to educate clients, their families, and the community on a variety of health-awareness issues, including the dangers of smoking, alcohol and drug abuse, HIV and AIDS.

### Nurse teacher

Nurse teachers are being encouraged to link with health care service areas, not only to provide support to student nurses in training, but increasingly as resource people to marry the theoretical aspects with clinical practice.

### Ward manager

In many hospitals the title of ward sister/ charge nurse is being replaced with the title ward manager, which aims to reflect their responsibilities within a resource management environment.

Ritter (1989) cites Ever (1977), who concluded that 'the ward sister has central responsibility for integrating and strengthening interprofessional relationships and communication.' This is still true, however, there is a real danger that the ward manager's role will increasingly reflect the needs of general management, with an emphasis on managing the physical environment and managing a budget, rather than on the direct clinical nursing care of clients.

It is important for senior nurses in the community and at ward level in the hospital to maintain their primary role of being the clinical nurse leaders for planning and implementing nursing care through primary nursing.

What the sister/charge nurse needs, perhaps, is a ward clerk or a business manager who is accountable to them for administrative/managerial duties. This would ensure that the sister/charge nurse retains full responsibility for the ward as in the past, but frees them from unnecessary day to administrative/management tasks. They can then continue to work with nurses and other clinical staff to meet individual patient's clinical care needs.

## OCCUPATIONAL THERAPIST

Occupational therapists are responsible for activity programming, including the assessment of clients' domestic and work skills, which is crucial in the process of rehabilitation. Occupational therapy does not necessarily begin and end in the hospital. Increasingly it is being recognized that a skilled occupational therapist has much to offer in supporting the client at home and in day-care settings in the community. Often a key role of the occupational therapist in the community is to ensure that the client has access to educational services, which may form an important part of the rehabilitation process.

## SOCIAL WORKERS

Social workers are accountable and responsible for family casework and social placement. If they have approved status under the Mental Health Act (1983), they have statutory duties in respect of people with mental health problems. The Children Act (1989) specifies the statutory duties of social workers in the care of children. Social workers are also often likely to undertake the case/care manager role in relation to community care.

## PSYCHOLOGISTS

Psychologists are responsible for psychological assessment and testing, and psychological treatments.

If the roles and responsibilities of the team members are not clarified and agreed, conflicts may arise, with the crossing of professional boundaries resulting in role ambiguity and role conflict. Some overlapping of roles is desirable and in the client's interest, but there are inherent dangers in viewing each team member as being the same.

An effective team will respect and value each member's area of expertise, and recognize when another member of the team or a referral to another service would be in the best interests of the client.

## EDUCATION

Staff need to be treated as individuals in order to better understand their needs and aspirations and promote the awareness that management cares. Planned staff development programmes can broaden knowledge and develop the nurse's clinical and professional skills. A number of national initiatives for continuing professional education are presently being implemented.

Community Education and Practice Report (UKCC, 1991) and PREPP (1989) set out proposals for the future of community education and practice in response to the following changes:

- to ensure education for community practice meets contemporary health care needs and the needs of health services;
- to ensure that the professions are prepared to meet the demands of changes in service provision (following legislative change such as the National Health Service and Community Care act 1990 and the Children Act 1989);
- to eliminate unnecessary duplication and fragmentation of post-registration nursing education.

The two reports are designed to develop a coherent and comprehensive framework to develop and enhance standards of education and practice, and to improve standards of care by securing a firm link between the needs of patients and clients and the preparation required for practice. Continuing professional education is the way in which quality of care can be achieved and sustained.

To further promote the benefits of teamwork in delivering a quality service, multidisciplinary training courses for health care professionals should be promoted. This, perhaps, is the key to developing role appreciation across functions and enhancing teamwork.

## MANAGEMENT DEVELOPMENT

Changes in the delivery of health care services present a number of opportunities for nurses to develop their skills, both clinically and managerially.

For those nurses who wish to develop their management skills, it is worth contacting your local college of further education or university, which are likely to run several types of management courses. The Royal College of Nursing also provides management training courses at certificate and diploma level.

The level and type of course will depend on individual circumstances and career goals. It is desirable for all trained nurses to obtain at least a diploma in management studies. This will prove invaluable in taking on new responsibilities in a resource management environment and ensure that nurses can be appointed to senior management positions in the future.

## CONCLUSION

The changes that have taken place will do much to improve health care services to clients, and present real opportunities for nurses to take a lead role in clinical care as well as in the management and provision of services.

Project 2000 and the framework of the United Kingdom National Boards for continuing professional education will help to ensure the future quality and expertise of the nursing profession.

A profession which really fulfills its potential shares knowledge, experience, and the findings of research within its membership and with the community it serves. This requires nurses continuously to extend their understanding, to update their practice and to communicate their experience as widely and as cogently as possible.

## REFERENCES

Best, G. (1987) The future of NHS general management: where next? report; King's Fund College, London.

Carr, P., Butterworth, A., Hidges, B. E. (1980) *Community Psychiatric Nursing*, Churchill Livingstone, Edinburgh.

Disken, S., Dixon, M., Halpern, S. *et al.* (1990) Models of clinical management. IHSM, London.

Ham, C. (1991) *The New National Health Service*, Radcliffe Medical Press, Oxford.

Hardiman F. W. (1985) The psychiatric nurse's viewpoint. *Nursing Mirror*, Nov.

HMSO (1989) *Caring for People*, HMSO, London.

HMSO (1989) *Working for Patients*, HMSO, London.

Kotler, P. (1976) *Marketing Management*, (3rd edn), Prentice-Hall, New Jersey.

Kotler, P. (1991) Silent satisfaction. *Marketing Business*, Dec/Jan.

Maxwell, R. J. (1984) Quality assurance in health. *British Medical J.*, 288, 1470–2.

McFarlane, J. (1980) The multidisciplinary team, in *Multidisciplinary Clinical Teams* (eds I. Batchelor, J. McFarlane) Kings Fund Centre, London.

Millar, C. (1990) Continuity and change. *Insight for Managers in the Community*, 5, 6.

Murray, R. B. and Huelskoetter, M. W. (1983) *Psychiatric Mental Health Nursing: Giving Emotional Care*, Prentice-Hall, New Jersey.

Nelson, M. J. (1989) *Managing Health Professionals*, Chapman & Hall, London.

Pearson, A. (1988) *Primary Nursing*, Croom Helm, London.

Richardson, A. (1991) Making a clear case for care. *The Health Service J.*, Aug.

Ritter, S. (1989) *Bethlehem Royal and Maudsley Hospital Manual of Clinical Psychiatric Nursing Principles and Procedures*, Harper and Row, London.

Sharpe, D. (1982) GPs' views of community psychiatric nurses. *Nursing Times*, 78.

Simmons, S., Brooker, C. (1991) *Community Psychiatric Nursing*.

Stuart, G. W., Sundeen, S.J. (1991) *Principles and Practices of Psychiatric Nursing*, Mosby, St. Louis.

Sugden, *et al.* (1985) *A Handbook for Psychiatric Nurses*, Harper and Row, London.

Townsend, P. (1982) *Inequalities in Health, The Black Report*, Pelican, Harmondsworth.

Tyler, P. (1984) Psychiatric Clinics in general practice: an extension of community care. *British J. Psychiatry*, 145.

## FURTHER READING

Bridges J. (1991) Working with doctors, distinct from medicine. *Nursing Times*, 87, 27.

The Children Act (1989)

DHSS (1975) *Better Services for the Mentally Ill*, HMSO, London.

DHSS (1985) *Community Care: Government Response to the Second Report from the Social Services Committee*, 1984–5, Cmnd. 9674.

Griffiths, R. (1983) *NHS Management Enquiry Report*, DHSS, London.

Hardiman, F.W. (1985) Mental health nursing – quality is the prime concern. *Nursing Times*, Sept.

Hardiman, F.W. (1984) Mental health nursing – patients at risk. *Nursing Times*, Sept.

Harker, P., Leopoldt, H., Robinson, J.R. (1976) Attaching community psychiatric nurses in general practice. *J. Roy. Coll. Pract.* 26.

The National Health Service and Community Care Act (1990)

RCN (1991) *Clinical Directorates and Nursing*, Royal College of Nursing, March.

Taylor, P. (1984) *Understanding the NHS in the 1980s*, Office of Health Economics, London.

UKCC (1991) *Community Education and Practice Report*.

Wilkinson, G., Freeman, H. (1986) *The Provision of Mental Health Services in Britain: The Way Ahead*, Roy. Coll. Psych., London.

## WORKING PAPERS

No. 1 (1989) *Self-Governing Hospitals*, HMSO, London.

No. 2 (1989) *Funding and Contracts for Hospital Services*, HMSO, London.

No. 3 (1989) *Practice Budgets for General Medical Practicitioners*, HMSO, London.

No. 4 (1989) *Indicative Prescribing Budgets for General Medical Practitioners*, HMSO, London.

No. 5 (1989) *Capital Charges*, HMSO, London.

No. 6 (1989) *Medical Audit*, HMSO, London.

No. 7 (1989) *NHS Consultants: Appointments, Contracts and Distinction Awards*, HMSO, London.

No. 8 (1989) *Implications for Family Practioner Committees*, HMSO, London.

No. 9 (1989) *Capital Charges: Funding Issues*, HMSO, London.

No. 10 (1989) *Education and Training*, HMSO, London.

No. 11 (1990) *Framework for Information Systems: Overview*, HMSO, London.

**USEFUL ADDRESSES**

The Institute of Health Service Management
75 Portland Place,
London W1
071 580 5041

The British Institute of Management
Africa House
63-74 Kingsway
London WC2B 6BL
071 497 0580

The Chartered Institute of Marketing
Moor Hall
Cookham
Berkshire SL6 9QH
(06285) 24922

The Institute of Personnel Management
IPM House
Camp Road
Wimbledon, London SW19 4UX
081 946 9100

DISTANCE-LEARNING COURSES

The Open College
781 Wimslow Road
Didsbury
Manchester M20 BRW
061 434 0007

The Open University
PO Box 625
Milton Keynes MK1 1TY

# PART EIGHT

# IN THE BEST INTERESTS OF THE CLIENT?

*David Carpenter*

What is the duty of the nurse? This would appear to be the first and most fundamental question to ask when attempting to analyze the role of the mental health nurse from legal and ethical perspectives. There are, however, other questions to consider, such as, what precisely is a duty? Are legal duties the same as moral duties? Are the duties of a nurse different to those of other citizens? Are the duties of the mental health nurse different from those of other nurses?

A tentative answer to the first question might be that the duty of the nurse is to act in such a way as to benefit the client in her care, and to avoid actions or omissions that might result in harm to the client. In other words, to act always in the best interests of the client; or, to 'Act always in such a way as to promote and safeguard the well-being and interests of patients/clients.' (UKCC, 1984).

Although this answer might appear to be entirely satisfactory, it assumes general agreement as to what the best interests of any individual might be. Agreement, however, is unlikely; a client's perception of what is best for him might easily be in conflict with the perceptions of those responsible for his care and treatment. It is this very conflict that characterizes ethical and legal concerns within mental health nursing practice. Mental illness can impair an individual's capacity to determine what his own best interests might be; similarly, it can lead others to assume they know what is best for him. Much of this chapter is devoted to the consideration of how the best interests of a client might be

determined, and the duty of the mental health nurse to attempt to do so. This can most effectively be examined in relation to particular groups of clients.

## CLIENTS WHO WANT WHAT OTHERS SUGGEST THEY NEED

These people have identified a need for help, and have voluntarily sought that help. Their perceptions of their problems might well coincide with those of the professionals who are assessing them, and there is agreement in respect of appropriate care and treatment. They may well be fully autonomous and competent, legally speaking, to make personal decisions, including those related to health care; this is recognized in that no treatment can lawfully take place without their consent. Such clients are in a similar position to the fully autonomous person who enters a general hospital for cold surgery: in the absence of unusual circumstances, there are no fundamental legal or ethical problems.

It is important to distinguish between those clients who truly want what others suggest they need, and those who merely agree with the recommendations of others because they feel under pressure to do so.

## CLIENTS WHO WANT WHAT THEY DO NOT NEED

It should be immediately clear that satisfying the best interests of such a client might well lead to frustrating his personal desires, or simply doing something to or for him in the face of his protests. Perhaps the most dramatic example would be someone who is suicidally depressed. For the client who *wants* to die, is it in his best interests to allow him to take a lethal overdose of drugs? If by 'best interests' we mean best medical interests, it certainly is not. On the other hand, is the nurse entitled to prevent the suicide in the face of the client's protests? If it is the nurse's duty to intervene, what authority is there for doing so? Much will depend on whether the client is autonomous or not.

## CLIENTS WHO NEED WHAT THEY DO NOT WANT

It is not difficult to think of clients in this category. Consider, for example, the anorectic who needs food, or the psychotic who needs neuroleptic drugs, or, rather more controversially, the continuing-care client who needs contraceptive pills.

All of these clients are likely to protest when a nurse attempts to satisfy their real needs. Is she entitled to satisfy needs on the basis that the client's best interests are being served? If she is entitled, from where does the power come enabling her to do things to people against their wishes?

Clients in this and the previous category may well be suffering from some impairment of autonomy as a result of illness; in other words, they might be unreliable determiners of their own best interests. Does this in itself allow the nurse to simply ignore the clients' protests, dismissing them as symptoms of illness?

## CLIENTS WHO DO NOT DESIRE THEIR OWN ACTIONS OR THOUGHTS

Clients in this category exibit behaviour that occurs in spite of their better judgment; their behaviour is 'unwilled'. It is not difficult to imagine, for example, a person who is suffering from a compulsive illness. He knows

that the behaviour is not necessary, but he nevertheless is 'obliged' to continue it.

Another possible interpretation of this category is that the behaviour might follow the thought and be willed, yet not be the willed behaviour of the client in normal circumstances. Imagine, for example, a person in a state of automatism, literally acting as a robot, perhaps following an epileptic fit; here there is a real sense that he is 'not his usual self'. If the person committed a crime while in this state he might reasonably claim that 'he' did not do it, although accepting that he did do it 'bodily'; he simply did not desire that which he did.

Clients in the first group are likely to be competent, and their autonomy will be at the most only marginally impaired. They are likely to be the best assessors of their own needs, and it is likely that they will seek the help of the nurse in attempting to reinstate willed action.

Clients in the second group will be fully autonomous as soon as they have returned to consciousness. The biggest question here may be whether the client should be held responsible for his action.

## CLIENTS WHO DO NOT ACT ACCORDING TO THEIR DESIRES

Here, the client's actions appear to be completely dislocated from both thought and will. The most obvious example are those suffering from dementing illnesses, in which during the latter stages, the behaviour of the client appears to be completely 'mindless'. These clients will have seriously impaired levels of autonomy, and will almost certainly be incompetent to make decisions in respect of ongoing care and treatment.

These five categories are all based on interrelationships of the same concepts: autonomy, needs, desires, wants, and competence. All of these are legally and morally significant, and are relevant in considering the duties of the mental health nurse.

## NEEDS *VS* WANTS

Nurses generally are preoccupied with the needs of clients. Some would argue that this is a good thing, and almost certainly morally desirable; surely a nurse ought to endeavour to satisfy a client's needs? Her task is made that much easier by the many nursing models that are based on the identification of needs. The nurse is often urged to identify problems and needs when assessing clients in the pursuit of systematic approaches to care. It is clear, however, that an individual is not normally preoccupied by his own needs – he is far more likely to be in touch with his desires or wants. We all know what we want; what we need might be seen as something for the expert to decide, at least in the context of health care. Confusion between wants and needs is common in everyday life; consider the person who claims that he really needs a holiday – it is far more likely that he actually wants one.

People do not always want what they need, nor need what they want. This is a feature of all people, not only of mental illness. It is not unusual, for example, for a person to need to lose weight, but not want to; or to want to smoke tobacco or drink alcohol, but it would be odd to suggest he needs to do either.

Needs tend to be identified by health professionals, particularly nurses, who see the satisfaction of needs as fulfilling their obligation to do what is best for the client. The satisfaction of needs can be viewed as an attempt to maintain some sort of bio-psycho-social equilibrium. People ought to have balanced diets, adequate respiration, mobility, a meaningful occupation, and so on. Notice, however, that the 'ought' signals a value judgement, and raises the likelihood of an ethical issue that might benefit from closer examination: do nurses know what is good for a person, and, if they do, are they entitled to thrust the goodness upon him?

There is no reason in principle why nurses should not know what is good for a person in the sense of maintaining optimum health. It might be argued that this is fundamental nursing knowledge. What, however, should the nurse do about the client who slouches in an armchair, thus causing breathing difficulties; or the client who eats plates of fatty food, and spends all day twiddling his thumbs? Or the client who continually enters into relationships that cause a great deal of stress and pain? While she can give the client the benefit of her knowledge, if he thanks her kindly – or for that matter tells her to mind her own business – there is probably not much else she can do.

This sort of situation is frustrating, but it demonstrates the priority of wants over needs. The wants of any client can only be established by talking with him, which is a good reason to always plan care with him as a partner. It is possible to plan care based on need in isolation from the client, but he might reject it. In the event of conflict between needs determined by the nurse and wants determined by the client, a working partnership would at least facilitate negotiation.

There are, then, practical reasons for acknowledging the client's wants, but, more importantly, there are also ethical reasons: the nurse who acknowledges the client's wants is basically respecting his autonomy, which is one of the most fundamental moral duties of the nurse.

## RESPECT FOR AUTONOMY

Autonomy is literally self-rule; it is our capacity to think, act, and make decisions for ourselves. It is this capacity that distinguishes man from other members of the animal kingdom. It is certainly significant in understanding man as a moral agent, as no person can be either morally praiseworthy or blameworthy unless their actions can be seen as resulting from autonomous deliberation. It would be ridiculous, for example, to praise a robot for its generosity, as it does not have the capacity to choose its actions.

In this respect, autonomy is related to other concepts such as responsibility and culpability, and can be understood as intimately related to human freedom. The fact that a person can decide for himself is a step towards the further considerations that, firstly, he ought to decide for himself, and, secondly, others ought not to interfere with his freedom to decide for himself. The latter obligation is the principle of respect for autonomy. To respect autonomous agents is to recognize their right to self-governance by affirming they are entitled to such autonomous determination, free of imposed limitations (Beauchamp *et al.* 1989).

The principle of respect for autonomy has been supported by a range of moral philosophers who would, arguably, agree on little else. Kant (Paton, 1969) argued that respect for autonomy is a logically necessary feature of being a rational agent, respecting the rights of other persons to make decisions for themselves supports a claim to a similar right ourselves. Mill argued that respect for autonomy is necessary to ensure an overall maximization of human happiness which, in part, results form individuals freely exercising autonomy. In *On Liberty*, (Acton 1983) Mill stated,

> ...the sole end for which mankind are warranted, either individually or collectively, in interfering with the liberty of action of any of their number, is self protection. The only purpose for which power can rightfully be exercised over any member of a civilised community against his will is to prevent harm to others. His own good, either physical or moral is not sufficient warrant.

Respect for autonomy, however, does not mean allowing a person absolute freedom. One person's autonomy ends where the next person's begins; we are free to make our own decisions insofar as we allow others to do likewise. A person is not free to steal from another, since this would compromise his freedom to do as he wishes with his own property. No one is free to interfere with the liberty of another except for self-protection; the welfare of the other person is not a sufficient justification to interfere with his liberty.

Not all people are fully autonomous. Small children, some mentally handicapped people, some people suffering from serious mental illness, and, of course, unconscious people, all suffer some impairment of autonomy. As there can be no obligation to respect autonomy unless the capacity for autonomous actions exists, if a person is not fully autonomous it will at times be necessary to make decisions on his behalf.

However, almost every person is capable of making at least some decisions, and autonomy should be respected as far as any individual's capacity allows; even an unconscious person is autonomous insofar as he has the latent capacity to be so – the limitation lies in his ability to exercise his autonomy. It is possible to consider the case of an acutely mentally ill person in a similar vein. It would be odd to refer to a sleeping person as non-autonomous: he has the capacity but is not exercising it, and when he wakes the capacity will be in evidence. A similar description may be made of an acutely mentally ill person: on recovery he will, again, be able to exercise his autonomy. It might similarly be possible to respect the autonomy of a mentally ill person, as long as it can be known with reasonable certainty what decisions he would have made for himself had he been able. It might thus be argued that the ultimate goal of any caring interventions include the restoration and maximization of autonomy.

## LEGAL REQUIREMENTS IN CONSENT

The moral obligation to respect autonomy is recognized in the legal requirement to obtain consent before any 'touching', including medical treatment. It is a person's right to decide whether to accept any intervention which might be proposed; the fact that care or treatment might be in a client's best interests is not sufficient in itself to impose treatment without his consent.

For the client's consent to be real, it must represent an autonomous decision – he must be competent to make that decision. In addition, real consent requires that the client's decision be sufficiently informed and voluntarily given. If any health professional imposed care or treatment without the client's consent, he invites a legal action in battery (Chapter 28). It would be unlawful, for example, to force drugs upon a client in the face of his protests, and it would equally be unlawful to give similar treatment to an incompetent client, since he would lack the capacity to decide for himself. Although he might not protest, his acquiescence would hardly count as consent.

The law assumes that all persons over 18 years of age are autonomous, and they alone can accept or decline any care or treatment offered. If the client is a minor but nevertheless has the capacity to make decisions *vis à vis* proposed treatment, his consent is equally valid. If he lacks the necessary capacity, then proxy consent can be obtained from parents or guardians.

While the law protects persons from undesired medical intervention, unless some provision is made available, it effectively denies care and treatment to those unable to decide for themselves. Provision exists partly in statute law and partly in common law, which is intended to benefit incompetent people: those who have suffered some impairment of autonomy, or who have achieved majority but remain not fully autonomous, for example, severely mentally handicapped people.

The Mental Health Act (1983) makes provision for the treatment of mental illness of those people who by virtue of their illnesses would not be competent to seek and consent to treatment. It is not a license to either hospitalize or to treat people against their wishes if those wishes are autonomously expressed. It should be viewed as a mechanism to ensure that people gain, and hopefully benefit, from care and treatment that they are unable to demand for themselves. This is perhaps an unusual explanation of the role of the Act, but it is the most appropriate way of expressing the spirit of the statute (Chapter 32).

Common law power permitting the treatment and care of incompetent adults, notwithstanding inability to consent, has only recently been clarified (Dimond, 1990). It has been clear for some time that treatment can be given out of necessity to an incompetent person, but the case of F. *v.* West Berkshire Health Authority, 1989 established precedent for the giving of treatment deemed to be beneficial rather than absolutely necessary. Lord Bridge stated:

> It seems to me to be axiomatic that treatment which is necessary to preserve the life, health or well-being of the patient may lawfully be given without consent. But, if a rigid criterion of necessity were to be applied to determine what is and what is not lawful in the treatment of the unconscious and the incompetent, many of those unfortunate enough to be deprived of the capacity to make or communicate rational decisions by accident, illness, or unsoundness of mind, might be deprived of treatment which it would be entirely beneficial for them to receive.

## THE PROBLEM OF ASSESSING COMPETENCE

It is both legally and morally desirable to provide care and treatment to those people who but for their incapacity would have given consent. It is important, however, to differentiate this group from those who are fully autonomous but wish to decline such intervention as might be available. Some test of competence will need to be applied when it is not clear to which of the two groups the client belongs. Tests of competence are peculiarly difficult to develop. Roth, Meisl, and Lidz (Kennedy, 1989) state:

> The search for a single test of competency is a search for a Holy Grail. Unless it is recognized that there is no magical definition of competency to make decisions about treatment, the search for an acceptable test will never end... Judgements of competency go beyond semantics or straightforward applications of legal rules; such judgements reflect social considerations and societal biases as much as they reflect matters of law and medicine.

Despite such difficulties, it is possible to provide examples of unreasonable tests of competency, and it is possible to describe current practice. Often, competency is a matter of status accorded by others (Kennedy, 1989) rather than a capacity decided on objective criteria. Unfortunately, it is those with the power to accord such status that equally act on the basis of it.

Health care practitioners usually decide competency, and they may also impose care or treatment in the face of apparent protests if they can establish incompetence. There have also been attempts to suggest that certain statuses entail incompetence. Obvious candidates include minority, mental illness, and mental handicap. It is far from obvious that age or diagnosis in itself should be a reliable indicator of competence. A further attempt can be found in the form of the 'outcome approach'. Here, competence is decided on the basis of the quality of the client's decisions; if he chooses rationally he is considered competent. The problem lies in the precise understanding of the word 'rational', which may amount to little more than 'in agreement with the health practitioners concerned'.

There is no reason to suggest that an irrational decision is *de facto* an indication of incompetence. Decision-making, whether rational or otherwise, is the prerogative of the autonomous person; one of the virtues of being autonomous is the opportunity to behave irrationally if a person so wishes. We are all familiar with the autonomous decision to 'do something crazy'; in some real sense it is our very autonomy which licenses irrationality.

The most reliable indication of competency is probably the client's ability to understand the proposed intervention. This at least has the benefit of concurring with the law of consent, which states that no one can be said to consent to treatment unless he has the capacity to understand its general nature and purpose.

It perhaps seems strange to describe the law as protecting clients from undesired treatment, or, for that matter, suggesting that overriding autonomy *vis à vis* decisions regarding treatment is unethical. After all, treatment is generally perceived as a good thing. Does it really matter what the client thinks about it? The reason why it does is because there is a fundamental moral duty to respect autonomy.

There are, however, occasions when respecting autonomy conflicts with other duties; notably the duty of beneficence which is the duty to as far as possible do good to others. While it might be counter-argued that it can never be beneficent to ignore the autonomous wishes of the client, many health professionals find it difficult to accept a client's decision if in their opinions it is not in accord with his best interests. This difficulty is sometimes evidenced in a tendency to deprive the client of opportunities to make decisions for himself, instead making them for him on the basis of 'we know best'; such an approach is paternalistic and is generally not acceptable.

There may be occasions where there might be defensible reasons to deny a client choice, but these will be rare. The all too common practice of intervening without the client's real consent on the basis that he will be grateful in the long term is both unethical and unlawful. Furthermore, it is mistaken to assume that treatment is intrinsically good; treatment becomes a good thing when it is desired; if it is not desired, it is simply not good. This is best understood by the analogy of the Boy Scout who is so keen to help a blind person across the road that he fails to hear his protests that he is taking him in the opposite direction to which he wants to go.

## CASE EXAMPLES

Having considered the issues of autonomy, competence, and paternalism, let us return to the categories of clients outlined earlier and consider them in greater depth.

### CLIENTS WHO WANT WHAT OTHERS SUGGEST THEY NEED

If we assume that clients are autonomous, then legal and ethical issues should be relatively minimal. Good nursing practice includes a requirement to work as a partner with the client in planning care; this can also be understood from an ethical point of view as demonstrating respect for client autonomy.

There is both a professional and an ethical basis for seeking the client's agreement to, and active participation in, care and treatment. This general principle is perhaps more important in mental health nursing than any other branch of the profession.

Most nursing and medical interventions in mental health care aim to change the ways in which a person views himself or the world in which he lives. Consider, for example, the plight of the phobic person who seeks treatment to change his perception of the object of his phobia; or the anxious person wishing to be relieved of symptoms that deleteriously affect his life. Seeking changes such as these is a considerable issue and might well have a fundamental impact on the life of the individual. They therefore should not be affected without his full and informed consent. It is not uncommon to find clients whose lifestyles have been so affected by treatment that in some cases relationships change to the point of disintegration. Marriages, for example, can thrive in circumstances where one partner is mentally ill; restoration of health can result in the collapse of the marital relationship. Treatment can bring harm as well as benefits.

Even clients who might be judged to be fully autonomous might not have considered the potential harms that might follow treatment. While any harm is usually outweighed by benefit, this in itself is no reason to deprive a client of relevant information. On being informed of potential harm, some clients may choose to reject the offer of treatment and care. Acknowledging a client's right to choose is a demonstration of a respect for autonomy. While there is a basic obligation from an ethical point of view to inform clients of risks associated with treatment, in some cases nurses are disinclined to give frank accounts of the risks involved. Consider the following case.

> John is suffering from depressive illness, and has been prescribed electroconvulsive therapy. He understands the treatment in general respects, and has given his consent. John asks the nurse, Linda, whether any client has ever reported adverse effects associated with the treatment. John is anxious about the treatment and is looking for reassurance. It is likely he will withdraw his consent if he is not reassured by the answer he receives.

It is likely that Linda will be aware of several clients who in the past have reported adverse effects of such treatment. While the majority of the clients concerned were eventually benefited, rather than harmed, as a result of the treatment, the truth remains that harms were suffered. She thus has several choices: she could tell John the bald truth; she could tell a lie; she could be 'economical' with the truth, perhaps suggesting that while minor adverse effects have been reported, all clients have gained some considerable benefit.

Linda's choice of response will be influenced by the effects it might have on John's decision regarding his treatment. It will also be influenced by anticipated reactions from her colleagues. She knows that on the one hand telling the truth is a fundamental moral requirement, but on the other, telling the truth might result in the client refusing treatment from which he might benefit.

Moral theory can help when attempting to deal with problems such as this. It is unlikely to provide the perfect answer, since it is concerned with values rather than facts, but it will help in analyzing the relative merits of potential responses.

Looking to the consequences of one's actions to determine their moral significance is in effect desiring the benefit for the greatest number of people who might be affected by any decision made. Duty-based theories require one to consider one's duty regardless of consequences. Here, certain fundamental moral duties must be accepted regardless of the consequences; truth-telling is among these. Health care professionals tend to be duty-orientated, as evidenced in the statement of duties within various codes of professional conduct.

How, then, ought Linda respond to John's question? Telling a lie appears to be fundamentally morally wrong. It is not difficult to imagine how hard life would be if lying was commonplace. One of the main reasons why people should receive honest answers to their questions is in order to ensure they can make decisions based on those answers. From a more moral point of view, lying can be seen as a basic abuse of trust, a point confirmed by the UKCC (1989). It would appear that the fundamental duty of the nurses is to tell the truth.

Should Linda lie in order to achieve what might be best for John? While it might be argued that in the short term a lie might be justified, if the longer-term considerations are taken into account, it becomes clear that lies are not morally defensible. For example, if John or other clients discovered the lie, this would prejudice any future relationships; if it became known that mental health nurses were not to be trusted, many clients would suffer because they would be reluctant to accept any care or treatment offered. Relationships founded upon deceit are unlikely to succeed.

If lying is not acceptable, should Linda then tell the bald truth? Most nurses would be reluctant to respond in such a way that causes a client to refuse potentially beneficial treatment; the truth therefore appears to be best avoided.

We are then left with the economical-truth option, which is probably the most commonly used. Is it defensible? The answer is closely related to the intentions of the nurse using such a strategy. An economical truth is no different to a lie if the intention is to deceive the client. If, for example, Linda used an economy of the truth to lead John to believe that there are no risks attached to the proposed treatment, she would clearly be deceiving him. She has also ensured the same end result as from telling a lie. Even if Linda deceived John with his best interests in mind, she would nevertheless seriously damage a caring relationship. If Linda was to deceive John in order to protect herself from, for example, the criticisms of her colleagues, such a deceit would also be totally indefensible.

Economies of the truth can be morally defensible: it is possible to impart the truth in such a way as to not deceive the client, but to minimize anxiety and maximize autonomy. An anxious client will find it hard to maintain his autonomy: the nurse should seek to establish the client's autonomous decision regarding any proposed care or treatment. Maintaining autonomy is vital. This might be best achieved by imparting truths in manageable 'portions', which might be argued as being a well-intentioned economy of the truth. It would of course be essential to ensure that clients such as John are in possession of all the relevant information before they make any final decisions, even though this information would have been given piecemeal and with due care.

Linda's answer to John, then, must be the truth, but she should take care in the way she chooses to impart it. If John refuses the treatment when he is in full possession of the facts, then his rights to do so should be respected. If he is competent to make such a decision – and it should be assumed he is in the absence of evidence to the contrary – his decision should be accepted. John may choose to have no treatment at all, or he may wish to consider alternatives. The fact that treatment is refused gives no support to the suggestion that the client must therefore be incompetent to make the decision.

Sometimes clients appear more than willing to accept any treatment proposed, but such willingness requires further analysis; do they really want what others suggest they need? Nurses and other health care professionals are often viewed as authority figures by clients, and authority carries considerable power. Many clients might not question their care and treatment because they feel overpowered by the professionals concerned.

Advocacy, pleading the cause of another, is a clear duty of the nurse, and requires the nurse to ensure that all the client's questions are answered. Because these questions will include those that are not explicitly stated, the duty of advocacy will entail helping clients to express any concerns they might have, and, if necessary, anticipating them. Clients can only be described as wanting care and treatment if their pertinent concerns have been considered.

What of the related assumption that acceptance of treatment is an indication of competence? Imagine that John had welcomed the opportunity to receive ECT, claiming he was delighted since it would improve his mind-reading abilities. John would either have been mistaken, or incompetent. On balance, the latter would appear most likely.

It would be wrong to suggest that John wanted the treatment in terms of any reasonable understanding of a 'want'. In circumstances such as this, however, a signature on a consent form is often taken as sufficient warrant to proceed with treatment. It is not. Treatment given in these circumstances is unlawful and immoral, since it is based on 'consent' obtained by deception, or it is effectively being given with no consent at all.

## CLIENTS WHO WANT WHAT THEY DO NOT NEED

Some clients' 'wants' may be seen in sharp contrast with their needs, as perceived and determined by mental health professionals. At the most dramatic extreme, some clients want their own deaths; others may wish to continue abusing drugs or alcohol. The professional practitioners, however, perceive a clear need to stop.

Beside the issue of nursing accountability (Chapter 28), there are further legal and ethical considerations to examine. The desire to end one's life is not in itself a reflection of impaired autonomy or mental illness. Indeed, it might be argued that suicide is the ultimate expression of autonomy. Many suicidal people, however, are not autonomous; their apparent desire to end their own lives is symptomatic of mental illness, rather than a real desire.

If a person autonomously chooses to attempt suicide, do others have a duty to prevent it? Since the enactment of the Suicide Act (1961), suicide has not been a crime. Even if it was, there might be no legal obligation to prevent it, or for that matter to report it, as there is no legal obligation to prevent or report crimes. There is power in common law to prevent a person from committing suicide. While it is generally unlawful to interfere with the liberty of others, it would not be difficult to argue in court that such an intervention could be defended on public policy grounds, as would be the case in preventing a crime from being committed.

While there are no clear legal duties to prevent the suicide of another person, most people would agree that there are moral grounds for doing so; after all, not many people would stand idly by while a person killed himself.

A moral duty to prevent the suicide of another person is not clearly defensible. If the suicidal person is autonomous, then any decision to prevent his suicide is likely to be based on an evaluation of the conflicting duties to save a worthwhile life, and to respect autonomy. It is clearly impossible to follow both duties, a problem that has been considered by many mental health professionals and philosophers. Perhaps the most comprehensive analysis is that provided by Glover (1977), who argues that while autonomy should generally be respected, preventing a suicide might be defensible on the basis that it gives the person an opportunity to reconsider his plans. It might also be argued that the act of suicide has an impact on the lives of other people and their freedom to exercise autonomy. There may, therefore be grounds for preventing a suicide insofar as it does harm others.

Is suicide immoral? People who uphold the sanctity of life doctrine believe it is because it can be seen as an offence against God, who divinely determines the end of life. While this argument will gain little support from those not sharing the relevant religious beliefs, there are counter arguments in any case. Hume (Singer, 1979) argued that if the determination of the end of life was God's sole prerogative, then interventions designed to save lives would be as immoral as suicide.

It is difficult to establish any clear argument that suicide is in itself immoral; it does, however, challenge normal reasoning: how can we improve our lot by destroying ourselves?

Often, a decision to commit suicide is not the result of autonomous reasoning, but a reflection of impaired autonomy resulting from mental illness. In this case, preventing a suicide is not an infringement of the liberty of the person concerned. There is a real sense that the person does not desire his death at all, since his desires are not the free expressions of autonomous thinking. Thus, the care and treatment of clients who are suicidal as a result of mental illness are founded on an attempt to restore autonomy, not to override it.

People who autonomously choose to continue abusing drugs or alcohol while fully appreciating the need to cease have every right to continue their behaviour unimpeded. As they are able to understand the consequences of their actions, they maintain responsibility of their behaviour and any effects it might have on others. Most people in these circumstances, however, do not want to continue to abuse the substance concerned – not, at least, in the real sense of 'want'. Many seek the help of mental health professionals in an attempt to regain the autonomy that has been substantially impaired by drug or alcohol abuse.

## CLIENTS WHO NEED WHAT THEY DO NOT WANT

The most striking examples of clients in this group are seen in the context of acute physical illness. Consider, for example, the clients who refuse potentially life-saving treatment on the grounds of religious beliefs – the Jehovah's Witness who refuses blood, or the Christian Scientist who refuses any form of orthodox treatment. Again, any autonomous client has the right to refuse treatment, no matter how beneficial it might be. There are some clients, however, whose refusal of treatment is not the result of deliberate autonomous thought, but a reflection of the illness from which they are suffering: why should any person who believes himself to be perfectly well accept treatment?

If a person is mentally ill and that illness is susceptible to treatment, there are provisions within the Mental Health Act (1983) to give such treatment, if necessary in the face of protest (Chapter 32). This mechanism exists in recognition that the protests are most likely to be symptomatic of illness rather than true refusals. It should be emphasized that the Act only makes provisions for the treatment of mental disorder.

Until recently, if a mentally ill person was not competent to consent there was not any clear legal basis for providing treatment of physical illness that was anything less than life-threatening. There is now clear authority for providing treatment of physical illness, where that treatment is seen to be in the best interests of the client – as opposed to absolutely necessary (Re. F, 1989). The most recently published guidance on consent includes details of new consent forms to be used in the event of providing beneficial treatment to incompetent clients (DOH, 1990).

The provision to treat incompetent clients might be a mixed blessing. While it does mean that clients previously denied treatment as a result of legal restrictions can now receive treatment from which they might gain benefit, it also means that clients who were previously protected from such controversial interventions as abortion and sterilization have lost that protection.

It is likely that the provision will largely be used for those clients who neither protest nor consent. It could, however, be used for providing treatment in the face of protests if it could be argued that the protests were the result of mental disorder. It is noteworthy that under this common-law power, a second opinion is not necessarily required before treatment is provided.

The role of the mental health nurse as an advocate is important in ensuring that those clients who are incapacitated by mental illness gain beneficial treatment. The nurse will also need to advocate for those clients who may be subjected to treatment that others determine as beneficial, but which the client might have declined had he been competent.

Advocating for a client requires the nurse to present the client's interests as he himself might do – it is not merely an opportunity for the nurse to add her view of what she thinks is in the best interests of the client. As the UKCC states:

> The practitioner must be sure that it is the interests of the patient or client that are being promoted rather than the patient or client being used for the promotion of personal or sectional professional interests. Professional conduct envisages the role of patient or client advocate as an integral and essential aspect of good professional practice.

## CLIENTS WHO DO NOT DESIRE THEIR OWN ACTIONS OR THOUGHTS

A person's autonomy might be so substantially affected by mental illness that it would be inappropriate to hold him responsible for his actions. Criminal law includes provisions for such eventualities. Although the relevant aspects of criminal law are complex, it is important to consider a basic overview, as most mental health nurses encounter clients who have been sent to hospital following the commission of a crime. Mental health nurses equally meet with clients who have committed homicide, but who have been considered to be victims of diminished responsibility.

### Diminished responsibility

If a mentally ill person commits a crime and there is a direct relationship between that crime and his mental illness, there would appear to be good grounds for not finding him guilty of the particular crime. To be found guilty of a crime, it is necessary to prove that the person concerned consciously and deliberately meant to effect the crime in question.

A defence of diminished responsibility is only available in the case of a person who has committed homicide. While it might be clear that the person was guilty of the crime, it might equally be clear he was suffering from mental illness and was incapable of forming the necessary intention to be guilty of murder. A successful defence of diminished responsibility effectively 'reduces' a charge of homicide to manslaughter; in this way, while the person is still considered to be guilty, the judge can exercise discretion in sentencing. For example, in the case of murder, the judge must sentence the person to life imprisonment, but a verdict of manslaughter means the judge can demand appropriate care and treatment for the person, as opposed to imprisonment.

## Automatism

The law recognizes the concept of automatism, which means acting like a robot. If a person is in a robot-like state, it would be difficult to consider him guilty of any crime he might commit.

Automatism is subdivided into insane and non-insane categories. The former is pleaded by people whose crimes can be seen as attributable in some respects to mental disorder; the latter is pleaded by those who commit crimes while in a state of temporary automatism, for example, following a blow on the head. These subdivisions are far from clear and are surrounded by considerable debate. In both cases the person will be found not guilty, but a successful defence of insane automatism is likely to result in an indeterminate 'sentence' in a special hospital such as Broadmoor or Rampton, whereas a successful plea of non-insane automatism will result in the person leaving court completely acquitted.

The special verdict of 'not guilty by reason of insanity' is returned in the case of a person successfully pleading insane automatism. The plea is assessed against the M'Naughten rules which require that,

...at the time of committing the act, the party accused was labouring under such defect of reason from disease of the mind, as not to know the nature and quality of the act he was doing, or, if he did know it, that he did not know he was doing what was wrong.

The insanity plea is rarely used, given the possible outcome of an indeterminate 'sentence'. If the accused person has committed murder, it is more beneficial to plead diminished responsibility. For most other crimes, a plea of guilty is often regarded as preferable to 'insanity'.

Non-insane automatism is a popular plea, but it cannot be accepted unless insane automatism is ruled out, which will be based on a judgement as to whether the person's 'defect of reason' could be attributable to 'disease of the mind'. A 'disease of the mind' is conceived in law rather differently to professional mental health practice, being seen as an internal state leading to a defect in reason, an understanding that has led to surprising conclusions. States of automatism following epileptic fits (R *v.* Sullivan [1983]); cerebral arteriosclerosis (R *v.* Kemp [1956]); and diabetic hyperglycaemia (R *v.* Hennessy [1989]) have all been legally defined as examples of insane automatism. An accused person is generally well advised to change his plea to guilty rather than to adopt the insanity plea following rejection of sane automatism.

Until recently (Fenwick, 1989), sleepwalking was seen as an example of non-insane automatism, and people committing crimes while sleepwalking could be acquitted. Sleepwalking is increasingly regarded in law as a 'disease of the mind', since it can be argued as attributable to the internal psychological makeup of the individual rather than to the effects of external factors such as stress. Sane automatism can only be used as a plea by those who have suffered some defect of reason as a result of some external factor, such as the effects of drugs like insulin (R *v.* Quick [1983]) and trauma. Automatism resulting from the effects of drugs will only be considered as a defence if those drugs have been taken according to medical directions; a diabetic who became hypoglycaemic as a result of not eating following insulin would be regarded as reckless and would not escape appropriate punishment.

## CLIENTS WHO DO NOT ACT ACCORDING TO THEIR OWN DESIRES

It is very difficult to promote the best interests of clients who are unable to express their own desires. Clients suffering from dementing illnesses, for example, will be unable to express personal wishes, particularly in the latter stages of the illness. While statutory and common-law powers are available to ensure that clients suffering from mental disorder gain beneficial care and treatment, there are further legal and ethical issues to be considered in the case of people suffering substantial impairment of autonomy.

The ethical duty of the mental health nurse is to respect the autonomy of clients; but what should the nurse do in the case of a client who can no longer exercise autonomy? While it might be tempting to label the client non-autonomous and make all relevant decisions on his behalf, such a response would ignore the possibility that the client might not actually want what is best for him.

It is likely that before becoming ill the client had views of how he might wish to be treated and cared for should he become incompetent as a result of illness or trauma. If these views can be established, it will be possible to respect the autonomy of a client suffering a substantial impairment. This adds weight to the requirement to gain a detailed nursing history, which also is ethically desirable. Such a history will provide some guidance in respect of the decisions the client would have made had he been competent; relatives may also be a valuable source of information. As some of the decisions that need to be made in the cases of incompetent clients are literally life and death. If the client's previously expressed wishes can be established, it will be far easier to make morally defensible decisions on his behalf.

## Advocacy

If the client's previously expressed autonomous decisions are to be respected, he will require an advocate. Many clients will have relatives who will act as advocates, but some relatives may be more concerned with their own interests than those of the client; for example, it is a sad fact that some relatives welcome the early death of the client in order to take advantage of inheritances. It is also true that many clients will have no obvious advocate; the mental health nurse is an obvious choice, given her professional duties.

Ideally, an advocate should be able to represent the client as he would do himself, and should be able to voice the client's words for him, protecting his interests as he would himself. This model of advocacy is often referred to as 'substituted judgement', and is probably the most morally desirable form of advocacy. An advocate will have a vital role in some major decisions, for example, in the case of a seriously demented person suffering from a chest infection, and the prescription of potentially life-saving antibiotics. Other decisions may well be less dramatic, but nevertheless very important, for example, ensuring that the client maintains his normal dietary choices, particularly in circumstances where diet is related to religious or moral beliefs.

The moral desirability of advocacy is clear, but advocates do not have powers that are enforceable in law other than managing financial affairs of incompetent clients, if they have enduring power-of-attorney. Decisions in respect of care and treatment are ultimately the prerogative of professionals acting on the basis of professional judgement within the constraints of the law. For example, if an advocate knew that as a Christian Scientist a particular client would refuse any conventional treatment, the advocate would represent this view, but would have no power to ensure it was respected. Similarly, an advocate who knew that in the event of becoming incompetent a client would not wish to receive any life-prolonging treatment would have no power to prevent such treatment taking place.

## Living wills

Considerations such as the above have led to a recent interest in living wills. A living will is a statement made by a person specifying how he would wish to be treated in the event of becoming incompetent. It is an example of self-advocacy, aiming to ensure that personal wishes are respected rather than being subjected to decisions made on the basis of general principles. In theory, it is possible to specify which treatment would or would not be acceptable. It is also possible to appoint a surrogate decision-maker.

Living wills have legal force in some US jurisdictions; they are subject to statutory regulation; and health care professionals are obliged to respect them. The situation in the UK is not clear. Some writers (Kennedy, *et al.*, 1989) take the view that living wills might have legal status on the basis of common-law principles, but there are as yet no cases that firmly establish such legal status. It is likely that interest in living wills will be maintained, and their precise status will be established in the near future.

## Ethical dilemmas

Living wills may have a significant role in the future, but currently there are many ethical problems in respect of treating and caring for incompetent adults. One major issue is concerned with life-prolonging, or sometimes life-saving, treatment. Many nurses express concern when treatment is not given and clients are left to nature to take her course; other nurses become concerned when a client's life is prolonged yet that life is perceived as being of poor quality. Some nurses will argue that in cases where the quality of an individual's life is particularly poor, active euthanasia is morally defensible.

Letting nature take its course may be a morally defensible position, but closer analysis express an obvious flaw: why should health professionals spend much of their time stopping nature from taking her course by providing treatment and care, yet choose in some cases to abandon the client? Letting nature take her course would appear to be a fundamental abrogation of duty.

Similarly, it is far from obvious that people suffering from dementing illnesses are either in pain, or, in the normal understanding of the concept, terminally ill. Many clients suffering from dementing illnesses appear happy and show no obvious signs of pain. It is not possible to be sure how they really feel, but it would be odd to assume they would welcome a release from pain and suffering when there is not any evidence of such. On the other hand, it might be argued that a life of confusion, amnesia, and gross intellectual impairment will be of such limited quality that its prolongation will be a pointless, if not immoral, exercise.

Ideally, decisions should be based on an understanding of the person concerned; quality of life is a matter of subjective judgement: some people would wish to continue living a life that others would see as devoid of any worthwhile qualities.

Some have argued convincingly that letting clients die is morally equivalent to killing them since both have the same outcome and both share similar intentions – that through either one's acts or one's omissions the life of another person will be foreshortened (Kuhse *et al.*, 1985). If letting a person die is morally equivalent to killing them, and the reason for letting a person die is to reduce pain and suffering, then, surely, that pain and suffering might be further reduced by killing the person. It might also be argued that, if moral equivalence is accepted and it is agreed that killing is wrong, then letting people die is wrong. Clearly the practice of letting clients die is questionable.

Despite such arguments, there are some clients for whom life-prolonging treatment is not indicated. It is unlikely that many people, while incompetent, would welcome the prospect of merely being kept alive as long as possible; it is surely right that some people, in some circumstances, should be 'allowed' to die.

In part, problems are caused by the language we use, and that concepts like witholding or withdrawing treatment run counter to a normal understanding of the roles of health care professionals. It is unlikely that any nurse would agree that there are some clients from whom care should be withdrawn or withheld; treatment and care should continue until the client's death. There are some clients who require care and treatment for dying as opposed to living. Treatment for dying is practically different to merely letting someone die; it is not just a matter of semantics. If a client is being treated for dying, then life-prolonging treatment is neither indicated nor ethical. Moreover, it would probably be considered negligent to save the life of a client being treated for dying.

Other ethical issues concerned with the care of incompetent adults include that of the reasonable use of restraint. Conflicts between maximizing a confused client's freedom while protecting him from harm are commonplace. Incompetent clients are vulnerable and require protection; protection from abuse as well as protection from themselves. Sadly, it is often the most vulnerable people who are most likely to be the victims of abuse; tales of abuse by relatives as well as health professionals are all too common.

While physical and psychological abuse are to be deplored, there are other equally abhorrent forms of abuse that are less obvious, for example, over-protection. All clients could be protected from harm if they were to be kept

in beds, heavily sedated, yet this would be an obvious violation of autonomy. It is unlikely that many nurses would seriously advocate this for clients who are able to enjoy mobility and freedom, but similar practices abound. Many hospital wards for elderly, confused clients are either locked or have such complex systems of door handles that they might as well be. Some chairs appear to be deliberately designed to ensure that their occupants are unable to leave them. It is a rarity to find elderly clients residing in hospital wards who have outdoor clothing and shoes. All of these effectively limit the freedom that clients might otherwise enjoy.

When nurses are challenged in respect of such practices most argue that forms of restraint are required in order to ensure client safety. There is little doubt that abandoning confused, elderly clients to their own devices would be negligent, particularly if doing so resulted in harm suffered by the clients concerned. Often, however, restraint of various descriptions is not utilized in the best interests of clients – it is used as an expedient measure to protect the interests of staff. It is easier to manage the 'care' of confused clients if there really is no chance of them coming to any harm.

In the pursuit of good practice, the nurse should be prepared to take calculated risks with the interest of the client in mind. Sometimes, even the most carefully calculated risk will materialize, perhaps with tragic results, but this in itself is no good reason for never taking risks. The skill of the professional mental health nurse should enable her to maximize the freedom enjoyed by confused clients; negligent exposure to risks of serious harm over-protects as well as compromising real freedom.

In many ways, legal and ethical considerations in respect of the issue of restraint are secondary to matters of good nursing practice. The task of the mental health nurse includes maintaining as far as possible the lifestyle enjoyed by the client before he became ill; many people enjoy aimless wandering as part of normal life; why should opportunities to continue the habit be denied should a person be victim of dementing illness? On the other hand, many people lead entirely purposive lives and gain security from routine and self-imposed 'boundaries'; it would be quite wrong to leave such a person wandering aimlessly. Freedom, then, is not necessarily being free from constraints – it is to be found in opportunities to continue living life as one would choose, even when the capacity to make significant choices has long faded. The rightness or wrongness of restraint in respect of any client probably lies in the motives for the restraint: in whose best interests is it?

## SUMMARY

Some of the most significant legal and ethical issues in mental health nursing practice have been addressed within a framework constructed from the related concepts of autonomy, needs, wants or desires, competence, paternalism, and freedom. While it is not possible to address every specific issue in detail, the principles addressed can be applied in the context of other ethico-legal issues, and the reader is urged to utilize the framework and its underlying concepts in the pursuit of further analysis.

## REFERENCES

*The Living Will* (1988) Age Concern/King's College, London.
Beauchamp, T. L. and Childress, J. F. (1989) *Principles of Biomedical Ethics* (3rd edn) Oxford Univ. Press, Oxford.
Dimond, B. (1990) Common law powers for health professionals. *Bulletin of Medical Ethics*, April.
DoH HC (90)92 *Patient Consent to Examination or Treatment*.
Fenwick, P. (1989) Automatism and the law. *Lancet* Sept.
Glover, J. (1987) *Causing Death and Saving Lives*, Penguin, Hardmondsworth.
Hume, D. (1988) Of suicide, in *Applied Ethics* (P. Singer), Oxford Univ. Press, Oxford.
Kennedy I. and Grubb, A. (1989) *Medical Law: Text and Materials*, Butterworths, London.
Kuhse, H. and Singer, P. (1985) *Should the Baby Live?* Oxford Univ. Press, Oxford.
Mill, J. S. (1972) (ed. H. B. Acton) *Utilitarianism, On Liberty and Considerations on Representative Government*, J. M. Dent, London.
M'Naughten (1843) 10 Cl & Fin 200, HL.
Paton, H. J. (1969) *The Moral Law: Kant's Groundwork of the Metaphysic of Morals*, Hutchinson Univ. Press, London.
UKCC (1984). *Code of Professional Conduct for the Nurse, Midwife and Health Visitor*, UKCC, London.
UKCC (1989) *Exercising Accountability*, UKCC, London.

## STATUTES

Mental Health Act (1983)
Suicide Act (1961)

## CASES

Re F. [1989] 2 All ER 545
R *v.* Hennessy *The Times*, 31 Jan. 1989
R *v.* Kemp [1956] 3 All ER 249
R *v.* Quick and Paddison [1973] 3 All ER 347
R *v.* Sullivan [1983] 2 All ER 673

## FURTHER READING

Bavidge, M. *Mad or Bad?* (1989) Bristol Classical Press, Bristol.
Bloch, S. and Chodoff, P. (1981) *Psychiatric Ethics*, Oxford Univ. Press, Oxford.
Brazier, M. (1987) *Medicine, Patients and the Law*, Penguin, Harmondsworth.
Brody, A. B. (1988) *Life and Death Decision-Making*, Oxford Univ. Press, Oxford.
Buchanan, A. and Brock, D. W. (1990) *Deciding for Others*, Cambridge Univ. Press, Cambridge.
Callahan, D. (1987) *Setting Limits: Medical Goals in an Aging Society*, Simon & Schuster, New York.
Campbell, R. and Collinson, D. (1988) *Ending Lives*, Blackwell, Oxford.
Campbell, T. (1988) *Discrimination and Mental Illness*, Dartmouth, Aldershot.
Cavadino, M, (1989) *Mental Health Law in Context: Doctors Orders?* Dartmouth, Aldershot.

Carrier, J. and Kendall, I. (1990) *Medical Negligence: Complaints and Compensation*, Gower, Aldershot.

Cohen, M. *et al.* (1982) *Medicine and Moral Philosophy*, Princeton Univ. Press, Guildford and Princeton, New Jersey.

Downie, R. S. and Calman, K. C. (1987) *Healthy Respect: Ethics in Health Care*, Faber, London.

Dyer, A. R. *Ethics and Psychiatry: Toward Professional Definition*, Amer. Psych. Press Inc., Washington.

Edwards, R. B. (ed.) (1982) *Psyhchiatry and Ethics*, Prometheus, 1982, New York.

Gilhooly, M. (1990) *Legal and Ethical Issues in the Management of Dementing Elderly*, Dartmouth, Aldershot.

Gillon, R. (1986) *Philosophical Medical Ethics*, Wiley, Chichester.

Harris, J. (1985) *The Value of Life: An Introduction to Medical Ethics*, Routledge, London.

Hirsch, S. R. and Harris, J. (1988) *Consent and the Incompetent Patient*, Gaskell.

Kennedy, I. (1988) *Treat Me Right: Essays in Medical Law and Ethics*, Clarendon Press, Oxford.

Kennedy, L. (1990) *Euthanasia: Counterblast 13*, Chatto and Windus, London.

Knapman, P. and West, I. (1989) *Medicine and the Law*, Heinemann, Oxford.

Lewis, C. J. *Medical Negligence: A Plaintiff's Guide*, Frank Cass and Co., London.

Lockwood, M. (1985) *Moral Dilemmas in Medicine*, Oxford Univ. Press, Oxford.

Mason, J. K. and McCall Smith, R. A. (1987) *Law and Medical Ethics* (2nd edn), Butterworths, London.

Radden, J. *Madness and Reason*, George Allen and Unwin, London.

Seedhouse, D. (1988) *Ethics: The Heart of Health Care*, Wiley, Chichester.

Skegg, P. D. G. (1989) *Law Ethics and Medicine*, Clarendon Press, Oxford.

Veatch, R. M. and Fry, S. T. (1987) *Case Studies in Nursing Ethics*, Lippincott, New York.

# PART NINE

# THE MENTAL HEALTH ACTS: THE UNITED KINGDOM AND EIRE

# THE MENTAL HEALTH ACTS – THE UNITED KINGDOM AND EIRE

*Seamus Killen*

Mental health legislation has existed in various forms for over 200 years. By current standards many of the early laws were extremely repressive, but, as with all legislation, they were intended to provide for the safety and protection of both the patient and society.

In the nineteenth century, the Asylum Act of 1890 governed the treatment of mental illness; A Mental Treatment Act of 1930 permitted voluntary admissions and temporary admissions without court orders; by the 1940s voluntary admissions had become widespread, and by the 1950s the majority of admissions were voluntary.

The law relating to mental illness and mental deficiency was examined by the Royal Commission, set up in 1954, whose report in 1957 made far-reaching recommendations that resulted in the Mental Health Act of 1959, which repealed all existing legislation on mental illness and mental deficiency. It incorporated the principles that no one should be admitted to hospital if care in the community is more appropriate, and where admission to hospital is required, compulsion should be a medical matter instead of a judicial procedure.

The considerable changes in mental health services and practice during the 1960s made it necessary to review the Mental Health Act in the mid-1970s. After wide consultation over a period of seven years, the Mental Health Act 1983 received the Royal Assent. It made substantial amendments to the 1959 Act, as well as introducing new powers relating to the treatment and discharge of mentally disordered patients.

## THE MENTAL HEALTH ACT (1983)

### SECTION 2 – ADMISSION FOR ASSESSMENT

Where admission to hospital is considered necessary and the patient is willing to be admitted informally, this should be arranged. Compulsory admission should only be considered when a patient's current mental state, together with reliable evidence indicates a strong likelihood that he will change his mind about informal admission before admission to hospital, with a resulting risk to his own health and safety, or to other persons.

Section 2 of the Act (Admission for Assessment) authorizes compulsory admission of a patient to hospital for assessment and for detention for this purpose for up to 28 days. An application for admission for assessment may be made in respect of a patient on the grounds that he is suffering from mental disorder to a degree that warrants his detention in a hospital for assessment, and that he ought to be detained in the interests of his own and others' health or safety.

An application under Section 2 can be made by either the patient's nearest relative, or by an approved social worker. The nearest relative cannot prevent an approved social worker making an application, but he must be informed that the application is to be made. An application for admission for assessment also has to be founded on the written recommendations of two registered medical practitioners. The approved social worker has overall responsibility for co-ordinating the process of the assessment, and where he decides to make an application, for implementing that decision.

## SECTION 3 – ADMISSION FOR TREATMENT

Under Section 3 of the Act (Admission for Treatment) a patient may be admitted to a hospital and detained there for a period allowed under the provisions of the Act: an initial period of up to six months, renewable for a further six months, and thereafter renewable at yearly intervals. It is possible for a patient to be granted leave of absence from hospital during this time.

An application for admission for treatment shall be founded on the written recommenda-tion of two registered medical practitioners, including in each case a statement that in the opinion of the practitioner the conditions set out in the Act are complied with. An applica-tion for admission for treatment can be made by either the patient's nearest relative, or by an approved social worker.

Section 3 is often used where a patient who has been admitted in the past is considered to need compulsory admission for the treatment of a mental disorder already known to his clinical team, and has been assessed in the recent past by that team.

It can also be used where a patient already admitted under Section 2, who is assessed as needing further medical treatment for mental disorder under the Act at the conclusion of his detention under Section 2, is unwilling to remain in hospital informally and to consent to the medical treatment.

Where a patient is detained under Section 2 and the assessment points to a need for treat-ment under the Act for a period beyond the 28 days detention, an application for detention under Section 3 is made, which should not be delayed until the end of Section 2 detention.

## SECTION 4 – ADMISSION FOR ASSESSMENT IN CASES OF EMERGENCY

Under Section 4 (Admission for Assessment in Cases of Emergency), a patient may be admitted to hospital and detained for a period of up to 72 hours.

This Section has been used far more frequently than was initially envisaged, and during the 1970s it became the most widely used form of compulsory admission. An application under Section 4 cannot be renewed at the end of the 72-hour period. If compulsory detention is to be continued, the application must either be converted into a Section 2 application, in which case the patient can be detained for 28 days beginning with the date of his admission, or an application for treatment should be made under Section 3.

## SECTION 5 – APPLICATION IN RESPECT OF PATIENT ALREADY IN HOSPITAL

Section 5 permits an 'application for admis-sion' to be made in respect of those patients who are already informal inpatients.

This Section provides for applications to be made for compulsory detention under Section 2 or 3 of the Act. It also sets out the proced-ures that can be used if it is considered that a patient might leave the hospital before there is time to complete an application.

### Section 5(2) – doctor's holding power

A doctor may authorize the detention of an informal patient for up to 72 hours, but this can only be used where the doctor in charge of an inpatient's treatment concludes that an 'application for admission' is appropriate. This power cannot be renewed. Any patient detained under this Section should be dis-charged from the order as soon as an assess-ment is carried out and a decision taken, or when the doctor decides that no assess-ment for a hospital admission needs to be carried out.

## Section 5(4) – nurse's holding power

This subsection provides for a Registered Mental Nurse or a Registered Nurse for Mental Handicap to evoke a holding power in respect of a patient for a period of not more than six hours or until a doctor arrives, whichever is the earlier. The use of the holding power is the personal decision of the nurse, and she cannot be instructed to use it by anyone else.

The nurse's holding power can only be used if a patient is indicating either verbally or otherwise that he wishes to leave the hospital. It should not be used to restrain or seclude patients who are not indicating they wish to leave the hospital.

The holding power lapses upon the arrival of the doctor, or after six hours if no doctor has attended; this is the maximum, and non-renewable, period during which a patient can be detained.

## SECTION 7 – GUARDIANSHIP

The purpose of guardianship is to enable patients to receive care in the community where it cannot otherwise be provided without the use of compulsory powers. Care outside hospital should be on the basis of persuasion to accept help and advice, and should take advantage of arrangements for a socialization such as employment, recreation, and training. Where a person is unwilling to receive such help, it would be appropriate to place him under guardianship if this offered the prospect of success.

This Section specifies the circumstances whereby a patient aged 16 or over may be received into the guardianship of a local social services authority, or a person who is acceptable to that authority. A patient ceases to be subject to guardianship if an order for his discharge is made by his responsible medical officer, by the responsible local social services authority, or by his nearest relative. Discharge by the nearest relative cannot be barred by anyone.

A patient can seek his own discharge from guardianship by making an application to a mental health review tribunal. He may be kept under guardianship for an initial period of up to six months from the day on which the application was accepted. The authority for guardianship may be reviewed for a further period of six months, and then for yearly periods. If a patient under guardianship is admitted for psychiatric treatment as an informal patient, he will remain subject to the guardianship order unless he is discharged from it.

## SECTION 8 – POWERS OF THE GUARDIANSHIP

Under Section 8 the guardian has the power to require the patient to reside at a place specified by the authority or the guardian; and to require the patient to attend at places and times so specified for the purpose of medical treatment, occupation, education, or training. The guardian has also the power to give authorized persons access to the patient, at any place where the patient is residing. This includes any medical practitioner, approved social worker, or other person specified.

Where a patient is placed under guardianship, a comprehensive care plan is required that identifies the services needed, including care arrangements, appropriate accommodation, treatment, and personal support requirements, as well as those who have responsibilities under the care plan. There should be a commitment on the part of all concerned that care should take place in the community.

## SECTION 11 – GENERAL PROVISIONS AS TO APPLICATIONS AND RECOMMENDATIONS

This Section contains general provisions relating to applications for admission for assessment; applications for admission for treatment; and guardianship applications.

Although the responsibility for checking that statutory forms have been completed correctly rests with the applicant, hospital managers and local social services authorities should each designate an officer to scrutinize the documents as soon as they have been completed, and to take any necessary action if they have been improperly completed. In many circumstances the managers' obligation to receive documents is delegated to nursing staff, usually the nurse in charge of the ward.

There is a difference between receiving documents and scrutinizing them. The managers should have a clear policy and procedures for the receipt and scrutiny of admission documents. Those delegated to scrutinizing documents must be clear about what kinds of errors on application forms and medical recommendation can and cannot be corrected. Managers should also ensure that those delegated to receive and scrutinize admission documents understand the requirements of the Act, and if necessary, receive appropriate training.

## PART 3 – PATIENTS CONCERNED WITH CRIMINAL PROCEEDINGS

This Part of the Act deals with patients under the order of a court, or who have been transferred from penal institutions on the direction of the Home Secretary. The circumstances relating to patients admitted or detained in hospital on the order of a court are contained in Sections 35–55.

### REMANDS TO HOSPITAL

Section 35 of the Act gives courts the option of remanding an accused person to hospital for the preparation of a report on his mental condition. The remand can last for a maximum of 12 weeks, but the court may terminate the remand at any time.

An accused person who is in custody awaiting trial and who is suffering from mental illness may be remanded by the court to hospital for treatment for a maximum of 12 weeks. This power, under Section 36, can be used in cases in which if the defendant could receive treatment in hospital for a period it might be possible to proceed with the full trial. The courts also have the power to make a hospital or guardianship order as an alternative to a penal disposal for offenders who are found to be suffering from mental disorder at the time of sentencing. The effects of such orders are dealt with under Section 40 of the Act.

In making a hospital order, the court is placing the patient in the hands of the doctors, foregoing any question of punishment, and relinquishing from then onwards its own control over the patient. When the doctor or the mental health review tribunal thinks it right, the patient will be discharged. If it appears quickly that the patient does not need inpatient treatment, or that he has no intention of co-operating, he may be discharged. District health authorities and local social service authorities have a duty to provide aftercare services for hospital-order patients who cease to be liable to be detained and leave hospital (Section 117).

### Restriction orders

Having made a hospital order under Section 37, the Crown Court has the power to make a further order restricting the patient's discharge, transfer, or leave of absence from hospital for a specified or unlimited period without the consent of the Home Secretary. A restriction order can only be made where it is necessary to protect the public from serious harm. The order is to protect the public from the inappropriate release of patients from hospital where there remains a real risk of further and serious crime being committed. These powers are dealt with under Section 41 and 42.

## PART 4 – CONSENT TO TREATMENT

Section 56–64 form Part 4 of the Act, which clarifies the extent to which treatment for mental disorder can be imposed on detained patients in hospitals. It provides for two categories of treatment that have different legal consequences; the first concerns the most serious treatments, which require the patient's consent and a second opinion; the second concerns other serious treatments, which also require the patient's consent or a second opinion. Treatments that do not come within either of these categories can be imposed on a detained patient who understands the nature and purpose of the treatment but expressly withholds consent.

This part of the Act only applies to treatment relating to the patient's mental disorder. Everyone involved in the medical treatment for mental disorder should be familiar with the provision of Part 4 of the Act, but it is for the doctor in charge of treatment to ensure that the Act's provisions relating to medical treatment are complied with. Treatments include the use of electroconvulsive therapy (ECT), the administration of drugs, and psychotherapy.

'Consent' is the voluntary and continuing permission of the patient to receive a particular treatment, having been given an explanation in simple terms of the nature, purpose, and effect of the proposed treatment. The patient must be given the necessary information to enable him to understand what will be done to him, why it is being done, and what is likely to happen when the treatment is given.

The fact that a person is suffering from a mental disorder does not mean he is incapable of giving consent. A person is more likely to be able to give valid consent if the explanation is appropriate to the level of assessed ability. The capacity of a particular patient to consent should be assessed with regard to the treatment proposed. Before the doctor issues his certificate, he must consult with two other persons who have been professionally concerned with the patient's treatment, one of whom must be a nurse.

## Treatment requiring consent and a second opinion

Section 57 applies to medical treatments involving the surgical operation of brain tissue, and the surgical implantation of hormones for the purpose of reducing male sexual drive. This Section applies to informal patients as well as to patients who are liable to be detained. If a patient is given treatment under this Section, his responsible medical officer must provide the Mental Health Act Commission with reports on the treatment and the patient's condition.

When ECT is proposed, valid consent should always be sought by the patient's doctor. If the patient consents, the doctor should complete the necessary form and include the proposed maximum number of applications of ECT. Such information should also be included in the patient's treatment plan. Where the patient's valid consent is not forthcoming, an independent medical practitioner should certify that either the patient is incapable of giving his consent, or that he should receive the treatment even though he has not consented to it.

Section 57 of the Act applies to the administration of medicine to a patient, by any means, if three months or more have elapsed since the first occasion when medicine was administered to him for this mental disorder. At the end of the three-month period, the patient's doctor should personally seek the patient's consent to continuing medication, and such consent should be sought for any subsequent administration of medication. If the patient's consent is not forthcoming, the doctor must comply with the safeguard requirements of Section 58.

## Withdrawal of consent

Section 60 provides for the patient to withdraw his consent to treatment, at any time before the completion of the treatment. Even though the patient has withdrawn his consent, the treatment can be continued if the patient's responsible medical officer considers that discontinuance of treatment would cause serious suffering to the patient (Section 62).

## Urgent treatment

Under this Part of the Act, provision is made for urgent treatment that is immediately necessary to save the patient's life to be administered. There is also provision for a review of treatment requiring a report on the patient's condition by the responsible medical officer.

Nurses have a specific responsibility under this Part of the Act to be consulted by the 'second-opinion' doctor. The nurse, who must be qualified, should be professionally concerned with the patient's care; the nurse has to decide if she is in a position to fulfill this function.

## MENTAL HEALTH REVIEW TRIBUNALS

Psychiatric patients are provided with a safeguard against unjustified detention or control under guardianship. This is provided by means of an independent review of their cases, from both medical and non-medical points of view. The review is undertaken by a local tribunal, which consists of medical and non-medical members selected from a panel of suitable people. The panels came into effect with the Mental Health Act 1959, and are known as mental health review tribunals.

The function of a tribunal is to review the justification for the patient's continued detention or guardianship at the time of the hearing. If the patient considers his admission to be unlawful, he can attempt to secure his release by making an application to the High Court for a writ of habeas corpus. An alternative course of action for a person who considered that he has been wrongfully detained would be to apply to the High Court for judicial review.

Part 5 of the Mental Health Act (Sections 66–79) deals in detail with applications and procedures for mental health review tribunals. The tribunal has the power to discharge patients from hospital or guardianship if the specified criteria are satisfied, however, it has no general discretion to order the discharge of a patient restricted by a court or by the Secretary of State.

## REMOVAL AND RETURN OF PATIENTS WITHIN THE UK

Part 6 of the Act provides powers under which certain categories of detained patients may be moved between England and Wales and other parts of the UK, the Channel Islands, and the Isle of Man while remaining under detention or guardianship. The patient may be re-taken in those places when absent without leave from hospitals or institutions. It also provides powers for moving mentally ill patients who are neither British nor Commonwealth citizens with the right of abode here, from hospitals in England and Wales to countries abroad.

## MANAGEMENT OF PROPERTY AND AFFAIRS OF PATIENTS

This part of the Act is concerned with the powers of the Court of Protection over the management of the property and affairs of persons incapable by reason of mental disorder of managing their own affairs. The Court of Protection has extensive powers over the patient's property and all affairs except for his or her management or care. The Court can transfer and invest money, sell or purchase property, release money to pay debts, make and execute wills, and arrange for someone to carry on a patient's business. An application to the Court of Protection can be made by the patient's nearest relative, a doctor, a social worker, a solicitor, a nurse or a friend.

There is no automatic review whether the court's continued intervention is required. If the patient recovers his mental capacity, he could either ask a solicitor to apply to the Court to determine the proceedings, or he could write to the Court making the request and giving the name of a doctor who will support the application with medical evidence of recovery.

## APPROVED SOCIAL WORKERS

Section 114 of the Act requires local authorities to appoint sufficient numbers of approved social workers to carry out the functions given to them, by the Act. Only social workers who have been approved by authorities as being competent can be appointed. In October 1984 approved social workers replaced the mental welfare officers who were appointed under the 1959 Act.

## AFTERCARE

Section 117 of the Act imposes a duty to provide aftercare services for certain patients who have ceased to be detained and leave hospital. The purpose of aftercare is to assist a patient to return to his home, and to minimize the chances of him needing any future inpatient hospital care.

The Act requires health authorities and local authorities, in conjunction with voluntary agencies, to provide aftercare for certain categories of detained patients. Procedures should be agreed for establishing proper aftercare arrangements. The responsibility for a discharge care plan rests with the

doctor. The process of discharge requires the efforts of a multidisciplinary team, who should assess the patient's needs before discharge. This part of the Act applies to any patient who has been receiving hospital treatment for mental disorder for six months or more. Before such a patient is discharged, the hospital managers must send written notification of the date of discharge to the health authority and the local social services authority for the area in which the patient is to live.

## MENTAL HEALTH ACT CODE OF PRACTICE

Section 118 of the Act imposes a duty on the Secretary of State to prepare, publish, and from time to time revise, a code of practice for those concerned in the admission and treatment of mentally disordered persons. The Code of Practice offers much detailed guidance on how the Mental Health Act 1983 should be implemented. It imposes no additional duties on statutory authorities, managers, and professional staff working in health and social services, but offers advice on how they should proceed when undertaking duties relating to the Act.

The Code needs to be read in the light of the following broad principles, that people being assessed for possible admission under the Act, or to whom the Act applies should:

- receive respect for and consideration of their individual qualities and diverse social, cultural, ethnic and religious backgrounds;
- have their needs taken fully into account, though it is recognized that within available resources it may not always be practicable to meet them;
- be delivered of any necessary treatment or care in the least controlled and segregated facilities practicable;
- be treated or cared for in such a way that promotes to the greatest practicable degree their self-determination and personal

responsibility, consistent with their needs and wishes;
- be discharged from any order under the Act to which they are subject, immediately it is no longer necessary.

This means that individuals should be fully involved as practicable, consistent with their needs and wishes, in the formulation and delivery of their care and treatment. Where linguistic and sensory difficulties impede such involvement, reasonable steps should be taken to attempt to overcome them. It means that patients should have their legal rights drawn to their attention, consistent with their capacity to understand. Finally, it means that when treatment or care is provided in conditions of security, patients should be subject only to the level of security appropriate to their individual needs, and only as long as it is required.

The Code of Practice is not mandatory, in that professionals carrying out functions under the Act are not legally obliged to follow its advice. However, a failure to have regard for the Code could be used in court and disciplinary proceedings as evidence of bad practice. The Code can also specify forms of treatment that give rise to special concern, and should not be given without the patient's consent and an independent second medical opinion.

## THE MENTAL HEALTH ACT COMMISSION

The Mental Health Act Commission works as a special health authority that carries out certain functions on behalf of the Secretary of State. The commissioners aim to visit each of the psychiatric hospitals in England and Wales at least once a year. During their visits, they make themselves available to detained patients who wish to see them, and ensure that staff are helping the patients to understand their legal position and rights. The commissioners will look at patients' records of admission and renewal of detention, and at records relating to treatment. They will also ensure that detained patients are satisfied with the handling of any complaints they may make. Commissioners do not have to give notice of their intention to visit a hospital, but it is their normal practice to do so.

Other functions that the Commission perform on behalf of the Secretary of State include:

- appointing medical practitioners and other persons for the purpose of providing a second opinion and verifying consent to treatment;
- receiving and examining reports on treatment given under the consent-to-treatment provisions;
- keeping the Act under review, and visiting patients and investigating complaints;
- submitting proposals for the Code of Practice.

The Commission does not have the power to discharge a patient. The Commission can be directed to keep under review the care and treatment of informal patients in hospitals.

## OFFENCES COMMITTED UNDER THE MENTAL HEALTH ACT

Section 128 of the 1959 Mental Health Act was not repealed by the 1983 Act. This Section makes it an offence for a man on the staff of a hospital of a mental nursing home to have extramarital sexual intercourse with a woman who is receiving treatment for mental disorder in that hospital either as an outpatient or an inpatient, and for a man to have extramarital sexual intercourse with a woman who is subject to his guardianship or is otherwise in his custody or care. No offence is committed under Section 128 if the man did not know, and had no reason to suspect, that the woman was a mentally disordered patient.

### OTHER OFFENCES

It is also an offence to either forge or make false statements in applications, recommendations, or other documents made under the Act. Ill-treatment or wilful neglect of a patient who is receiving treatment either as an inpatient or outpatient is also an offence. Helping a patient to escape from custody or to absent himself from hospital without leave, or to harbour or prevent the recapture or return to hospital of such patients can lead to criminal proceedings.

## INFORMAL ADMISSION OF PATIENTS

Section 131 provides that a patient can enter hospital for treatment on an informal basis, or remain in hospital on an informal basis once his detention has come to an end. Admission is on the same basis as to a general hospital, with no special formalities. Informal patients can leave hospital when they like, providing Section 5 of the Act does not apply (page 412). About 90% of current admissions to psychiatric hospitals are on an informal basis. Once an informal patient has been admitted to hospital, there is no legal obligation to inform him of his status.

## THE DUTY OF MANAGERS TO GIVE INFORMATION

Managers of a hospital are required under Section 132 of the Act to inform a detained patient of his legal position and rights. Unless the patient request otherwise, the information must also be given to the patient's nearest relative. A failure to provide information may be referred to the Mental Health Act Commission for investigation. The patient should also be told about any legal-aid schemes that could help him to obtain representation for a court appeal, and the patient should be provided with information about welfare benefits.

In carrying out their statutory responsibilities, the managers should devise a system that ensures the correct information is given to the patient; the information is given in a suitable manner; a record is kept of the information given; and a check is made that information has been properly given to each detained patient.

The managers need to ensure that staff know that information is to be given, and that they have received sufficient training and guidance to enable them to give it. The managers should ensure that a member of staff is designated to check the patient's records regularly, to ensure that all information has been given at the appropriate times, and that it has been repeated as necessary. This officer should also be available to give advice to those whose job it is to give information.

## MENTALLY DISORDERED PERSONS FOUND IN PUBLIC PLACES

Under Section 136 of the Act, a policeman may remove a person from a public place to a place of safety if he considers the person to be suffering from mental disorder and is in immediate need of care or control. A place of safety is normally a hospital or a police station. Section 136 is not an emergency admission Section, but enables an individual who falls within its criteria to be detained in a place of safety for up to 72 hours so that he can be examined by a doctor and interviewed by an approved social worker, and any necessary arrangements be made for his treatment or care. The police do not have to complete any statutory form under this Section.

Good practice depends on the establishment of a clear policy between the local social services authority, the district health authority, and the police. Such a policy should define the responsibilities of the police officers, the doctors, and the approved social workers so that a competent and speedy assessment can be carried out. The local policy should also ensure that police officers have no difficulty identifying whom to contact.

## MANAGEMENT PROBLEMS

Whether detained or informal, patients may behave in such a way as to disturb others around them, or present a risk to themselves or to others, including the staff responsible for their care. While the majority of people do not behave in a disturbing way, such disturbed behaviour many occur at any time and in any place.

Behaviour that can give rise to managerial problems can include:

- refusal to participate in treatment programmes, e.g., refusing medication;
- prolonged verbal abuse and threatening behaviour;
- destructive behaviour;
- self-injurious behaviour;
- physical attacks on others.

### RESTRAINT

The purpose of restraint is to contain or limit another person's freedom. It may take many forms, and vary in degree from giving instruction to seclusion. The basic principle that should underlie methods aimed at reducing and eliminating unwanted behaviour is intervention. Any restraint must be reasonable in the circumstances and it must be the minimum necessary to deal with the harm that needs to be prevented. Staff should review regularly any intervention as part of the patient's agreed treatment programme relating to his particular managemnet problem. Staff who work in areas where control and restraint might be necessary should attend an appropriate course run by a qualified instructor. Health authorities should have clear written policies on the use of restraint.

Physical restraint should be used as little as possible, and only as a last resort; it should be used in an emergency where significant harm might occur if intervention was withheld. Any initial attempt to restrain aggressive behaviour should as far as the situation will allow be non-physical.

Where such methods have failed, or the incident is of such significance to warrant immediate action, the person in control of the incident may decide to restrain the person physically. In doing so they should ensure that no weapons are visible, and should aim at restraining the patient's arms and legs from behind, if possible. They should constantly explain the reason for their action to the patient, and enlist support from him for voluntary control as soon as possible.

### SECLUSION

Seclusion is the supervised confinement of a patient alone in a room that may be locked for the protection of others. It should only be implemented as a last resort and for the shortest possible time, when all reasonable steps have been taken to avoid its use. Seclusion should not be used as a punitive measure or to enforce good behaviour. It is not a treatment technique, and should not be used as part of any treatment programme. It should not be used because of staff shortages or because equipment or furniture is being damaged. It should never be used where there is a risk that the patient may take his own life or otherwise harm himself. Clear guidelines containing instructions on the roles and responsibilities of members of staff should be issued to ensure the safety and well-being of a patient in a dignified and humane environment.

The decision to use seclusion should only be made by an experienced nurse in charge of the ward or by a doctor or a senior nurse. Where the decision is taken by someone other than a doctor, then the necessary arrangements must be made for a doctor to attend immediately. A nurse should be by the room at all times throughout the patient's seclusion, and be present at all times with a patient who has been sedated. The aim of observation is to ascertain the state of the patient and to assess how soon seclusion can be terminated. If seclusion needs to be continuous, a review should take place every two hours carried out by two nurses in the seclusion room, and every four hours by a doctor. Detailed records should be kept in the patient's casenotes of any use of seclusion, the reasons for its use, and subsequent activity.

## DUTIES AND RESPONSIBILITIES OF THE NURSE

### ADMISSION TO HOSPITAL

Admission to hospital can be an anxiety-provoking experience for any person, even when they understand and agree to the necessity for admission. It is sometimes necessary to admit a person under the provisions of the Mental Health Act 1983 who is neither willing nor comprehending of the reasons for compulsory admission.

As with any person admitted to hospital, each individual who is detained under the Mental Health Act will have their own needs determined by their particular circumstances, to which the nurse must respond. Their needs will be influenced by their views and feelings about their detention, how they react to being detained, and their need to understand their legal rights.

### Arrival on ward

Wherever possible, the approved social worker should ensure that the patient is expected by the ward and inform staff of an approximate time of arrival. He should also ascertain to whom the admission documents should be delivered. The appropriate person should receive the documents either before or on arrival of the patient.

The approved social worker should attend the hospital and ensure that the documents have been correctly received at the time of the patient's arrival. All relevant information should be passed on to the nursing staff by the social worker, who should be satisfied that the patient has been detained in a proper manner before leaving the hospital.

If the nearest relative has made the application and an approved social worker is not involved, then the other professionals involved in the admission should be prepared to give advice and assistance to the nearest relative. If the patient has been sedated before being conveyed to hospital, then they must be accompanied by a nurse or doctor.

### THE DUTY TO PROVIDE INFORMATION

Hospital managers are directed to give particular information to detained patients under Section 132. Although the managers have the ultimate responsibility for complying with the statutory requirements, the responsibility is usually delegated to a member of the multi-disciplinary team, and the primary nurse or keyworker may be designated to give the information.

Nurses should be aware what information is to be given, and have received training and guidance to enable them to carry out their duties. The information should be given both verbally and in writing; information leaflets are available from the Department of Health for this purpose.

Such steps that are practicable must be taken to ensure patients understand their rights and the effect the detention has upon them. It should be ascertained whether the patient understands the information as soon as practicable following the commencement of their detention. It is good practice to make a record when an attempt has been made to assist the patient to understand his rights and the assessment of his comprehension.

It cannot be prescribed precisely, how, when, or what information should be given at a particular time. This must be a matter of professional judgement. An attempt to mechanistically read the relevant information to a seriously disturbed person may not be conducive to developing a sound therapeutic relationship.

## Type of information to be given

The following information must be given to the patient:

The provision of the Act under which he is being detained, and the effect of the provision. This should include the reason why he is being held and on whose advice, the duration of the Section, and the role of the responsible medical officer regarding discharge or renewal of the detention. The effects of leaving hospital without permission should also be explained.

Patients should be informed of their right of appeal to the mental health review tribunal, the role of tribunal, and when application can be made. The patient must be given every opportunity and assistance to apply to the tribunal if he wishes, and help should be given in obtaining representation and legal advice.

He should be informed of his right to appeal to the hospital managers who authorize discharge, and be given details of where to apply. When renewal of patient's detention is being considered, the patient should be told of his right to appeal to the managers.

The patient must understand his rights regarding consent to treatment. He must understand the nature, purpose, and likely effects of any treatment proposed. He must also understand his right to withdraw consent to treatment at any time, and whether the doctor can order the treatment to be given against the wishes of the patient. Some treatments require both consent and a second opinion from an appointed doctor. Other treatments such as ECT or the administration of medicine beyond three months require consent or a second opinion. These complex provisions should always be explained by a member of the medical or nursing staff.

The role of the Mental Health Act Commission should be explained to the patient, and the appropriate address for him to correspond with the Commission if he so wishes.

The patient should be made aware of the Mental Health Act Code of Practice, and have access to a copy if he wishes.

The patient must be asked if he has any objection to the above information being given in writing to his nearest relative. He must also be advised whether the nearest relative may request that the patient should be discharged, and their right to apply for a tribunal if appropriate.

If the patient has any questions or complaints for which he feels he has not been given satisfactory answers or explanations, he should be given the name of the appropriate officer to make complaints to. Patients who wish to make a complaint should not be discouraged from putting their criticisms in writing, as well as discussing these with the staff. Organizations such as MIND or the Community Health Council can assist patients who are unable to complain on their own account.

Because of the complexity of the information to be given to the patient, especially when they are detained under several different Sections during an episode in hospital, the policy for information-giving should be viewed as a continual process. Checks should be made periodically to ensure that the patient has understood the information given to him, and whether he wishes to exercise any of his rights.

In addition to the above information, patients detained under Part 3 of the Act (under court order) should be advised to consider whether they wish to appeal to the court against being held in hospital. They should be encouraged to discuss this with their legal representative.

## NURSES' SIX-HOUR HOLDING POWER

The 1983 Act made it possible for a nurse to detain a patient lawfully until either the responsible medical officer or their nominated deputy arrived to assess whether the patient required detention under Section 5. Section

5(4) (page 413) enables a nurse of a prescribed class to detain a patient for up to six hours under strictly specified circumstances.

The following criteria must be met before a nurse may implement the holding power:

- the nurse must be a first-level nurse trained in nursing people suffering from mental illness or mental handicap, (RMN, RNMH);
- the patient must be already being treated for mental disorder as an inpatient;
- it appears to the nurse that the patient is suffering from mental disorder to such a degree that it is necessary for his health or safety, or for the protection of others for him to be immediately restrained from leaving the hospital; and
- it is not practicable to secure the immediate attendance of the appropriate practitioner.

A person may not be dealt with under the Act as suffering only by reason of promiscuity or other immoral conduct, sexual deviance, or dependence on drugs. This means there are no grounds for detaining a person in hospital because of drug or alcohol abuse alone, but it is recognized that alcohol or drug abuse may be accompanied by, or associated with, mental disorder. Therefore, an informal patient being treated for alcoholism who returns to the hospital severely inebriated may not necessarily satisfy the criteria for use of Section 5(4), and would have to therefore be managed without invoking the nurse's holding power.

## Responsibilities of the nurse with holding power

The decision to implement the nurse's holding power is both a personal and professional responsibility. The nurse cannot be instructed by another person, either a medical practitioner or a more senior nurse, to carry out the holding power. The use of the holding power neither increases nor decreases the duty of care that a nurse has towards a patient. The UKCC Code of Conduct for nurses states:

Each registered nurse, midwife and health visitor is accountable for her practice and, in the exercise of professional accountability, shall ensure no action or omission on her part or within her sphere of influence is detrimental to the condition or safety of the patient/client. Provided the nurse exercises her judgement rationally and according to the reasonable standards of the profession, she should not fear any civil action or false imprisonment. However, any evidence of malice and unreasonableness would place her at risk of a civil action.

Conversely, a decision not to implement the holding power unreasonably or maliciously could also result in disciplinary or legal action. It is preferable, but not a legal requirement, for the nurse to have previous acquaintance with the patient. A nurse who does know the patient is obviously in a better position to make a more considered decision whether to detain or not than a nurse who does not know the patient.

In extreme circumstances, it may be necessary to invoke the holding power without carrying out proper assessment. This may occur when no RMN is available, or the RMN has to be called from another area, or has just arrived on duty. The suddenness of the patient's determination to leave and the urgency with which the patient's attempts to do so should alert the nurse to potential serious consequences if the patient is successful in leaving.

There are no recommendations that the RMN has to be of a certain grade before they can implement the holding power. The restriction of use of the holding power to senior grades by certain health authorities is not considered to be good practice, and could cause practical difficulties which the legislation was originally drafted to overcome. However, a senior or more experienced member of staff may be able to persuade a patient to stay, where an inexperienced member of staff could encounter great difficulty. If this is the case, then a more senior or experienced person should be asked to assist without hesitation.

If there is disagreement among the nurses responsible about whether the patient wishing to leave the hospital should be detained or not, the most senior nurse must take responsibility and decide whether or not to implement the holding power. She should, however, be mindful of the opinion of the other nurses involved in the care.

There may be occasions in some health-care establishments when there is neither a medical practitioner or an RMN who can be called upon. If an emergency occurs and it is necessary for ward staff to detain a patient, they must rely upon commonlaw powers. This could mean detaining a patient if there are reasonable grounds to believe he is a risk to himself or others due to mental disorder, or if there would be if he were to leave the hospital.

### Definition of 'inpatient'

The Mental Health Act Code of Practice states that for the purposes of Section 5 an 'informal patient' is one who has understood and accepted the offer of a bed, who has freely appeared on the ward, and has co-operated in the admission procedure.

### Factors to be considered before using the holding power

The Code of Practice states that before using the power the nurse should assess:

The likely arrival of the doctor, against the likely intention of the patient to leave. Most patients who express a wish to leave hospital can be persuaded to wait until the doctor arrives, to discuss it further. Where this is not possible, the nurse must try to predict the impact of any delay on the patient.

The immediate consequences of the harm that might occur to the patient or others, taking into account:

- what the patient says he will do;
- the likelihood of the patient committing suicide;
- the patient's current, and in particular any changes in usual, behaviour;
- the likelihood of the patient behaving in a violent manner;
- any recently received messages from relatives or friends;
- any recent disturbance on the ward, which may or may not involve the patient;
- any relevant involvement of other patients.

Also, the patient's known unpredictability, and other relevant information from other members of the multi-disciplinary team.

### GUIDELINES

When an informal patient expresses a wish to leave hospital, the nurse should discuss with the patient the reasons why he wishes to leave. She should encourage the patient to remain in hospital at least long enough to be seen by a member of the medical staff. If the patient agrees to this, then a doctor should be informed immediately.

If the patient is unwilling to stay following discussion with the nurse, and a doctor is not immediately available, with the power to implement the provisions of Section 5(4) the nurse should assess whether the patient meets the criteria for detention under the Act. Once the nurse's holding power has been implemented, attempts to contact the doctor must be made until he has been informed of the implementation. If an appropriate doctor is immediately available to see the patient, the responsibility to detain then rests with the doctor and not the nurse.

The holding power starts after the nurse has recorded her opinion on the statutory Form 13. Once the nurse has recorded her opinion she cannot reverse the decision; the holding power ends either six hours later, or on the arrival of the doctor entitled to make such a report under Section 5(2).

Consideration should be given to adjusting the patient's care plan. The nurse should compile a comprehensive written report, giving a full account of the patient's behaviour and reasons for having evoked Section 5(4), which should include:

- an account of the patient's behaviour;
- why it was necessary to detain; what other measurers were taken to prevent detention, i.e., resolution of disputes or complaints;
- how the patient was restrained from leaving;
- the name of the doctor contacted;
- the time he was contacted;
- the time he arrived and reason for any delay in attending and further action taken.

As soon as practicable, the nurse in charge should ensure that all staff on the ward are aware of the patient's new legal status and future care, including observation requirements and treatment.

The nurse should ensure that the patient is fully informed of his rights, providing him with Leaflet Number 1, reading it to him, and ensuring as far as possible that he understands what has been said. If the patient has no objection, the nearest relative should be informed both verbally and in writing, explaining the action which has been taken. As soon as the power to detain has lapsed, the prescribed nurse should complete Form 16. In the event of the nurse initiating the holding power having ended duty, the prescribed nurse who has taken over may issue Form 16.

If the doctor cannot be contacted, or, if in the nurse's opinion they have taken an unreasonable amount of time to arrive at the ward, the nurse should inform the senior nurse or manager responsible for the unit. The Code of Practice states that the use of Section 5(4) is an emergency measure and the doctor should treat it as such, arriving as soon as possible. If the doctor has not arrived within five hours, the nurse should contact the consultant or the unit general manager and one of the managers should be informed.

Either the unit general manager or the manager should supervise the patient's leaving after six hours if no doctor has attended.

If on arrival the doctor decides to detain the patient under Section 5(2) for a period of up to 72 hours, this would commence from the time the six-hour holding power was implemented.

Documents 13 and 16, (nurse's reports) and document 12 (doctor's report), if completed by a doctor, should be sent to the hospital manager as soon as possible. Form 15 (receipt of doctor's report) should accompany Form 12. These documents should be sent by a reliable means, by hand if necessary.

Where the six-hour holding power spans more than one duty period, the original decision to detain a patient continues and cannot be repealed by any other prescribed nurse.

In incidents where the patient is considered potentially violent, the nurse should make every attempt to ensure that facilities are available so that the situation can be managed safely. If necessary, a senior nurse or other senior manager should be contacted for advice. Staff should refer to their policy document on the prevention of violence and management of challenging behaviour. To detain the patient safely, consideration may have be given to requesting extra manpower; locking the ward door; transferring the patient to a more appropriate environment.

CASE STUDY – ALAN

Alan has been an inpatient in an acute psychiatric unit for two days. He was divorced from his wife approximately a year ago, and has a young son, Tim, who is four years old. He has a long history of mania and depression. At the moment, Alan is agitated, interfering, and very angry. He refuses to discuss how he is feeling with staff except in a very hostile and indirect manner.

During a busy period on the ward, without warning Alan runs off the ward towards a busy major road. Due to the speed with which he left the ward, nobody could have prevented him leaving. The nurse in charge of the ward asks one nurse to follow Alan, and contacts the other wards within the unit to obtain staff to accompany this nurse. The nurse from Alan's ward and another nurse arrive in time to see Alan, who is standing on the pavement with his eyes closed, jump into the path of an oncoming car. The car manages to swerve round Alan, and fortunately there are no casualties.

The two nurses try to persuade Alan to come back to the hospital, but he is resistant and refuses. In view of the likelihood of traffic coming along, the two nurses take one arm each and take Alan back on to the pavement. They release his arms, but stand in a way that prevents him from directly running on to the road. This results in one of the nurses being head-butted on the side of the face. The nurses feel they have no alternative but to take Alan by force back to the hospital. They are fortunately able to take him back to the hospital grounds, where they are met by the nurse manager and another member of staff who have been called for assistance.

- Under what authority did the nurses restrain this patient?
- Is it appropriate here to use Section 5(4) of the Mental Health Act 1983?
- Could the nurses be accused of assault?
- If Section 5(4) of the Mental Health Act is used, what time should be stated on the document?

CASE STUDY – LILY

Lily White is a slight, 68-year-old woman who has been admitted to hospital following a recent serious attempt to take

her own life, and is considered to be at risk. She has attempted to leave the ward, and a doctor has been informed. The nominated doctor, however, is busy on another ward dealing with a medical emergency, and directs the nurse to use her holding power by implementing Section 5(4). It is estimated that he will arrive at the ward within the next 15 minutes. Although Lily cannot be persuaded to stay, she is prevented from leaving the ward by the staff nurse standing in her way. Lily will not attempt to force her way past the staff nurse, which is probably due to their relative sizes rather than a lack of desire to leave the ward. The nurse is conciliatory, and explains that it is in Lily's best interest to remain on the ward.

- Has a doctor got the authority to direct the nurse to implement Section 5(4)?
- Should this nurse implement Section 5(4)?

CASE STUDY – JANE

Jane is a patient on a rehabilitation unit within a large psychiatric hospital. She has a diagnosis of chronic schizophrenia, but has not had any overt florid symptoms for over one year. She is being encouraged to make choices regarding her personal life, and to take responsibility for her behaviour. She has developed a relationship with a young man of a similar background, from another ward in the hospital. Her mother's views are well known regarding this relationship, being strongly disapproving. Her mother telephones the ward and says she suspects the young man and Jane are having a sexual relationship. She insists that the nurses detain Jane if she attempts to leave the unit that evening. It is nearing the time when Jane would normally leave the unit to go out for the evening.

- Is it appropriate to use Section 5(4)?

## CASE STUDY – KEVIN

Kevin has been an inpatient for eight weeks in a local psychiatric hospital. He has a diagnosis of chronic schizophrenia, but is much improved since his admission. A discharge plan has been formulated, and Kevin is expected to be discharged to a rehabilitation unit in the community during the next week. For the past five years he has lived in bedsits, and has had various admissions to other psychiatric units within the region. One evening there is serious disturbance between two other patients on the ward, during which a lot of objects are thrown around the day-room. This greatly upsets Kevin, who demands to leave the ward. He says he has some money, and he is going to find a bedsit and will go there rather than stay in the ward any longer.

- Should Kevin be allowed to leave the ward?
- Would it be appropriate to use Section 5(4) of the Mental Health Act 1983?

## THE MENTAL HEALTH (SCOTLAND ) ACT 1984

### SECTION 24 – EMERGENCY ADMISSION TO HOSPITAL

In cases of urgent necessity, a recommendation may be made by a medical practitioner, usually a GP, who is of the opinion that the patient is at risk to themselves or others and should be in hospital for a period of assessment. The doctor should gain the consent of the next-of-kin or a mental health officer (approved social worker), or state why he has not done so.

The period of detention is 72 hours from the time the patient is admitted to the ward. Once in hospital, the patient is informed of his rights, which are those of any individual, with the exception of being allowed to leave hospital.

In some circumstances, nursing staff may be required to withhold outgoing mail if an individual has stated they do not wish to receive letters from the patient.

Section 24 cannot be applied consecutively, and at the end of 72 hours the patient either becomes informal or goes on to further detention.

### SECTION 25(1) – DETENTION OF PATIENTS ALREADY IN HOSPITAL

This order has the same provisions as Section 24 except that it applies to a patient already in hospital who wishes to leave but is deemed to require detention.

### SECTION 25(2) – NURSES' HOLDING POWER

A nurse who is Registered in Mental Illness or Mental Handicap may detain an informal patient, if it is necessary under the criteria, for a period of two hours in the absence of a doctor. Once applied, nursing staff must make every attempt to get a doctor to see the patient within the two hours. Nurses' holding power cannot be used consecutively, and at the end of two hours the patient either becomes informal or is detained under Section 25(1), invoked by a doctor making an emergency recommendation.

### SECTION 60-76 – PATIENTS CONCERNED IN CRIMINAL PROCEEDINGS

Tried and untried prisoners may be detained under the Criminal Procedures Act (Scotland) 1975. The relevant parts of the Act have equivalent applications under the Mental Health Act (Scotland) 1984, and are similar to the Mental Health Act 1983 for England and Wales.

### CONSENT TO TREATMENT

Patients on Section 24 have the right to refuse treatment, but may be treated in cases of emergency, i.e., if they become an immediate and severe risk to themselves or others.

## SECTION 26 – SHORT-TERM DETENTION

This may follow on from Section 24 after the expiry of 72 hours, and cannot be applied independently. Section 26 is a detention order lasting for up to 28 days, which a senior psychiatrist can apply with the consent of the nearest relative or a mental health officer. The order can be rescinded at any time by the responsible medical officer.

## SECTION 18 – ADMISSION AND DETENTION OF PATIENTS TO HOSPITAL

This may follow on from a Section 26, or it may be sought independently to bring someone who is chronically unwell in the community into hospital for treatment. Application for Section 18 is made by a nearest relative or a mental health officer, and founded on two recommendations by a senior psychiatrist and another doctor who knows the patient, usually a GP. In addition, the Section must be approved by the sheriff. The patient has the right to attend the sheriff's hearing to contest the application of the Section. Once applied, the responsible medical officer reviews the patient at four weeks, three months, six months, and then annually to determine whether continued treatment and/or detention is necessary.

Once treatment is established, patients may be allowed to return to the community or be granted leave of absence and be regularly reviewed as an outpatient. If circumstances change, the patient may be readmitted against their will at any time.

Patients on Section 18 must accept treatment that does not require formal, informed consent, for a period of up to three months. If after three months the patient continues to refuse treatment, then a certificate of second opinion must be sought from the Mental Welfare Commission, which will give clearly

defined boundaries of the treatment that may be given to the patient without his consent.

## SECTION 35 – RIGHTS OF APPEAL

All formally detained patients have the right to appeal against their detention and treatment in hospital. Any patient may ask the Mental Welfare Commission to review their care at any time. In addition, patients detained under Section 26 and Section 18 may appeal to the sheriff on one occasion at every renewal of detention. Nursing staff should give patients all the assistance they require to appeal.

## MENTAL WELFARE COMMISSION

This is a statutory body similar to the Mental Health Act Commission in England and Wales. The main function of the commission is to protect the rights of all psychiatric patients and their families. In addition, they produce an annual report.

Any member of staff, patient or relatives may contact the Commission (anonymously, if desired) and ask them to investigate any aspect of care and treatment. The Commission may visit the hospital at any time unannounced and request unlimited access to all documentation relating to individual patients, and to interview any member of staff. They have the power to order the discharge of individual patients, and to make recommendations on any sphere of hospital functioning that impinges on direct patient care.

## NURSING DILEMMAS

### Nurses' holding power

A nurse, having already applied the holding power, asks a doctor to examine the patient. The doctor arrives within two hours, but does not know the patient, who agrees to stay informally. The doctor leaves, and the nurses holding power is terminated. The patient decides to leave the ward.

- Can the nurse reapply the holding power?

## Medication and the detained patient

A middle-aged woman was admitted under Section 24 Mental Health Act. Her family stated she had been behaving oddly for some time, neglecting her personal hygiene, shouting at things and people who were not there, having arguments with her family, breaking things at home, and spending large amounts of money. Her family was exasperated. On admission, the woman was well dressed, clean, and neat. Her manner was aloof, her speech was appropriate, although her conversation was superficial.

After 72 hours, she was further detained on Section 26 Mental Health Act. She was angry at this, requesting to know why. She stated she had remained in hospital to be assessed, behaved appropriately and cared for herself. She felt having been assessed she should be allowed to go home. Her family insisted she was unwell, although after assessment no symptoms were observed. She was then prescribed depot medication as she was thought by the doctor to be suffering from a psychotic illness. The nurses did not agree, and expressed unwillingness to administer the medication. Although the woman may have appeared odd, their observations and assessment showed no sign of psychosis. A family meeting was held with nurses, doctors, patients, and family. Following this, Section 26 was rescinded and the woman was discharged home.

- Were the nurses within their rights to refuse to give the prescribed medication?

## MENTAL HEALTH LEGISLATION IN EIRE

The legal provisions for mentally ill patients in Ireland are contained in the Mental Treatment Act 1945, amended in 1961. Further amendments were proposed under the Health (Mental Services) Act 1981, but these were not enacted by the Oireachtas. A further review of the legislation is proposed, but no date has been set.

### CLASSES OF PATIENTS

There are two main classes of patients received into mental hospitals: voluntary patients and non-voluntary patients. Non-voluntary patients are those who have to be compulsorily admitted and detained. They are divided into two groups - temporary patients and persons of unsound mind. A temporary patient is a person who needs detention but is believed to require for his recovery not more than six months suitable treatment. A person of unsound mind is a person who is certified to need detention and to be unlikely to recover within six months.

### ADMISSION TO A MENTAL HOSPITAL

#### Section 184/185 – temporary patient

An application for admission can be made by a husband or a wife or a blood relative. The relative should then ask a doctor to complete Part two, which is a medical certificate that the patient is suffering from mental illness and requires treatment. If the doctor completes Part 2 of the certificate, he then returns the form to the applicant, who may present the form to the appropriate medical officer in the district mental hospital. The hospital medical officer then completes Part 3 of the admission form, which authorizes him to admit the patient to hospital within seven days.

The applicant is obliged to inform the patient of the nature of the medical certificate, and the fact that the patient may request a second medical examination. If the patient requests a second medical examination, he may not be removed to hospital unless the second examination has been made, and the second doctor has signified in writing that he agrees with the first certificate.

### Section 162/163 – person of unsound mind

Where it is desired to have a person received as a person of unsound mind in a district mental hospital, form Number 4 must be completed. This form consists of four parts. Part i is a statement of particulars regarding the patient. Part ii is an application for recommendation for reception. Part i and ii should be completed by a suitable applicant. The form should then be presented to a doctor for completion of part iii, which provides for a recommendation that the patient should be received as a person of unsound mind. Alternatively it provides for a refusal to give such a recommendation. If he considers he should give the recommendation, he should complete the appropriate portion of part iii and return the form to the applicant, who may then remove the patient to the district mental hospital.

On arrival of the patient at the hospital, the form should be presented to the appropriate medical officer of the hospital, who, if he is satisfied, will complete Part iv. A person of unsound mind may be detained until his removal or discharge by proper authority or his death. These periods of detention are all subject to the safeguards laid out in the role of the chief medical officer.

### SAFEGUARDS

The patient has several safeguards contained in the Mental Treatment Act against wrongful detention of patients. The main ones are:

- The patient has a right to have a letter forwarded, unopened, to the Minister, the High Court, the Mental Hospital Visiting Committee, or the Inspector of Mental Hospitals. As a result, an independent examination of the patient may be required.

- Any person may apply to the Minister for an order for the examination of a detained patient by two medical practitioners.
- The Act specifically requires that a patient who has recovered must be discharged.
- The inspector of mental hospitals must visit all mental institutions, at stated intervals. He has a duty to give special attention to the state of mind of any patient detained where the propriety of detention is doubtful, or where he is requested by the patient himself to do so.
- Any relative or friend of a person detained may apply for the discharge of a patient and has the right of an appeal to the Minister.
- Every mental hospital authority must appoint a visiting committee, whose duties include a requirement to hear the complaints of any patient and to see him in private.

### OTHER ISSUES

The powers of the Gardai (police) are fairly extensive, and include the power to make an application for reception and to provide escort when a doctor makes a recommendation. Provision is made within the Act for persons who commit criminal offences. The removal of a patient from one hospital to another is also accommodated within the Act.

The Act does not specify any holding powers for nurses, but the chief medical officer can detain a voluntary patient for up to 28 days if that patient becomes incapable of expressing himself, or is not willing to remain in the institution.

### MENTAL HEALTH LEGISLATION NORTHERN IRELAND

Legislation in Northern Ireland is governed by the Mental Health (Northern Ireland) Order 1986. The Department of Health and

Social Services in Northern Ireland has also produced a guide for staff who are involved in the procedures for the compulsory admission of mentally disordered people. This is an extremely helpful document as it dispenses with much of the legal jargon. Unlike the rest of the UK, the various paragraphs are referred to as articles and not sections.

## ADMISSION TO HOSPITAL FOR ASSESSMENT

Unlike the 1961 Act, which had two ways by which a mentally disordered person could be compulsorily admitted to hospital – the normal procedure and the emergency procedure - there is now only one procedure under the Order. Central to this procedure is the requirement that all patients who are compulsorily admitted to hospital will be held initially for a period of assessment for up to 14 days before being detained for treatment. Patients will be examined on admission or within 48 hours by a consultant psychiatrist, and before they can be detained for treatment they must be examined by a consultant psychiatrist on two or more occasions.

The application for admission for assessment is similar to those in England and Wales, involving the patient's nearest relative or an approved social worker, followed by the medical recommendation.

In respect of a patient already in hospital, an application for assessment can be made in the same way as for a patient outside hospital. Under Article 7(2) a doctor has the power to restrain a voluntary patient from leaving hospital for 48 hours by furnishing a report to the Board. This is to allow time to have an application form and medical recommendation completed.

## ARTICLE 7(3) – NURSES' HOLDING POWER

A first-level nurse trained in nursing people suffering from mental illness and mental handicap may detain a voluntary patient, who is already being treated for mental disorder as an inpatient, for up to 6 hours. The criteria and the procedure are similar to England and Wales.

## ARTICLE 12 – DETENTION TREATMENT

During the second seven days of the assessment period, the patient must be examined by a doctor to decide whether it is necessary to detain him for treatment beyond that period. If the patient's condition has improved during the assessment period, he may be given the opportunity to remain in hospital as a voluntary patient or to receive treatment as an outpatient.

If as a result of the examination a doctor is satisfied the patient should be further detained on the grounds that he is suffering from mental illness; that he is very likely to cause serious harm to himself or others; and that no other methods of dealing with the patient are available, the patient may then be detained for up to six months beginning with the date of admission so that he can receive the treatment he needs.

Patients in hospital for assessment or detained for treatment may be discharged at any time by the responsible medical officer, the responsible board, or the nearest relative. The responsible medical officer has a duty to discharge a patient if he is satisfied that the criteria for detention are no longer satisfied.

The regulations for guardianship and consent to treatment are similar to those for England and Wales. There are a number of differences relating to procedure, which require reference to the Act, if a nurse is involved in dealing with detained patients in Northern Ireland.

**REFERENCES:**

DoH (1986) *Mental Health Act (1983)*, HMSO, London.

DoH (1990) *Code of Practice (MHA 1983)*, HMSO, London.

DHSS (Northern Ireland) (1985) *Mental Health (Northern Ireland) Order 1985*, Belfast, HMSO.

DHSS (Northern Ireland) (1986) Guide to Mental Health Order 1985, Belfast, HMSO.

An Roinn Sláinte (1961) *Mental Treatment Acts 1945–1961* Dublin, SO.

Oireachtas (1981) *Health (Mental Services) Act 1981* Dublin, SO.

Department of Health (1986) *Mental Health Act (Scotland)* 1984 Edinburgh, HMSO.

# PART TEN

# THE RANGE OF THERAPEUTIC FACILITIES

*David B. Cooper*

This chapter gives an overview of some of the facilities available that can be used in the development of appropriate care packages for the client. They will of course vary within different health authorities.

Over the last 20 years, there has been a gradual move away from an institutional approach to care towards a holistic, community-based service, and there are many more facilities available to the client than those offered by the NHS. The commercial and voluntary sectors may well be able to provide the help the client needs in the process of recovery from mental health problems. As well, the development of well-managed and organized self-help groups, run by people who have had life experiences of mental health problems, have proved to be a major resource to those working within the health care professions.

There will be an increasing need for more community service facilities with the introduction of the recently published White paper *Caring for People* (1989), in which it is made clear that the aim of each district health authority should be to develop community services:

> The aim of health authorities should be to ensure that community health services are available to enable people to live in their own homes for as long as possible. Health authorities are therefore expected to continue to develop their community health services in line with this objective.

The Paper goes on to stress the importance of the nurses' role:

Community nursing services including Health Visitors (HVs), Mental Handicap Nurses (MHNs), who bring to their work a variety of skills and expert knowledge. They are able to assist people with social, psychological and health care problems which may affect the quality of life. As community workers, nurses are in touch with the network of help available in a neighbourhood and can mobilize resources to respond sensitively to people's needs.

Generally speaking, in each health district therapeutic facilities are offered by the voluntary, commercial, or public sectors, which have developed in response to an identified need. The GP is often the first point of contact, or the service user. Most agencies inform the GP of new services available to the client.

All the services available in a health district should be identified. The best way to assist the client is by using the following process: phone–meet–talk–index, for each organization. This is time-consuming initially, but well worth the effort.

The local phonebook often lists services under the 'useful numbers' section, and many local papers list daily or weekly contact numbers for both public- and voluntary-sector services. In contacting the Community Health Council, the Citizens' Advice Bureau, and by talking to colleagues, local and other areas of health care, a composite picture is built up. For example, a health visitor may be able to tell you the location of the mother and toddler group and the Well Women Clinic. The client himself may also have information on useful services, including self-help groups.

When this information has been gathered, it is helpful to meet the personnel to get a clear idea of the people involved and the service they offer. Leaflets giving information about the service and its access are often available. It is useful at this stage to index the organization, recording the phone number, an overview of the service, and a contact name on a card index system or computer.

There are national agencies such as The Commission for Racial Equality, MIND, Good Practices in Mental Health, Alcohol Concern and Narcotics Anonymous which may be able to guide the nurse to a suitable local group, or a service most appropriate to the client's needs. The information collated will help to prevent inappropriate referrals and ensure the correct use of services. (At the end of the chapter, there is a list of useful addresses and further reading.)

## PUBLIC-SECTOR SERVICE PROVISION

### ACUTE ADMISSION MENTAL HEALTH UNITS

Since the early 1970s, an increasing number of acute admission mental health units have been built or developed within the grounds of district general hospitals. At the same time, the equivalent facilities within the grounds of large psychiatric hospitals have closed. This is a move away from the traditional asylum or institutional approach to care that recognizes the need to provide those with mental health problems with appropriate services within their own communities.

These, often purpose-built, units contain mixed-gender admission wards. Some offer an additional continuing care ward to assist in short-term rehabilitation following an acute episode; some have an elderly severely mentally ill ward attached. Integrated within these units are occupational therapy areas and a day hospital. Some units still maintain

a small ECT suite, usually staffed on two days per week by the day hospital. A team of nurses, doctors, consultants, social workers, occupational therapists, CPNs, psychotherapists, and psychologists usually work from and in these units, providing a mixture of skills.

Until recently, all referrals would be from GP to consultant, or consultant to consultant. Now, referrals may also come from community mental health teams, GPs, social workers, CPNs, and others, without direct need for individual consultant involvement.

The introduction of multidisciplinary approaches to care and the primary nurse system has enhanced the quality of care offered to those with mental health problems, with many units now running multidisciplinary quality-control groups.

The client may undergo several interventions during admission, which may include individual counselling with a psychologist or a nurse; groupwork, which may be general or specific depending on need; occupational therapy; home assessment; and recreational activities. All of these may be included on an individual's care plan, which is discussed and agreed with the client and all those involved in his or her care. Ongoing review and update is implicit to the success of the care package offered.

### ELDERLY SEVERELY MENTALLY ILL (ESMI)

ESMI units are mainly purpose-built within the grounds of a general hospital, though in some forward-thinking health districts, large houses within the community have been adapted to produce small, six-to-twelve bedded units within the client's home locality. These are staffed by multidisciplinary teams, which may include consultants and other doctors, nurses, social workers, psychologists, occupational therapists, and CPNs in the larger units, with additional services from physiotherapists and chiropodists, delivered as needed.

The smaller units are usually manned by nurses or other care workers, with perhaps a GP offering daily cover. These units have access to other services such as social workers, occupational therapists or CPNs. The smaller units are funded by the district health authority or the social services, and some have joint funding.

The wards are of mixed gender, and have 15–20 beds, on average, per ward. The majority of units have two medium, long-stay wards and two acute admission wards, as well as day hospital facilities.

In addition to intensive physical and mental nursing care, and individual and group activities, reality-orientation programmes are undertaken. Most units offer holiday-relief beds to enable relatives to take a much-needed break.

Admission is usually arranged by a consultant, other doctors, the GP, social worker, occupational therapist or a CPN (elderly services), and occasionally by the community elderly team if it is available in the district.

## DAY HOSPITALS

These offer an intermediary care package, providing a mixture of approaches for those with mental-health-related problems. The hospitals can either be attached to a given admission unit, or based in the community. Some districts provide satellite day hospitals in health centres or village halls. Day hospitals may be funded by district health authorities, social service department, or voluntary-sector organizations such as MIND or Age Concern. Some are jointly funded by all three, or a combination of these organizations.

Attendance can vary, based on need, from sessional (for a given group or activity), to attendance for one day weekly, several days per week, or for a whole week. Day hospitals normally open from 8–5, Monday–Friday. A few offer weekend care, or operate during extended Bank Holidays.

There are three types of day hospital facility covering acute mental health, rehabilitation mental health, and elderly mental health. In many areas a single day hospital may offer services to each of the three groups. The team may consist of nurses, social workers, care assistants, doctors, and occupational therapist. Community psychiatric nursing, physiotherapy, chiropody and other services may be provided as required.

The emphasis of care will depend on the client group at any given time, within all three types of day hospital. Depending upon client group, care ranges from washing and meal preparation, the use of household equipment, budgeting, and the use of transport, to individual counselling, groupwork, and occupational therapy. An assessment is made of any disability, and appropriate aids are provided. General nursing tasks may also be undertaken, such as bathing, medication reviews, and monitoring of medical conditions. Day hospitals may also provide leisure facilities for clients and their families. They can be seen as important stepping-stones from residential to community care.

## COMMUNITY MENTAL HEALTH SERVICE PROVISION

Community services offered to those with mental-health-related problems have seen rapid changes and development over the last 20 years. Nurses have been at the forefront, and in many cases have pioneered new community services for this client group, often modifying and increasing their training to accommodate new specialities.

The early 1970s saw the introduction of the CPN, who, working from a hospital ward, would visit the client at home to monitor progress and medication, or administer depot injections. Most referrals originally were from consultants, but as nurses developed their skills, their work expanded to accept referrals from GPs, health visitors, social workers and other professionals, and included, for example, home assessments, family interviews, counselling and groupwork.

Gradually, community nursing teams were established, which today coexist with the developing community mental health teams, which are often based at mental health resource centres, community rehabilitation teams, and community elderly teams. Each one is a multidisciplinary team specializing in acute, rehabilitation, or elderly mental health care within the community.

Some of these services are joint funded by social service departments and health authorities. Other facilities are funded wholly by either the health authority or social service departments, with the holders of the staffing budget for each professional group providing finance, e.g., the employment of nurses is provided for from within the nursing budget, and that of psychologists from the psychology budget, and so on. Currently, health authorities are the primary funders of community mental health provision.

Although some of the services offered by CPNs and community teams are similar, they are described separately below in order to distinguish them.

## COMMUNITY PSYCHIATRIC NURSES (CPNS)

Many CPNs have tended to be hospital based, working from a mental health unit within a general hospital or large psychiatric hospital. However, increasingly they are based in a variety of community settings, for example, mental health resource centres, day hospitals, and GPs surgeries. From such places they undertake their work in clients' homes, in their own bases, or other health authority premises.

CPNs are often employed in specialist teams, such as generic teams dealing with acute and chronic mental health problems; teams working with the elderly; alcohol and drug misusers; and child and adolescent services. Services for the elderly mainly commence at 65–70 years, but some health districts have their own policies. Services are also provided on the basis of local needs. Each CPN may have additional specialist expertise, e.g. anxiety-related problems, solvent abuse, suicidal behavior, group therapy, psychotherapy, and AIDS/HIV.

CPNs can be contacted at their work base. Some CPN departments advertise in the phone book under the useful numbers section, and most GPs carry information about the service. Libraries also keep information on services, as do Citizens' Advice Centres and Community Health Councils.

Three-quarters of referrals originate from the medical profession, nearly half from psychiatrists and half from GPs. Any health professional, voluntary service, relative or client can refer direct to the CPN for advice, information, assessment, or intervention. The CPN will inform the GP of his/her involvement, as a matter of professional courtesy and to facilitate communication. If the referral is from a hospital source, the involvement of the CPN has sometimes been prearranged by a multidisciplinary team. It is important to remember that the client has a right of choice, and must agree before the CPN becomes involved in his care.

Most CPNs operate a 9–5, Monday–Friday service, with some flexible work outside these hours, depending on the needs of the client. A few departments may offer an emergency on-call system over the weekend, which may be accessed directly through a duty senior nurse, or via an answerphone system, which the CPN contacts from home several times a day. If this system is in operation, it is important that prospective clients or referrers are invited to leave a clear message, giving a name and a contact number where they can be located by the CPN. On no occasion should details about the client and his location be given, as this would breach confidentiality. A phone call may allow a quick response, but it is usual to follow this up with a written referral, either on a referral form or by letter.

## COMMUNITY MENTAL HEALTH TEAMS (CMHTS) AND MENTAL HEALTH RESOURCE CENTRES (MHRCS)

The development of CMHTs, often based in MHRCs, has taken the care of those with mental health problems one step further by transferring the base from which care is provided, into the community.

The MHRC is often a house or office located within the area it serves, providing general and other office space, a reception area, a resource room, interview, group, and other meeting rooms. Most teams offer a 9–5, Monday–Friday, 'shop-front' service, that is, anyone can call in for general information and/or advice between these hours, or to make a referral. This is also a base for the CMHT members from which to work. CMHTs are multidisciplinary bodies consisting of a consultant, doctor, community psychiatric nurses, social worker(s), psychologist(s), and occupational therapists(s).

Some CMHTs or MHRCs provide a rapid access team, which operates an out-of-normal-hours service, in addition to providing assessment and treatment during normal working hours.

Phone numbers and addresses can normally be obtained from the GP, libraries, and so on. The number may also be found in the phone book under 'useful numbers'.

As with referrals to CPNs an open referral system operates, enabling a rapid response. The service offers preventative as well as interventionist provision. Urgent referrals assessed by a rapid access team, which is multidisciplinary in structure, and will undertake a crisis visit. Subsequent care may be by a given member of the team, for example the psychologist, nurse psychotherapist, or social worker. The client may attend group therapy at the centre, or hospital admission may be arranged, depending on need.

The link between the hospital and the team is strong, with the client moving between services as his needs dictate. A recommendation for admission from the team is normally accepted without the need for further assessment or delay.

The following services may be provided by the community psychiatric nursing team, the CMHT, or the MHRC.

### Satellite clinics

These operate in rural areas in order to improve access for those with mental-health-related problems. They open for one or two days or half-days each week, offering drop-in facilities, groupwork, individual counselling, behavioural and cognitive treatments, or a depot clinic, depending on the needs of the individual and the client group.

Satellite clinics are based in health centres or other community facilities; church or village halls, for example. The centres improve access to mental health service to those areas more remote from the MHRC.

### Crisis intervention teams

These were developed in the early 1970s; Napsbury Hospital, St Albans, was one of the pioneers of this approach (Fairwell, 1976). The teams operate very much like today's rapid access teams. Many provide a rapid response to mental-health-related crises on a 24-hour basis, in the client's home environment. The team usually consists of a consultant psychiatrist, social worker, and/or a CPN.

Access at the time of crisis is via the GP, the social services or the service user, friends, or family. The team travels to the client's home, or other location to undertake an assessment. The objective is to bring the crisis to a controllable level. By spending time with the individual or family in crisis, it is often possible to deal with the presenting complaint within the home environment, containing the problem and thereby making treatment and other interventions more effective. If admission to hospital is required, it can be arranged quickly.

## Depot clinics

Although outmoded, depot clinics still function in some health districts, often operating from health centres or other satellite facilities.

Depot clinics are organized by CPNs. The aim is to enable those who work or have other difficulties in attendance or access to attend a clinic in the evening, in order to receive long-acting intramuscular injections of the prescribed psychotropic drugs. At the same time, clients' general mental and physical health are assessed, and counselling or other interventions are arranged as needed. Difficulties with any side-effects of medication are also monitored and reviewed. Referral to consultant or other services can be made, for example, to the disablement resettlement officer. Most depot clinics operate on an appointment basis.

## Other groups/activities

Most CPNs, CMHTs, and MHRCs either run, or participate in a variety of groups. These may include: relaxation; anxiety management; phobic management, tranquillizer withdrawal; bereavement; post-natal; mother and toddler, and support groups.

The development of these groups usually arises from identified demand, and operate at varying levels of intensity and structure. The duration of the therapeutic intervention is dependent on the client group and the model used by the group leader.

By contacting the CPNs, CMHT or MHRC (also the social service department or probation office), one is able to find out which groups are operating at that time, and the mode of referral. There are many self-help groups that address associated mental health problems, including, for example, stress management.

RISK ASSESSMENT TEAMS

Some districts now operate a risk assessment team. These work closely with district general hospitals, especially the accident and emergency department and the emergency admission ward.

The team may consists of several members, or just two. Working a rota to cover weekends and evenings, they aim to assess, and offer early intervention to, anyone admitted following self-injury. People admitted overnight are seen the following day, or, if the need is considered urgent, are referred through normal duty doctor channels.

The extent of the team's involvement is based on client need, and may include referral to the acute mental health admission unit or the CMHT; the offer of individual counselling; or referral to another voluntary or statutory service.

FAMILY SUPPORT GROUPS

These are sometimes organized by acute admission wards and CMHTs or by the voluntary sector. The rehabilitation and elderly service teams may also operate such groups for their clients. These are much needed, and their development is an important contribution to client care. They normally operate as open groups, allowing people to join and leave as they please. They offer advice, information, and group support to the client's relatives.

It cannot be stressed enough that support for relatives, which reduces their sense of isolation, is an important and integral part of any care package offered. Such groups are often advertised on notice boards within the hospital, mental health resource centre, and GP practices.

COMMUNITY REHABILITATION TEAMS

These newly developed, multidisciplinary teams are similar to the CMHTs. The client group consists of those who have either been resident in the long-stay wards of psychiatric hospitals, or who suffer from chronic mental health problems, but reside in group homes, or in the community.

The aim is to offer a support and intervention network of care, assisting the clients' eventual integration into the community. This may include help with housing or group home accommodation, and maintaining the individual's well-being, while personal control is regained by the client of his own life and destiny.

As with the CMHT, groupwork, individual counselling, and the administration and monitoring of prescribed medication are all part of the team's role. Regular reviews are held, and include assessment, planning, implementation, and evaluation of any care the client may need.

## COMMUNITY ELDERLY TEAMS

Some multidisciplinary teams do exist, but this provision currently is mainly organized by CPNs specializing in the care of the elderly who link into ward and day hospital multidisciplinary teams. They tend to be based in elderly severely mentally ill units, or day hospitals for the elderly. As a general rule, clients aged over 65–70 years are referred to this service for mental health care.

Working along similar lines to the CMHT or CRT, the CPNs for elderly services often work in the client's own home, and with the family as a whole.

## ALCOHOL AND DRUG TEAMS

The alcohol and drug teams now tend to be integrated, and offer a joint service that operates from a shared community base.

These specialist teams often work within the client's home, but also function from a town centre located base and satellite clinics. The teams mostly consist of specialist nurses but others have social workers, psychologists, occupational therapists and, occasionally,

probation officers attached to them. A few have consultant psychiatrists, but on the whole, this provision is fulfilled by a consultant who has a special interest in alcohol- and drug-related problems.

Referrals to the team may be from any source, including self-referral. The centres operate a 9–5 service, with drop-in facilities either daily or on given days per week. The teams usually work a flexi-time system to allow evening visits to clients who work.

The teams offer advice, information, education, counselling, home detoxification, groupwork, and referral to dry hostels or hospital units, either statutory or voluntary, as needed. Many projects also conduct research.

The introduction of outreach workers has greatly assisted drug teams. Working directly with the client in his own environment, contact is usually made with a user via a snowball effect, that is, one user introduces the outreach worker to a friend, and so on. The worker slowly increases his contacts offering help to each individual as required.

Health education is an important part of the work of both teams. They provide information, advice, and help to occupational health departments in both the private and statutory sectors, to employers and the employees, to schools and through many other public relations events and activities.

## NEEDLE-EXCHANGE SCHEMES

Often this is organized by either the health promotion department or the community drug team. Satellite clinics are established around each district. Drug users can exchange their 'dirty works' (needles and syringes) for clean material. In some districts, chemists offer this facility.

These schemes operate in the strictest confidence. Their aim is to reduce the risk of infection from AIDS or Hepatitis B. However, help and advice on other matters, including the management of the habit, is available to the user if required.

The health promotion or drug and alcohol team will be able to provide nurses with contact times and other information for their clients.

## CHILD AND ADOLESCENT SERVICES

Most health districts provide or have access to child and adolescent services, also referred to as child and family services, or family services.

### Hospital-based services

These operate like normal hospital facilities, providing residential care for adolescents between the ages 11–17. They usually include classroom facilities, used by the education department during school term. Teachers are mainly funded through the local education authority budget. Staffing consists of consultants, nurses, social workers, an educational psychologist, occupational therapists, teachers and CPNs who specialize in this area of care.

The units tend to be mixed, with 12 or so beds. They will have recreation rooms, classrooms, group rooms, single bedrooms, and dormitory areas, administrative offices, and interview rooms.

### Child and family guidance teams

Based in the community, these teams work closely with the education system, dealing with behavioural issues, school phobias, and other problems including quite severe difficulties with relationships, and the physical and sexual abuse of children.

Teams often include a consultant child psychiatrist, CPNs educational and clinical psychologists, social workers, and child psychotherapists. These teams may be jointly or separately funded by district health authorities and/or social services departments. The treatment offered will depend on the identified needs relating to the individual and his or her family, but may include individual and group psychotherapy, family therapy and special needs education. The system of referral is usually open.

## THE HEALTH PROMOTION DEPARTMENT

Depending on the district, the department is either referred to as health education or health promotion. In this chapter they will be referred to as the latter.

The departments are separately funded district authorities, monies being allocated from the Health Education Authority (HEA). In many cases the director of health promotion (often a doctor), sits on the district management board and is accountable to the district general manager.

Health promotion departments provide information and promotional material to the public. They also undertake health promotion activities in schools, offices, and factories. Anyone can request their help. The publicity material for 'National No-Smoking Day', 'Drinkwise Day', or the 'Look After Your Heart' Campaigns stem from this body.

Typical staffing would consist of a director, health promotion officers, administrative staff, and specialist trained in art and design. Specialist health promotion officers deal with issues such as, AIDS/HIV, alcohol/drugs or other significant threats to health, for example, heart disease.

They operate Monday–Friday, 9–5, enabling access to the department for literature, leaflets, audio-visual aids, and posters. One can also seek advice and assistance in the design and publication of health education material. It is possible to borrow slides, videos, and teaching aids such as manuals, models, and handouts.

## VOLUNTARY- AND COMMERCIAL-SECTOR SERVICE PROVISION

### COMMUNITY RESOURCES (INCLUDING SELF-HELP)

There are many commercial- and voluntary-sector resources available within the community that have expertise that is of value to our clients. Directory enquiries offer a useful service in providing the phone number of local services. The local library will also have many lists of helpful organizations. They also carry an extensive stock of national phone directories. The phone book also has 'useful numbers' section.

### The Samaritans

With a base in nearly every town, the Samaritans offer a 24-hour counselling service and a help-line for those in need of help. The service is manned by trained counsellors, all of whom are volunteers. This service is not only (as sometimes thought) for those feeling suicidal, but is also for those with other problems.

### RELATE (formerly The Marriage Guidance Council)

RELATE have some 400-plus counselling centres around the country. They have entries in the directories under both 'Marriage Guidance' and 'RELATE'. The organization helps those with relationship difficulties, including partnership and family problems. Counsellors do not necessarily need to see both partners, but often prefer to do so. All counsellors are well-trained and supervised.

### National AIDS Helpline

These were established to answer questions and to deal with anxieties that any individual may have about AIDS. The phone call is free and confidential. Anyone can request literature, which is dispatched free. For personal advice and counselling, the caller can talk directly to a trained advisor. The advisor can also put people in contact with a local specialist agency.

### CRUSE bereavement care

CRUSE offers support and counselling services for those who are bereaved. This is provided by trained bereavement counsellors, who may have been bereaved themselves. They provide phone support as well as self-help groups.

### Citizens' Advice Bureau (CAB)

CAB offer a free, confidential, information service. They operate a computerized, national information system. The main enquiries tend to be related to social security, money matters, consumer problems, housing, family, personal, employment, and justice issues. They also deal with other problems related to living in the community today.

### Age Concern

This voluntary body has its own social services, home help, and occupational therapy facilities, as well as offering advice, counselling, social, and recreational services to the elderly in their own localities. Age Concern also runs day-centres and groups for elderly people in many towns.

### Community Health Councils

Community Health Councils look after the interests of those who come into contact with the health services. As well as dealing with complaints, they are usually active in the development of new services representing the public interest. They can give information about these as well as general advice relating to health care issues.

### Alcoholics Anonymous/Gamblers Anonymous/Narcotics Anonymous

These self-help groups are organized and run by people who have drug-, alcohol-, or gambling-related problems. Anyone can attend the meetings, as long as they 'have a desire to stop drinking' (or gambling, or taking drugs). They offer individual and group support at a local level.

## Al-Anon/Al-Ateen and Families Anonymous

Al-Anon and Al-Ateen offer support and self-help groups to the families of those with drink-related problems. Families Anonymous is for the families and friends of those with drug-related problems. The groups are run on the same lines as AA and NA, by people who have had first-hand experience of close relationships with substance abuse.

## British Association of Counselling

Nurses and members of other professional groups with counselling skills may joint this organization. It aims to promote good practices in counselling and offers a counselling resource to the public. The organization produces two directories; one of training resources and one of counselling resources. They also provide a geographical directory of counsellors to members of the public. They are a membership and training organization for counsellors.

## CONCLUSION

It is important that the transition from one area of care to another is smooth and well planned, and that the client is involved in making any choices throughout this process. The client should be adequately prepared for the eventual withdrawal of nursing involvement, and full preparation for the client's discharge should be made well in advance of the planned finishing date. It may seem self-evident, but it is wise to avoid discharging the client home on a Friday, when many of the services they might depend upon for support are closed.

The time spent assessing the availability of voluntary and statutory sector community resources is a good investment when organizing a care package.

Many churches and voluntary bodies organize friendship clubs or support groups for the elderly client. Village coffee mornings still take place, and can be a good source of companionship for those living in rural areas.

The GP's surgery, parish clergy, or parish magazine, are all useful points of enquiry. The local council may provide meals-on-wheels, home-helps or provide aids (such as bath seats, zimmer-frames, or toilet seats with a support frame). They may also have information about volunteer taxi schemes to assist in the transportation of the client to and from appointments.

The network of information is complex and varies between geographical areas. There is no specific point of departure when compiling information about community provision. Anywhere is a good place to start, and the information obtained will snowball from there. Once gathered, the resources can be used to their optimum and the information shared.

## REFERENCES

Caring for people (1989) Community care in the next decade and beyond. *Caring for the 1990s*, HMSO, London.

Farwell, T. (1976) Crisis Intervention. *The Nursing Mirror*, 143, 60–1.

## FURTHER READING

Alcohol Service Information Pack (1989) Alcohol Concern.

Goldie, N., Pilgrim, D., Rogers, A., *Community Mental Health Centres: Policy and Practice*.

*Crisis Intervention Pack* (1989), (ed. J.Renshaw)

Housing Information Pack: *Ordinary Housing for People with Major Long-Term Psychiatric Difficulties* (1985)

*Information Pack on Day Care* (1989).

*Mental Health in Primary Care: A New Perspective* (1989).

Morris, B. (1989) *The Islington Forum*.

Sherlock, J. *At Home in the Community*, Directory, GPMH.

All the above are available from:
Good Practices in Mental Health (GPMH),
380-384 Harrow Road
London, W9 2HU

Lodge, B.(1981) *Coping with Caring*, MIND.
Norman, A. (1982), *Mental Health in Old Age: Meeting the Challenge*, Centre for Policy and Ageing.
Brandon, D..(1981), MIND. *Voices of Experience - Consumer Perspectives of Psychiatric Treatment*

These books are available through:
MIND,
National Association for Mental Health
22 Harley Street
London, W1N 2ED

## USEFUL ADDRESSES

ACCEPT Clinic
Tranquillizer and Alcohol Support Groups
200 Seagrave Road
London SW6

Age Concern
4 Frampton Street
Lisson Grove
London NW8 4LF

AIDS Helpline:
Personal advice and counselling 0800 567 123
For literature and free publicity pack 0800 555 777
Minority and cultural groups 071 992 5522
Hard of hearing 0800 521 361

Al-Anon.
Al-Anon Family Groups
61 Dover Street
London SE1 4YF

Alcohol Concern
275 Gray's Inn Road
London WC1X 8QF

Alcoholics Anonymous
PO Box 514
11 Redcliffe Gardens
London SW10

British Association of Counselling
1 Regent Place
Rugby CV1 2PJ

Childline: 0800 1111

Commission for Racial Equality
Elliot House
10-12 Allington Street
London SW1E 5EH

Compassionate Friends
(Support group for those who have lost a child of any age.)
2 Norden Road, Blanford, Dorset

CRUSE Bereavement Care
CRUSE House
126 Sheen Road
Richmond Surrey TW9

Families Anon
88 Caledonian Road
London N1

Gamblers Anonymous
17-23 Blantyre Street
London SW10

Good Practices in Mental Health
380-384 Harrow Road
London W9 2HU

MIND
National Association for Mental Health
22 Harley Street
London W1N 2ED

Narcotics Anonymous
PO Box 246
London SW10

National Association of Citizens' Advice Bureau
115-123 Pentonville Road
London N1 9LZ

National Schizophrenia Fellowship
79 Victoria Road
Surbiton, Surrey

Parents' Advice Line
Box 161
Rode
Bath BA3 4QE
Helpline: 0898 333 002

RELATE
Marriage Guidance
Herbert Gray College
Rugby CV21 3AP

Tranquillizer Withdrawal Support
160 Tosson Terrace
Heaton
Newcastle NE6 5EA

Westminister Pastoral Foundation
23 Kensington Square
London W8 5HN

# PART ELEVEN

# THE RANGE OF THERAPEUTIC APPROACHES

*Gary Rolfe*

Individual approaches in mental health nursing – those interventions where one nurse works with one client – are one of several methods that include group, milieu, and family therapies. The choice of approach may be based, first, on theoretical considerations, for example, the theory that psychiatric problems have their origin in the family and thus the whole family must be treated; second, on ideological grounds, for example, that individual therapy is elitist and disempowering, and should therefore be rejected; or, third, on practical grounds, for example, that the cost of group therapy is far less than that of individual work. In practice, most psychiatric nurses find themselves involved in a variety of approaches to treatment, and most teams employ a wide range of therapeutic interventions, often with the same client.

Unless the unit in which the nurse is working is extremely specialized, such as a formal therapeutic community, she will almost certainly be called upon to make individual, one-to-one interventions with her clients. Furthermore, in the past, many teams relied in part on the therapeutic benefits of the ward milieu, or simply on providing sanctuary from the stresses and strains of the outside world. However, with the move towards care in the community, many clients never see the inside of a psychiatric hospital. The nurse therefore has to rely increasingly on her own qualities as a therapist, often being required to respond to on-the-spot situations without the immediate resources of other team members. For these reasons, it is important that the nurse

has some knowledge and skill in the theory and techniques of individual approaches to therapy.

When she comes to make a choice of which approach to pursue, however, she is often faced with a bewildering array of alternatives, many claiming to be the best and most effective. Some approaches have been in use for a century or more, others have been developed during the last decade. Some are placed within complex theoretical frameworks, often extending beyond psychiatry to a whole philosophy of life, while others borrow unashamedly from a wide variety of approaches and philosophies. Some grew naturally out of clinical practice, whereas others are practical extensions of psychological and sociological theory.

Some of these approaches have become established as broad theoretical schools of thought, and include a variety of methods and techniques within a specific model of psychiatry. Four such schools presented here are the **analytic**, the **behavioural**, the **person-centred**, and the **cognitive**. Other approaches stem from one of the above, or else are less widely accepted as schools of psychiatry in their own right.

The dangers and limitations of working without any theoretical framework must be stressed. Firstly, it is difficult to adopt a systematic approach to working with clients without an underlying theory of the nature of psychiatric disorder and treatment. Secondly, the nurse who is working entirely intuitively runs a great risk of *countertransference*, that is, of failing to recognize that the feelings the client has towards her may belong to some other significant person in his life, and may respond back to the client on the basis of those feelings. Thirdly, unless the working methods of the nurse are grounded in theory, they are unlikely to be accessible to other members of the therapeutic team.

A further reading list, and information about relevant organizations and training for each of the therapies appears at the end of the chapter (page 483). Terms in **bold type** are explained more fully in the Key Concepts Sections.

## ANALYTIC PSYCHOTHERAPY

### HISTORY

The term 'analytic psychotherapy' covers a broad range of therapeutic interventions, all deriving from the theories of Sigmund Freud. Classical psychoanalysis was first outlined by Freud in the late nineteenth century, and grew out of his work with patients suffering from hysterical neurosis (Freud, 1895). Through experiments with hypnosis, he came to explore the notion of the unconscious and the importance of dreams (Freud, 1900). Later Freud postulated a structural theory of the human mind, introducing such terms as **ego**, **id**, and **super-ego** (Freud, 1923). Many other of his concepts have found their way into general use, such as the oral, anal, and phallic **phases of development**, the Oedipus complex and **defence mechanisms** such as repression, projection, and sublimation.

Freud's theories on infant sexuality and the **libido** as the primary motivating force led to early splits within the psychoanalytic movement, with both Carl Jung and Alfred Adler going their separate ways to form schools of their own. As orthodox Freudian theory became subject to greater critical analysis, it was modified by theorists and practitioners into the diversity of approaches found today, which include the schools of Fromm, Horney, Rank, Sullivan, Winnicott and Klein. As a broad approach to therapy, the general school of thought is often referred to as 'psychodynamic' to distinguish it from other approaches such as the behavioural, cognitive, and humanist.

Although psychoanalysis and other analytical treatments continue to be practised by psychiatrists and psychoanalysts, their rigorous training programmes and lengthy and often costly treatments make them prohibitive to most prospective clients and therapists alike. However, many nurses, psychologists, psychiatrists, and social workers employ the theories of analytic psychotherapy in a more creative and eclectic way, and it is on this broad psychodynamic approach that attention will be focused.

### PHILOSOPHY

The psychodynamic approach to therapy is based on three broad assumptions. Firstly, that psychological problems in adult life derive largely from childhood experiences; secondly, that these psychological (and sometimes physical) problems are manifestations of underlying unconscious conflicts; and thirdly, that the relationship between therapist and client is an important tool in uncovering, and hence dealing with, those conflicts.

Unlike the behaviourists, for whom the presenting behaviour *is* the problem, psychodynamic therapists believe that the overt behaviour of the client is either a symptom, often in symbolic form, of a deep-rooted conflict that has been removed from consciousness due to its painful or threatening nature, or else a maladaptive **defence mechanism** – a technique employed by the ego to protect itself from a reality that is too painful to face. However, in protecting the client from a painful reality, the defence mechanism may itself cause as many problems as it seeks to prevent. Removal of the symptom thus is not in itself sufficient, since the underlying problem will simply re-emerge in a different form. Rather, it is necessary to trace the problem back to its childhood origin.

Psychoanalytic therapy is therefore the attempt to bring unconscious material into consciousness. There are several ways by which this can be accomplished. Freud believed that unconscious material filters through into consciousness when the defences are weakened. Freud found that one way to reach the subconscious was through hypnosis, a technique which he experimented with early in his career but later abandoned for methods such as **dream analysis** and **free association**. He also believed that our unconscious intentions and motivations make themselves known to ourselves and others through everyday occurrences such as, for example, slips of the tongue, or forgetfulness. (Freud, 1901).

By forming a **therapeutic alliance**, the therapist and client together work on the material derived from the client's unconscious. A powerful tool in their work is the use of **transference**, in which the feelings belonging to significant people in the client's past are felt by the client towards the therapist. Such feelings originally were suppressed into the unconscious because they were too painful or dangerous to be acknowledged, thus they reappear in a symbolic form as feelings towards the therapist. For example, for most of us it is probably more acceptable to have strong feelings of hatred towards a therapist than, say, towards our mothers. One of the main tasks of the therapist is to recognize when and how the transference is taking place, and to offer the client an **interpretation** of it. It is easy to see why the importance of supervision for the therapist cannot be overemphasized, since without it, she may not recognize that transference is taking place, and may develop countertransference feelings towards her client, that is, feelings that really belong to someone other than the client (Chapter 25).

In simple terms, then, the aim of analytic psychotherapy is to uncover defence mechanisms and to interpret the symbolic or disguised symptoms presented by the client and trace them to their roots in childhood. Once the true cause of the presenting problems has been uncovered to the client, he develops insight, which is the beginning of a resolution. In formal psychotherapy this process may take years, but significant breakthroughs and progress may be made more quickly by using analytic psychotherapy techniques.

KEY CONCEPTS

### Ego, id, and super-ego

Freud's subdivisions of the mind: the ego mediates between external reality and the inner psychic world; the id is the biological instincts, including the sexual and aggressive drives; and the super-ego represents the moral conscience.

### Phases of development

Freud believed that as we grow and develop, we pass through several clearly delineated phases, known as the oral stage, the anal stage, the phallic stage, and latency, before emerging into the genital stage. If we have difficulties in negotiating these stages, or if a traumatic incident occurs during one of them, we may become 'stuck', or fixated, at a particular stage, or regress to it during times of stress.

### Defence mechanisms

When the ego feels under threat, it may respond by defending itself in one of many ways. For example, **projection** is the attributing to others of unacceptable personal thoughts, feelings, or behaviours; **repression** is the barring of unconscious thoughts from consciousness; and **introjection** is the internalizing of desirable traits in others.

### Libido

The libido is the sexual or life force, and is one of the basic drives or impulses.

## Dream analysis

Freud believed that dreams reveal our unconscious wishes and desires in symbolic form; he thus placed great emphasis on their interpretation as a means to understanding the unconscious.

## Free association

Another attempt to gain access to the unconscious, free association is the reporting to the therapist whatever comes into the client's mind, without censure or interpretation.

## Therapeutic alliance

The working agreement between therapist and client, in which the client commits himself both to treatment and to the ethos of the approach being used.

## Transference

A therapeutic situation whereby the client responds to the therapist as if she were a significant other in his life, often a parent.

## Interpretation

Material that has been repressed into the unconscious usually resurfaces in a disguised or symbolic form. One of the main tasks of the therapist is to interpret the material so that it becomes meaningful to the client.

## CASE STUDY – RICHARD

Richard is a 21-year-old single man living at home with his mother, who has received treatment in the past for alcoholism. His father left home when Richard was five, and has since died. Richard misbehaved at school, where he was described as a shy, introverted boy, and left school with five 'O' levels. He now works as a policeman, and was recently referred to the acute psychiatric service by his occupational health doctor, suffering with obsessional hand-washing, which was beginning to affect his work.

### Assessment

At the referrals meeting of the acute team, Susan, an experienced psychiatric nurse, was allocated to work with Richard. She wrote to him offering an appointment at the day hospital, which he duly kept. On their first meeting, Susan explained that she used a psychodynamic approach in her work, and that she believed that his current problem could be seen as a symptom of an underlying psychological conflict from his past. She proposed that in order to effectively treat the obsessional hand-washing, they would have to explore Richard's childhood to discover the roots of the problem. Richard was a little surprised at the thought that the past might have such an influence on his current behaviour, and felt anxious at the prospect of unearthing painful memories, but eventually agreed to do whatever was necessary.

Susan spent the remainder of the session assessing Richard to determine whether he was suitable for analytic psychotherapy, or whether he would be better helped by some other approach, for example a behavioural intervention. This involved not only exploring his current life situation and difficulties, but also obtaining a comprehensive history of his life, going back as far as he could recall. Richard was an active participant in this process, and was allowed to direct the course of the session, since Susan believed that much valuable information could be gained by the way Richard prioritized his problems – by the material he chose to leave out as much as by what was included.

### Formulation

By the end of the first hour, Susan had gathered enough information from Richard to feel confident that a psychodynamic approach would be beneficial. She hypothesized that the two major factors contributing to his obsession were his mother's alcoholism and his father leaving home when Richard was five. At this stage in treatment, it was difficult for Susan to discern exactly the connection between those events and the excessive handwashing, but she felt this would become clear as therapy progressed.

## Planning

By this stage, Susan had accomplished the first and most essential requirement for analytic psychotherapy. Richard not only appeared committed to working hard to resolve his problem, but as the first session progressed, he became more interested in the approach being taken. He was eager to continue the exploration of his past, showing great insight and ability to make connections with the present. Thus, Susan felt that a therapeutic alliance had been forged between them. She explained to Richard that it might take many months, or even years, to fully resolve his difficulties, and would mean much hard work on his part. He said that he no longer wanted to sweep his problems under the carpet, and was ready to face them. They arranged to meet regularly at the day hospital for one hour each week, with a review in three months.

## Implementation

As the sessions progressed, it became apparent that Susan's initial hypothesis was correct. Richard's mother had drunk heavily throughout his childhood, although she had always managed to care for his physical needs. He described her mood as unpredictable, alternating between being dominant and overstrict some of the time, and submissive and tearful at other times. Richard gradually began to realize the effect this upbringing had had on him. He recalled a recurrent dream from

his childhood, which began shortly after his father left home, in which he, Richard, drove his father out with a large stick, resulting in his mother turning to drink, and dying.

Susan was quick to recognize the symbolic content of the dream, but chose to focus on the fact that Richard felt in some way that he was the cause of his parents' actions. At first Richard denied that he had ever felt responsible for his parents' breakup and his mother's drinking, but Susan detected some resistance to her suggestions, and gently persisted, attempting to give Richard permission to express his true feelings. Eventually he began to cry, recounting how as a child he would misbehave at school because he felt he needed to be punished. Susan encouraged him to continue expressing his feelings, and the tears turned to anger as Richard began to realize the implications of the guilt he had been carrying with him, and how it was continuing to affect his life today. At first this anger was directed towards himself, but over the weeks it began to turn outwards to his parents.

## Evaluation

Susan noticed that Richard's attitude to her was changing. Previously, he had been extremely pleasant towards her, and seemed eager to please. However, as he began to direct anger at his parents, she sensed that his feelings for her were also becoming hostile. She wondered whether a transference was taking place, and suspected they had reached a significant stage in Richard's therapy. In her next meeting with her supervisor, Susan decided on a full case review. Her supervisor, Margaret, gave a fresh analysis of the situation, which confirmed to Susan that she was making progress with Richard. Margaret attempted to show the case diagrammatically (Figure 34.1).

Susan could now clearly see how Richard's early life experiences were continuing to affect him in the present, and how his use of defence mechanisms led to his obsessional

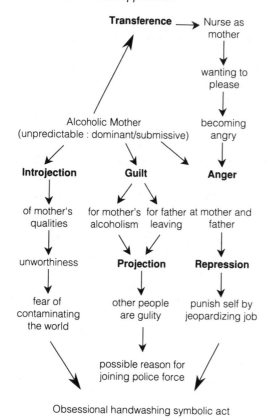

Figure 34.1 Case diagram of Richard

behaviour. She realized that hand-washing was for Richard both a symbolic act and a confirmation of his unworthiness. He was attempting to wash away his guilt and contamination; at the same time he was continuing his childhood pattern of needing to be punished, first at school and now at work. It also clarified his behaviour towards Susan, who could see that a transference relationship was forming. Margaret hypothesized that Richard dealt with his mother's unpredictable behaviour by constantly trying to please her, and that his feelings for her had become transferred to Susan. Because Susan presented to Richard as safe and consistent, he could gradually express his feelings of anger at his mother towards Susan without fear of the consequences.

Therapy had now been ongoing for two months, and Susan was just beginning to make links between Richard's past and present. Her task in the months ahead was to present the above hypothesis to him in a gradual and non-threatening way, to explore new directions, and to employ the transference relationship therapeutically and constructively. By coming to understand his own motivations and behaviours, Richard would eventually be able to give up his destructive methods of coping and replace them with other, less-intrusive defence mechanisms. Only by exploring the cause of the problems rather than the symptoms, does true healing come about.

## BEHAVIOURAL PSYCHOTHERAPY

### HISTORY

Behavioural psychotherapy derives from the school of psychology known as behaviourism, and the psychological theories of **classical conditioning** (Pavlov, 1928) and **operant conditioning** (Watson, 1913). Behaviourism was developed as a reaction against the earlier introspective approach, and sought to establish psychology as a 'hard' science on the same footing as physics and chemistry. For this reason, the notion of internal mental states was rejected as being unverifiable and hence unscientific, and behaviourists concentrated on deriving and testing theories on observable behaviour.

Many behaviourists took the next logical step, rejecting not only the internal functionings of the mind, but also the workings of the brain as being unobservable, and instead postulated a 'black-box' approach, whereby the brain was conceived as a sealed unit whose workings were unimportant. All that was required of psychologists was that they measured or recorded the inputs to the black box (stimulus) and the outputs in the form of behaviour (response).

The 1920s and 1930s saw behaviourism established as the dominant school of psychology, but it was not until after the Second World War that it made an impact in psychiatric circles. This was due partly to the massive increase in demand on the mental health services, combined with the realization that psychodynamic and humanistic therapies were slower and less effective than initial expectations; and partly due to an expansion in the role of behaviourally trained clinical psychologists in the US to include psychological treatment. Although the term 'behaviour therapy' was first used by the American psychologist B.F. Skinner in the 1950s, it was established as a school of therapy at the Maudsley Hospital in Britain by Joseph Wolpe, together with psychiatrists and psychologists such as Isaac Marks and Hans Eysenck.

During the late 1960s and the 1970s, the limitations of the simple behavioural model began to be recognized, and more sophisticated alternatives were devised. Thus, Bandura postulated a social-learning theory approach, which placed far greater emphasis on human relations and internal processes. Later, Meichenbaum and Seligman both argued convincingly for the inclusion of cognitive concepts into the vocabulary of the behaviour therapist, and the adoption of a 'talking treatment' approach to therapy, which was formally recognized by a change in title to 'behaviour psychotherapy'. However, the traditional behaviour-modification approach, employing operant conditioning techniques, is still employed in some treatment centres.

PHILOSOPHY

In its pure, or 'radical', form, behavioural psychotherapy rejects the basic tenets of both the medical model and the psychodynamic therapies. The medical model distinction between symptoms and underlying pathology is considered false, since, according to Eysenck (1960), if you 'get rid of the symptom...you have eliminated the neurosis'. Similarly, the focus in behavioural treatment is on the current interaction between behaviour and the environment, rather than the Freudian concern with past events and unconscious motivations. The emphasis is thus on the here-and-now behaviours of the client rather than on any supposed underlying pathology. Furthermore, it is argued that these disorders of behaviour have been learnt by the client, and therefore have the potential to be unlearnt. Four broad behavioural approaches have been identified.

**Behaviour modification** stems from Skinner's (1953) radical behaviourism, and is based on operant conditioning techniques such as **reinforcement, aversion,** and **extinction.** As Skinner suggests, this approach is radical because it adopts the purist view that cognitive processes have no place in scientific analysis, and are thus dismissed as irrelevant, or, in extreme cases, as non-existent.

A modified or **neo-behaviouristic model** (Wilson, 1984), based on classical and avoidance conditioning, considers internal processes as hypothetical constructs, and particularly emphasizes the importance of anxiety. Techniques employed in this model include **systematic desensitization, flooding,** and the use of imagery and relaxation techniques.

**Social learning theory,** most often associated with Bandura (1977), places even greater emphasis on internal cognitive processes. Whereas the Skinnerian view of people is that their behaviour is beyond their control and shaped entirely by the environment, Bandura stresses the importance of free will, and the capacity for self-directed behaviour change, often modelled on the behaviour of others.

**Cognitive behaviour modification** covers a range of therapeutic interventions such as Ellis's rational emotive therapy, and is sufficiently far removed from the original concept of behaviour therapy to warrant separate consideration.

These four approaches are representative of a continuum ranging from a Skinnerian view – in which people are little more than stimulus-response machines, differing from the lower animals only in their degree of complexity – to the cognitive view - in which people are rational, thinking beings, able to gain insight into their own psychic workings.

The therapies deriving from this latter view are considered beyond the accepted definition of behavioural techniques, and there is good reason for also rejecting the techniques based on Skinner's radical behaviourism from our discussion. Firstly, whatever the merits or demerits of the operant conditioning approach, it does little to warrant the title behavioural *psychotherapy*. Secondly, many of the techniques involved are extremely specialized and require a carefully controlled environment. They are thus considered to be beyond the scope and experience of most nurses. There are specialist units where an operant conditioning approach is employed, for example in the treatment of anorexia nervosa, but attempts by the nurse to practise these techniques in a standard clinical environment, with no specialist backup and without the support of the whole clinical team, are unlikely to prove effective.

KEY CONCEPTS

## Classical conditioning

A theory deriving from the work of Ivan Pavlov, a Russian physiologist, who 'taught' dogs to salivate at the sound of a bell by repeatedly linking the sound with the presentation of food. The unconditioned response of salivating when presented with food was thus replaced by the conditioned response of salivating at the ringing of the bell.

## Operant conditioning

Based on work by behavioural psychologist B.F. Skinner, who found that he could shape the behaviour of rats and pigeons by rewarding or reinforcing desired behaviour and ignoring undesired behaviour. In this way, pigeons could be conditioned to perform elaborate dances or recognize shapes, and rats could learn to run mazes.

## Reinforcement

Reinforcement can be defined as anything that increases the likelihood of a behaviour being repeated in the future. Positive reinforcement is the act of rewarding behaviour that the psychologist or therapist wishes to encourage, whereas negative reinforcement is a means of encouraging behaviour by the avoidance or removal of an unpleasant event. Reinforcement schedules are continuous if the behaviour is rewarded every time it is performed, and intermittent if it is not.

## Extinction

The gradual dying-out of reinforced behaviour when the reinforcement regime is discontinued. Extinction takes longer when behaviour has been reinforced intermittently.

## Systematic desensitization

A technique for eliminating unwanted behaviour by counter-conditioning. Developed by Joseph Wolpe (1958), it is based on the theory of reciprocal inhibition, which argues that the client cannot be both anxious and relaxed at the same time. Thus, the client is asked to construct a hierarchy of anxiety-provoking situations, and to work through them in his imagination, while at the same time practising relaxation techniques. In this way, the association between the anxiety-evoking situation and the anxious response is weakened. A typical use of systematic desensitization is in the treatment of phobias.

## Flooding

In contrast to systematic desensitization, flooding is prolonged exposure, often several hours at a time, to the situation that evokes the maximum anxiety in the patient. Extinction occurs over the period of exposure, and this method is fast but extremely stressful. It is particularly important that the client has no escape from the situation, or negative reinforcement may take place. It has been shown to be the most effective treatment for phobias (Marks, 1981a) and is often used where a rapid response is required.

## Aversion therapy

Unwanted behaviour is eliminated by associating it with an unpleasant stimulus such as electric shocks or nausea and vomiting. This technique has been used successfully with alcoholics (Wiens *et al.*, 1983), and, more controversially, with homosexuals, transvestites, and sadomasochists (Marks, 1981b).

## Token economy

Tokens are secondary reinforcers which are given for socially desirable behaviour, and which may be exchanged for primary reinforcers such as cigarettes, watching television, or anything the client identifies as pleasurable. Token economies have been successfully employed in the treatment of chronic schizophrenia within a highly controlled living situation (Walker, 1984).

CASE STUDY – MARY

Mary is a 47-year-old housewife who lives on a large council estate three miles from the nearest town. Since moving to this house two years previously, she has had difficulty travelling more than one stop on the bus due to feeling 'panicky', which has prevented her from getting out to shop or visit friends. Her husband works during the day, and she has two teenage sons living at home, both unemployed. Recently things have become worse, and her GP was called out to visit her following a panic attack in the street. The doctor referred her to the local psychiatric hospital for assessment. Peter, a community psychiatric nurse, has arranged to visit her at home.

## Assessment

On the morning of the first visit, Peter found the home clean and tidy. Mary's husband was at work, and her two sons were in their room listening to records. Mary appeared relaxed and welcoming. The first ten minutes were spent in general conversation, while Mary made coffee for Peter and herself. Peter then said that he felt from the doctor's referral letter than the prospect of his being able to help Mary with her problem was good. He explained that if she agreed to therapy he would first need to talk to her to determine her condition before treatment started, which he referred to as her 'baseline behaviour'. He told Mary that one of the techniques he proposed to use would involve her identifying the situations she found anxiety-provoking, and arranging them in order. Then, with the help of relaxation training, she would imagine being in those situations one by one, beginning with the one that caused the least anxiety. Once she could imagine being in that situation with little or no anxiety, she would progress to the next one, and so on down the list. Peter told Mary that this treatment programme was based on a technique known as 'systematic desensitization'. Although Peter was not trained in behavioural techniques, he was supervised closely in his work by a qualified behavioural nurse therapist.

Peter began the baseline assessment by asking Mary to identify the situations that caused her anxiety, and to operationalize them by stating them as observable behaviours. She was then asked to rate each behaviour on a scale of 0–8, depending on the amount of anxiety it produced. A shortened version of Mary's list was:

| | |
|---|---|
| Leaving the house | 2 |
| Waiting at the bus stop | 3 |
| Seeing the bus coming | 4 |
| Stepping on to the bus | 6 |
| Paying the fare | 8 |
| Sitting down on the bus | 8 |

Mary felt apprehensive at the thought of even imagining some of the more anxiety-provoking situations, but was reassured by Peter that these would not be tackled without adequate preparation.

## Formulation

Peter's formulation was that Mary was suffering from a form of claustrophobia, a fear of being in enclosed spaces, which produced feelings of panic. This phobia was negatively reinforced by the rapid reduction in anxiety brought about by getting off the bus after only one stop. Peter had several hypotheses about the cause of the phobia, but considered these to be of secondary importance to dealing with the immediate cause of distress.

## Planning

A treatment programme of two visits per week was planned. The initial three weeks would be spent teaching relaxation techniques, before progressing to the systematic desensitization programme of imagining performing the hierarchy of tasks. Once the most anxiety-inducing situation of sitting for long periods on a bus could be imagined in a relaxed state, it was planned that Peter would accompany Mary on bus journeys, where he could act as a model for her behaviour.

## Implementation

During the first three weeks of visits, Mary was taught to relax both at home with the aid of a special tape, and also when she was out and felt a panic attack beginning to start. She was encouraged to practice everyday. Once she felt confident about her ability to relax, the desensitization programme began. Mary was asked to imagine engaging in the first task on her list, leaving the house. Peter told her to describe the scene in order to make it as realistic as possible. She was then asked to rate it on the 0–8 scale for anxiety, and Mary

rated it at 1. She then performed her relaxation techniques, and her anxiety quickly fell to zero. Mary then moved through the list. After imagining each behaviour on the list, she rated it on the scale and used her relaxation techniques until the behaviour could be imagined with a tolerable degree of anxiety. After four sessions, Mary could imagine sitting on a bus for 20 minutes with an anxiety level of 2, which she considered to be acceptable.

The next phase of the treatment was to work through the list in real life, with Peter as a model. The target was to take the bus to the shops and back, a ride of about 15 minutes each way. At each stage, Peter asked Mary to rate her anxiety level and to use the relaxation techniques to reduce that level when necessary. On the first attempt, Mary had a strong desire to get off the bus after three stops, but Peter felt that it was important that she followed the task through to avoid negative reinforcement, and persuaded her to continue to the end of the journey.

## Evaluation

Behavioural programmes are relatively easy to evaluate, since the goals of therapy are clearly stated at the outset in terms of observable behaviour. Thus, this particular programme was successful in that Mary achieved her goal of travelling to the shops and back by bus with an acceptable level of anxiety. Whereas in a radical behavioural regime, Mary's internal psychological state would be dismissed as irrelevant, Peter chose to focus on her level of anxiety throughout the programme. Theoretically, her anxiety could have been 'scientifically' measured by monitoring her pulse rate or galvanic skin response (GSR), but Peter chose to utilize Mary's subjective rating on a 0–8 scale.

At this point in treatment, Peter chose to review the goals to include travelling to the shops alone, and at the same time began the gradual process of disengaging from Mary.

Up to this point, the treatment had been very effective, and had taken only 12 sessions.

## PERSON-CENTRED THERAPY

### HISTORY

The person-centred approach was developed by Carl Rogers, an American psychologist. Born the son of a minister in Chicago in 1902, Rogers trained as a clinical psychologist and worked as a counsellor and director of the Rochester Guidance Centre, New York. He became disenchanted with the authoritarian stance he was expected to adopt as a psychodynamic therapist, and left Rochester in 1940 to become professor of psychology at Ohio State University. He published his first book, *Counselling and Psychotherapy*, in 1942, which outlined the non-directive counselling approach. With the publication of his second book, *Client-Centred Therapy*, in 1951, he became a major force in the world of psychotherapy, but it was not until the mid-1960s that his ideas were first studied in depth in Britain.

The 1960s marked a period of extensive research for Rogers and his colleagues in an attempt to validate his theories. The 1970s saw the broadening of the client-centred approach to related fields such as teaching, marriage guidance, politics, and management, leading to a change in name from client-centred to person-centred therapy, reflecting the wider role the theory now embraced. Rogers claimed the approach was valid in any interpersonal situation in which personal growth was the goal.

Carl Rogers died in 1987, but person-centred therapy has continued to grow and diversify, and is now established as one of the main schools of counselling and psychotherapy.

### PHILOSOPHY

The philosophy underlying person-centred therapy is in direct contrast to the assumptions of analytic psychotherapy. Whereas the psychoanalytically oriented therapist is concerned with the self-centred, asocial, and often destructive impulses of human beings, the person-centred therapist sees people as motivated by positive rather than negative forces. That is not to deny the existence of emotions such as jealousy, hostility, and aggressiveness, however, from the person-centred perspective these are not basic, spontaneous impulses, but rather reactions to the frustration or blocking of positive strivings towards love and belonging.

The basic human tendency is for growth and development, towards becoming what Rogers described as a **fully functioning person.** The person can be seen as analogous to a plant: given the right conditions and appropriate care, a plant will develop and grow to its full potential; if planted in poor soil, or if starved of light or water, the plant will adapt to its environment, often resulting in stunted or abnormal growth. So too with a person: in an environment of love and acceptance, people will flourish and grow, becoming loving and well-adjusted human beings; when starved of such growth-enhancing conditions, people strive to meet their needs for love and acceptance in distorted or negative ways.

The aim of person-centred therapy is to enable the client to become fully functioning, to reach his full potential. In order to do this, the therapist must create a climate in which growth can take place. In fact, Rogers believed this is all the therapist needs to do. Given the right psychological conditions, the client will no longer need the maladaptive coping mechanisms previously used to meet his needs, but will be free to strive towards his true potential. For Rogers technique is of little importance: the therapist does not need to push her client towards psychological wellness; all that is necessary is that she provides the right conditions for growth.

These core conditions take the form of attitudes that the therapist holds towards her client, and are best summarized in a paper written by Rogers (1957) entitled 'The necessary and sufficient conditions of therapeutic personality change'. These conditions, or attitudes, are genuineness, acceptance, and empathy. As the title of the paper suggests, Rogers believed them to be necessary in that they must all be present for therapeutic change to take place, and sufficient in that no other conditions are required. Thus, as Rogers (1961) said:

> When I hold in myself the kind of attitudes I have described, and when the other person can to some degree experience these attitudes, then I believe that change and constructive personal development will inevitably occur.

The implication of Rogers philosophy is that in order for the client to become fully functioning, he must work with a therapist who is herself a fully functioning person.

KEY CONCEPTS

## Genuineness

The condition or attitude of genuineness is also referred to by Rogers as realness, authenticity, and congruence. It is the desire by the therapist to become fully emotionally involved in the relationship by the expression of her genuine feelings, rather than hiding behind a uniform or a professional role. Rogers spoke of the therapist becoming transparent, so that her client could metaphorically see through her outer façade to her real self. This involves a close matching, or congruence, between the therapist's verbal and non-verbal expressions, between what she says and what she does. It is an attitude of openness and honesty.

## Acceptance

The condition of acceptance, prizing, or unconditional positive regard is an attitude of non-possessive, non-judgemental caring. It is unconditional because no strings are attached to the therapist's positive feelings towards her client. The therapist is not judging the behaviour of her client, nor is she using her praise as an enticement to change. She is accepting him as he is in the here and now. She is not, however, condoning his antisocial or destructive behaviour, but valuing him despite that behaviour. She is saying, in effect, I accept and respect you for what you are, warts and all.

## Empathy

Empathy is the sensing of the feelings being experienced by the client, and the communication of those feelings back to him. As Rogers points out, when the therapist is functioning best she is so much inside the private world of the client that she can clarify not only the meanings of which the client is aware, but even those just below the level of awareness. It is a condition of experiencing the world as if she was the client, but without losing the 'as if' quality.

## Client

The word 'client' is deliberately used rather than words like 'patient' in order to emphasize the person's self-responsibility and self-determinism. The term 'client-centred', later broadened to 'person-centred', implies that the client is an active participant in his own therapy, and largely directs the course of that therapy.

## The fully functioning person

Each individual has a tendency towards self-actualization, towards growth and the fulfilment of his or her potential. When this self-actualizing tendency is allowed to develop to its maximum, the individual can be said to be fully functioning, and is in a state of optimum mental health. Rogers outlined three characteristics of the fully functioning person: openness to experience; an existential mode of living; and the organism as a trustworthy guide to satisfying behaviour.

The fully functioning person actively seeks out new experiences, seeing them as growth enhancing. He lives in the present, savouring life to the full, the bad and painful as well as the good and pleasurable, and he relies on his instincts and gut-feelings when making decisions. To function fully in this way is the goal of psychotherapy.

## CASE STUDY – MICHAEL

Michael is a 28-year-old man whose wife of seven years recently left him. After appearing to cope fairly well for a week, he was admitted to the accident and emergency department of the local hospital in the middle of the night after taking an overdose of sleeping tablets and calling for an ambulance. Following a gastric lavage, Michael was seen by the duty psychiatrist, who felt the suicide attempt was not serious, but nevertheless admitted Michael to the psychiatric ward for assessment and observation. The following morning, Michael was assessed by the ward doctor, who found no signs of clinical depression. However, Michael maintained that he was still suicidal, and was referred to the nursing team for counselling.

### Assessment

Later that day, Anne, a staff nurse, introduced herself to Michael and explained she would be working with him to help him resolve his current difficulties. She told him that their time together would be for Michael to use in whatever way he chose. She began by asking him to recount the events leading up to his admission to hospital, and listened without comment, encouraging him to continue whenever there was a long pause. Michael dwelt on the fact that his wife had every right to leave him, that he was unworthy of her,

and stressed that he was very depressed and frightened of making another attempt on his life. Anne concentrated her efforts on building an atmosphere of trust and acceptance. She did not disagree with Michael when he expressed his feelings of unworthiness, nor did she challenge his suicidal thoughts, but rather attempted to understand the situation from his perspective, to empathize with him.

### Formulation

By trying to understand how Michael was feeling, and following discussion with the ward team, Anne acknowledged Michael's negative self-image and depressive, suicidal thoughts. She also took into account the ward doctor's impression that Michael was not suffering from clinical depression, and her own intuitive feeling that he was suppressing a great deal of anger. Her formulation was thus that Michael's strong feelings of anger towards his wife for leaving him could not find direct expression due to his low self-esteem. His attempt at self-harm was therefore viewed partly as punishment for being an unworthy person, and partly as an act of aggression towards his wife by making her feel guilty for leaving him.

### Planning

This phase was undertaken together with Michael in the second meeting. When asked what he wished to accomplish in therapy, he said he wanted to feel less depressed, although he felt this would not be possible. Anne replied that she could understand how it must feel for him to have lost someone so close, and that in addition to feeling hurt, his pride must have taken a battering. Michael acknowledged he had a low opinion of himself, but said he deserved everything that had happened to him. Together, Michael and Anne planned a series of 12 sessions over a six-week period in order to work on his low self-esteem. Anne emphasized again that the time was for Michael to use as he wished, and explained that the sessions would be confidential between Michael, Anne, and her supervisor.

## Implementation

Anne's main objective in the early sessions was to build up an atmosphere of trust. She did this by listening actively and accepting what Michael was saying without contradicting him or being judgemental. She found this difficult, particularly when he was expressing thoughts of unworthiness. She attempted to display unconditional positive regard towards him by letting him know, both verbally and non-verbally, that whatever his view of himself, she still thought well of him. She was particularly troubled by his continued threats of self-harm, and told him she was worried by what he was saying, but that she believed he would come through the crisis unharmed.

This trusting, caring, non-judgemental approach was continued by the ward staff outside formal sessions. Concern was expressed about the suicide threats, and although most staff felt there was no serious risk of harm, Michael was treated in a serious, caring way when he made such threats. However, some of the nurses on the ward had difficulty adopting a person-centred approach to Michael, finding it difficult to refrain from actively doing things for him, and seeing their role as nurses under threat.

Anne's feeling that Michael was suppressing anger towards his wife steadily grew, and in the sixth session she said to him, 'I know you say you still love your wife, but I sense you feel quite angry towards her. I respect you for wanting to keep it to yourself, but some emotions are better let out.' At this point, Michael became very hostile towards Anne, and told her she had no idea how he felt. Anne realized that his anger was not intended for her, and allowed him to continue. He eventually began to cry and apologized, saying she was right, and that his suicide

attempt had been to make his wife suffer. What really annoyed him was that she had not even bothered to contact him while he was in hospital.

## Evaluation

This was to be a turning-point in Michael's treatment. The suicide threats stopped, and following discussion between Michael, Anne, and the ward doctor, he was discharged home after four weeks in hospital. He continued to visit the ward for his remaining sessions, and began to rebuild his self-confidence. At the end of the agreed series of 12 sessions, Michael was asked to evaluate his current situation and future goals. He still admitted to feeling low at times, but could now identify the reason for those feelings. He felt he still needed to work on his self-esteem, and enrolled in assertiveness classes at a local college. He could see he still had a long way to go, but he now knew which direction he was moving in. A year after finishing treatment, he wrote to tell Anne that he had met another woman, and that life was going very well. He particularly thanked her for understanding him when he could not understand himself, and for respecting him when he had no self-respect.

### COGNITIVE THERAPY

#### HISTORY

Cognitive approaches grew out of a discontent with the mechanistic notions underlying the practice of behaviour therapy in the 1960s. However, rather than reject the tenets of behaviourism, early cognitive theorists such as Ellis (1962) extended it to include cognitive states such as thoughts and feelings. Thus, for Ellis internal states were 'covert behaviours', subject to the same principles of modification as 'overt' behaviours. Many other behaviourists were also beginning to recognize the limitations of a theory which in its pure form rejected internal states, and Bandura's work on modelling (Bandura *et al.*, 1968) was particularly influential in drawing attention to the importance of cognitive factors in behaviour therapy.

Cognitive therapies were developed more fully during the late 1970s, initially to complement behavioural approaches in treating cases that did not respond well. Thus Beck (1976) devised a treatment for depression; Bandura (1977) worked with phobic states; Meichenbaum (1977) with social inadequacies; and Wolpe (1982) with obsessions and compulsions. By the 1980s and 1990s, cognitive therapy had emerged as a school of therapy in its own right, and has diversified to produce effective treatments for a wide range of psychological disorders.

PHILOSOPHY

Cognitive therapy grew out of behaviourism, but whereas behavioural approaches seek to change behaviour directly, without the mediation of internal states, cognitive theory argues that behaviour is controlled by thinking. Thus, in order to influence maladaptive behaviour, the underlying maladaptive thinking must be challenged and altered. Ellis (1977) offers a simple model of this process, known as the 'ABC' framework: **activating events** are situations that are misinterpreted by the client due to false **beliefs**, which can be either inferences about the situation, or evaluations based on the inferences, which in turn lead to emotional and behavioural **consequences**.

Wessler's (1986) definition of cognitive therapy as a 'collection of assumptions about disturbance and a set of treatment interventions in which human cognitions are assigned a central role' makes the further point that cognitive therapy embraces a variety of approaches.

Rational emotive therapy (RET) (Ellis, 1962; 1973) sees the client's interpretation of his situation as the root of neurotic disorder. Psychological distress occurs when misfortune, such as failure at work, comes into conflict with an irrational, non-empirically based belief such as 'a person must be perfectly competent, adequate, and achieving to be considered worthwhile'. Thus, even the most trivial and inconsequential failure becomes a major trauma, since it violates the client's deeply held conviction that he must be perfect in everything he does.

Ellis identified eleven such irrational beliefs, such as, 'It is essential that a person be loved or approved by virtually everyone in the community'; and 'Past experiences and events are the determinants of present behaviour; the influence of the past cannot be eradicated'. The role of the therapist is to demonstrate to the client how to challenge and dispute his irrational beliefs. In the event of failing at work, for example, the client is encouraged to ask himself, 'Why is it awful that I failed? Who says I must succeed? Where is the evidence that I am a worthless person if I fail or get rejected?'. This, as Ellis (1962) points out, can lead to a new set of more realistic beliefs that:

- 'It isn't awful, but only very inconvenient, if I fail';
- 'I don't have to succeed, though there are several good reasons why I'd like to';
- 'I'm never a worthless person for failing or being rejected. And if I never succeed or get accepted, I can still enjoy myself in some ways and refrain from downing myself.'

Self-instructional training (SIT) was developed by Meichenbaum (1977) from RET as an anxiety-reducing technique. It applied Ellis's techniques to the behavioural theory of systematic desensitization, and brings about behaviour change by altering the instructions that the client gives to himself. This is done firstly by teaching him to identify negative inner verbalizations such as, 'It would be terrible if I dried up in front of this large audience'; and 'I am starting to feel nervous and my mind is going blank'. The second stage is a modification of the desensitization procedure, in which the client is taught to relax and to imagine successfully coping with the stressful situation. Finally, the client is taught to develop new coping self-statements and plans for behaviour change, and to rehearse them in a safe environment before trying them out for real.

Thought-stopping (Wolpe, 1982) is an extension of SIT developed for cases of severe anxiety, particularly obsessive-compulsive problems which the client knows to be irrational. He is taught to give the subvocal command 'stop' to his obsessive thoughts, by first hearing the therapist shout the command, then by shouting it himself, and finally by silently 'saying' it to himself.

Cognitive therapy (Beck, 1976) was originally applied to the treatment of depression, but was later extended to cover a wide range of emotional disorders. Beck refers to **negative schemata**, or thought patterns, which are maintained by errors in logic, and these errors are challenged both verbally and behaviourally. Beck's cognitive therapy has a great deal in common with Ellis's RET, although they have different starting points. Thus, Ellis might initially respond to the man who did badly at work by saying 'So what? You made a mistake, but that doesn't mean that you are no good at your job. It is irrational to be depressed about making a mistake at work.' Beck, on the other hand, might first challenge the evidence that the man has done badly, for example, who says he has? Is that person's judgement to be trusted? Beck would also encourage the man to actively test out the assumption that he is no good at his job, perhaps by asking others, or by making a note of when he does things wrong.

KEY CONCEPTS

One of the aims of cognitive therapy is to demystify the therapeutic process and enable the client to understand his own thoughts, emotions, and behaviours. For this reason, it is usually presented in a clear and easily understood form, employing little or no technical language.

### Activating events, beliefs, and consequences (ABC)

An activating event – for example, being awarded a low mark for an essay – produces a set of beliefs about the event. Some of these beliefs may be inferences about the essay mark, such as 'The marker thinks I am stupid', and 'I am far worse than everyone else on the course'; and some will be evaluations such as, 'It is bad to be so stupid.' These beliefs may lead to emotional consequences such as depression, and behavioural consequences such as giving up the course. If the beliefs can be exposed as false or illogical, then more positive consequences may result.

### Automatic thoughts

The name given by Beck to thoughts and images occurring involuntarily as we go about our daily business. The client is taught by the therapist to detect such thoughts and examine their validity, since negative automatic thoughts lead to negative emotional states.

### Self-fulfilling prophesies

If negative thoughts continue, they will eventually cause the client to behave negatively, bringing about the very situation he falsely believed to be the case in the first place. For example, in the case of the student who received a bad mark for an essay, his negative thinking will lead him to believe he is worse than the rest of the class, and he will begin to avoid lectures and get behind with his work. Thus, when his next essay is not up to his usual standard, his fear that he is at the bottom of the class begins to become a reality.

### Chaining

The beliefs connecting activating events to emotional and behavioural consequences typically occur in long, connected chains of inferences and evaluations, so that the client may see little connection between an event and his feelings about it. By exposing the chain, the therapist helps the client to see the illogical connection between the two.

## Disputing

Once the inferences and evaluations have been exposed, the therapist then challenges or disputes their validity. In its simplest form, a dispute will take the form of the question: 'What is the evidence for X?' Thus, in the case of the student who did badly on an essay, the question may be, 'What is the evidence that you are at the bottom of the class?' (disputed inference); or, 'Why is it so bad even if you are?' (disputed evaluation). There are other, more sophisticated, forms of disputing, based on the principles of scientific experimentation.

## Dependency beliefs

As therapy nears termination, a common concern of clients is that they will not be able to cope without their therapists. Such beliefs are disputed in the same way as other false beliefs. One way might be for the client not to see his therapist for a while in order to prove to himself that he can manage without her. Another way might be to recall a time when the client coped before he knew his therapist. In either case, the resolution of dependency beliefs is vital for successful outcome of therapy, since otherwise it could lead to the self-fulfilling prophesy that the client cannot manage without his therapist.

CASE STUDY – JANE

Jane is a 38-year-old single woman who lives alone in a small flat and works as a legal secretary. She had been seeing her doctor for several months complaining of lack of appetite, feeling listless, and no longer enjoying her work. After exhaustive tests revealed no physical abnormal-

ities, her GP concluded the problem to be psychological, and suggested she be seen for a psychiatric assessment. Although initially reluctant, Jane eventually agreed, and was assessed by the consultant psychiatrist at the local day hospital. He diagnosed mild depression, and prescribed a course of medication. Jane was reluctant to take the tablets, and enquired whether there was any alternative. Stephanie, one of the psychiatric nurses in the hospital team, had received training in cognitive therapy, and agreed to see Jane.

## Assessment

Stephanie and Jane met at the day hospital the following week. Stephanie began by assessing Jane's symptoms and current life problems. She learned that Jane had always felt different and isolated from other people, but that things had become worse over the previous few months, following a date with a work colleague. Jane had never got on very well with men, and could see nothing in herself that men would find attractive. She had thus resigned herself to remaining single, and had arranged her life accordingly. When David, a solicitor with whom she worked, asked her out for a meal, she felt flattered and immediately agreed. However, on reflection, her decision seemed hasty, and she felt convinced he had only asked her out of pity. Her doubts were confirmed on the date, when she acted clumsily and could think of nothing interesting to say; and at work the next day, when David was pleasant but made no attempt to ask her out again.

Since that time, Jane had found difficulty talking not only to men, but to women also. She felt that work colleagues were talking about her behind her back, and that she was completely unlikable. At home, her two main hobbies of music and gardening both suffered. She had been a keen violin player, but found she no longer had the desire to play, and her garden, once her pride and joy, was suffering from neglect. An accomplished cook, she now had little appetite, and ate only frozen meals and takeaway food. Her lack of energy, coupled with her conviction that people did not like her, made it an effort for her to get up in the morning and go to work.

Stephanie then turned from current problems to explore the possible origins of Jane's condition. She learned that Jane had been adopted at the age of three following the breakup of her parents' marriage. The family into which she was adopted consisted of a couple in their 40s with two children of their own, aged 10 and 12. Jane felt her new parents did not really want her, but had only adopted her out of duty, and that her new siblings resented her. She reported an unhappy childhood in which she was loved by no one, a condition which had continued into the present, and which seemed to hold no solution in the future.

### Formulation

Stephanie outlined her formulation of Jane's case diagrammatically (Figure 34.2).

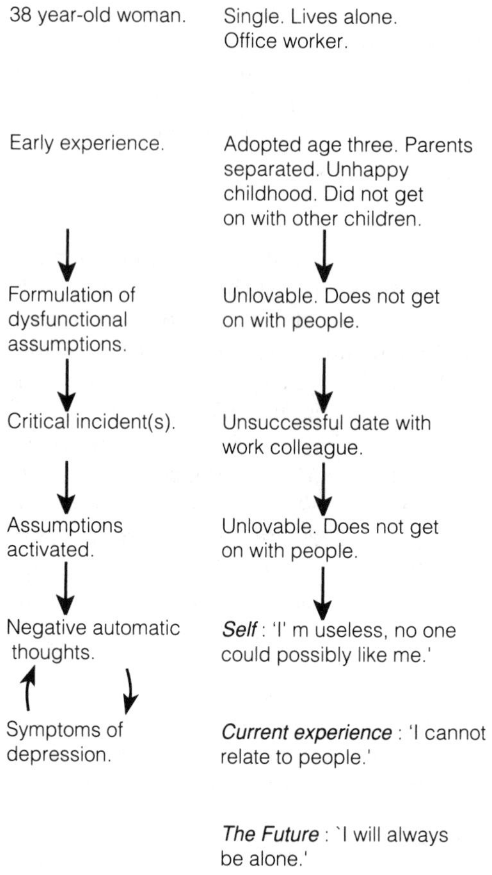

### Planning

A second session was arranged for the following week, which Stephanie used to plan the treatment programme and gain Jane's commitment to cognitive therapy. The first stage in planning was for Jane to make a list of her current problems. Her list included: not being liked by other people; not getting on with others; having no interest in life.

The second stage, called goal definition, involved Jane defining how she would like things to be different in each problem area, and to imagine how her life would change if that was the case. The third stage was for Stephanie to put forward the treatment rationale. This involved three elements.

Firstly, presentation of the main principle of cognitive therapy, of a vicious circle in-

| 38 year-old woman. | Single. Lives alone. Office worker. |
|---|---|
| Early experience. ↓ | Adopted age three. Parents separated. Unhappy childhood. Did not get on with other children. ↓ |
| Formulation of dysfunctional assumptions. ↓ | Unlovable. Does not get on with people. ↓ |
| Critical incident(s). ↓ | Unsuccessful date with work colleague. ↓ |
| Assumptions activated. ↓ | Unlovable. Does not get on with people. ↓ |
| Negative automatic thoughts. | *Self* : 'I'm useless, no one could possibly like me.' |
| Symptoms of depression. | *Current experience* : 'I cannot relate to people.' |
| | *The Future* : 'I will always be alone.' |

**Figure 34.2** Case diagram of Jane

volving negative thinking and low mood. Stephanie introduced the concept of negative automatic thoughts, and explained how Jane's low self-esteem, which had its roots in her childhood, was confirmed by the experience of her recent date, and which in turn lowered her self-esteem still further. This led to various symptoms of depression, such as lack of interest in other people and paranoid thoughts, which deepened the depression, and so on, in a downward spiral. Second, to convince Jane that change is possible, that she could break out of the vicious circle. Third, to outline a practical plan of action that included the number, frequency, and duration of sessions, and the concept of homework assignments. Jane and Stephanie agreed on a series of eight weekly meetings, each lasting one hour.

The session ended with the identification of a target for immediate action. Jane had bought some bulbs for her garden some weeks previously, and her homework assignment was to tidy the garden and plant the bulbs before the next session. The aim of this intervention was to demonstrate to Jane that she had the power to change her life, albeit on a simple level, and that by changing her behaviour she could alter her mood.

## Implementation

As the weeks passed, Jane noticed that the sessions followed a logical pattern. Stephanie would begin by reviewing the previous week, including any particular difficulties that had arisen since the previous meeting, a report on the homework assignment, and an opportunity for Jane to ask questions and clarify any points she was not sure about.

The main focus of each session was a major topic, which Jane and Stephanie chose together. For example, the third session looked at the difficulties that Jane was experiencing in relating to men. They had already identified various automatic thoughts, such as Jane's conviction that she was unlovable, and Stephanie now proceeded to challenge that assumption by logical questioning. This involved tracing the thoughts back to their roots in Jane's childhood, and exposing them as irrational. Stephanie pointed out that the fact that her parents gave her up for adoption did not necessarily mean they did not love her, and even if that was the case, it made no sense to assume that because her parents did not love her, then neither would anyone else. Similarly, her perception of her date with David might be different from his view of it. She had no evidence that it was a disaster apart from her own feelings, and there may have been other reasons why he had not asked her out again.

The sessions would end with feedback and a homework assignment related to the current problem being tackled.

## Evaluation

Ongoing evaluation is an integral part of cognitive therapy, and is included in each session. However, as Jane's last meeting with Stephanie grew closer, she became worried that the gains made during therapy would be lost, and that she would be unable to cope by herself. Stephanie treated this example of negative thinking in the same way as all the others. Jane was encouraged to test out her assumption that she could not cope without Stephanie's help by reviewing the progress she had made during their sessions, and in practical ways in her homework assignments as their meetings became spaced further apart.

Evaluation in cognitive therapy is therefore more than a final phase tacked on to the end. It is a dynamic, continuous process by which the client comes to realize that the progress she has made has been through her own hard work, and that it will continue long after therapy is over.

## GESTALT THERAPY

### HISTORY

Gestalt therapy was developed by Friedrich (Fritz) Perls, a German psychoanalyst who studied under Wilhelm Reich and knew both Freud and Jung. Perls left Germany in 1934 during the rise of Hitler for South Africa, where he established the South African Institute for Psychoanalysis, and later moved to the US, where he co-founded the New York Institute for Gestalt Therapy in 1952. He began writing on Gestalt therapy in the 1940s, his two most popular books being *Gestalt Therapy Verbatim* and the autobiographical *In and Out of the Garbage Pail*, both published in 1969. Following Perls's death in

1970, there was an upsurge of interest in Gestalt therapy in Britain. Initially, seminars and courses were run by visiting therapists from the US, but as demand for training grew, and more therapists became established in this country, a wide range of training opportunities has become available nationally.

## PHILOSOPHY

Gestalt therapy is based on the concepts of self-actualization and holism. Self-actualization refers to the potential and drive experienced by the individual towards psychological, emotional, and spiritual growth. For Perls, this occurs through a series of situations requiring completion or resolution: 'Life is practically nothing but an infinite number of unfinished situations – incomplete gestalts. No sooner have we finished one situation than another develops.' (Perls, 1969).

The word *gestalt* means pattern, integration or whole, and refers not only to the completion of unfinished business, but also to the integration of the personality into a self-actualizing whole. Gestalt psychologists often use the figure-and-ground diagram (Figure 34.3) to illustrate the concept. The whole, or gestalt, can be perceived either as a white vase on a black ground, or as two black faces on a white ground. Each relies on the other for its existence, and neither makes sense in isolation.

The concept that human beings are unified wholes is termed 'holism'. There is not an I that *has* a mind, soul or body, but rather a whole that is a thinking, feeling, acting being. This whole person is in a state of homoeostasis or balance, which is constantly under threat, either externally from the environment or from internal needs. These needs emerge from the gestalt to become figures against the background of life. Once the needs are met, the gestalt becomes a whole and the figure merges once more into the ground, only to be replaced by other needs. 'The dominant need

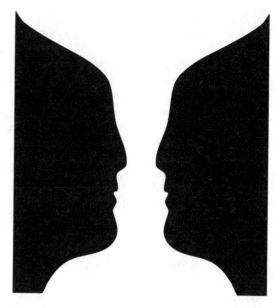

**Figure 34.3**

of the organism, at any time, becomes the foreground figure, and the other needs recede, at least temporarily, into the background.' (Perls, 1973).

If needs are frustrated for any reason, homoeostasis will be upset and the individual will be unable to function in an integrated way. According to Perls, there are four basic ways or mechanisms by which this frustration may become apparent.

Firstly, by introjection whereby concepts, beliefs, and attitudes of significant people in the individual's life are accepted uncritically. These take the form of 'should's' and 'should not's' and inhibit the development of the subject's own personality. Secondly, by projection, where parts of the person which are unacceptable are disowned or attributed to somebody else. Thirdly, by confluence, where the individual feels no boundaries between himself and his environment. This is experienced in states of ecstasy or deep concentration, but is pathological when it continues for any length of time. Fourthly, by retroflection, in which projections on to the outside world are redirected back at their originator. Thus, narcissism is retroflected love, and suicide is retroflected murder.

Perls (1973) sums up the four mechanisms as follows:

> The introjector does as others would like him to do, the projector does unto others what he accuses them of doing to him, the man in pathological confluence doesn't know who is doing what to whom, and the retroflector does to himself what he would like to do to others.

The mechanisms are necessary for normal functioning, but become pathological when used inappropriately or when their use becomes chronic.

THERAPEUTIC INTERVENTION

If psychological and emotional problems are the result of stunted growth and imbalance caused by unmet needs, then the aim of gestalt therapy is to enhance growth and restore homoeostasis. Thus 'the object of every treatment... is to facilitate organismic balance, to re-establish optimal functions' (Perls, 1947).

Gestalt therapy is not concerned with the 'whys' of the client's problem or with his past, but with the here and now. Although problems may have their roots in the past, they are causing difficulties in the present, and it does not help to explore why they arose in the first place. Rather than the client merely recounting past unfinished business in the attempt to understand it intellectually, the gestalt approach advocates re-experiencing it so that it can be resolved in the here-and-now.

There are many techniques designed to accomplish this aim. Awareness of the here-and-now is facilitated by ensuring that the client remains rooted firmly in the present throughout therapy, perhaps by asking him to concentrate on his breathing, gestures, feelings, emotions and voice, or by requesting that he begin sentences with the statement, 'Now I am aware....'.

At the same time as focusing on awareness, the client is required to take responsibility for his actions. This can involve rephrasing questions as statements, or using the word 'I' rather than 'you' or 'it' when referring to himself or parts of his body. For example, when referring to his stammer, a client might say, 'Don't you find it lets you down at awkward moments?' He would then be asked to repeat the assertion, this time saying, 'I let myself down at awkward moments', thus taking responsibility for his own actions.

Although Perls believed that the above methods are in themselves sufficient to bring about recovery, he considered them to be too slow for most clients, and enhanced them with a number of other techniques and exercises. Many of these were designed for groupwork, but can be employed effectively in one-to-one situations. These include the empty-chair technique, unfinished business, reversals, exaggeration, repetition, offering a sentence, staying with a feeling, and dreamwork. Greater understanding of these methods may be gained by reading Perls' own texts, but it may be of benefit to briefly examine two of the most widely used examples.

**Empty-chair work**

Empty-chair work involves the client moving back and forth between two chairs that are facing one another. The technique can be employed to work on conflicts between the client and another person, in which case the client will play himself when sitting in one chair, and the other person when sitting in the other chair. In this way dialogue is facilitated, and the client can perceive the whole situation, or gestalt. The technique can also be used to explore intrapersonal conflict, in which case the chairs will represent different elements of the same person.

## Dreamwork

Gestalt therapists have a unique way of working with dreams in which the client's dream is viewed as a representation of himself. Thus, if a client reports a dream in which he is knocking on the door of an empty house wanting to be let in, the therapist will ask the client to imagine himself as each element of the dream. As well as describing how it feels in the here-and-now to be knocking on the door, the client will also be asked to imagine being the door and the house. The empty-chair technique may be employed to facilitate a dialogue between the dreamer and the door, with the door describing how it feels to be knocked on; or between the door and the house, with the house reporting the feelings of wanting to be entered, but being prevented by the door. In this way, different aspects of the client are able to get in touch with one another.

## TRANSACTIONAL ANALYSIS (TA)

### HISTORY

TA was devised by Eric Berne, a Canadian living in California. Berne trained first as a surgeon and then as a psychoanalyst under both Paul Federn and Erik Erikson, and developed TA as an extension of Freudian psychoanalysis during the 1950s. In 1962, the first course in TA in Britain was established at the University of Leicester, and in 1964, Berne published his best-selling book *Games People Play*. Following Berne's death in 1970, TA flourished in both Britain and the US, and has become widely accepted as a method of treatment by psychiatrists, social workers, and psychiatric nurses.

### PHILOSOPHY

As its name suggests, TA is concerned in its basic form with analyzing the transactions or communications between individuals. Berne took as his starting point Freud's notion of the ego as the conscious part of the personality, which is in touch with and capable of dealing with reality, and divided it into three parts, or ego states, known as the Parent, the Adult, and the Child (note the use of capital letters).

The Child ego state comprises the feelings, thoughts, and behaviours of the child that we once were, accumulated and stored during the first few years of life; it can be further broken down into the Free or Natural Child, and the Adapted Child. The Parent is the collection of rules, commands, and injunctions absorbed during the same period, usually from our parents, and comprises the Critical Parent and the Nurturing Parent. The Adult is the reasoning part of our conscious mind, the part concerned with making decisions based on objective facts. Thomas Harris (1973) referred to the three ego states as the felt concept, the taught concept, and the thought concept, respectively.

Berne asserted that during our entire waking life, one or other of these three ego states has executive control over our thoughts, feelings, and behaviour. The human personality thus can be neatly packaged as the sum of the three states (Figure 34.4).

Berne believed that under normal circumstances we can move quickly and easily from one state to another, with the Adult state maintaining overall control. In our everyday dealings with the world we spend much of our time in our Adult state, analyzing information, solving problems, and going about our work. When appropriate, we might slip into our fun-loving Child state, or our Nurturing or Critical Parent state.

To a large extent, the state in which we are functioning at any one time will depend on

Figure 34.4 Ego states

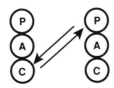

**Figure 34.5** Alan/boss transaction

our interactions with the people around us. For example, Alan, a 30-year-old engineer, might spend most of his time at work in the Adult state, thinking rationally and attempting to solve problems with his colleagues. However, when confronted by the boss, in his own Critical Parent state, who criticizes Alan for making a mistake, Alan might revert to his Adapted Child (Figure 34.5).

At lunch with his colleagues, Alan relaxes in his Free Child state, laughing and making jokes. Later in the afternoon, he enters his Nurturing Parent state when giving first-aid to an injured workmate (Figure 34.6).

Difficulties arise when transactions become crossed, that is, when the ego state to which a communication is being directed is not the same ego state from which the response is coming. Thus, Alan's boss admonished him in a critical way for making a mistake (Parent-Child), and Alan responds by attempting to point out that, as far as he is concerned, it was

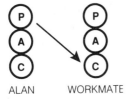

ALAN          WORKMATE

**Figure 34.6**

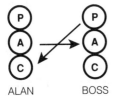

ALAN          BOSS

**Figure 34.7**

not an error (Adult-Adult). The boss was expecting Alan to admit his mistake and apologize (Child-Parent), but instead the transactions became crossed (Figure 34.7).

Berne points out that in the case of crossed transactions, one of two things can happen: either the transaction will end in silence, or in an argument; either way, communication breaks down.

## THERAPEUTIC INTERVENTION

There are several ways in which TA can be of help in detecting and treating psychiatric problems. Structural analysis, the analysis of ego states, may uncover one of two pathological conditions. Firstly, one state might be contaminating another. For example, if the Child contaminates the Adult, delusions or hallucinations may result, since irrational fears or grandiose ideas from childhood will distort the Adult reasoning capacity. Secondly, one state might be excluded or decommissioned, so that the person is effectively functioning with only two ego states. Thus, an excluded Parent might result in a sociopathic personality whose Adult successfully puts into action his Child's antisocial wishes without the restraining influence of his conscience in the form of the Parent.

Game analysis can help uncover repeated patterns of transactions known as games that end in a payoff, often negative. Some games are harmless, some cause distress, and some are dangerous. At best, games can lead to frustration and arguments in relationships, at worst, to serious injury or death.

Berne (1968) gives an interesting example of using game analysis in uncovering the dynamics of a psychiatric problem. He describes a game titled, 'If It Weren't For You (IWFY)', in which 'Mrs White complained that her husband severely restricted her social activities, so that she had never learned to dance'. On eventually going along to dance classes, however, she discovered that 'she had a morbid fear of dance floors and had to abandon this project'. After trying and abandoning many other similar projects, it became clear that she had a deep-rooted phobia of social situations, and, according to Berne, 'out of her many suitors had picked a domineering man for a husband. She was then in a position to complain that she could do all sorts of things 'if it weren't for you'. Contrary to her complaints, however, 'her husband was performing a very real service for her by forbidding her to do something she was deeply afraid of, and by preventing her from even becoming aware of her fears.' (Berne, 1968) This was one reason that her Child had shrewdly chosen such a husband. A cleverly concealed phobia, hidden even from the client, had been uncovered, and could now be treated.

Script analysis goes deeper than game analysis, and seeks to uncover the unconscious life-plan that each of us formulates as children. As Berne (1972) states:

> Each person decides in early childhood how he will live and how he will die, and that plan, which he carries in his head wherever he goes, is called his script. His trivial behaviour may be decided by reason, but his important decisions are already made: what kind of person he will marry, how many children he will have, what kind of bed he will die in, and who will be there when he does. It may not be what he wants, but it is what he wants it to be.

Scripts are programmed by our parents, by the messages they give us, even by what we are named. They often closely resemble Greek myths, fairy-tales or the lives of famous people, and they dominate our lives thereafter. Some are positive, winning scripts ('Florence [Nightingale] or See It Through'): some are negative, losing scripts ('Sisyphus or There I Go Again'). Winning scripts usually lead to happy, fulfilled lives, negative scripts to misery or consistent failure in whatever is attempted.

Berne considered all psychiatric problems as explicable in terms of TA, and treatment is basically the same in all cases. During the first stage of treatment, which is educational, the therapist teaches the client the basic theory and terminology of TA. The client is also taught to identify his own ego states, along with any destructive games he might be playing. These games are disrupted by the therapist by refusing to play her part in them; by playing an unexpected role; or by using psychodrama techniques in which other people act out the client's game roles.

Scripts can be identified and revised. Harris (1985) reports a client suffering from depression who uncovered two conflicting messages: always be best, and always be nice. His long-term depression had been due to attempting to carry out both injunctions at once. In some cases, Berne found that simple script reversal messages were sufficient. For example, after gaining the trust of a suicidal client, Berne would simply say, 'Do not kill yourself', the counter-injunction to an earlier parental message such as 'drop dead'.

In more deep-rooted cases, Berne prescribed re-parenting, a technique in which the client is regressed in a supportive residential environment, followed by directive, positive re-parenting by the therapist. This approach was found to be particularly effective with otherwise untreatable schizophrenics.

The aim of TA therapy is for the client to have a healthy, functioning Adult which has executive control, but which feels secure enough to hand over to the Child or Parent at appropriate times.


## EXISTENTIAL PSYCHOTHERAPY

### HISTORY

Existential psychotherapy is derived from a philosophical tradition of twentieth-century Western European thought. It has its roots in two schools of philosophy: the phenomenological approach of Edmund Husserl, and the existentialism of Kierkegaard and Jaspers.

Phenomenology argues that all knowledge is subjective, and that we must examine our preconceptions and assumptions about the world before we can even attempt to understand it. Later existentialists such as Jean Paul Sartre incorporated the subjective approach of phenomenology into a view of the human experience as essentially alienated and alone in a godless universe. Sartre, a Marxist and French Resistance fighter, popularized existentialism more than any other philosopher, mainly through his novels and plays. His philosophical works, like those of most existentialists, are difficult to comprehend and require extensive study, but he left one short work, *Existentialism and Humanism* (1973) which is both clear and simple.

Although Rollo May and Irving Yalom in the US, and Victor Frankl, an Austrian who studied under Freud, attempted to apply some of the theories of existentialism to psychotherapy, it was British writers such as Laing, Berke, and Cooper who took the existentialism of Sartre to its logical and radical conclusion in the 1960s and 1970s by actively living out its tenets. Although still practised today, the value of the existential approach is more in terms of its historical contribution to the evolution of therapy than as a practical approach that has immediate contemporary relevance.

## PHILOSOPHY

Most writers point out that existential psychotherapy is not a unified school, but more a general approach to therapy, and this observation is itself very much in the subjective spirit of existentialism. The existential philosophy of Sartre takes as its starting point the view that for most material objects in the world essence precedes existence. That is to say, their use of purpose is predetermined before they are made. Sartre gives the example of a paper-knife, made by a craftsman who referred to the concept of what a paper-

knife is, and manufactured it in a certain way and with a particular use in mind. Similarly, God is conceived of as a superior sort of craftsman who made human beings according to a preordained plan and for a predetermined purpose.

Even atheists usually have a notion of human nature, which is the concept of the human. However, Sartre claims that if God does not exist, and there is no logical reason for us to suppose that He does, then for human beings, existence precedes essence. First of all, we exist, and only afterwards do we define ourselves. Thus, we can be whatever we choose, and we are responsible for the choices we make, as Sartre (1973) states:

> Man is nothing else but what he purposes, he exists only in so far as he realizes himself, he is therefore nothing else but the sum of his actions, nothing else but what his life is.

When we become aware of the enormity of the choices we are making, the result is anguish, sometimes referred to as existential angst. While 'there are many, indeed, who show no such anxiety', this is because 'they are merely disguising their anguish or are in flight from it' (Sartre, 1973). The denial that we are free to fashion our own lives as we choose is referred to as 'bad faith'. Living in bad faith is to deny our freedom and to refuse to accept responsibility for our destiny. Its opposite, authenticity, is the realization that there is no rule-book for life, that we must go through life facing up to choices and making decisions.

Existential anxiety is 'an ontological characteristic of man, rooted in his very existence as such' (Boss, 1957). This anxiety can be the result of the choice between being and non-being, that is, the realization that we will all eventually die and can choose to do so at any time; the result of a feeling of aloneness or alienation from the world; or the result of existential neurosis (Frankl, 1973), the realization that there is no external, imposed meaning to life.

The three main concerns of the existential psychotherapist therefore are death, alienation, and meaninglessness, and the aim of therapy is to restore a sense of freedom and control over our destiny.

## THERAPEUTIC INTERVENTION

The existential psychotherapist, living an authentic existence, rejects any rules, guidelines, or techniques imposed by others. Existential psychotherapy is more a description of the orientation or philosophy of the therapist than of a set of therapeutic techniques, as May *et al.* (1984) state:

> The existential therapist begins with presuppositions about the sources of the patient's anguish and views the patient in human rather than behavioural or mechanistic terms. He may employ any of a large variety of techniques used in other approaches insofar as they are consistent with basic existential presuppositions and human, authentic therapist-patient encounter.

To a large extent, existential psychotherapy is similar to the person-centred approach, since both stress the importance of the client-therapist relationship. However, whereas person-centredness maintains that this relationship is sufficient in itself to bring about change, the existential psychotherapist adopts an eclectic approach to technique, borrowing from a wide variety of sources.

Arguably, it is the approach of R.D. Laing and his colleagues at Kingsley Hall during the 1960s that came closest to the true spirit of existential therapy, since they attempted to live their therapeutic approach. Kingsley Hall was a large community centre in the East End of London, which Laing, along with David Cooper and Joseph Berke, converted into a kind of therapeutic community after becoming disillusioned with the restraints of the state psychiatric system. These self-styled 'anti-psychiatrists' created a microcosmic society in which the roles of therapist and client became so blurred that people sometimes crossed from one to the other; where people came to stay as 'guests', contributing what money they could afford; and where they could experience or work through their madness without fear of compulsory detention or unwanted treatment.

Kingsley Hall survived for five years until its lease expired, during which time it was home to over 100 guests, the most famous of whom was Mary Barnes. Mary, a psychiatric nurse tutor, suffered a full psychotic breakdown while at Kingsley Hall, and later wrote a book about her experience along with Joseph Berke. Even Berke and his colleagues stopped short of allowing Mary the ultimate existential choice – that of choosing not to be. Unlike Binswanger, another existential psychotherapist, who claimed that one of his clients had been helped existentially, even though her choice was suicide, Berke saved Mary's life by force feeding her when she became dangerously close to death from starvation.

Although the Kingsley Hall experiment represents a brave attempt at fully implementing the existential approach, it is not a viable choice for most nurses working within the confines of the NHS. A practical alternative, albeit requiring extensive training, is derived from the work of Viktor Frankl, an analytically trained psychotherapist who studied under Freud. Frankl's logotherapy differs from Freudian theory in that the basic human drive is neither the life instinct nor the death instinct, but the 'will-to-meaning', or *logos*. If that will is blocked, then the client manifests neurotic symptoms of existential frustration, which may develop clinically into anxiety neurosis.

Frankl's most famous and successful technique for combating these conditions was paradoxical intention, or prescribing the symptom, and he cites many cases where this method of treatment was successful. For example, a client with a fear of bacteria that led to an obsession with scrubbing and cleaning was instructed to wipe her hands on the floor, making them as dirty as possible; a client with an obsession about collapsing in the street and dying from a heart attack was told to try as hard as possible to make his heart beat faster and have a heart attack right on the spot; a lawyer with a fear of making mistakes at work, which totally incapacitated and hospitalized him, was instructed to make as many errors as possible and get sued at least three times a day; finally, a client with a phobia about hair growing on her face – to the extent that she could not go near a mirror or even pronounce the word 'hair' – was told by her therapist to wish that a single hair would grow on her cheek (Frankl, 1973):

> The woman nearly fainted. She looked at him as if she were seeing a monster. Ten minutes later he was able to lead her to a wall mirror. For the first time in years she looked closely in the mirror and she chose the place on her cheek where she wished one hair to grow.

Frankl quotes many other cases where paradoxical intention has proven to be an extremely quick and effective treatment, and the underlying factor in each example is humour. In every case, the client is encouraged to ridicule his or her symptoms, and in every case the client began to smile or laugh when the feared consequences, which he or she had invested so much energy in trying to avoid, would not manifest themselves despite enormous effort. Thus, the lawyer referred to above was told by his therapist on every visit, 'For heaven's sake, are you still around! I've been looking through the newspapers hoping to read about the big scandalous lawsuit', at which point the client would burst into laughter. In another example, a young woman who wore dark glasses because of a compulsion to look at the genital region of any man she met, was instructed to remove her glasses and actively carry out her compulsion:

For a moment, the patient looked as though she were paralyzed. Then she slowly took off her glasses and broke into a smile. She claimed that she felt more relaxed than she ever remembered. Over the next few days she not only learned to apply paradoxical intention, but actually started to enjoy using this method. It made her somewhat euphoric. In two weeks she reported that her compulsion had disappeared completely.

Paradoxical intention is successful because it exposes the essential meaninglessness of life and the absurd lengths we go to in the attempt to impose our own meaning on it. If, as the existentialists suggest, we choose to make our lives what they are, to give them their meaning, then why make things more difficult than they need to be? If life is an absurd, meaningless joke, then let us laugh at it rather than torturing ourselves with it. It is important to note that paradoxical intention is only one of a range of techniques employed by the logotherapist, and as with any theory of psychotherapy, it should be viewed within the context of the school of thought from which it is derived. Thus, it should only be used by those who have had special training, or under the supervision of someone who has had, such training.

## NEURO-LINGUISTIC PROGRAMMING (NLP)

### HISTORY

NLP began in the early 1970s as a study of famous and successful therapists such as Fritz Perls, Virginia Satir, and Milton Erickson. It was devised by linguist John Grinder and mathematician and gestalt therapist Richard Bandler, initially as an attempt to discover how a variety of therapists and schools of therapy could all produce similar results using different techniques. The result of this study was Bandler and Grinder's first book (1975).

Only in 1976 was the approach seen as a method of therapy in its own right, and the name NLP given to it. A series of workshops was run during the next few years, and in 1978 the Society for Neuro-Linguistic Programming was formed, offering training and certification on three levels. In 1979, Gene Early, a student of Bandler, first presented a paper on NLP in Britain, and in 1982 the UK Diploma in NLP was launched.

PHILOSOPHY

If existential psychotherapy is a theory without specific techniques, then NLP is a set of techniques without a theory. More precisely, it is a methodology from which techniques are generated: 'We never had the intention of starting a new school of therapy, we wished rather to start a new way of talking about it' (Grinder *et al.*, 1976). The approach was to model existing therapies with the aim of producing similar outcomes; as Grinder noted, a theory has to address what is real and true, whereas a model merely has to produce the same results as the therapy being modelled.

NLP is not merely a model, it is a meta-model – a model of how we make models. It concentrates in particular on how we make models of the world, on how we make sense of our experiences. It argues that it is physically impossible to be aware of the full richness and complexity of the world, and therefore our nervous system has to act as a filter. Thus, what we experience with our senses is not the world as such, but a **primary representation** of the world. Our experience of the world is further filtered when this primary representation is expressed in words as a **secondary representation**.

We have five primary representation systems: visual (V), or sight; auditory (A), or hearing; kinesthetic (K), or feeling (sensation and emotion); gustatory (G), or taste; and olfactory (O), or smell. We are born with an equal awareness in all five systems, but as adults we usually have a preference for either V, A, or K. This preference can be detected by eye movements, and by expressions of speech such as 'I see what you mean' (V); 'I hear what you're saying' (A); or 'That feel's right' (K) – all of which have the same meaning of 'I understand you.'

It is thought that eye movements to the left or right when thinking correspond to the functioning of the left or right hemisphere of the brain, usually associated with logical thought and creativity, respectively. Similarly, upward eye movements are thought to correspond to the visual system, ahead to the auditory system, and downward to the kinesthetic system. For example, if a normal, right-handed individual is asked to make up a tune in his head, we would expect his eyes to look horizontally (auditory) to the right (creative); whereas if we asked him the colour of his bedroom walls,

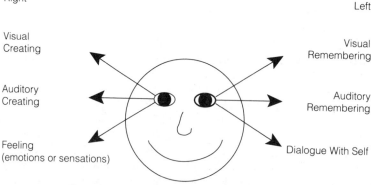

Right                                                        Left

Visual Creating                                    Visual Remembering

Auditory Creating                                    Auditory Remembering

Feeling (emotions or sensations)                  Dialogue With Self

Straight ahead and de-focused is also visual

**Figure 34.8**

he would probably look upward (visual) to the left (remembering). The complete range of eye movements and their corresponding states is represented in Figure 34.8

Complications arise when we attempt to translate material from our primary representation system into our secondary representational of system of language, since a great deal of the information is filtered out in the process. In particular, there are three ways in which information may be lost or distorted:

- Deletion, or selectively paying attention to certain things and leaving others out, for example, believing 'I'm no good' because I can't spell, but forgetting that I'm exceptionally gifted at arithmetic.
- Generalization, or selecting certain thoughts or experiences and applying them to all situations, for example, believing 'I'm no good at cooking' because I have difficulty in making cakes.
- Distortion, or applying thoughts and experiences to situations out of context, for example, believing 'I'm no good because my teacher doesn't like me', as though the disapproval of a significant person somehow causes me to be no good.

Thus, we are restricted and handicapped by our model of the world. As Bandler *et al.* say (1975), people 'are not bad, crazy, or sick – they are, in fact, making the best choices available to them in their model'. The aim of therapy is to add choices and extend the client's model of the world, to help the client realize he already has the resources to solve his problem – he just doesn't know it!

THERAPEUTIC INTERVENTION

Since NLP represents a model for therapeutic change rather than a self-contained, cohesive theory, it is not surprising that it borrows both philosophy and technique unashamedly from all the major schools of psychotherapy. From analytic psychotherapy comes the notion of an unconscious part of the person, which influences behaviour and which can be reprogrammed by the therapist using hypnosis or subliminal suggestions. From behaviourism comes the assertion that behavioural change should be the goal of therapy, and the subsequent rejection of the importance of insight and the influence of the past. From person-centred approaches comes the importance of building rapport with the client, and the techniques of pacing and tracking. And from cognitive therapy comes the notion of psychological distress being the result of cognitive misinterpretations of the environment in the form of deletion, generalization, and distortion. Some therapeutic techniques associated with each of these approaches are outlined below.

The first step in NLP is to build **rapport** with the client. This is achieved by the therapist adjusting her physical systems to those of the client, for example, by adopting his posture and gestures, by matching his voice tone and tempo, and by breathing at the same rate. The therapist should note which representation system the client tends to use – either visual, auditory or kinesthetic – and **track** him by employing the same system in her speech; and she should **pace** him by going along with all his belief systems, thus avoiding resistance.

Once the therapist is synchronized with her client, she can subtly influence him by changing her own systems. For example, when working with an over-active person, the therapist should first match his posture, breathing, rapid speech, and so on, even to the extent of running alongside him. Then, by gradually slowing down and speaking more quietly, she can calm him down until his physical system has returned to normal.

The next step, borrowed from both behavioural and cognitive therapies, is for the client to state his **desired outcomes** in well-formed, behavioural or experiential terms. Dilts *et al.* (1979) suggest five questions the therapist could ask to help the client state his outcomes:

- What do you want? (Note the use of the positive – we generally find it much easier to say what we do not want.)
- How will you/I know you have got it? (The outcome should be stated in terms that can be recognized by both parties.)
- When and where do/don't you want it? (It is important to recognize situations in which the change is not wanted.)
- What do you need to get it?, and the related question, What stops you from getting it? (There is no point in stating an outcome the client has no power to bring about.)
- What will happen if you get it? (The client should examine the negative aspect of the outcome and the problems that it may cause. He may find that he does not really want it after all!)

The proposed changes should fit harmoniously with the life of the client, that is, they should be ecological.

The next step is therapeutic intervention. The interventions employed by the NLP therapist are many and varied, and are freely borrowed from a variety of schools of therapy. For example, the use of **trance states** and **metaphor**, both adapted from psychoanalyst Milton Erickson, rely heavily on the therapist gaining access to the unconscious part of her client. In the latter case, the therapist relates a simple story to which the client responds at an unconscious level, without the interference of conscious processes. Other techniques, such as **anchoring**, are behavioural and operate at a stimulus-response level. In this case, complete representations of experiences are associated with a touch, word, or visual cue (depending on the representation system employed by the client), so that they can easily be recalled to consciousness at a later time.

Many of the therapeutic methods are derived from cognitive therapy. For example, the NLP concept of **strategies**, which are loops of bad feelings and perceptions, is very similar to the cognitive therapist's notion of automatic thoughts and self-fulfilling prophesies, and the intervention of challenging those feelings and perceptions is also similar. Another technique reminiscent of cognitive therapy is **reframing**, which seeks to reinterpret behaviour seen by the client as negative in a positive light, either by reframing its meaning or the context in which it is being displayed. As an example of the former, a child whose parents always want to know where he is going, and insist that he is home by ten o'clock every evening, are perceived by him as being fussy and over-protective. However, that perception could be reframed as caring enough about him to want to know where he is and worrying if he is late. As an example of the latter, the above parental behaviour may seem inappropriate towards a 17-year-old boy in a quiet suburb, but would be very sensible towards a ten-year-old girl in an inner-city.

Successful outcome of NLP is easy to detect, since the criteria for success will have been defined at the onset of therapy. The main advantage of NLP over other forms of therapy is its speed. Major changes often begin in the first or second meeting, and it is usual for the therapeutic intervention to last only about four or five sessions.

## COUNSELLING

### HISTORY

Counselling originated from the person-centred approach of Carl Rogers. It was a term he first used in the 1930s and 1940s, because at the time psychologists were not allowed to practice psychotherapy in the US. He later used the terms 'counselling' and 'psychotherapy' interchangeably, which contributed to the confusion surrounding them. When Rogerian therapy began to be used in Britain in the mid-1960s, many practitioners chose to call themselves counsellors rather than therapists, emphasizing the non-directive aspect of their work, and in a genuine attempt to demystify what they were doing.

Counselling became established as an intervention separate from person-centred therapy with the publication of Gerard Egan's book *The Skilled Helper* in 1975. Egan took Rogers's work as a starting point, but emphasized and developed the skills component in such a way that made it quick and simple to teach. Following the book's publication in Britain in the following year, courses in counselling sprung up throughout the country.

Egan's model of counselling reached a wider audience with two series of television programmes entitled 'Principles of Counselling', leading the British Association of Counselling (BAC) to invite Egan to run workshops for counselling trainers. Of particular significance for nurses is the fact that in 1978 the tutor responsible for counselling training at the Royal College of Nursing (RCN) visited Egan in Chicago, and the RCN has since been heavily influenced by his model.

## PHILOSOPHY

Arguably, counselling is the foundation of all the forms of psychotherapy discussed in this chapter, and indeed, 'all the skills involved in the counselling process are also relevant to any nurse/patient relationship of any depth' (Burnard, 1985). There is, however, some confusion over exactly what counselling is, and how it differs from psychotherapy on the one hand, and with helping on the other. For example, Parry (1975) distinguishes between therapists – which includes doctors, nurses, social workers, clinical psychologists, and occupational therapists; and counsellors – including ministers of religion, lawyers, marriage guidance workers, and Samaritans. Nelson-Jones (1988), on the other hand, refers to members of the helping professions as counsellors, and those using counselling techniques as part of an otherwise non-caring role, as helpers.

For our purposes, the term 'counselling' will be used to distinguish it from other systematic, helping interventions that usually fall loosely under the heading of psychotherapy.

While all writers appear to agree that counselling is largely skills-based, it is more than just the application of a set of techniques. Munro *et al.*(1983) refer to it as the various skills and principles of helping, claiming it also includes a set of ethical conditions, including confidentiality, and an emphasis on personal responsibility for one's own behaviour. Nelson-Jones (1988) offers six criteria that must be present for counselling to take place; that it:

- is a relationship based on Rogers's therapeutic conditions for growth (page 460);
- involves a repertoire of skills;
- emphasizes self-help and responsibility;
- emphasizes the need and ability of the client to make choices;
- focuses on problems of living;
- is a fluid and interactional process.

## THERAPEUTIC INTERVENTION

Egan (1982) identifies three stages of the counselling relationship, which can be simplified as exploring, understanding, and acting. Each stage requires different skills from the counsellor. Burnard has divided these skills into two categories, namely listening and attending skills, and counselling intervention skills. Listening is distinguished from hearing by being an active process that requires deep concentration and attention. It involves being aware of one's own gaze, expression, posture and gestures, and is mostly non-verbal. The behaviours involved in active listening can be recalled by remembering Egan's acronym 'SOLER', which stands for:

S   sit **squarely** in relation to the person being listened to;
O   maintain an **open** position, with uncrossed arms and legs;

L   **lean** slightly towards the client, showing warmth and interest;

E   maintain reasonable **eye** contact;

R   **relax**.

The counselling intervention skills are mainly verbal, and have been categorized by Heron (1989) as:

- prescriptive – making suggestions and recommendations;
- informative – giving information and knowledge;
- confronting – challenging restrictive beliefs, attitudes, and behaviour;
- cathartic – helping to express emotion and release tension;
- catalytic – encouraging self-discovery and problem solving;
- supportive – affirming worth.

These categories represent the full range of possible therapeutic interventions, and the aim of the counsellor should be to distinguish between them, be competent in the use of all six categories, and be able to move freely and smoothly between them as necessary. Burnard (1985) offers a useful application of these interventions to nursing situations.

Another way of categorizing counselling interventions is according to the skills employed in them. Some of those skills are as follows.

## Questioning

Questions are usually categorized as 'open' or 'closed'. A closed question elicits a one-word reply, whereas an open question invites the respondent to expand on his answer. Open questions may be employed to clarify situations about which the counsellor is unsure, for example: 'What did you mean when you said. . .?', or to encourage the client to explore further, for example, 'How did you feel when that happened?'

## Reflection

Another way of encouraging the client to say more is by reflecting back, or echoing, the last few words that he said. For example, in reply to the client's statement, 'When my wife left me, life just didn't seem worth living', the counsellor might reply, 'Life didn't seem worth living', thus encouraging the client to continue. This is a very effective technique, but one which should be used sensitively to avoid it sounding mechanical.

## Focusing

Often, the client will make a seemingly innocuous remark in the middle of a longer statement, on which the counsellor may wish to focus. For example, the client might say, 'When my wife first left me, I felt so depressed that I didn't leave the house for weeks, but I feel much better now. Why, only the other day...' He clearly wants to give examples of how much he has improved, but the counsellor suspects he may not be fully recovered from the depression. Therefore, she might say, 'You felt depressed', or, more directly, 'Can you say some more about the depression?', thus focusing on what she considers to be an important area that would otherwise have been glossed over.

## Restating

As a way of checking that she understands the client's meaning, the therapist may occasionally summarize the conversation by saying, for example, 'Let me just sum up what you've been saying. . ., or, 'Have I got this right? You are saying that. . .' This is not only a useful check for the counsellor that she fully comprehends what the client is trying to say, but also communicates to the client that she is attending, and that she has a desire to help.

These are just some of the many skills involved in being a counsellor, but it is important to emphasize once more that counselling is more than just the application of technique. It is first and foremost about the relationship between the two individuals, which must be based on trust, warmth, and non-judgemental understanding if it is to be therapeutic. Furthermore, counselling, like all forms of therapy, often involves the disclosure of sensitive information, and should therefore be based on a code of ethics such as that issued by the BAC.

## CHOOSING AN APPROACH

Having read this chapter, the mental health nurse will hopefully realize the benefits of adopting a systematic approach to her individual work with clients. However, she may well feel bewildered by the vast range of possible interventions, most of which are very different, and all of which profess to be the best and most effective form of treatment. Which should she choose? Clearly, she would want to work in a way that will prove beneficial to her clients, but all the therapeutic approaches discussed in this chapter make that claim.

Which is the most effective? This is a difficult question to answer, and one that has stimulated a great deal of research over the years. The basic difficulty in attempting to compare the number of successful outcomes of different schools of therapy is the simple observation that different therapies have different measures of success. For example, to the behavioural psychotherapist the presenting problem is simply the sum of the client's symptoms, and therefore successful therapy involves the eradication of those symptoms. The analytic psychotherapist, on the other hand, will see the symptoms as a manifestation of a deeper problem, usually originating in childhood, and will argue that it could be dangerous to attempt to remove them without first addressing the underlying problem. Furthermore, if the underlying problem is brought to the surface of consciousness, the symptoms will usually resolve themselves.

For the analytic psychotherapist, then, successful therapy involves insight.

A further difficulty in comparing outcomes of different schools of therapy is the question of whether the subjective internal state of the clients should be taken into account. Should the eradication of symptoms be the sole guide to success, irrespective of whether the client feels better following therapy? Or, alternatively, should success be measured by whether the client reports feeling happier, regardless of whether he continues to display his original symptoms? Thus, although Garfield *et al.* (1978), in a review of outcome studies, were able to conclude that 'these findings generally yield clearly positive results when compared with no-treatment, wait-list and placebo or pseudotherapies', nevertheless, 'difference in outcome between various forms of intervention are rare'.

There are various other considerations when choosing a therapeutic approach:

- Client-centredness – choosing an approach that suits the client and his problems and needs. Certain therapies are thought to be more effective in dealing with specific problems, for example, cognitive therapy for depression, behavioural therapy for certain phobias.

- Nurse-centredness – choosing an approach that is:
  - suited to the nurse's personality, training, and experience. Corsini (1984) has noted a correlation between various therapeutic approaches and the personalities of their innovators, suggesting that the personality of the therapist is an important factor when choosing a therapeutic approach;
  - suited to the political and ethical outlook of the nurse and the organization, including issues of power, control, and authority; this has particular relevance for nurses wishing to pursue a therapeutic approach with obvious political and ethical implications, such as existential therapy;

– suited to the nurse's views of humankind, for example, does the nurse consider that people are basically good or bad, altruistic (Rogers), self-interested (Freud), or blank slates (Skinner)?

- Agency-centredness – choosing an approach that fits with the philosophy of the team, department, or whole organization of which the nurse is a part.

- Practical – choosing an approach that considers the resources of the client, for example, some approaches assume a certain intellectual capability, whereas others are more feeling or practically oriented.

Ideally, the nurse should develop an eclectic approach that involves an understanding of all the major therapeutic interventions; and skill and expertise in a useful range. Thus, the nurse will be able to assess and evaluate the most appropriate intervention for each client, and either offer therapy herself, or refer the client to a team member with the necessary skills.

## REFERENCES

Bandler, R. and Grinder, J. (1975) *The Structure of Magic*, Science & Behavior Books, Palo Alto.

Bandura, A. (1977) *Social Learning Theory*, Prentice Hall, Englewood Cliffs, New Jersey.

Bandura, A. and Menlove, F. L. (1968) Factors determining vicarious extinction of avoidance behavior through symbolic modelling, *J. Personality and Social Psychology*, 8, 99–108.

Beck, A. T. (1976) *Cognitive Therapy and the Emotional Disorders*, New American Library, New York.

Berne, E. (1968) *Games People Play*, Penguin, Harmondsworth.

Berne, E. (1972) *What Do You Say After You Say Hello?*, Corgi, London.

Boss, M. (1957) Daseinanalysis and psychotherapy, in *Progress in Psychotherapy*, (eds. J. H. Masserman and J. L. Moreno) Grune & Stratton, New York.

Burnard, P. (1985) *Learning Human Skills: A Guide for Nurses*, Heinemann, London.

Corsini, R. (1984) *Current Psychotherapies* (3rd edn), Peacock, Itasca, Illinois.

Dilts, R. B., Grinder, J., Bandler, R. *et al.* (1979) *Neuro-Linguistic Programming* (Vol. 1) Meta Publications, Cupertino, California.

Egan, G. (1982) *The Skilled Helper* (2nd edn), Brooks/Cole, Monterey.

Ellis, A. (1962) *Reason and Emotion in Psychotherapy*, Lyle Stuart, New York.

Ellis, A. (1973) *Humanistic Psychotherapy: The Rational-Emotive Approach*, Julian Press, New York.

Ellis, A. (1977) The basic clinical theory of rational-emotive therapy, in *Handbook of Rational-Emotive Therapy* (ed. A. Ellis and R. Grieger), Springer, New York.

Eysenck, H. J. (ed.) (1960) *Behaviour Therapy and the Neuroses*, Pergamon, London.

Frankl, V. E. (1973) *The Doctor and the Soul*, Penguin, Harmondsworth.

Freud, S. (1895) *Studies on Hysteria*, Penguin, Harmondsworth.

Freud, S. (1901) *The Psychopathology of Everyday Life*, Penguin, Harmondsworth.

Freud, S. (1900) *The Interpretation of Dreams*, Penguin, Harmondsworth.

Freud, S. (1923) *On Metapsychology*, Penguin, Harmondsworth.

Garfield, S. L. and Bergin, A. E. (1978) *Handbook of Psychotherapy and Behaviour Change* (2nd edn), Wiley, Chichester.

Grinder, J. and Bandler, R. (1976) *The Structure of Magic II*, Science & Behavior Books, Palo Alto.

Harris, T. A. (1973) *I'm OK-You're OK*, Pan, London.

Harris, A. and Harris, T. A. (1985) *Staying OK*, Pan, London.

Heron, J. (1989) *Six Category Intervention Analysis* (3rd edn), Human Potential Research Project, Univ. Surrey, Guildford.

Marks, I. (1981a) *Cure and Care of Neurosis*, Wiley, Chichester.

Marks, I. (1981b) Review of behavioural psychotherapy. 2: sexual disorders. *American J. Psychiatry*, 138, 970–6.

May, R. and Yalom, I. (1984) Existential psychotherapy, in *Current Psychotherapies* (ed. R. J. Corsini) Peacock, Illinois.

Meichenbaum, D. (1977) *Cognitive-Behaviour Modification*, Plenum, New York.

Munro, E. A., Manthei, R. J., Small, J. J. (1983) *Counselling: A Skills Approach* (rev. edn), Methuen, New Zealand.

Nelson-Jones, R. (1988) *Practical Counselling and Helping Skills* (2nd edn) Cassell, London.

Parry, R. (1975) *A Guide to Counselling and Basic Psychotherapy*, Churchill Livingstone, Edinburgh.

Pavlov, I. P. (1928) *Lectures on Conditioned Reflexes*, International Publishers, New York.

Perls, F. (1969) *Ego, Hunger and Aggression*, Random House, New York.

Perls, F. (1969) *Gestalt Therapy Verbatim*, Real People Press, Lafayette, California.

Perls, F. (1969) *In and Out of the Garbage Pail*, Real People Press, Utah.

Perls, F. (1973) *The Gestalt Approach*, Science and Behavior Books, Palo Alto.

Rogers, C. R. (1942) *Counselling and Psychotherapy*, Houghton Mifflin, Boston.

Rogers, C. R. (1951) *Client-Centred Therapy*, Houghton Mifflin, Boston.

Roger, C. R. (1957) The necessary and sufficient conditions of therapeutic personality change. *J. Consulting Psychology*, 21, 95–103.

Rogers, C. R. (1961) *On Becoming a Person: a Therapist's View of Psychotherapy*, Constable, London.

Sartre, J. P. (1973) *Existentialism and Humanism*, Eyre Methuen, London.

Skinner, B. F. (1953) *Science and Human Behaviour*, Macmillan, New York.

Walker, S. (1984) *Learning Theory and Behaviour Modification*, Methuen, London.

Watson, J. B. (1913) Psychology as the behaviourist views it. *Psychological Review* 20, 158–177.

Wessler, R. L. (1986) Conceptualizing cognitions in the cognitive-behavioural therapies, in *Cognitive-Behavioural Approaches to Psychotherapy* (eds W. Dryden and W. Golden) Harper & Row, New York.

Wiens, A. N. and Menustik, C. E. (1983) Treatment outcome and patient characteristics in an aversion therapy program for alcoholism. *American Psychologist*, 38, 1089–96.

Wilson, G. T. (1984) in *Current Psychotherapies*, R.J Corsini, Peacock, Illinois.

Wolpe, J. (1959) *Psychotherapy by Reciprocal Inhibition*, Stanford Univ. Press, California.

Wolpe, J. (1982) *The Practice of Behavior Therapy* (3rd edn) Pergamon, New York.

# FURTHER READING

## GENERAL

Corsini, R. J. (ed.) (1984) *Current Psychotherapies* (3rd edn), Peacock, Illinois. Well written, for a professional readership.

Dryden, W. (ed.) (1984) *Individual Therapy in Britain* Harper & Row, London. A clear and detailed account of the main therapeutic approaches, written by major British practitioners.

Kingston, B. (1987) *Psychological Approaches in Psychiatric Nursing*, Croom Helm, London. A simple account of applying a variety of therapeutic methods to psychiatric nursing, including chapters on behavioural, psychodynamic and psychosocial approaches.

Kovel, J. (1978) *A Complete Guide to Therapy* Penguin, Harmondsworth. An excellent introduction to the psychotherapies. Written as a consumer's guide, but equally useful to the practitioner.

## ANALYTIC PSYCHOTHERAPY

Brown, J. A. C. (1961) *Freud and the Post-Freudians* Penguin, Harmondsworth. A critical account of the works of Freud and his followers. Worth the effort.

Freud, S. (1962) *Two Short Accounts of Psycho-Analysis*, Penguin Harmondsworth. A good introduction to the writings of Freud. An outline of basic psychoanalytic concepts written for the lay reader.

Jacobs, M. (1988) *Psychodynamic Counselling in Action*, Sage, London. A practical, casework-based guide takes the reader through two cases from beginning to end.

Sandler, J., Dare, C. *et al.* (1973) *The Patient and the Analyst*, Maresfield Library, London. A straight-forward and detailed account of the basic concepts used in the understanding of the psychoanalytic process.

Stafford-Clark, D. (1965) *What Freud Really Said*. Penguin, Harmondsworth. Wide-ranging and readable. An excellent introduction to Freudian theory.

## BEHAVIOURAL PSYCHOTHERAPY

Barker, P. J. (1982) *Behaviour Therapy Nursing*, Croom Helm, London. A practical and readable book that presents behaviour therapy from a nursing perspective. Includes useful appendices on assessment, ethical implications, and relaxation training.

Bellack, A. S. and Hersen, M. (eds) (1988) *Behavioural Assessment* (3rd edn), Pergamon, New York. A more advanced text which provides both an overview of assessment strategies, and a series of individual approaches to different problems.

Butler, R. J. and Rosenthall, G. (1978) *Behaviour and Rehabilitation*, John Wright, Bristol. Gives psychiatric nurses working with long-term patients in hospital settings a sound, basic understanding of the procedures involved in behaviour modification.

Skinner, B. F. (1953) *Science and Human Behaviour*, Macmillan, New York. A good introduction to the basic theory of radical behaviourism, from one of its founders.

## PERSON-CENTRED THERAPY

Kirschenbaum, H. and Henderson, V. L. (eds) (1990) *The Carl Rogers Reader*, Constable, London. A broad selection from the lifetime work of Carl Rogers. A good starting point for the prospective person-centred therapist.

Rogers, C. R. (1951) *Client-Centred Therapy* Houghton Mifflin, Boston. The first major exposition of the person-centred approach. Includes a client's perspective of therapy, and useful chapters on play therapy, group-centred approaches, and student-centred teaching.

Rogers, C. R. (1957) The necessary and sufficient conditions of therapeutic personality change. *Consulting Psychology*, 21, 95–103. This short paper is probably the clearest outline of Rogers's core conditions for therapeutic change

Rogers, C. R. (1961) *On Becoming a Person: a Therapist's View of Psychotherapy*, Constable, London. A useful and readable book on the philosophy and practice of person-centred therapy. Includes a section on the applications of person-centredness to everyday life

## COGNITIVE THERAPY

Ellis, A.(1962) *Reason and Emotion in Psychotherapy* Lyle Stuart, New York. The first book to present the theory of RET. Valuable reading, not only for practitioners, but also widely used as a self-help handbook.

Ellis, A. and Grieger, R. (1977) *Handbook of Rational Emotive Therapy*, Springer, New York. A sourcebook of classic RET writings, with sections on theoretical and conceptual foundations, and techniques and processes of RET.

Hawton, K., Salkovskis, P. M., Kirk, J. *et al.* (eds) (1989) *Cognitive Behaviour Therapy for Psychiatric Problems*. Univ. Press, Oxford. A more advanced

work aimed at psychiatrists and psychologists as well as nurses, presenting a detailed and indepth analysis of a variety of psychiatric conditions from a cognitive perspective.

Trower, P., Casey, A., Dryden, W. (1988) *Cognitive-Behavioural Counselling in Action*, Sage Publications, London. A simple and practical guide for the beginning cognitive therapist. A useful text for nurses who wish to incorporate elements of cognitive-behavioural counselling into their work.

## GESTALT THERAPY

Houston G. (1982) *The Red Book of Gestalt*, The Rochester Foundation, London. Although written as a guide to setting up and facilitating a self-help Gestalt group, the book contains a wealth of exercises that can be used in individual therapy situations.

Perls, F (1947) *Ego, Hunger and Aggression*, Allen and Unwin, London.

Perls, F. (1969) *In and Out of the Garbage Pail*, Real People Press, Utah. Perls's autobiography, written the year before he died. Provides a rich and valuable insight into his character.

Perls, F., Hefferline, R. F., Goodman, P. (1972) *Gestalt Therapy*, Souvenir, London. Comprises a series of experiments and exercises, followed by a theoretical outline of Gestalt therapy. Difficult, but essential reading.

Perls, F. (1973) *The Gestalt Approach*, Science and Behaviour Books, Palo Alto. Perls's last and clearest outline of Gestalt therapy.

## TRANSACTIONAL ANALYSIS

Berne, E. (1968) *Games People Play*, Penguin, Harmondsworth. First published in 1964, this eminently readable book includes a concise theory of TA, followed by a thesaurus of games.

Berne, E. (1975) *Transactional Analysis in Psychotherapy*, Souvenir Press, London. An entertaining account of TA in action, and an essential handbook for the practitioner wishing to apply the principles and techniques of TA to their clinical work.

Harris, T. A. (1973) *I'm OK – You're OK*, Pan, London. Along with its sequel, *Staying OK*, this book offers a useful self-help guide to TA.

Stewart, I. (1989) *Transactional Analysis Counselling in Action* Sage, London. A practical guide to the use of TA in counselling, aimed at counsellor trainers and their trainees, as well as practising counsellors and nurses who are interested in developing TA skills.

## EXISTENTIAL PSYCHOTHERAPY

Barnes, M. and Berke, J. (1971) *Two Accounts of a Journey Through Madness*, MacGibbon and Kee, London. Mary Barnes's stay at Kingsley Hall seen through her own eyes and through those of Joseph Berke, her therapist. A usefully subjective view of the schizophrenic process.

Frankl, V. E. (1973) *The Doctor and the Soul*, Penguin, Harmondsworth. An outline of the philosophy, theory, and major therapeutic techniques of Frankl's logotherapy.

Laing, R. D. (1965) *The Divided Self*, Penguin, Harmondsworth. Subtitled 'An existential study in sanity and madness', Laing offers the view of schizophrenic as outsider.

Sartre, J. P. (1973) *Existentialism & Humanism*, Eyre Methuen, London. A transcript of a lecture, this is a basic and easy-to-read introduction to Sartre's existentialism.

Yalom, I. D. (1980) *Existential Psychotherapy*, Basic Books, New York. A comprehensive clinical overview of the American school of existential psychotherapy.

## NEURO-LINGUISTIC PROGRAMMING

Bandler, R. and Grinder, J. (1975) *The Structure of Magic*, Science and Behavior Books, Palo Alto. The first of a series of books, this presents NLP in embryonic form. Interesting background reading.

Bandler, R. and Grinder, J. (1979) *Frogs into Princes*, Real People Press, Utah. Transcripts from a series of workshops given during the late 1970s, with sections on representational systems, anchoring, and reframing.

Bandler, R. and Grinder, J. (1982) *Reframing*, Real People Press, Utah. Advanced reframing which continues where *Frogs into Princes* left off. Contains chapters on working with couples, families, alcoholics, and drug abusers.

Lankton, S. (1980) *Practical Magic*, Meta Publications, Cupertino, California. A basic beginner's manual to NLP.

## COUNSELLING

Burnard, P. (1985) *Learning Human Skills: A Guide for Nurses*, Heinemann, London. Part One is theoretical and looks at self-awareness and experiential learning. Part Two is a set of exercises based around Heron's six-category intervention analysis. There are also useful sections on group skills and self-awareness methods.

Egan, G. (1982) *The Skilled Helper* (2nd edn), Brooks/Cole, Monterey. A practical, skills-based introduction to counselling, in which Egan outlines his three-stage helping model.

Munro, E.A., Manthei, R. J., Small, J. J (1983) *Counselling: A Skills Approach* (rev. edn), Methuen, New Zealand. A book of exercises that takes the prospective counsellor from first principles (discussing the reasons for wanting to be a counsellor), to terminating the relationship and beyond (process-recording, supervision, consultation work).

Nelson-Jones, R. (1988) *Practical Counselling and Helping Skills* (2nd edn), Cassel, London. A more advanced but user-friendly text that takes an eclectic approach to counselling, borrowing from, among others, Rogerian therapy, behaviour psychotherapy, and cognitive therapies.

## OPPORTUNITIES IN TRAINING

## ANALYTIC PSYCHOTHERAPY

The British Association of Psychotherapists offers a three-year training in Freudian, Jungian, and child psychotherapy at reasonable cost. Applicants must have a university degree in medicine, psychology, or social science, or an equivalent professional qualification, and some experience of working with disturbed people. They should also currently be in therapy with an approved training therapist. For further details, contact:

The British Association of Psychotherapists
121 Hendon Lane
London N3 3PR

Nurses might also be interested in the ENB courses in psycho-dynamic techniques. Further details from:

The English National Board for Nursing Midwifery and Health Visiting

Victory House
170 Tottenham Court Road
London W1P OHA

## BEHAVIOURAL PSYCHOTHERAPY

The ENB offer courses for nurses in adult behavioural psychotherapy and rehabilitation in residential settings. Further details from:

The English National Board for Nursing, Midwifery and Health Visiting
Victory House
170 Tottenham Court Road
London W1P 0HA

## PERSON-CENTRED THERAPY

Person-Centred Therapy (Britain) offers a two-and-a-half-year part-time course recognized by the British Association for Counselling. No formal academic requirements are necessary, and course members should ensure opportunities for counselling experience with statutory or voluntary agencies. For further information, contact:

PCT Britain,
C/O Dave Mearns
Psychology Department
Jordanhill College of Education
Glasgow G13 1PP

## COGNITIVE THERAPY

The Institute for Rational Emotive Therapy run a series of practical workshops for people interested in finding out more about RET. For further information, contact:

The Institute of Rational Emotive Therapy (UK)
39 Bignor Road
Wadsley Bridge
Sheffield S6 1JD

## GESTALT THERAPY

Information on training in the UK can be obtained from:

The Gestalt Centre
7 Parliament Hill
London NW3

Metanoia offer a variety of courses, including a diploma course in Gestalt psychotherapy for professionals in medicine, counselling, psychother-

apy, and others in the helping professions. Further details from:

Metanoia
13 North Common Road
London W5 2QB

## TRANSACTIONAL ANALYSIS

The Institute of Transactional Analysis co-ordinates training throughout the country. Beginners start with an introductory course. Details of training opportunities can be obtained from:

Institute of Transactional Analysis
BM Box 4104
London WC1 3XX

Metanoia offers a part-time, three-year course in Transactional Analysis Psychotherapy, as well as a variety of short courses, and can be contacted at:

Metanoia
13 North Common Road
London W5 2BQ

## EXISTENTIAL PSYCHOTHERAPY

The Philadelphia Association was founded in 1964 by R.D. Laing and his colleagues, and was active in setting up Kingsley Hall. It currently offers two training programmes – in individual psychotherapy and community therapy – as well as a one-year introductory course in phenomenology and psychoanalysis. The training consists of four parts: attendance at seminars and clinical presentation; own psychotherapy; seeing patients under supervision; involvement in Philadelphia Association households. Further details from:

The Philadelphia Association
4 Marty's Yard
17 Hampstead High Street
London NW3 1PX

## NEURO-LINGUISTIC PROGRAMMING

There are now a number of institutions offering training courses recognized and approved by both the Society of Neuro-Linguistic Programming (US) and the Association for Neuro-Linguistic Programming (UK). International Teaching Seminars provide a variety of courses, from open evenings and two-day seminars to full practitioner training.

They can be contacted at:

International Teaching Seminars, 1 Mulgrave Road, London NW10 1BS

## COUNSELLING

There are a large number of training schemes in counselling on offer throughout the country. Be selective, and choose one that appeals to your particular therapeutic orientation. If in doubt, find a course that has been accredited by the BAC. They can be contacted at:

British Association for Counselling
37a Sheep Street
Rugby
Warwickshire, CV21 3BX

*Ruth Davies*

As in any other setting, the nurse working in a group needs certain skills and qualities as the basic tools of her trade. This chapter addresses the knowledge, skills, and attitudes the nurse needs to work effectively with groups.

There are many types of group in which a client might become involved as part of the therapeutic programme. This array of activities might leave the nurse uncertain as to what groups are; how they differ; how they work; the role and leadership style of the staff; and even as to whether or not the groups play a part in therapy.

## WHY WORK IN GROUPS?

Human beings are born into and live in groups. Our interactions with other people are the source of emotional satisfaction and growth, but also of unhappiness and trauma. We need the love of others, and contact and co-operation with them in order to live a relatively happy and fulfilled life. It is often the quality of our relationships and/or lack of relationships with others that distresses us, resulting in defensive behaviours being used that we learnt as children, and that do not serve us in adult life.

Some of the main indicators of mental illness are the inability to fulfil social roles, contribute to society, and care for ourselves and others on a functional basis. To change this we may have to learn new ways of relating. It makes sense, then, to enter a group in order to explore our relationships with other people, and to explore new ways of

making contact and enjoying that contact with others.

A person might say, 'My problem is with person 'X'. How will a group help me?' One of the principles of groupwork is that the group is representative of the outside world, which is brought inside by the members. Thus, problems we experience with particular individuals or types of behaviour are likely to recur within the group, and can then be worked through in a safe setting, whereas it might not be possible, or desirable, to do this directly with the person who is the main focus. It is also possible that although the presenting issue might be with person 'X', this may be a repetition of patterns, such as an inability to sustain relationships, or to deal with conflict constructively. These patterns may recur in the group, and can then be made conscious, explored, and relived in a more healthy way.

## TYPES OF GROUPS

There are many types of group, based on different theories, models of practice, and therapeutic orientation. It is important that the group staff members have a clear idea of the purpose of the group. This enables boundaries pertaining to content and process to be clarified, and safety to be enhanced.

There is likely to be a difference between the content and process of a social skills training group and a small analytic group, although the individual may find it useful to take material raised in one to the other in order to practise responses, or to explore an issue in more depth. This may only be possible within residential or day units, where a comprehensive group programme is available.

Some groups may have guidelines or ground rules, perhaps written by the members for the benefit of existing and new members. A statement such as 'We're here to talk about ourselves and our relationships with each other' may be simultaneously very meaningful and very meaningless, but it does indicate what it is appropriate to talk about.

Some words or phrases used to describe groups can be usefully defined. Although much of the theory and practice of group-work applies to all kinds of groups, each type will have its own structures and boundaries within which it operates.

## OPEN AND CLOSED GROUPS

Groups are often described as open or closed. Generally speaking, an open group is one which replaces members as they leave the group, thereby maintaining a consistent size. Sometimes these groups run within out-patient services and have 'terms', with new members joining at the start of each term and others leaving at the end. Some people may be referred to such a group while in hospital, and discharged home to attend the group at an appropriate time. These groups usually meet once or twice weekly, and are run by one or two therapists over a considerable period of time, often years. The therapists themselves may change as their circumstances dictate, and a replacement will be found so that the group may continue. Sometimes these groups continue for years, with a slowly but ever-changing membership.

An extremely open group is one that people attend when possible, and may also be open to visitors. A group with a fluctuating membership works differently from an intensive, small group. An example might be that of the ward meeting.

By contrast, a closed group has a fixed membership, and often meets for an agreed period of time or number of sessions. Members who leave are not replaced. Examples of this type of group might be those established for a specific purpose, often to do with social skills training, where there may be a structured programme; or for training purposes for trainee therapists; or for contractual purposes.

## LARGE AND SMALL GROUPS

Groups may also be referred to as large or small. Groups in inpatient units may be referred to as the large group – also known as the community or ward meeting – and the small group – often an intensive therapy group.

A newcomer to the unit may wonder if there is any difference between the groups other than that of size. There is. The size of the group is likely to influence people's willingness and ability to share or disclose their thoughts and feelings with others. There is no fixed rule about the optimum size of a small therapy group, but eight to ten members is thought to be best in order that all members can relate to each other; it is both big enough for variety, and small enough for intimacy. However, some therapy groups will have 15 members, whereas in some small units this would represent all the community. Large groups commonly have over 15 members, and may have 100 or more if a unit is part of a larger community.

## VERBAL AND ACTION-BASED GROUPS

Groups may also be referred to as verbal or action-based. Some groups, notably traditional, analytic therapy groups, are verbal in their mode of conduct; others, perhaps using more recently developed techniques, may include a structured exercise, or an appropriate activity, for example art therapy, social skills training, psychodrama, Gestalt, and psychosynthesis. Many self-awareness or consciousness-raising groups are activity-based, and use techniques such as relaxation, guided imagery and visualization, mono-drama and regression, any of which may be experienced by the individual at a variety of levels, ranging from social to educational to therapeutic.

## Psychodrama

Psychodrama is a powerful way of working in groups. It has a particular format. The member working (the protagonist) is helped by the therapist (the director) to recreate a conflict he or she experienced in the past or experiences currently. Other group members enact roles in whichever situation is chosen. It is then acted through, as in a play or drama, with the protagonist being encouraged and helped to try out different or new behaviours, express thoughts and feelings that previously had been contained, reverse roles, or to observe while someone else plays his part, any or all of which may be in some way therapeutic. After the enactment of the drama, the group processes what happened and how they all felt as participants and observers, and help the protagonist to consolidate his learning from the experience.

The leader is directive and visible, and must be sensitive at all times to the individual and to the group as a whole. There is some safety in working in a structured way, but a climate of trust needs to be established in order for therapeutic change to occur. Because the protagonist will move between roles, he or she needs to have a sense of self and to know who he or she is. Psychodrama is not a technique for people with fragile ego bound-aries, who experience depersonalization, or other thought disorders such as delusions and hallucinations.

Other action-based groups use techniques such as structured exercises (games, art, problems to solve in a group); and fantasy (imaginary journeys or guided daydreams);

role-playing and re-enactment of situations. These all help the individual to explore and express feelings and thoughts. There is an emphasis on the here-and-now in the group, on spontaneity and taking risks, and open, honest feedback is encouraged between members. Other such groups include Gestalt, encounter, psychosynthesis, tran-sactional analysis, art therapy, and sensitivity training groups, all of which work on similar lines, the group facilitator drawing from the pool of techniques avail-able to her. Psychodramatic method is used in a variety of forms in many of the eclectic and action based groups (Chapter 34).

## ANALYTICALLY BASED GROUPS

In groups based on psychoanalytic principles the group itself is seen as the therapeutic medium. The conductor helps members to become aware of processes as they occur in the group, and of possible underlying parallel communications. The conductor is non-directive in order to allow collective, uncon-scious group processes to surface, which can then be explored. The term 'group processes' refers to patterns of interaction and relation-ship. For example if one person raises on issue and another changes the subject, this is 'process material'. An exploration of what happened, why, and how members feel about it can provide much material to work on.

## INTERACTION-BASED GROUPS

This type of group is based on the work of Yalom (1985). Known as interactional group therapy, it lays greater emphasis on conscious process and behaviour. Members are encour-aged to view the group as a safe environment, a venue in which new solutions may be ex-plored and enacted. There is no need for members to describe interpersonal problems, because sooner or later they will surface within the group as living relationships. Self-disclosure and honest feedback are key elements, and there is less emphasis on the unconscious group processes than in groups based on analytic principles. These groups may be seen as eclectic, at times paying attention to unconscious processes, at others being relatively active and directed.

## EDUCATIVE, SUPPORT, AND SELF-HELP GROUPS

The educative, support, and self-help groups provide perhaps the earliest model of group therapy. Providing information and advice about a problem, whatever its nature, and encouraging mutual support is the key feature of such groups. The role of the conductor is to maintain a non-threatening and cohesive atmosphere by setting limits on the level of personal disclosure and the amount of confrontation. The group might also have a set format by which it works. The conductor need not be professionally qualified, as is often the case in self-help groups. Examples of such groups include social skills training groups, Alcoholics Anonymous, Narcotics Anonymous, and support groups of various kinds that deal with specific problems, ranging from weight loss, to cancer, to phobic anxieties.

### Social skills training groups

The term 'social skills' covers a range of issues, from basic self-care and presentation to how people communicate with one another. It may also include stress management and self-awareness.

While the early years of life are crucial in the development of social skills and self-esteem, some remedial work can be done and gaps filled by working in groups that focus on the development of relationship skills. Often these will include theory and modelling of a skill, with practice and feedback.

While social skills training groups are usually structured and task-related, it is acknowledged that there may be deep psychological roots to some members' problems in relating to others. Such problems can be explored, if appropriate, in other settings.

A framework or programme is offered, and the group may meet for eight or ten sessions at a time, exploring and practising such skills as how to get to know each other, communicate clearly, be assertive, and deal with conflict. Much of the programme is focused on daily living skills, for example negotiating to watch a preferred television programme, or dealing with a demanding partner. After practice or a role-play, the experience is discussed in the group and key features are identified, such as what worked and what did not, how might a new skill be used in the actual setting, and how might the individual sabotage his own efforts, and the support he may need while trying to change.

The conductor in such a group is visible, directive, and gives information, while endeavouring to act as a role model for the members. Education and information processing is important, as is the opportunity to try out new behaviours in a safe setting, and to give and receive feedback after the exercises. As the group develops, members will engage in more complex levels of activity, and are likely to feel increasingly free to take risks. This process cannot be hurried; some groups will always work on a behavioural, dependent level that is to be determined by the members of the group as an unconscious process.

Whatever the type of group, all may be therapeutic for the client, and selection is important to suit the client to the type of group. Whatever the orientation of the group, the therapist should pay attention to group process and development, and work to bring about the emergence of therapeutic factors. The orientation of the group will guide the style of the conductor and the interventions made, but ultimately it is the group conductor who has to be sensitive to and aware of individual and group process, and act accordingly.

Some people find they work better in a particular type of group, whether this be analytic or action-based, although a prime factor in any therapeutic activity is the relationship with the therapist.

## THE GROUP STAFF MEMBER

Traditionally, the term 'conductor' or 'convener' is used within group theory to refer to the staff member. 'Leader' is a name given to one of the possible roles individuals might take in a group and is therefore mobile. The conductor or convener will have a leadership role in the early, dependent stages of the group and during subsequent crises, but otherwise the leader will come from the group itself.

## WHAT HAPPENS IN GROUPS?

This section outlines the stages of group development, group defensive processes, and how groups help people. These processes, phenomena, or factors occur in all groups, whatever their orientation, background, or purpose, and whether they are therapy groups or not. For example, the group leader in any group has to pay attention to helping the group develop a safe climate in which to work. All groups – therapeutic, managerial, or social – develop through the same stages or phases.

## STAGES OF GROUP DEVELOPMENT

Tuckman (1965) reviewed and summarized the findings of over 50 studies dealing with group development in various types of group. On the basis of this, he proposed a four-stage developmental model, which can be usefully applied to groups in all kinds of settings. He named these four stages **forming, storming, norming,** and **performing**. A fifth stage, **termination**, has been suggested by some authors (Levene, 1979). This model of group development is simple, and provides a

framework within which to reflect on and inform practice as a therapist. If this model is taken in conjunction with the work of other authors such as Bion (1961), greater depth of analysis can be gained.

## FORMING

How, then, do groups develop? How do they come about? If we consider a brand new group, like an intake of students entering training, or outpatients at the start of a closed group, some similarities are apparent. The process leading to this point will have included a referral agency, and some contact with the institution and the group conductor or his representative. Basic information will have been sought and exchanged, and a place offered and accepted. The biographical details asked of a prospective student will also be asked of a prospective patient, and hopes and insights will be explored with both individuals.

What happens when a group meets for the first time? Consider what you experienced when you started training and met for the first time; or when you get a new clinical placement, with a new group of people.

Typically, this first phase of group life is characterized for the individual by emotions such as anxiety, fear, anticipation, and excitement; curiosity also features, as we try to find out who is who, where they are from, and if they are likeable ('Will I like them?'; 'Will they like me?') Other questions may arise, such as: 'What am I supposed to do?' 'Who will tell me what to do?' 'Do I want to be here?' Behaviours may range from sitting quietly in a corner waiting to be noticed and approached, to being noisy, highly visible, and organizing contact and activity, or trying to do so. Both the behaviours, and the range in between, are individual methods of dealing with the anxiety of being in a new group and needing to be noticed by the conductor (parent figure), while not standing out too much.

The forming stage may last for several meetings. Over a period of time, the individual will probably begin to feel more like a member of the group than previously. This is also a time when there is a relatively high loss rate, with people leaving the group for a variety of expressed reasons. In relation to the conductor, this is a time of dependency, with members expecting that she will tell them what to do, how to do it, give permission, answer questions, solve problems, and keep the group safe.

While the conductor always has a responsibility to maintain safety, this may not be apparent when she reflects questions back rather than answering them. This may leave the questioner feeling uncomfortable, dissatisfied, or even hurt. The conductor has to strike a balance between allaying anxiety and helping the group and its members to develop a sense of safety, while simultaneously resisting the fostering of unhealthy dependence. Independence and self-direction are central to healthy functioning in adult life, as is the ability to develop attachments, which are not dependencies: we can love people and be separate from them.

Some authors refer to this early phase of group life as orientation (Yalom, 1985). Introductions are likely to be made; the conductor might model behaviours that later will be taken up by the members, for example, attempting to bring in people who are silent, and asking questions to encourage people to continue speaking.

Often at this stage the conductor is experienced as wonderful or awful, neither of which is probably true, and the conductor must be sensitive in the way she makes interventions in the group, while remembering that she is not personally responsible for the reactions of others. In psychodynamic terms, the group will regularly react unconsciously to the conductor as a parental figure rather than as the person she actually is. This 'transferential material' that emerges may or may not be worked on depending on the

setting. The conductor must be aware of these unconscious processes, and exercise choice over the use she makes of them. This is useful material, for example, in a therapy group, but is far less likely to be addressed in an educational group or social skills training, or when the group is still forming, and trust between members and the conductor is yet to be established.

During any stage of group life, discussion may be about 'outside' issues such as the environment, work, or family, and this often bears some relationship to what is not being discussed in the group. A comment such as 'Our rooms are really cold' might be brought inside the group as 'You say your rooms are cold. How do you feel in this room, right now?' This might open up a discussion on how people feel in the group, experiences of warmth, or being included or shut out, which are directly relevant to the group and the way its members interact with each other. This means people have to talk and express themselves, activities which, in the early stages of group life, will be undertaken tentatively, with only snippets being disclosed.

Little work in terms of the formal group task is done at this stage. People do not really hear what the other is saying, and are not willing, generally, to disclose much about themselves or their lives, and are too scared to give and receive interpersonal feedback. This is normal: trust has to be built and respect earned, and this is a time for testing the constancy and predictability of care within the group. It is worth exploring this process, as very often we expect clients to relate to us immediately and to tell us everything, and yet in a similar situation we also would be immobilized by anxiety and would disclose minimally, although sometimes people disclose precipitately, anxiously trying to replace discomfort by getting down to personal problems and issues.

The conductor can do much to make people feel safe, if for example, she can intervene to help to create a climate where people feel able to talk and express their anxieties. She can also hold and provide time and room boundaries, such as starting and finishing promptly, or keeping the same room available for the group each time it meets. Attentive listening and gently stopping precipitate self-disclosure also will contribute greatly to feelings of safety, as will being patient and non-judgemental.

Some action-based groups may use 'ice-breakers' or accelerating exercises at this stage, such as 'getting-to-know-you' games. Initially these may be useful in providing structure and some security, but also may act purely as an active diversion from anxiety and be relatively meaningless. Some people may be so anxious that they do not listen to others and are unable to introduce them to the group because they have not taken in what they were told. The conductor of a verbal group would not introduce such an activity, choosing to comment on the process as it happens, and to let the group make its own introductions in its own way. Some groups using exercises progress quickly, others do not. The same is true of verbal groups, and much depends on the individuals who make up the membership of the group.

STORMING

'Stormy' is an apt word for the next phase, which may be characterized by competition, hostility, and defensiveness. Members experience feelings such as fear, rage, anxiety, love, hate, inclusion, and rejection. It is a stage of establishing a pecking order: who is most and least liked, clever, intelligent, attractive, healthy, and sick. The pecking order is different for each individual, as each member projects different aspects of themselves on to others. **Projection** is the process by which we put on to others aspects of ourselves, for example, we might see someone as being very intelligent, and forget that we, too, are intelligent.

In this phase, subgroups may form and re-form, people may collude with each other, and disagree with each other. It is a stage of conflict as members try to sort out what each wants from the group and its process. Personal goals will be revealed that will conflict with those of others. For example, in an educational group personal goals may vary from, 'I like to have notes dictated' to, 'I don't want any lectures'; in a therapy group the equivalent might be, 'I won't say anything until I feel ready, and I don't know when that will be', to the individual who wants to start working on deep issues immediately, discloses a great deal of personal information in the early stages of the group, and scares most other members in the process, which the conductor may acknowledge as a defence against the anxiety generated by getting to know each other.

There may also be competition for roles within the group – often student representatives are elected while a group is still forming; a business meeting may elect a chairperson early on, and then by the storming phase he or she may find their ideas and leadership challenged. Equally, the authority of the conductor in a therapy group may be challenged and questioned.

People jostle for position in terms of influence and power, position, and attention, and many repeat roles that are already part of their repertoire: organizing, taking notes, joking, being obedient, or feeling responsible. One or two members may be scapegoated and blamed for everything that happens, and it may at times feel safer to blame the conductor or an outside authority than each other. However, to attack the conductor is also felt to be threatening: a group without a conductor, or one without authority, is ultimately frightening.

The role of the conductor here is to be aware of both the content and the underlying process, and to intervene to prevent any destructive events occurring. The balance to achieve is one of allowing people to state their feelings without blaming or making others feel responsible for them. For example, members might be encouraged to say, 'I feel cross' rather than, 'You make me cross'; 'I disagree' rather than, 'You're wrong'.

This stage may be uncomfortable for both members and conductor. As a conductor it can be difficult at times not to get caught up in the group and unconsciously collude with some of the processes. It is also important for the conductor to help the group to weather the storm rather than to calm things down. An essential part of groupwork is the development of an ability to be aware of and honest about feelings and other people, – to prevent healthy argument is not useful. Of course, intervention, containment, and saying 'stop' may also be necessary, and in this the conductor needs experience, knowledge, and skill.

Minimal work at a deep level is accomplished at this stage, but the working-through of these early difficulties will provide a solid base for the resolution of future difficulties and will aid group cohesion. Healthy relationships enable the group to tolerate and resolve conflict, and having done so once makes it easier to do so again in the future.

## NORMING

The third phase, 'norming', is one of setting behavioural rules and the establishment of belief systems. At this stage the individual begins to experience a sense of belonging and achievement, and that the group is cohesive and is beginning to accept individual differences. It is very human to want to be part of a group and to identify with it, while also wishing to remain individual and not to be taken over: to conform but still be valued for one's differences.

The group develops a way of working in order to achieve its objective, with members starting to talk more freely about themselves, offering disclosures, and support. By this stage, people begin to feel more confident. They are more readily accepting of themselves and others, and feel more accepted by others in turn.

Another 'norm' might be about the level of disclosure, for example, the group might tell a member it has heard all it can tolerate; others may be invited to participate more fully. Those who have never been in such a group before may feel anxious that sooner or later they will be expected to talk about themselves. The disclosure of a similar piece of information may be easy for one person but impossible for another because of the associations and history that go with it. Here, the role of the conductor is to be supportive of all members, and to mentally note what is happening: the verbal content and the underlying process and dynamics; who speaks and who is quiet; how members react, verbally and non-verbally. She does this at all stages, and feeds back to the group what is useful and relevant. She may find that as the group develops its own way of working, she intervenes less and less, and may occasionally address comments to help individuals and the group to progress.

## PERFORMING

In Tuckman's final stage, the group, having done the necessary work of the previous stages, gets on with its deeper tasks. This may be described as a mature group or a 'work group' (Bion, 1961.) The members feel they are a group, can relate and give direct feedback to each other, and can care for each other on a deep level, where personal liking is relatively unimportant. At this stage, roles may vary as people do what suits them best. The leadership and other roles may be identified with various participants depending on the task in hand.

This is a therapeutic stage, when insight and the ability to work through develops, and constructive self-change begins to occur. For example, in a small therapy group, as they have learned that the group offers an opportunity for help rather than judgement and punishment, members may feel safe and cared about enough to risk disclosing 'secret' information. Often people are eventually able to share feelings and experiences which they have never felt able to speak of before. Feelings of rejection, anger, sadness, memories of abuse, or the admission of deviant behaviour may all be revealed at this stage. Accompanying the verbal disclosure intense emotions may be experienced, and perhaps for the first time in his or her life, the individual may be able to express these feelings rather than hold them in. To be able to cry or to be angry is in itself a great release and can be therapeutic; to find that others support you in doing it can be a tremendously freeing experience.

The conductor's role here is to follow the process and to help it unfold. People may need to cry for the duration of the group, and perhaps longer, but the conductor nevertheless should keep to time, while also helping other members to share their feelings before the group finishes. Many may be touched by what they have heard, and may also identify with the situation or the feelings. The balance the conductor tries to achieve is between the individual and the group, with the needs of both being respected. The group should finish at its set time, and the last few minutes should be spent winding down, with either the members or the conductor bringing attention to the time available.

Being in a performing or working group can be both exhilarating and exhausting, freeing and frightening. A taste of insight and catharsis provides plenty of energy to do more, but the individual must be helped to consolidate what he has done before moving on, which takes a tremendous amount of energy. Other people may be scared by the depth of work they have witnessed or participated in, and hold back for a while. Often a group which works deeply one session will hold back the next. Some task-centred groups, for example, experience a tremendous sense of achievement when they produce what is expected of them, but choose never to repeat the challenge, turning down the next project offered them.

TERMINATION

Groups come to an end either because they were established for a fixed time or because members move on. When endings and departures are known about, this period of notice allows the opportunity for the ending to be worked through, However, this does not always happen: individuals may begin to close down, to be silent and participate less than they did earlier, giving many reasons such as 'There isn't enough time left', or, 'We'll never meet again', even when there are several sessions left.

The last few weeks of a group is not the best time to bring up deep issues, so reticence is understandable. However, such profound issues are sometimes placed before the group by its members, often as part of a denial that the group is ending. Both the reticence and inappropriate disclosure may be understood as defensive.

There may also be idealization during this stage, for example, 'This group was the best ever; we loved each other right from the start', which is probably not true. Also, people might discuss future plans rather than stay in the present. Members may exchange addresses and phone numbers in an attempt to recreate the group after it finishes. Equally, many members use the ending stage and work through it. It may also provide an arena for working through earlier losses and separations in a therapeutic way, rather than denying past and present sadness. Termination issues do not only occur at the end of groups, but can be provoked by other separations – holiday breaks, for example, or the absence of a group member.

Some people cope with endings by leaving first, failing to turn up to the final few groups, or booking a holiday for the last week and thereby avoiding the pain of ending. Some people will need a lot of support at this stage, and may need to proceed to further therapy; this may be the case if the group has been relatively short term, and issues have been raised but not fully explored. A person might wish to enter individual therapy, for example, or a long-term group.

While the conductor cannot make people attend or work, she can point out the processes as they occur, and help the group by offering exploratory and supportive interventions, while remaining firm that the group will end, and that extensions are not possible.

## THE LIFE OF THE GROUP

A group may work one week and then use the following session to renegotiate norms, and seem not be performing. This regressive move happens often when there is a threat of some sort; perhaps the task is too difficult, or there is a change coming up, such as a holiday break, or members leaving or joining, which might mean the group has to re-form. A single new member may be incorporated into the group relatively easily, while three or four may change the group so radically that a new group is created, perhaps with some 'culture carriers' who know the rules – or think they do. Control over timing the admission of new members is much easier in an outpatient setting than on an admissions ward, where it can be difficult to refuse to admit someone who needs residential care. One or two floridly disturbed people can influence the whole ward atmosphere, and the groups within that ward.

## DEFENSIVE PROCESSES IN GROUPS

Bion (1961) writes about two types of group: the work group, which is similar to the performing group, and the basic-assumption group. The latter occurs as an unconscious group defence to a threat, and may take the following forms:

- dependency on the leader – whether the formal or an informal leader;
- fight or flight – i.e., confrontation and challenge within the group among members or of the conductor, and flight into the past, the future, or the outside world;
- pairing – here, the communication is between couples, and members may be encouraged to work, to discuss, or to dominate the group in some way. Bion describes the unconscious fantasy that a Messiah will be produced who will rescue the group from its current state. This is often referred to as the 'messianic fantasy'.

Using the model of Tuchman and Bion, the nurse has two complementary frameworks of group life, one of developmental stages and the other of unconscious defences. She can then begin to describe and analyze what happens in groups by identifying the processes that occur, and that often account for events and behaviours within the group. The experienced practitioner can hold this framework during a group and intervene appropriately.

Someone new to groupwork may find this difficult to achieve, and will need to develop skills of internal (personal) supervision or self-monitoring. All group conductors need to review their groups in a supervisory setting so they might reflect on what happened, and consider their own interventions once the group has finished. This is good practice as it allows for blocks and collusions to be explored, new strategies to be discussed, and teaching to occur.

## THERAPEUTIC FACTORS IN GROUPS

It is useful to look at how groups work, and to examine the knowledge and skills needed to enhance the likelihood of a therapeutic outcome. A vast literature exists on groupwork; here we will introduce some basic concepts, one of which is therapeutic, or curative, factors (Bloch, 1985; Yalom, 1985), which are what people report as conditions or mechanisms within a group that have helped them to change in some way for the better.

How can a nurse help a group to create conditions for change? She must realize and believe that she alone, or the rest of the staff involved, are not able to control the unconscious life of the group and the group's process; she alone cannot make people speak during a silence, or share problems or opinions, which will happen when the group is ready and not before. She can note what is happening and perhaps share her thoughts, but she cannot make a group do what it is not ready to do.

Few people will speak in a group when they feel threatened, afraid, and unsure, or imagine they will be judged or rejected. The conductor cannot make things easier for each group member. She can, however, intervene to help people to introduce themselves; comment on how anxious individuals and the group seems to be; and invite them to speak rather than to stay silent. She might also interpret the process of which the silence is a part. Speaking in a new group, or as a new member entering an existing group, takes courage, and this needs to be acknowledged. Frequently, people are afraid of being rejected in some way if they were to say how they feel; this anxiety has to be tested by each member in order that confidence can be enhanced.

Yalom (1985) describes eleven therapeutic factors, briefly outlined below. Some are **mechanisms of change**, others are **conditions for change**.

### Instillation of hope

Some clients may benefit from the conductor's confidence that she and the group are able to help, and from hearing other members tell their stories and how they have come through.

### Universality

This refers to the discovery that one is not alone in one's feelings, thoughts, or experiences. Sharing information about oneself may be very difficult, but the discovery that others have similar problems or feelings can bring about a great sense of relief, changing the previous feelings of isolation.

### Imparting information

It is helpful at times to give instruction or advice to clients, either to structure the group, as in action-based groups, or to explain what might be happening with individuals or in the group as a whole. This information may quite appropriately be given by other group members – it is not necessarily the responsibility of the conductor alone.

### Altruism

At times clients may gain by giving to others. Feeling that one has helped or been useful to someone, for example by listening or giving advice, may increase the self-esteem of the client, especially if he experiences feelings of worthlessness. Altruism is also the process of doing something because it is right rather than because of an expectation of personal gain. The experience of selfless generosity as either recipient or donor may address many issues, for example, greed, jealousy, envy, suspicion, and even a deeper paranoia.

### Development of socializing techniques

Clients who have not learnt how to relate to others may benefit tremendously from practising social skills and receiving feedback from others on their behaviour. Some groups address social skills training as their main task, others include such feedback when it spontaneously arises.

### Imitative behaviour

This refers to benefit gained by copying the behaviour of a group member or the conductor which seemed to work for them; it also refers to observing someone else work with a problem and gaining insights from it - so-called 'vicarious therapy'.

## Corrective recapitulation

Problems with others are likely to be re-enacted within the group, and the emphasis here is that they are re-lived or re-experienced in a corrective manner, that is the old family patterns are explored, and opportunities for change occur.

## Interpersonal learning

Yalom writes extensively about three areas of learning between or from people: the importance of interpersonal relationships; the corrective emotional experience; and the group as a social microcosm.

## Group cohesiveness

This concept is difficult to define, but refers to the group's 'attractiveness' to its members. A cohesive group is often experienced as one with a high rate of attendance and level of commitment, wherein members want to meet and work together; members care about, support, and accept each other. People often describe the experience of being able to be themselves in such a group, and may feel, perhaps for the first time in their lives, that they belong.

## Catharsis

The experience and expression of feelings is often described as helpful, especially when they have been withheld for a long period of time. Emotional expression alone, however, is not enough. Therapeutic change comes about from a combination of catharsis and cognitive processes, such as insight or sense-making, alongside other factors, such as working through and re-experiencing.

## Existential factors

This refers to a sense of accepting or recognizing that sometimes life is the way it is; acknowledging that we cannot change our past; and that the future will not be assuredly problem-free. It also relates to a developing ability to take responsibility for oneself. This may be experienced at a deep or central level as a form of acceptance of ourselves and our life experience.

These therapeutic factors do not occur in isolation or in any particular sequence. It may be that the feelings of belonging, or cohesion, result in an individual being able to express how he feels, catharsis, with gains achieved from the processes of universality and information-giving all contributing to a therapeutic experience. An understanding of therapeutic factors can also inform the practice of the conductor, when they are taken in conjunction with an understanding of group developmental processes and defensive processes.

## THERAPEUTIC COMMUNITIES

Many currently established practices in mental health settings are rooted in or derived from therapeutic communities, which can be seen almost as a perpetual group. There is a wide literature on therapeutic communities, which defines what they are and what they are not (Kennard, 1986). The debate centres on therapeutic communities 'proper', which are by definition residential; and therapeutic community 'approaches', which are used in a variety of settings, not necessarily residential, and which may not be regarded as therapeutic communities because they fail or choose not to follow all the precepts that define a therapeutic community.

Rapoport (1960) identified four main principles of therapeutic community practice: democracy, permissiveness, reality confrontation, and communalism. Adherence to these principles will enable the community and its members to reflect on and analyze all aspects of life within the community, and to learn from social, as well as overtly therapeutic, settings and events.

The practice of democracy means residents are encouraged to be independent and responsible for themselves. For example, staff do not necessarily make decisions, these being negotiated among the whole community or representatives of it. Some communities have 'senior residents' who have particular roles, which in other settings might be undertaken by staff alone, such as selection of new residents and staff.

Permissiveness and reality confrontation go hand-in-hand: much behaviour is permitted and tolerated with the intention of exploring it. The individual retains responsibility for his behaviour and its effects on the community. Emergency community meetings may be called if, for example, a person cuts himself or gets drunk, in which the community as a whole will explore what happened, and decide what if anything should be done, and which sanctions if any apply.

Communalism means that everything within the community is shared. This includes housekeeping and the maintenance of the setting, and the living and learning that occurs. Just as residents have groups, so do staff, which are used for exploring their relationships to each other in terms of support and supervision rather than for therapy.

Underlying these principles is one of openness of communication, of making explicit what is implict, and stating what is being withheld. Only in this way can a community or group begin to examine and resolve problems and difficulties, whether they be inter- or intra-personal.

## THERAPEUTIC COMMUNITY APPROACHES

Many mental health nurses might usefully question their practice with the intention or understanding the underlying principles that guide their work. This would include an exploration of boundaries: how much responsibility do I want to give my clients, and how much can I realistically give them, given the setting in which we work, the wider institution, or community? In other words, how can mental health units be made more democratic and less authoritarian? On a personal level, how much do I need to be in control? Do I feel responsible for other people's behaviour? Also, permissiveness – in the sense of seeking immediate gratification – is not fashionable at the moment, and what we do as nurses is influenced by the outside world.

## THE WARD OR COMMUNITY MEETING

Perhaps the most problematic group in general inpatient psychiatry wards is the ward meeting, which may also be called the community meeting, or business meeting, or large group, or morning group. These terms, and probably more, are used to describe a regular time when the ward community – patients, and staff – meet, whether daily, weekly, or somewhere in between.

Kennard (1983) suggests that the community meeting might fulfil several purposes. For example, people meet as a whole and are reminded they are part of that whole; information can be shared, decisions made, interpersonal difficulties aired, and possibly resolved. It certainly might be an arena in which democracy is increased and authoritarianism decreased by sharing decision-making or information-giving.

Each unit, ward, or residential setting can suggest its own guidelines for the community meeting. These will be influenced by the client group involved, and their ability to tolerate unstructured large groups. It is quite appropriate to have and hold guidelines for the ward meeting, and, paradoxically, to allow them to evolve with conscious awareness of this process. Certainly with disturbed people it is important to be able to provide a structure that can contain and hold until the client is able to do this for himself; the therapist's role is to be caring and therapeutic, not to further increase anxiety in already distressed people. Likewise, one would not wish to provide so formal a structure that it holds clients back and promotes an unhealthy dependency, as opposed to dependability and consistency.

We all need structures and frameworks within which to organize our lives, and it is a skilled and able person who can hold a structure while remaining flexible and responsive. It is important to ask ourselves the questions, 'Why do we have a ward or community meeting?'; 'What purpose does it serve?'; 'What purpose could it serve?'; What is relevant for discussion within the meeting?'; 'Should there be a chairperson and an agenda, or should it be unstructured?'; 'Who should attend?'; 'Is it acceptable for people to not attend?'

If these issues are discussed by staff and clients together, a shared feeling of ownership of the meeting may well emerge. It is then important to operate the meeting in the agreed way and to give it time to become established, and not just evaluate it after, say, one month, decide it is not working, and cancel the whole thing. Rather, thoughts and feelings must be shared and explored.

The therapeutic-community approach is useful in many settings, for example in rehabilitation units, group homes, and hostels, where it provides a model for promoting independence and responsibility for oneself and others. The social structure itself is therapeutic in a way of facilitating growth in clients and residents, and the diminishing of authority and power relationships allows all members of the client community to contribute to the whole.

## TRAINING

The vast majority of mental health nurses have most likely received insufficient training or experience in working in groups, when-

ever they qualified. Group analysis and group therapy have developed rapidly since the 1930s and 1940s, but this has not been significantly reflected in mental health nurse training and supervision. Many tutors are unable to facilitate learning about and experience in groups, having themselves never learned experientially about groups.

Mental health nurses are now realizing that groups are an important part of a therapeutic programme, but are being run by other staff. For example, occupational therapists frequently run social skills training groups, stress awareness and management, and anyone who has an interest, or has undertaken further training, in groupwork may be involved in running small, therapy groups.

There are many reasons why nurses have relatively less formal involvement in groups than other professionals. Until recently nurses had a relatively secure, prescribed role in institutional care, whereas psychologists, occupational therapists, and psychiatric social workers have sought to develop their roles and expertise. They have done this in specialized ways, and have seen and filled gaps in the previously existing therapeutic menu by offering groups as a way of working, and, quite appropriately, have claimed ownership of this.

How do nurses learn about groups? The best way of learning about groups is to be a member of one. Many colleges of nursing that prepare student mental health nurses for practice include group dynamics in the educational programme. However, this may cause problems, especially if one considers the irregularity of meetings and the confusion one may experience between being a student one minute and a client the next, and between being a teacher one minute and a group conductor the next. This muddies the therapeutic field, and may adversely influence the overall group and educational processes.

The inclusion of group dynamics in mental health nurse training may often be a limited, though well-intentioned exercise, which does not provide the nurse with the experience most clients gain of being a part of a regular, ongoing, discrete group. One alternative may be to provide an introductory, ongoing group for all students, with a facilitator who does not have teaching responsibilities. A further, more intensive group experience might be offered to those who wish to continue with personal work while they are students. All nurses should join a weekly support group as an expectation during training; as well, membership of seminar groups should continue after qualification as a prerequisite of professional practice.

Currently, the first-level registration programme is generalist, and rightly so. Further training in groupwork is available in many colleges of further and higher education and specialist training establishments (below).

A key feature of sound, reflective, professional practice is the mental health nurse's own supervision and possibly therapy. This is a requirement of any advanced professional training, but should also be available on a regular basis in the clinical setting for all nurses working with groups, whether or not they are undertaking further development.

## CONCLUSION

This chapter has addressed the rationale for working in groups, and has explored some basic concepts of group development, defensive processes, and how groups help people. Particular types of group have been described, and suggestions have been made for further training opportunities.

As in individual psychotherapy, the range of orientations is broad, from behavioural to psychoanalytic, and the degree of structure and the role of the therapist varies according to the underlying model. Ultimately, the quality of the relationship between all members of the group, and also their relationship with the therapist, is paramount in influencing the outcome of the group experience, whatever the orientation. Groups have a central part to play in current and future mental health nursing.

## REFERENCES

Bion, W. R. (1961) *Experiences in Groups*, Tavistock, London.
Kennard, D. K. (1983) *An Introduction to Therapeutic Communities*, Routledge, London.
Levene, B. (1979) *Group Psychotherapy: Practice and Development*, Prentice-Hall, New Jersey.
Tuckman, B. W. (1965) Developmental sequence in small groups. *Psychological Bulletin*, 63, 6.
Yalom, I. D. (1985) (3rd edn) *The Theory and Practice of Group Psychotherapy*, Basic Books, New York.

## FURTHER READING

Aveline, M. and Dryden W. (1988) (eds) *Group Therapy in Britain*, Open Univ. Press, Milton Keyness.
Bloch, S. (1985) *Therapeutic Factors in Group Psychotherapy*, Oxford Univ Press, Oxford.
Clark, D. H. (1981) *Social Therapy in Psychiatry* Churchill-Livingstone, Edinburgh.
Hinshelwood, R. D. and Manning, N. (1979) (eds) *Therapeutic Communities: Reflections and Progress*, Routledge, London.
Johnson, D. W. and Johnson, F. P. (1987) (3rd edn) *Joining Together: Group Theory and Group Skills*, Prentice Hall, New Jersey.
Kreeger, L. (1975) (ed.) *The Large Group*, Constable London.
Whitaker, D. S. 1985 *Using Groups to Help People*, Routledge, London.
Whiteley, J. S. and Gordon, J. (1979) *Group Approaches in Psychiatry*, Routledge, London.
Wright, H. (1989) *Groupwork: Perspectives and Practice*, Scutari, London.

## OPPORTUNITIES FOR TRAINING

The following organizations offer training in various aspects of groupwork, sometimes in regional centres.

The Association of Therapeutic Communities
c/o Peper Harow Foundation
14 Charterhouse Square
London EC1
071 251 0672

The Cassel Hospital
1 Ham Common
Richmond, Surrey

The Institute of Advanced Nursing Education
The Royal College of Nursing
20 Cavendish Square
London WM 1AB
071 409 3333

The Institute of Group Analysis
1 Daleham Gardens
London NW3 5BY
071 431 2693

The Lincoln Institute for Psychotherapy
Lincoln Tower
77 Westminster Bridge Road
London SE1
071 928 7211

The London Centre for Psychotherapy
19 Fitzjohns Avenue
London NW3
071 435 0873

The Tavistock Clinic
120 Belsize Lane
London NW3
071 435 7111

Westminster Pastoral Foundation
23 Kensington Square
London W8 5HN
071 937 9355/6956

# CREATIVE AND EXPRESSIVE APPROACHES

*Jean Simms*

There are myriad creative and expressive approaches to mental health nursing that are of value for their liberalizing and humanizing effect, and for developing human potential. Science may provide the mental health nurse with knowledge on which to base her nursing care, but art adds a dimension in stimulating creative, expressive, and imaginative ways of working. Creative and expressive approaches are more than ways of working; they are also ways of being – a form of humanism.

Humanism is a philosophy that 'asserts the intrinsic worth of humans and their capacity for fulfilment'. Art, literature, drama, poetry, and other forms of creative expression can all help in the understanding and alleviating of human distress as part of a holistic mental health culture.

The root of the word 'health' is the Greek *holos*, meaning whole. *Holos* is also the original meaning of the Anglo-Saxon word meaning 'well'. The word 'holy' also comes from the same root; so the healthy, well person is not only someone who is physically healthy, but also someone who is spiritually aware. There are therapies that concentrate on the mental, spiritual, and inner life, for example, psychoanalytic, psychodynamic, behaviourism, and humanistic approaches – the latter including psychosynthesis and transpersonal psychology. And there are body-orientated therapies, such as bioenergetics, biodynamic therapy, and biosynthesis.

This section explores ideas from the literature, and from people using creative and expressive ways of working with clients. It is not intended to be prescriptive, but rather to open up to the mental health nurse the possible approaches that could be incorporated into mental health principles and practices.

At an individual clinical level the possibilities are infinite, but it is also important to consider the context in which therapy takes place. In the present political and economic climate, ethical decisions may be influenced by organizational constraints where matters of cost-effectiveness are likely to be relevant. The pressure of using groups and time-limited therapy, as opposed to longer-term individual therapy, may be institutionally exerted, especially as long client waiting lists grow.

## THE NURSE/CLIENT RELATIONSHIP

What is so special about the relationship between the mental health nurse and the client? Is it that nursing can be quantified, with strict observance and conformance to methodology? – or is it an art, concerned with quality and the uniqueness of the individual? Brandon (1982), writing of this relationship believes:

> The art and science of psychiatric practice should be inseparable. In medicine practice in general, and in psychiatry in particular, the traditional concern is with the highly personal, intimate, and confidential relationship between the individual doctor and his/her unique patient. The emotional distress associated with psychiatric disturbance, the confessional element of the psychiatric consultation, and the time spent in face-to-face contact

does lead towards an unusually intense patient/doctor relationship. Within the relationship lies much of the art of medicine.

Historically, from the beginning of the century the mentally ill were cared for in custodial settings. Paternalistic attitudes were the norm, and the clients were often removed from society, with many institutions built away from towns and cities and apart from the ordinary population. In the 1950s and 1960s more liberal approaches were developed. These, together with the introduction of psychotropic drugs, became a turning-point in the care and treatment of the mentally ill.

During the past 20 years, there has been an increasing growth in rehabilitation, and a better understanding of the effect of institutionalization and of social factors. Psychiatrists like the American Harry Stack Sullivan influenced such changes by looking at patterns of communication between people. The core of Sullivan's work rests on the propositions that: a large part of mental disorder results from and is perpetuated by inadequate communications; anxiety interferes with the communicative process; and each person involved in two personal relationships is affected by the other, and is not a separate, personal entity.

Psychiatrists like Laing agreed with Sullivan about interpersonal, accurate communication. Writing in 1967, Laing stated that; 'theory is the articulated vision of experience.' Practice arises from being and working with the client. Laing believed passionately about physical, psychological and spiritual integration:

> Without inner reality, with just enough sense of continuity to clutch at identify - the current idolatry. Torn – body, mind and spirit – by inner contradictions, pulled in different directions. Man is cut off from his own mind, cut off equally from his own body – a half crazed creature in a mad world.

Laing, so pervasively humanistic, eloquently defined psychotherapy as 'an obstinate attempt of two persons to recover the wholeness of being human through the relationship between them'.

Mental health nurses are in a privileged position to make contact with clients/to bring about change, and to recover this 'wholeness' in both themselves and the clients they come into contact with.

The mental health nurse's main aim must be to maximize the time spent with clients. As potentially equal partners in this relationship – although issues of power and engagement need to be appreciated and worked through – each brings to such encounters their own personalities, styles of living, values, belief systems, and attitudes.

## WORKING CREATIVELY

By introducing creative and expressive ways into care, mental health nurses cannot only use the nurse/client encounter to bring about change, but also create a more accepting, caring culture. Working creatively and expressively in the context of the NHS may take courage, patience, sensitivity, and a great deal of perseverance, as succinctly stated by Hippocrates:

> Life is short, the art of medicine is long, time passes quickly, experience is fallacious, and judgement is difficult. It is not enough for the doctor to do the necessary, but the patient, his relatives, and the environment must play their part, and...if you can do no good, at least do no harm.

Many of the creative and expressive approaches require a matching of mental health nurse with client, and considering an eclectic way of working. Eclecticism comes in many forms, but working creatively and expressively should never mean working in a chaotic, muddled or mindless way.

Creative and expressive ways of working are aimed at empowering, enhancing self-esteem, and making interpersonal communication more meaningful. Many therapists believe that abreaction of catharsis – establishing contact with suppressed emotions and giving vent to them – and re-enactment of the traumatic event may help the healing process. Heron (1975) has little doubt that cathartic episodes can relieve the primary tensions of the human condition, for example, the longing for human closeness, the universal fact of separation, and the secondary tensions 'due to humans interfering with and hurting each other'.

Satir (1900) believes that increasing self-esteem is made possible by the willingness to be open to new possibilities. She has developed 'The Five Freedoms'. Living these freedoms is in Satir's opinion the strongest personal power one can have:

1. The freedom to see and hear what is here instead of what should be, was, or will be.
2. The freedom to say what one feels and thinks, instead of what one should.
3. The freedom to feel what one feels, instead of what one ought.
4. The freedom to ask for what one wants, instead of always waiting for permission.
5. The freedom to take risks on one's own behalf, instead of choosing to be only secure and not rocking the boat.

## TRANSPERSONAL PSYCHOLOGY

From a transpersonal perspective, ways of working with clients encompass, as Grof (1982) states, the 'increasing convergence of Western physics and Eastern metaphysics, of modern consciousness research and Eastern spiritual systems.'

'Transpersonal' was a world coined by Carl Jung, who severed connections, with Sigmund Freud and the psychoanalytical movement in 1914. In Jungian psychology, the whole personality is referred to as the psyche; the ego is the conscious mind, and co-existing with it is the personal unconscious. The personal unconscious is composed of experiences that have been suppressed, ignored, or forgotten; the collective unconscious consists of non-personal experiences, of universal archetypes or mental images. Operating within the psyche are a number of separate systems, such as the self, the 'shadow' – representing the darker side of human nature – and the 'anima' and 'animus', the feminine side of man's nature and the masculine side of woman's respectively; the 'persona' is the mask used to conceal thoughts and feelings.

Transpersonal approaches are concerned with altered states of consciousness, and work with three main theoretical assumptions. First, the collective unconscious – collective because it is the physical environment and the universal source of healing and energy. Past, present, and future are contained within it. It embraces all levels of awareness, from the instinctual to the transcendent; the fundamental building-blocks and patterns of the psyche, which Jung called archetypes, are found there. It may also be regarded as the continuum of energy and consciousness because it is a realm where fundamental life impulses to meaning, and wholeness and fulfilment reside.

One of the concepts underpinning transpersonal psychology is that life is a journey. Jung called this journey individuation, where the ego, after meeting crisis after crisis, eventually turns within to discover meaning. He wrote (1953):

> We can hardly help feeling that the unconscious process moves spiralwise round a centre, gradually getting closer, while the characteristics of the Centre grow more and more distinct. Or perhaps we could put it another way round and say that the Centre is itself virtually unknowable - acts like a magnet on the disparate material and processes of the unconscious and gradually captures them in a crystal lattice...Often one has the impression that the personal psyche is running around this central point like a shy animal, at once fascinated and frightened, always in flight, and yet, steadily drawing nearer.

Meditation is one way of working from a transpersonal perspective, a way of steadying the mind, and, according to Heron (1975), of 'witnessing primarily inner events, sensations, desires, moods, feelings, agitations, anxiety, images and ideas'. Attention can also be focused on some mental content, an image, a word, a concept, posture, or breathing. This practice is effective in stilling the mind and gaining access to a wide range of altered states of consciousness.

## DRAWING OUT THE PLEASURE AND THE PAIN

Art, so often the concern and practice of so few, is a powerful means of expressing ideas, thoughts, feelings, and emotions. Art therapy is a way of helping clients to express visually their deepest thoughts and feelings.

Richard Fuller has worked as an art therapist in the mental health services for the past 12 years. He believes the clients he works with fall into two categories: those who have chronic, long-standing problems, and whose lives are not going to change dramatically; and those who enter hospital for a few weeks with more acute problems. Fuller believes art can improve the quality of life for clients with intractable problems of living, and for those who may have to cope with depression, agitation, crisis, or a temporary inability to cope. For the more acutely distressed client, Fuller sees the task as enabling the client to work towards specific goals, and achieving a better state of mind in order to deal more effectively with their life.

When helping clients to make an image, Fuller tries as far as possible to let them work spontaneously; occasionally he will suggest a theme, and afterwards allow time for the client to reflect on what has been produced. It is the giving of form to their experience that remains, as a reminder accessible to them, 'like an entry in a diary, a personal communication'. The images produced may be private or generalized, and, at first, not evidence of much psychological content. For example, people who are not violent in their lives may produce work that evokes feelings of violence. Therapy provides a context, an atmos-

phere of safety where powerful feelings can be contained, faced, and worked through towards some kind of resolution.

Making images and symbols is a spontaneous activity many children freely engage in, but often give it up as they grow older and more inhibited. Much of the work within art therapy sessions is childlike, in the sense of being untutored and spontaneous. It can thus generate the primary emotions of early life, such as rage and frustration, the sort of rage that is felt by a child who says to her mother, 'I wish you were dead.'

Fuller tends to interpret the work as little as possible, because he feels his interpretation is not much use to the client if they do not see it for themselves. He does, however, use theoretical models, the three main ones being Freudian, which gives the background for the unconscious; Jungian, for the art of psychological thinking; and a phenomenological, or humanistic, framework for dealing with the present.

Freud (1916) acknowledged that images are important, likening them to dreams, and dreams to art. However, art is more permanent than dreams; Freud believed it helped to lead people from fantasy back to reality.

When an artist produces a piece of creative work, it is usually with a knowledge of what the subject matter is, how it will be produced, and what shape, form, and so on in which, it will be communicated. The creative act itself may be as important and therapeutic to the artist as the finished product. For the client using art as a way of communicating, there is a different reason for taking part in the creative act: it is a means by which the unconscious of the client is brought to a more conscious level. The role of the therapist/ nurse is to provide a safe context for this to happen in. As one client summed up a personal experience of art therapy:

Drawing was a tremendous way for me to release feelings and learn to get in touch with my inner life. At the very beginning, I used art simply to express my rage at the world – scrubbing at the paper with brush and crayon, using violent colours and movements. What a relief it was to get it on paper after all the time I had spent damping down my feelings with too much medication and too much repression – to share these feelings with someone I could trust, who listened and helped me to face whatever came up as a result of this process.

For Della, a mental health student nurse, art is one of the most powerful mediums for communication she knows:

I have used art ever since I can remember. For me it is a very personal, powerful medium. If there are situations in my life I feel unhappy about and cannot make sense of, I paint them out. Art is a spontaneous, active process. After working creatively, usually with paint because the materials are more readily accessible, I feel more in control. Through my art I can usually see things I have been avoiding. I know I can no longer go on avoiding them, but need to face whatever it is.

Not only does Della use art for herself, she has also used art with several clients. Lotte, for example, was a young girl with severe learning difficulties. She lived in a residential setting, and had become very institutionalized, isolated, and depressed. Verbal communication was limited, and Lotte seemed to have given up trying to make other people understand.

Della spent time trying to engage Lotte in a relationship. She used non-verbal ways, such as touch, and tried clay as a medium to enable Lotte to express herself. It took time for Lotte to hold the clay, squeeze it, and feel its texture, and then, slowly, to begin to make a shape. Recalled Della:

I wanted her to know I really cared about her and what she did mattered. I didn't want to make a judgement on what she was attempting to create with the clay, but just to show her I respected her, and

wanted her to express herself and share something of her world with me.

As the relationship progressed, Lotte began to let some of her defences down and feel she had the right to express her feelings and have control over her work with the clay: she was free to do what she liked with it – even if that meant destroying it.

Della hoped she could influence staff to use art in their interactions with clients. She was met with a mixture of hostility, scepticism, and curiosity:

Some of the staff displayed very defensive attitudes, and made assumptions about the work I was doing with Lotte. Initially they were very over-protective to her, and found me threatening. My way of offering time and space for Lotte raised issues for them, and it took time before they could see that I was not undermining their work with her in any way, but simply adding to it.

Another child Della used art with was a black boy who had a white mother. The little boy was very self-conscious of his colour, tended to polarize black and white, and was confused about his culture and identity. Della encouraged him to paint people, mixing and using a variety of colours. The mixing enabled him to see he could find a shade exactly like his own. He then went on to explore colour and the richness and diversity of the colours of different peoples of the world:

All these 'people paints', and the colours he used helped him to express some of his unspoken feelings, and have an increased awareness of his own identify. We used about ten colours, and he really began to be very exhilarated when we mixed them up in different ways. When he saw the lights and shades in the different colours, he gradually began to accept his own colour in a positive way.

The principles that apply to therapeutic relationships, such as respecting both the individual and the relationship, and the importance of warmth, genuineness, empathy, and unconditional positive regard, are vitally important:

> Whatever form it takes, art is neither good nor bad. It is people trying to express themselves, and their subjective experiences need to be accepted as real and important. My own artwork was once criticized for being fragmented. Although they were trying to make the point that something was not quite right in my painting, my critics could not see that it was just the way it was. At the time I was feeling fragmented, so why should my art be different from my feelings?

Della's own feelings, in keeping with many other professionals working in mental health settings, are that creative and expressive therapies should be part of the organization's culture, and not just confined to single therapy sessions.

In the setting of a long-stay ward, Della and a group of Project 2000 mental health branch students recently used art to encourage a group of clients, often seen as difficult and unresponsive, to get to know them better. It was an attempt to establish rapport, and through the medium of painting of providing a safe place. The encounter allowed time for sharing between nurse and client.

Like all such encounters, this was difficult for clients and students alike. There were many conflicting issues, such as the invasion of the clients' privacy, the unfamiliarity of the medium, the possibility of mutual rejection, and an inability of both parties to cope with inherent tensions.

The value of this experience can only be measured in terms of reviewing the authenticity and reality of such face-to-face encounters, and reflecting, acknowledging, and being aware and working on the feelings and resistance that are generated. For at least one student, it was the beginning of a longer-term relationship with a client.

In using art for teaching student nurses the nursing process, Carol Vestal Allen, (1990), an American nurse educator, described how she took a group of students to a art gallery. Each student was assigned a 'client' – a portrait 'frozen in time' – to observe, and then to apply the first three steps of the nursing process – assessment, nursing diagnosis, and planning.

The students had 40 minutes to write their care plans, and then to present them to their peer group. One student assessed Picasso's 'Melancholy Woman' (1902). The blue totality of the picture and the elongation of the figure conveyed a melancholy mood to the student, who wrote two nursing diagnoses. One was hopelessness related to abandonment, and the other was self-esteem disturbance related to loss of belief or loss of significant others. Describing the experience one student wrote: 'It helped in gathering the objective data because the client was not talking. It was easier to separate the objective data from the subjective data. Sometimes you just listen to the client and forget to look.'

## FUNCTIONAL ASPECTS OF ART THERAPY

In functional terms, art therapy has five aspects (Byrne, 1982):

- as a way of gaining self-knowledge;
- as catharsis – a way of acting our complex feelings;
- as a process which itself may be beneficial;
- as an artificial thing;
- as a diagnostic tool, in that images can sometimes correlate with dysfunctions.

Pine (1975) says of the potential of art:

> It is a universally pleasurable experience and therefore expansive of the self. It affords this most important and appropriate gratification, while at the same time it may be used to serve other functions. Creative experience allows for loosening of rigid defences, fosters integration, and

so provides the restoration of the whole-ness of the individual.

Many difficulties can undermine creative pro-cesses: the danger of the unknown; im-patience to achieve a result; the fear of self-disclosure, and the possibility of being misunderstood, and judged as being chaotic and disorganized.

Diane Waller (1983), art therapist and psychotherapist states that words can only describe part of experience at any one time, and an image or art object can serve the following function:

> It can lead to an exercise of choice, con-trol of the media, a chance to play. It can tell a story or be an element in a story. It can be loved, cherished, denigrated, or destroyed. It can be taken away, given to the therapist, hidden or displayed. In a group, it can serve these functions as well as acting as a 'holding form' while the group struggles to resolve the multitude of problems which its very existence creates.

She describes a client who was agoraphobic and dependent on alcohol, who painted a series of landscapes bereft of people. In so doing he had created a safe place for himself, hidden away within the picture, somewhere he could see but not be seen. Here was someone who could not verbalize feelings at the time, but the process of making images and being able to retain them as a permanent record enabled the client to bring to consciousness the symbolic content of the work. Creative needs are bound up in the basic need to be oneself and, as Kramer (1971) states: 'Art serves as a model of ego functioning. It becomes a sanctuary where new attitudes and feelings can be expressed and tried out, even before such changes can take place in daily life'.

In self-expression through art, right and wrong become immaterial, so the client has more chance of success. Creativity in art is not just an outlet for unconscious feelings and fantasies, but for feelings of disappointment and loss. It is possible for such feelings to stand alongside other feelings such as surprise, satisfaction, and happiness, with the recognition that all these feelings are part of the normal process of living, but if they are causing distress that they need to be dealt with. Jung believed that by creating some-thing through the unconscious, the unknown parts of the self are used, and serve to connect inner and outer reality.

When using art as a way of helping clients to express their innermost thoughts and feelings, there needs to be a clear contract. This is based on confidentiality, trust, and the shared understanding that the work under-taken is for the primary process of healing: the image is ultimately to give the client a better understanding of him or herself. When this is achieved, the image has served its purpose, although it could still be used as a reference point.

The value of this one-to-one relationship is that there is time and space for the client to try to express themselves. Fears of 'not being good at art' need to be overcome. Many adults remember negative criticism for a long time. Fran is one such person, and recalled:

> My art teacher at school told me my art was rubbish, and that all the faces and people I drew were 'pretty, pretty, silly, silly'. She showed them to the class and I remember they all sniggered. Years later when someone suggested to me I should use art I was convinced I couldn't – now I regret those wasted years. However, I'm making up for lost time, and drawing and painting for sheer pleasure and delight.

Often the images created may be unexpected, surprising, and sometimes disturbing. Over-simplistic judgement or interpretation should be avoided. The value in clients' work is as a vehicle for expression of their conflicts, fears, anxieties, and needs.

Rita Barton, a psychoanalyst and one of Britain's leading art therapists described how the drawing of monsters is often a recurrent theme in clients' drawings. She found such 'monsters' to represent the 'dark side' – the shadow – of human nature: 'They have value and significance, and tolerance of the monster on paper may well be the first step towards an inner reckoning with the dark side.'

There are also many and varied ways of working with art as a means of group therapy, for example, asking group members to draw 'symbolic portraits' of each other, using shapes, colours, and images to express the feelings associated with that person. Another way is to make individual masks or a group mask to represent the corporate group identity. It is not only the end product that is important, but the process of working together towards an agreed outcome as well, as a student nurse illustrates:

> When I was asked to take part in making a mask and image of myself I thought, 'what's the point', but as I got more into the task I found two aspects of myself emerging – the clown, always laughing and joking, and a more serious person. I actually made two masks representing those two different parts of myself. We took several sessions to complete the masks, and through this I realized how little we knew, not only our hidden selves but also about each other. We were more familiar with the masks portrayed than the actual person.

## ART AND THE NURSING PROCESS

The role of the nurse in using art therapy is to provide a safe physical place and psychological space for clients to make their images and to be creative. Knowing when and when not to intervene, and always allowing the client to describe what the images mean are essential. Nurses need not only to be receptive to the creative act, but also to be able to share and contain the feelings, projections, and fantasies evoked by the creative process and the images produced.

The importance of working creatively, and of knowing the limits of professional knowledge, competence, and expertise cannot be emphasized too much. The differences be-tween the role of a qualified art therapists and that of a mental health nurse in using art creatively and expressively needs to be respected. The goal of both, however, is for clients to recognize that creativity is not just an easy outlet for unconscious feelings and fantasies, but also feelings of conflict, helplessness, and discomfort, and all normal, acceptable feelings that are part of the human condition. If they are causing distress then they need to be dealt with. Waller (1900) believes that

> ...for many patients, an involvement with art therapy can provide them with a new and perhaps unexpected means of communication and discovery, ...I am also convinced that the art therapist must be a person who has a very sophisticated understanding of the language of the visual arts, and who is preferably familiar with the process of psychotherapy.

There are few art therapists in this country since this is a relatively small profession. Practising therapists are registered with the British Association of Art Therapists, and practise in hospitals, clinics, special schools, and see people individually or in groups. Registered art therapy practitioners are recognized by the NHS. They usually have either a post-graduate diploma or master's degree in art therapy, as well as a qualification or experience in art, craft or design

## DREAMS

Dreams are creative processes, a part of everyday life that concentrate on parts of self that are often ignored, glossed over, and neglected. Dreams, like art, are made up of symbols. For Freud, the verbalization of dreams and images was of primary importance, and so began the debate over the distinction between reason, emotion, and the description of images in words. Freud (1935) pointed out that 'all our dreams are preponderantly visual'. Much of the meaning of the dream is lost in the transition from images into words: the 'verbal' therapist deals with the translation of dream images; the art therapist deals with the reproduction of those images.

There are many ways of working with dreams: they can be talked through, drawn, acted out, or a record kept. Working with dreams commits the dreamer to remembering them, and to be more conscious of and more responsive to the inner life. McGlashan (1970) believes:

The dreaming mind, I suggest, in addition to all its other functions, is an instrument of liberation, capable of breaking up the conventional patterns of human perception, and releasing new forms of awareness. I invite you to regard the dreaming mind as a file smuggled into a space cell where man lies captive; a cell whose walls and ceilings are our five senses, and whose warders are the inflexible concepts of logic.

## DRAMA THERAPY

Historically, drama has its roots in religion, where Greek religious rituals were used as a way of teaching people about the gods. In mediaeval times, so-called mystery plays were introduced to teach biblical stories; later, morality plays were used to teach ethics also from biblical stories.

The idea of drama as a form of therapy came shortly after the end of the First World War. After observing children at play, Jacob Moreno launched the Theatre of Spontaneity, where professional actors took their cues from the audience and from current events to improvise a plot, action, and dialogue. The stage was open and situated in the centre of the room. Actors and audience were encouraged to portray their own dramatic situations. Moreno believed he had created a 'therapeutic theatre' that could heal the distresses and conflicts of the inner life by allowing people to act them out.

Psychodrama is a group process in which the problems and needs of one person, the protagonist, are the centre of activity. Moreno's belief was that people have roles and scripts in life; psychodrama is a way of changing and discarding unacceptable scripts and trying out new ones, as Langley *et al.* explain:

This is done by spontaneous scenes set up by the protagonist to look at himself and his relationships, and for the acting out of painful or desired situations. These situations are played for real, and the protagonist is supported by the 'double' who helps him to say and do things he finds impossible alone.

He is helped both to feel and express his emotions through a catharsis of feelings and thus ridding himself of emotions which may have built up over years. This flood of emotion can be a creative and extremely important experience, and is not what is commonly called 'acting out'.

Training is essential in the use of psychodrama, since it is about exposure to many role-play situations, and rigorous supervision is necessary to ensure safe and competent practice. It is essential to have training, experience, and specialist supervision when using psychodrama

Langley relates that drama can be used in two ways: first, for the pure pleasure and delight of having fun; second, for working towards specific goals, which might include rehabilitation, social skills, overcoming phobias, and role exploration. The powerful use of drama takes and examines experiences, situations, conflicts, and looks at alternative ways of dealing with them: 'By working through defences dramatically it is possible to uncover the problems involved. The client may have a vague idea about his illness/behaviour but the insight gained through drama can help him to see more clearly', Langley *et al.* explain.

The two examples they describe are of a group looking at fantasy roles in a creative way. The role of holiday-maker is considered and role-played, with the group exploring where to go on holiday and what may or may nor happen. The second example is of a group exploring their phobias and anxieties, and how phobias may possibly effect not only the sufferer but those around them.

There are other instances where role-play can be used to help clients to let go of the past. For example, Jo and her husband were divorced after many bitter rows and traumas. With the help of a supportive group and a skilled facilitator, Jo role-played saying good-bye to him. The goodbyes took many forms and were said with rage, remorse, and anger, but finally with acceptance and forgiveness. The acting out helped her to live more in the present, without the past contaminating her life with bitterness.

Drama therapy is generally performed in three stages. First, the warm-up, in which the group prepares for action and decides which member is going to work through a problem in the sessions. Second, the action stage, where the problem is acted through in a series of scenes, and third, the sharing of these experiences.

Many techniques are available. Blatner (1973) includes the 'action sociogram' where the star (the protagonist) presents what Blatner describes as his 'social atom' – the key people relevant to his experience – as if they were a group of sculptures. Members of the group become auxiliary egos, and portray these significant figures. The director helps the star to position them in characteristic poses that symbolically portray their essential relationship to the star. The star chooses someone to represent him/herself. The postures, directions in which each of the players face each other, and their distance from the protagonist may all represent the quality of their relationships. In the last part of the scene, the star gives each figure a charac-teristic sentence to speak to bring them symbolically back to life. The star then stands back, or enters the scene, and begins to relate to the group.

Another way is for the director to use physical objects to represent the social atom, for example, a chess set. The star is then instructed to identify the chessman of his choice with the people in his social atom. The choice of figure and its position can give some

insight into the dynamics of the star's social atom.

Drama at a group level may also be used to help clients improve and build on social skills, and to improve their ability to manage effectively changes and problems in everyday life. By working through many and varied problems over a period of time, the group members can give and receive constructive feedback, and generate alternative ways of dealing with situations.

Psychodrama and drama in all its many forms are ways of helping people to shed the masks they tend to hide behind – masks made up of mixtures of hope and anxiety, masks which portray bright, confident faces but may hide frightened selves. Drama is a powerful way of distinguishing between which parts of the personality are the mask, and which parts the true self, as Park (1927) wrote:

> In seeking to live up to a role we find ourselves in constant conflict with our-selves. Instead of acting simply and naturally as a child, we seek to conform to accepted models... In our efforts to conform we restrain our immediate and spontaneous impulses, and act, not as we are impelled to act, but rather as seems appropriate and proper to the occasion. Under these circumstances our manners, our polite speeches and gestures, our conventions and proper behaviour, assume the character of the mask.

The British Association for Drama Therapists state that skills from their perspective include techniques of theatre, dance, mime, psycho-drama and socio-drama, role-play, simula-tions, and improvization of verbal and non-verbal expression. Drama therapy is a coming together of many different ways of working with people. It is a flexible and action-based therapy, a way of using the imagination to make all things possible, of recalling past, current, or anticipated events, which can be explored for both the learning about and the expression of emotion.

A mental health nurse working with elderly clients described how he introduced

Perls's 'empty chair' technique (page 520) into his casework:

> I had role-played this in school and felt self-conscious while doing so. However, I was seeing this client whose husband had died suddenly. She never had time to say goodbye to him, so we used an empty chair for her to face, as if it represented her husband. She was a bit incredulous at first, but soon began to talk and say her farewells to him. She cried a great deal, and afterwards said what a moving experience it was, and how it helped her come to terms with his death. She continued to use this technique whenever she remembered things she would have liked him to have known.

## CREATIVE WRITING

Writing is another medium by which individuals can communicate – one whereby mental images and ideas can be committed to paper to become a permanent record. Writing can be a self-exploratory process, with endless and exciting possibilities. Writing is also a way of discovering and communicating feelings, values, and ideas in order to help clarify, analyze, and synthesize life experiences.

### WRITING AND THE THERAPEUTIC RELATIONSHIP

All interactions with clients, whether verbal or written, need to be carried out sensitively and authentically. A crucial element to be taken into account is the balance of power between the nurse and the client: the nurse is in a potentially powerful position and has the responsibility to use that power in the wisest possible way. In using the written word nurses especially need to apply care and sensitivity.

Below are some examples of how writing can be used to enrich one's own life and the lives of clients, to reflect on clinical practice and to enable the client to understand and explore thoughts and feelings within the context of the therapeutic relationship.

### SENTENCE COMPLETION

Sentence completion can be an effective way to focus on life experiences such as death and dying. The purpose of this exercise is to help the client face and attempt to overcome the anxieties and fears associated with these aspects of life by bringing anxiety-provoking issues to a conscious level, and then talking them through. More examples can be added to personalize them:

- My thoughts on death are …
- When I consider my own death I…
- My earliest experience of death was…
- When I hear of sudden, violent death I…
- If I were told I had six months to live, I would…

Because of the very personal nature of this exercise, time and space need to be given for reflection as the answers may contain intense self-revelations. It needs to be emphasized that these personal revelations must be treated with respect, confidentiality, and dignity.

### FACING THE PRO'S AND CON'S

When faced with an important decision to make, a useful device is to write down the arguments for and against on two separate sheets of paper. On completion, these should be talked through, and the possibilities and consequences explored from every angle. To add another dimension, another list can be made by ranking the pro's and con's in order of their importance.

### REVIEWING CRITICAL INCIDENTS

Critical incidents are snapshot views of daily life that can provide a focused description of a past event. The client is asked to describe these incidents, when they occurred, and to write down their importance to him or her.

> Joanne, a 30-year-old single parent of three children, was dying. She had no relatives, and was afraid her children would forget her and their life together. A mental health nurse helped the children to compile their 'life story' by making a record in words and photographs, so they would have something permanent to remind them of their mother, and of past times they shared.

These are useful in both remembered details and those which are initially omitted and only remembered in subsequent reviews. Again, time and space need to be allocated to discuss these events and their significance to each individual.

## KEEPING A DAILY/WEEKLY DIARY

Both nurses and clients can benefit from keeping and maintaining a diary. Diaries can be used as practical tools – for example, to record the amount of cigarettes smoked, drinks taken or food eaten throughout a given time span. Data collected can be valuable in planning, implementing, and evaluating client change, with the client very much involved in this process. Diaries can also be used to maintain a record of thoughts, feelings, and impressions. Reflecting on these over a period of time can be a valuable method of attempting to understand events with the benefit of hindsight.

## CREATING A PERSONAL JOURNAL

Recording details of daily living in an honest way through the medium of a personal journal is another valuable way of creatively using the written word. The journal can be a valuable resource, a place where the writer can be totally subjective. Re-reading the journal can be as valuable as writing it, as themes and signposts to personal growth and self awareness can be seen.

There are no right or wrong ways of keeping a personal journal, but anything that is emotionally charged or experienced needs to be included. First impressions on meeting new people or visiting new places can be equally revealing, especially when they are re-read after some time has elapsed. These impressions may be seen to be based on prejudice or stereotypical ways of thinking, which, in the light of time and reflection, may prove to be distorted and inaccurate. Since this is a personal journal, it is important to write down information for the eyes of the writer only. Information subsequently shared with another can be selected as the writer considers appropriate.

Self-observation and self-awareness can be enhanced in picking up themes, noting self-promises, decisions made, and their consequences, and recording dreams, as well as charting physical or bodily changes, like patterns of headaches and tiredness.

## USES OF AUTOBIOGRAPHY

Life histories can be complicated by time, and in struggling to make sense of the past by remembering and trying to justify it.

> Janet, a 28-year-old client found an autobiography a useful way of gaining insight. When she started to write about her life, she found she could not remember anything that happened to her before the age of eight, when she vividly recalled leaving home for school and returning home to find her mother had left. She never saw or heard from her again. Part of Janet's life was blank and, in time, she gradually began to remember and work through those earlier repressed emotional experiences.

The basic purpose of writing autobiographical material is to help put the past into perspective and to learn to get to know and care for the 'child within' so the adult can be free to reflect on the history and progression of their inner life; to help the person to live fully and vitally in the present without the memories of the past negatively, and sometimes, destructively making life miserable.

If the person is older, then an autobiography may be a way of helping to make sense of the past and give their life meaning, to re-encounter past experiences and re-evaluate them.

## WRITING LETTERS

Letters are useful ways of communicating, but they can sometimes be written in a moment of hurt and anger, full of subjective, uncensored, bitter feelings. This type of letter can be kept, locked away, and then re-read and acted upon at a later date. The writer may then have many options – to send it, or to symbolically destroy it by, for example, burning it.

This process has value in letting emotions have full range of expression and discharging them in a constructive way. Letters written and sent off in anger and undue haste may otherwise have a destructive effect on both the sender and receiver.

Dr Susan Forward, an internationally known therapist and writer, has devised a method of writing a confrontational letter to a dead parent and then reading it aloud at the parent's graveside. If this is not possible, then it may be read to a photograph of the dead parent, an empty chair, or someone who is prepared to stand in for the parent and hear the letter. This many sound difficult, but it can be powerful and intensely moving. Dr Forward writes: 'This gives you a strong sense of actually talking to your parent, and of finally being able to express the things you have been holding inside for so long.'

To use writing creatively is a skill and, like all skills, it can be abused. On the surface these techniques may seem simple, but they require sensitivity and care. Used cynically or carelessly they can only negate the dignity of the relationship between the nurse/client, and lose much of the potential for creative, life-enhancing care.

## DANCE

Dance is another way of discovering and integrating parts of the personality, and of balancing thinking, feeling, and sensation. The power of dance lies in sharing it with others. Whether classical ballet or simply moving to music for the sheer joy and delight of it, the same principles hold true. Space, and a trusting, supportive environment are created where people come together to share. A client who participated in a three-day dance workshop remembered afterwards:

> What made it a wonderful experience, was people coming together, starting off very awkwardly and then moulding and flowing together with the rhythm of the music. Sometimes in harmony, sometimes in conflict, but always being conscious of the time, space, and the relationship between mind and body. Added to all this was the excitement, the fear, the care, and the sense of wonder, that sometimes all came together, even for a small amount of time. It helped me to realize the value of creating space for myself and to let go.

Martyn Rudkin, the originator of Dancing Bodymind, believes:

> Dance can be a very good means of opening up communication between people and creating new insights into developing harmonious relationships. Let us not limit the meaning of dance to mean dance techniques or a series of steps, but to open up the word to mean bringing into play all aspects of ourselves, spiritual, mental and physical into the one expression. To me, dance can give a new perspective on how a person views the universe. It can create

a shift in attitude where people can discover new resources within themselves. Many psychological problems get frozen within a mind pattern, a whirling emotional mass that never gets grounded throughout the body. Dance can help to discharge those fixed patterns, dislodge a person from being stuck and create a new perspective.

Dance and body movement are about creating space where the person can explore movement–stretching, rolling, crawling, standing, walking and experimenting with different shapes and patterns to 'dance away pain'. As a result of working with many people in his workshops, Martyn Rudkin says:

> ...what is vital is that people rediscover and awaken the child within themselves and get in touch with that spontaneous gleeful spirit, that being joy. Unfortunately, this is not easy; there is so much in the way, a whole net of interference, a web of conditioning. The skills within the workshop is to gently and gradually remove blocks, so that people are left with their own selves and the security to know that it's OK to celebrate through dance.

## BODY-ORIENTATED THERAPIES

Body-orientated therapies originate mainly from the work of Wilhelm Reich, who trained with Sigmund Freud in Vienna and worked as a psychoanalyst. Reich moved away from Freudian thinking, however, on to considering the social conditions that contributed, created, and maintained client problems.

Reich became increasingly convinced that the key to health lay in utilizing life energy, and in finding ways of strengthening and releasing that energy. He writes:

> A new approach to the understanding or organic disease opens before us. We now

look at neuroses in a totally different way from the psychoanalysts. They are not only the result of unresolved psychic conflicts of childhood fixations. Rather, these fixations and conflicts cause fundamental disturbances of the bioelectrical system and so get anchored somatically. That is why we think it is impossible to separate the psychic from the somatic process.

Largely as a result of Reich's influence, 'bodywork' is now a term widely used in therapeutic work. The therapy works holistically with mind, body, and spirit, and focuses on breathing, touch, and movement to melt defensive and rigid patterns of behaviour and to allow energy to flow.

Bioenergetics is an example of this type of therapy – a therapy that evolved from Freudian psychoanalysis and Reich's understanding of 'character armour' and structure, for example chronic muscular tensions and the shape of the body. The first bioenergetics workshop was opened in London in 1975 by Alexander Lowen, who believes:

> The primary nature of every human being is to be open to life and love. Being guarded, armoured, distrustful and enclosed is second nature in our culture. It is the means we adopt to protect ourselves from being hurt, but when such attitudes become characterological or structured in the personality, they constitute a more severe hurt and create a greater crippling than the one originally intended.

Bioenergetics uses the language of the body to heal the mind (Whitfield, 1988). The major factors to be taken into consideration when working with clients include the following.

### Character analysis

This is fundamental to the therapy and based on the physical effects on the body by emotional trauma. An example is the collapsed, shrunken stance of a depressed person, whose drooping shoulders make the emotional statement, 'I can't', 'What's the use?', 'Give me support', 'It's all so hopeless.'

## Grounding

This is enabling clients literally to stand on their own: by strongly physically supporting their body they go on to discover their authority, stand their ground, and not lean on others for their support and well-being.

## Breathing

When breathing is made more effective, it can be developed to help to minimize the effects on the body of anxiety and tension, and to release feelings.

## Energy

This is visible in the body by the colour of the skin, the temperature, and the movement of the muscles. Stress blocks energy, and there is a lack of vitality.

## Discharge

This involves a variety of striking techniques – fists, arms, and different body postures, as well as verbal expressions are used to help release and give vent to blocked emotions.

Reichian therapy, bioenergetic, biosynthesis and biodynamic therapy are the most widely used body-orientated therapies. They all emphasize working with the body to release tensions and the conditioning of the past. In principle, all methods aim, with differing emphasies, to correct posture alignment, improve and deepen breathing, and to ease and relax tension and tightness in the muscles and joints. As body awareness develops, so feelings and emotions become more harmonized.

The goals of body-orientated therapies are to produce a sense of being alive, and to overcome resistances to the spontaneous energetic flow, so that energy is available to the body to help it to function in a vital and harmonious way.

The physical postures of clients living in psychiatric hospitals, who over the years have become institutionalized express their own histories.

> Hetti has haunted the hospital corridors for the past 20 years – for so long she has become part of the scene. She takes greetings from others but gives little in return. Her physical needs for food and clothing are met, but over the years the diagnosis and experience of schizophrenia, medication, and deprivation of emotional nourishment has taken their toll. She has adapted to survive the system.
>
> Hetti walks the long, echoing corridors of the hospital; her shoulders are bowed, her chest is shrunken and collapsed, and for most of the time her eyes are firmly fixed on the ground. Her hand movements are concerned with keeping a cigarette alight, her burnt fingers grasping it and putting it to her mouth as though her life depended upon it. Her clothes are ill-fitting, and her mannerisms add poignancy to her aura of isolation.
>
> The language of Hetti's stiff, bowed body, the way she holds her jaw, neck, head, and back reflect her tension patterns. All contribute to a life history that is a testament to illness – 'the destroyer of the beauty and the colour of the personality – institutionalization, and countless human rejections and indifferences'.

Any therapeutic approach must take into account the rights and needs of the individuals. Bodywork, if sensitively carried out, could help Hetti and those like her to be less passive and less resigned to the client role. Keleman (1985) eloquently writes:

The human anatomical form is distinguished by its uprightness and its flexibility. Uprightness is accompanied by an emotional history of parental bonding and separations, closeness and distance, acceptance and rejection. A person may stand with the compact density that reflects defiance, or the sunken chest that expresses shame. Human anatomy is thus more than a biochemical configuration; it is an emotional morphology. Particular anatomical shapes produce corresponding sets of human feelings.

Marina is a client who benefited from body-work being included as part of her nursing care:

> Marina was referred to a mental health nurse after her husband, who she had nursed throughout a long illness, died. Whilst she seemed to cope, several months after his death Marina still felt numb, unable to grieve, depressed and feeling that life had lost its meaning.
>
> Marina spoke with a clipped, staccato voice. She had a stiff-upper-lip attitude; her body was rigid, upright, and tense, and her movements were restricted, as though her emotional pain was trapped in her muscles and joints. Her face was tense and drawn, and her eyes appeared lifeless and dead.
>
> Marina was not used to asking for help: she could give, but found difficulty in receiving. All her life she had managed to keep her vulnerability away by denying its existence; she had been taught to stand on her own two feet, to be self-reliant and independent.
>
> Through many encounters with the mental health nurse, Marina began to verbalize her feelings, many of which had been repressed over the years. With the use of various physical exercises and techniques she was helped to ventilate her anger and sadness. Slowly she began to express her needs, frustrations, and deeper feelings.

> Over two years, Marina began to release her bodily tensions and to learn to relax. Through bodywork she explored her bereavement and sadness on the one hand, and her anger and rage on the other. Gradually her body softened, her breathing improved, and she became aware that her stiff, tense body was holding in past pains, hurts, and fears. As she released these tensions Marina became open to the energy circulating in her body, more alive and more able to cope with fear and anxiety. The frozen state she had existed in gradually melted away. For the first time in years she wept uncontrollably.
>
> Marina summed up her own experiences of therapy: 'I had not realized how my body, particularly my posture and my breathing, were affecting my emotions. It was often painful to confront those rigid attitudes in myself and unlearn much of the conditioning from the past. The first time the nurse asked me to hit a mattress with a tennis racquet I was reluctant, but as I gradually lost my self consciousness, I found I could rage, cry, and shout. These experiences helped to unfreeze me to breathe freely, to be more aware of my mind and body, and helped me to live more creatively in the present.'

There is no such thing as a 'cure' in many of the body-orientated therapies, but there is much value in learning to become finely attuned to how the body is held, how blocked feelings can be released, and how body energy can be used and life lived with more awareness and creativity.

In using creative and expressive approaches to client care, and in many relationships which purport to be therapeutic, there is value in negotiating a contract between mental health nurse and client. This needs to be based on specific needs of individuals, the amount of confidentiality and trust, and the shared understanding that the work undertaken is primarily for the process of healing.

Creative and expressive approaches are ways of working that strive to integrate mind, body, and spirit, aiming to alter the circumstances where clients may feel powerless, and where action can be taken to bring about change. Music, poetry, painting, drama, and dance have all been used in mental health nursing for their therapeutic effects. Nurse and client can share these experiences together; power and engagement in the relationship is equal. By using creative and expressive approaches, nurses can become more aware of mind and body; more aware of their enriching social, cultural, and communicative value, and also of their part in confronting reality.

Jackson *et al.* (1968) apply four criteria for the definition of creativity: novelty; appropriateness; transcendence of constraint; and coalescence of meaning, which happen when working and living creatively and expressively. The art and science of nursing are complementary; there is a place for both the intuitive, creative, and expressive, and the scientific way of working. All can become more powerful and valuable with each application, as they are purposefully interwoven to respond to human needs.

## REFERENCES

Allen, C. V. (1990) The art of communication. *Nursing Times* 86,

Blatner, H. (1973) *Acting In: Practical Applications of Psychodramtic Methods*, Springer, New York.

Brandon S (1992) *Art and Science in Psychiatry*, taken from a report of MIND's 1981 annual conference. National Association for Mental Health. London

Byrne, P. (1982) *Inscape- The Journal of The British Association of Art Therapists.*

Clarkson, P. (1989) *Gestalt Counselling in Action*, Sage Publications.

Feder, E. and Feder, B. (1981) *The Expressive Art Therapies*, Prentice-Hall, New Jersey.

Forward, S. (1989) *Toxic Parents*, Bantam Books, New York.

Freud, S. (1916) *Introductory Lectures on Psychoanalysis*, Penguin, Harmondsworth.

Freud, S. (1935) *The Psychopathology of Everyday Life*, Ernest Benn, London.

Grof, S. (1982) Presidential address to the 7th Annual Conference of the International Transpersonal Association, Bombay.

Heron, J. (1975) *Practical Methods in Transpersonal Psychology*, Human Potential Research Project, Univ. Surrey.

Jackson, P. W. and Messick, D. (1968) Creavity, in *Foundations of Abnormal Psychology* (eds P. London, D. Rosenhan), Holt, New York.

Jung, C. G. (1953) *Psychology and Alchemy*, Collected Works, Vol. 12, Routledge, London.

Keleman, S. (1985) *Emotional Anatomy*, Center Press, Berkeley.

Kramer, E. (1971) in *Developmental Art Therapy*, Williams Univ. Park Press.

Laing, R. D. (1967) *The Politics of Experience*, Ballantine Books, New York.

Langley, D. M. and Langley, G. E. (1983) *Drama Therapy and Psychiatry*, Croom Helm, London.

McGlashan, A. (1970) *The Savage and Beautiful Country*, Chatto and Windus, London.

Satir, V. (1976) *Making Contact*, Celestial Arts, Berkeley, California.

Sullivan, H. S. (1953) *The Interpersonal Theory of Psychiatry*, Norton, New York.

Waller, D. (1983) *Self and Society*. Vol. 11 Self and society, London.

Whitfield, G. (1988) Bioenergetics, in *Innovative Therapy in Britain*, (ed. J. Rowan and W. Dryden, Open Univ. Press, Milton Keynes.

William, S. K. (1984) *The Dreamwork Manual*. The Aquarian Press, Northhampton.

Worden, W. J. (1989) *Grief Counselling and Grief Therapy*, Springer, New York.

*Jean Simms*

During the past twenty years there has been increasing attention focused on alternative therapies. These therapies, once referred to as fringe therapies, are now becoming favoured, not so much as an alternative but complementary to traditional medicine.

A problem facing anybody trying to evaluate alternative therapies is that the term covers a wide range of varied and different practices. To help put these therapies into context, this chapter divides them into two main categories and reviews ways that the mental health nurse can incorporate these into existing practice. The intention is not that nurses become complementary therapists, but to help them to be more informed so they and their clients can both benefit and make wider choices in their lives.

## THE ORIGINS OF HOLISTIC MEDICINE

Centuries ago, medicine was a mixture of art, science, magic, superstition, and myths. It is easy to see why medicine gained credibility in the Western world, and why people surrendered responsibility for themselves so readily to the medical profession.

Contemporary Western science dates back to the seventeenth-century philosopher Descartes, who proposed that the human mind was the absolute basis for reality – 'I think, therefore, I am' – and from this established an analytical, scientific model for understanding the physical world. The approach here was that the human mind is separate from nature; reality is best understood by reducing matter and energy to their smallest, most elemental, forms and then constructing the physical world out of these discrete entities.

The Cartesian model proved very attractive. Its tendency to divide, analyze, and control is very different from the concept of holism, which was first popularized by Smuts (1926). Unlike Cartesian dualism, this perspective emphasizes the need to look at the whole rather than the parts.

Meanwhile, assumptions were made that diseases were organic, physical processes, caused by, for example, pathogens, viruses or toxins. The introduction of drugs like cortisone in the treatment of arthritis in the 1940s and 1950s gave hope that medicine could alleviate the suffering of thousands of victims of disease, and if medicine could not cure or halt the progress of disease, then advances in surgery could. Diagnostic techniques were also becoming more sophisticated and precise. Immunization procedures seemed to have largely eradicated epidemics of diseases such as diphtheria. It was widely believed that medical science was the answer to all ills.

Disillusionment and disenchantment gained ground in the late 1950s. For example, in the US, although it was acknowledged that more money was spent on health care than any other nation, it was found that Americans were dying younger (Inglis, *et al.* 1983). The thalidomide tragedy, when hundreds of babies were born deformed because their mothers had taken the drug during pregnancy, was a catalyst that brought home forcefully the potential price to be paid for such trust in medicine.

The crisis was highlighted by writers, like Illich (1975), who maintained that the medical establishment was becoming a major threat to health. The disabling impact of professional control over medicine had reached the proportions of an epidemic or, iatrogenesis, from *iatros*, the Greek for 'physician', and *genesis*, meaning origin.

The growth of alternative therapies came about with the recognition that many people were looking for answers other than medicine or surgery. Cure was not always possible, but quality, as opposed to quantity, of life could be. There was also an increasing awareness of psychogenic pain, pain that is brought on by psychological and physical disease, and of psychosomatic illnesses, bodily disease manifestations of psychological and physical suffering.

## THE HOLISTIC APPROACH

Holistic medicine is a state in which the individual is integrated at all levels of being – body, mind and spirit. Rather than looking only at the malfunctioning part of the body, it also explores the broader dimensions of a person's physical, nutritional, environmental, emotional, and spiritual lifestyle. The ultimate goal of holistic health is to foster the natural healing process.

Holistic approaches look to many philosophies, particularly Eastern, many authorities, and many resources to enable an individual to take responsibility for him or herself, and to bring about healing, by modifying unhealthy life styles, values, or attitudes.

The first category of alternative therapies is the complete healing systems, which includes acupuncture, chiropractic treatment, herbal medicine, homeopathy, osteopathy, and ayurvedic therapy. Practitioners of these systems have specific, often extensive training, and have continued to gain credibility and popularity. Many of these practices have existed for thousands of years, such as ayurvedic therapy. *Ayur* means 'life', and *'veda'* is the science of knowledge, therefore *ayurveda* means the science of life, and includes the art of living. It is an ancient Indian medical science that has been handed down from generation to generation.

The second category, the complementary therapies, is one that mental health nurses may find the most relevant to and useful in their work. It includes many self-help measures, like learning how to breathe more effectively, relaxation techniques, visualization, nutrition, touch and massage, reflexology, yoga, meditation, colour and aromatherapy. We will begin with touch, one of the most valuable ways by which people can convey meaning, and traditionally one which nurses have used throughout the ages.

## THE ART OF TOUCHING

Mental health nursing involves complex and intricate patterns of communication. While dialogue is relatively easy to record by using a tape- or video-recorder, it is more difficult to define and describe the non-verbal aspects of nursing, although research suggests that non-verbal communication is significantly more important than verbal in relationships.

It is with the initial encounter and greeting of the nurse and client that the nurse conveys her state of being, which can range from being preoccupied, troubled and distracted, to being alert and fully present with the client in the here-and-now. The quality and the perception of this greeting most certainly colours and influences the progress and the process of the ensuing relationship between nurse and client.

Mental health nurses are in a privileged position because they engage in a variety of complex relationships with each other and their clients. They can be in touch with their clients subjective experiences at an intellectual level as well as at an emotional level. Auditory, olfactory, oral, visual, tactile, kinesthetic, and visceral responses all come into play, and each can convey, even if only in fleeting moments, the quality and awareness of each other's consciousness.

Martin Buber wrote of the I-Thou relationship, which begins with the closeness of the mother and child. This gives all of us the memory of the experience of closeness, which we continue to seek throughout our lives. The 'I' is separate but merges with others, offering an authentic presence. With 'I-thou' relating, each person gains in awareness. This encounter between two human beings Buber maintains is the 'in-between'. Touch is a way of bridging that 'in-between' space to allow nurturing and healing to flow between two people. It not only enriches the receiver, but also the giver.

Touch is a universal language. From the moment of birth, babies need to be stroked and touched. All of the infant's early communication is by touch – the word 'infant' is derived from the Latin word *infans*, meaning incapable of speech. Studies of infants and children have shown that nothing is more important to early physical and mental growth than touch, through which the infant begins to feel affection and love, or lack of love. Warmth is conveyed through bodily contact, and touch helps to allay emotional distress and hurt. The early experiences of touch help the infant to have confidence in the world and to trust those around him or her. The foundations and issues of trust and mistrust stand or fall by those early relationships, and the denial or deprivation of early tactile experiences may impair the ability to learn or to establish meaningful relationships in later life.

In Western society there are many inhibitions about touching one another. Apologies are often made if two people accidentally touch, even when they are friends or close relatives. Despite touch being so important in the role of interpersonal relations, one elderly client recalled how, since her husband died five years ago, the only person who had touched her was her hairdresser; this is probably not uncommon.

Barnett (1972), on the concepts of touch as they apply to nursing writes, 'Touch is a means of expressing anger, frustration, excitement, happiness – any number of human emotions. By striking another person, an individual can express hostility. By patting another's shoulder or arm, he can convey solace and comfort.'

The communication between two persons may be governed more by physiological emotional reactions than by the content of the message, especially since the coding of the message may be warped or distorted by the emotional reaction of the sender. The quality or intent of a message, as contrasted with its content, may be conveyed by the emotional colouring, tone of voice, facial expression, gestures, or lightness or heaviness of touch, and the recipient may respond largely to this intent and quality. Thus small children often respond more to quality than to content, hearing the tone of voice more than the words spoken by a parent, and responding to the kinesic messages (Frank, 1957).

Many researchers have found that emotionally distressed people put their hands to their foreheads when faced with a situation that is hard to deal with emotionally. As the stress becomes more difficult, this gesture changes to the hand covering the brow; then, particularly if people are tearful, they cover their faces with the palms of their hands, fingertips resting of the forehead.

Touch can be a simple art of solace like a nurse's hand on the shoulder of a client waiting to go through some complex medical physical or psychological examination, or it can be more formalized like the use of therapeutic touch. Whether it is a simple, spontaneous gesture or a deliberate and structured activity, touch bridges the space between nurse and client, and, if it is effective, makes the nursing contact alive and meaningful.

The Canadian biologist Bernard Grad conducted a series of experiments to clarify some facts about healing. He concluded that some kind of energy transfer, not suggestion, was responsible for the effectiveness of touch in healing. Since this pioneering work, many others have reinforced Grad's findings, although there is still mystery surrounding what this energy may be.

Dolores Krieger (1963), who was also influenced by Grad, sought to promote the therapeutic use of touch because she believed the technique 'recaptured this simple but elegant mode of healing and mated it with the rigour and power of modern science.' She introduced her ideas into nursing in the 1960s, and now techniques of therapeutic touch are taught throughout the US. Kreiger expressed dissatisfaction with the modern practice of nursing: 'In our adulation of things mechanical, synthetic and, frequently, anti-human [the laying on of hands has come to be] all but forgotten in this scientific age.'

There is nothing new about the belief that some people have the ability to help the healing process in others. Hippocrates gives a description of the therapeutic effect that he and other doctors had observed to flow through their hands. However, what is new is the credibility of the practice that has been underpinned by scientific research.

Therapeutic touch does not require a trained practitioner; any two people can try it out on each other. Brennan (1988) describes simple exercises that provide the key to understanding the idea of therapeutic touch. Sitting comfortably in a chair, with the feet side by side and firmly on the floor, hold the hands outstretched so the palms face each other. The elbows should be away from the chest and the hands not touching. The hands are then cupped, and moved about ten centimetres away from each other, and then moved back again without touching. This action is repeated several times. Many people feel different sensations between the hands, including warmth, tingling, and pulsating feelings. This exercise can be done in a group of people holding hands, becoming aware of

the energy that passes from hand to hand around the circle. It can also be done in pairs, with each person sitting opposite each other and transferring this subtle form of energy from left to right and vice versa.

Dr Krieger's hypothesis is that nurses can help restore a healthy pattern to someone who is ill through the use of hands and the conscious intention to help. Therapeutic touch is practised by the movement of the hands three to five centimetres away from the skin's surface, in a head-to-toe direction. To assess the person's energy field, the hands are then run down each side of the body, feeling for signs of imbalance or congestion. Energy is directed to parts of the body where it is needed.

When people come into hospital, particularly those who do so dramatically and without warning, finding themselves in intensive care and surrounded by a vast array of complex electronic technology, they may potentially be overwhelmed by physical and mental pain. Anxiety is a common response, to threat to life, loss of control and self determination, and possible disfigurement. Touch can help lessen this fear and bridge the gap between the individual and environment.

Judith Ashton (1984) is an advocate of intuitive massage, and has gained firsthand experience of its healing powers when she took part in experimental work on people who had suffered from stress-related heart disease. They were given postoperative massage or a combination of massage and counselling. Says Ashtan: 'The deep relaxation that therapeutic massage induces is now being increasingly recognized for its contribution to the overall healing process.'

Many illnesses are caused by psychological stress. Feelings of anger, fear, or sorrow are locked in the body in the form of muscular tension, and touch is a way of releasing the flow of blood and lymph, thus relieving the tense muscles and the pain.

Marianne, a 60-year-old widow, was admitted to an acute admission ward in a depressed state. Her husband had died several years ago and she described her experience during her first night in hospital:

> I remember feeling very lonely, sad, and distressed. I was overwhelmed with confusion and fear, which seemed to come in spasms. I was struggling to try to keep control of my thoughts and feelings and not really succeeding too well. I cannot remember if I actually called out for help, but the night nurse came and just held my hand. I shall never forget the warmth and acceptance of that touch. I cannot remember very much about my early days in hospital, but I do remember the touch of her hand during that dreadful night.

Another powerful reminder of touch came from Joe, who was badly injured in a road traffic accident:

> I remembered lying in the road, feeling paralyzed with fear, not daring to move and wondering if I was going to die. An ambulance man came and stayed with me until I was admitted to hospital. I remember losing consciousness for a few seconds and then coming to again, but holding on to his hand gave me some sense of security by feeling the strength and power of that touch.

There are, however, instances in therapeutic encounters with clients in which the use of touch needs to be carefully considered; it may be that by engaging in touch the therapeutic process could be hindered. The psychodynamic approach, for example, is a verbal one and encourages full expression of thought and feeling. For the most part, physical expression is discouraged. Verbalization of even the most intense feelings is encouraged. Psychodynamic counselling might be likened to the theatrical stage, as opposed to the film set. In the theatre emotions are expressed through words, and rarely in action. The film set, or off stage, is the client's life outside the counselling session. On stage – in the counselling room – the vocabulary can be rich and expressive, but nevertheless confined to words.

An example of the consideration of touch comes from Patrick Casement, a British psychoanalyst, who describes a patient who reached a point where she could not go on with her analysis unless she could hold his hand if the reliving of an early trauma became unbearable. At the age of 11 she had been badly burned, and six months later her scars were operated on under a local anaesthetic. During the operation, her mother, who was holding her hands, fainted. By wanting to hold on to his hand, the client was appealing to Casement to be available to her as a mother, who would protect her from the transference experience of him as this surgeon. Casement reflected on this need of the client, but felt that conceding to her wish could be collusive and a way of avoiding the worst part of her experience. Instead he provided analytic 'holding' to enable her to remember the early trauma of not being held:

> ...her remembering (by re-experiencing that trauma in the transference) could be in the presence of someone against whom she could safely rage – as at a mother who had become absent through fainting ... It was vital to her that she had seen the evidence of my being truly in touch with the intensity of her distress, for it had been that which had contributed to her mother's fainting. But it had also been essential that I had managed to find a way of staying with her most difficult feelings of that trauma – that I had not deflected these by trying to be the 'better' mother.

Concepts of psychological holding and containment need more fully to be addressed, as the mental health nurse moves to a more specially orientated way of working.

## THE ART OF BREATHING

Breathing is something most people take for granted and do automatically, but it is an activity of daily living which mental health nurses can use more effectively, both for themselves and their clients.

Working as a community psychiatric nurse, I first used this with an elderly client, who had been referred after experiencing a series of panic attacks. His posture appeared shrunken, and he sat in a collapsed, defeated position in a large armchair. He could hardly speak, and his breath was shallow and rasping. It was difficult for him to articulate how he was feeling. I suggested we look first of all at his pattern of breathing and see if this would make any difference to him. Since there were no physical reasons for his condition, we looked at basic breathing techniques. We used one that measured the length of the breath by moistening the palm of the hand and holding it under the nostrils. As exhalation proceeds, the air blowing in the palm is felt and the evaporation of the moisture will cause a sensation of coolness. The hand is then slowly moved away until the exhaled air is no longer felt. In this way the approximate length of the breath is measured. From there we gradually explored different ways of working with the breath and techniques he could use to help him control his anxiety and feelings of dread.

At first he was resistant to try these breathing techniques, but he finally agreed and the results were almost immediate. He became more aware of his patterns of breathing by placing his hands on his chest, diaphragm, and abdomen to gradually help him to be freer in his inhalation and exhalation. Leboyer (1900) responds to the question of how to breathe in a special way. This is an example of a dialogue he uses to illustrate the art of breathing:

The secret of relaxation is a long, even out breath, letting the air out very slowly until you have emptied yourself completely.

*Letting the air out? Why! That is just the opposite of what we are taught.*

When you are tense, you hold your breath don't you?

*That's true.*

Any strong emotional situation comes to an end, finds its relief, its 're-solution' either in laughter or in tears: crying, sobbing?

*True.*

Both are exhaling, letting the air out, aren't they?

*Why of course!*

But such uncontrolled explosions, although they do relieve the tensions, leave you with your battery empty. Simply because you have been exhaling from your chest, where all the emotions are stored up. Once you are free from these emotions that come from your past, which are truly your past, the road is free for true breathing: not from the chest but from the stomach.

Breathing and touch are just two examples of activities of daily living which complementary therapies have developed and incorporated into many of their practices. A humane nurse, no matter what her clinical speciality, seeks to help clients to be free to use and maximize their inherent potential for growth.

Complementary therapies take, for example, colour and look at its effect on concentration, performance, and sense of physical and psychological well-being. There is increasing evidence that the use of colour in hospitals is influential, and for the stimulation of children with severe learning difficulties.

Colour affects all our lives in many ways. We tune into certain colours in our dress, our homes, and the environment. Colour therapy is an ancient art originally used in Ancient

Greece and in Ancient Egypt. Indians and the Chinese have held colour in high esteem for thousands of years.

Another revival of an ancient art comes in the form of aromatherapy – a combination of body and face massage using essential oils extracted from plants. Aromatherapy uses the touch and smell, very powerful but often neglected senses. This therapy also treats the whole person, and uses the body's own nerve pathways without becoming dangerous or addictive.

Dr Valnet, the founding father of modern aromatherapy, used essential oils to treat wounded soldiers in the Second World War. In the 1950s, biochemist Marguerite Maury discovered that when essential oils were combined with massage, they could clear up skin problems, delay the ageing process by speeding up cell regeneration, and relieve many ailments associated with stress.

Smell is also an evocative sense, and various fragrances have the power to trigger off many memories. Aromatherapy is not only a powerful therapy, but also a source of self-care and a way of refreshing the mind, body and spirit. The essences extracted from plants are complex natural oils with esters, alcohols, aldehydes, ketones and terpenes. When and where this ancient art began remains a mystery. Essential oils from plants are used in a variety of ways, but in Britain most are for massage treatments. However they can be inhaled, added to baths, or used for compresses. The medicinal use of plant oils is recorded in early Chinese writings and the ancient Persians also valued flower waters distilled from roses and orange blossom.

There are now an estimated 60,000 full and part-time healers and practitioners of these many therapies in Britain. Increasing numbers of doctors are referring their patients to alternative or complementary therapists, and nurses are seeking to incorporate or use their skills in complementary therapies in their nursing practice.

Whatever the approaches used in encounters with clients there needs to be unconditional positive regard. Trust and receptivity are necessary if growth, positive change, and conscious awareness are to be brought about as a result of the therapeutic relationships with the clients. Empathic responses facilitate growth. Carl Rogers's (1961) eloquent statement of empathy seems a fitting conclusion for this chapter and this book.

Being empathic means entering the private perceptual world of the other and becoming thoroughly at home in it. It involves being sensitive, moment to moment, to the changing felt meanings which flow in this other person, to the fear or rage or tenderness or confusion or whatever, that he/she is experiencing.

It means temporarily living his/her life, moving about delicately in it without making judgments, sensing meanings of which he/she is scarcely aware, but not trying to uncover feelings of which the person is totally unaware since this would be too threatening. It includes communicating your sensing of his/her world as you look with fresh and unfrightened eyes at elements of which the individual is fearful. It means frequently checking with him/her as to the accuracy of your sensing, and being guided by the responses you receive.

## REFERENCES

Barnett, K. (1972) A theoretical construct of the concepts of touch as they relate to nursing. *Nursing Research*, 21, 2.

Brennan, A. B. (1988) *The Hands of Light*, Bantam New Age Books.

Casement, P. (1985) *On Learning From the Patient* and *Further Learning From the Patient*, Tavistock, London.

Frank, L. K. (1957) Tactile communication, *Genet Psychology Monograph*, 56: 211–51.

Ilich, I. (1975) *Medical Nemesis*, Pantheon Books, London.

Inglis, B. and West, R. (1983) *The Alternative Health Guide*, Michael Joseph Ltd., London.

Leboyer, F. (1985) *The Art of Breathing*, Element Books Ltd., Dorset.

Smuts, Jan. C. (1926) *Holism and Evolution*, Viking, New York.

Teegarden, D. (1983) Holistic health and medicine in the 1980s in *The New Holistic Handbook*.

## FURTHER READING

The Academy of Traditional Chinese Medicine (1975) *An Outline of Chinese Acupuncture*, Foreign Language Press, Peking.

Alexander, F. M. (1941) *The Use of Self*, Gollanz, New York.

Annet, S. (1969) *The Many Ways of Being: A Guide to Spiritual Groups and Growth Centres in Britain*, London.

Assagioli, R. (1975) *Psychosynthesis: A Collection of Basic Writings*, Turnstone Press London.

Barlow, W. (1973) *The Alexandra Principle*, Arrow, London.

Bates, W. H. (1940) *Better Eyesight Without Glasses*, London.

Cho, Ta-Hung (1985) *Knocking at the Gate of Life:* (healing exercises from China: the official exercise manual from the Peoples Republic of China).

Clover, Dr Anne (1984) *Homeopathy – A Patient's Guide*, Thorsons.

Cummings, S. and Ullman, D. (1986) *Everybody's Guide to Homeopathic Medicines – Taking Care of Yourself and Your Family with Safe and Effective Remedies*. Victor Gollancz Ltd, London.

Griggs, B. (1982) *The Home Herbal*, London.

Grist, L. (1986) *A Woman's Guide to Alternative Medicine*, Fontana.

Grossman, R. (1986) *The Other Medicines: The Unique Treat Yourself Guide to Natural Remedies and Therapies*, Pan Books.

Hall, N. (1986) *Reflexology – A Patient's Guide*, Thorsons.

Hallowell, M. (1985) *Herbal Healing – A Practical Introduction to Medicinal Herbs*, Ashgrove Press.

Harvey, D. (ed.) (1986) *Thorson's Complete Guide to Alternative Living*, Thorsons.

Hastings A. C. (ed.) (1980) *Health for the Whole Person*, Boulder C A.

Hulke, M. (Ed) (1978) *The Encyclopaedia of Alternative Medicine and Self-Help*. Rider and Co.

Inglis, B. and West, R. (1984) *The Alternative Health Guide*, Mermaid Books.

Kadan, J. M. (1973) *Encyclopaedia of Medical Foods*, Thorson.

Kenyon, Dr. J. (1986) *21st Century Medicine – A Layman's Guide to the Medicine of the Future*, Thorsons.

Marcus, Dr. P. (1985) *Acupuncture – A Patient's Guide*, Thorsons.

Palaiseul, J. (1972) *Grandmother's Secrets: Her Green Guide to Health from Plants*, Penguin.

Passebecq, A. (1979) *Aromatherapy – The Use of Plant Essences in Healing*, Thorsons.

Pietroni, Dr. P, (1986) *Holistic Living – A Guide to Self-Care by a Leading Practitioner*, Guernsey Press, Guernsey.

Plesthette, J. (1986) *Cures that Work*, Century–Arrow, London.

Ross, G. (1976) *Homeopathy – An Introductory Guide*, Thorsons.

Stanway, Dr. A. (1980) *Alternative Medicine – A Guide to Natural Therapies*, Penguin, Harmondsworth.

Triance, E. (1986) *Osteopathy – A Patient's Guide*, Thorsons.

Werbach, M. R. (1986) *Third Line Medicine. Modern Treatment for Persistent Symptoms*. Routledge London.

Valentine, F. and C. (1985) *Applied Kinesiology*, Thorsons.

Valnet, Dr. J. (1980) *The Practice of Aromatherapy*, C. W. Daniel.

## USEFUL ADDRESSES

Institute of Complementary Therapies
21 Portland Place
London W1N 3AF

Human Potential Research Project
Adult Education Department
University of Surrey
Guildford, Surrey

Holwell Centre of Psychodrama
East Down,
Barnstaple, Devon

Laban Art of Movement Guild
Boynness
Hadley Common
Herts EN5 5QG

Natural Dance Association
14 Peto Place
London NW 4DT

British Association of Art Therapists
13c Northwood Road
London N6 5LT

British Wheel of Yoga
General Secretary
80 Lechampton Road
Cheltenham, Glous.

British T'ai Chi Chuan Association
7 Upper Wimpole Street
London W1M 7TD.

British Association for Psychotherapists
121 Hendon Lane,
London N3 3PR

# INDEX